AF813857

David M. Lichtman • Gregory Ian Bain
Editors

# Kienböck's Disease

## Advances in Diagnosis and Treatment

Springer

*Editors*
David M. Lichtman, MD
Rear Admiral (Retired)
US Navy
Adjunct Professor
Department of Surgery
Uniformed Services University of the Health Sciences
Bethesda, MD, USA

Adjunct Professor
Department of Orthopedic Surgery
University of North Texas Health Sciences Center
Fort Worth, TX, USA

Gregory Ian Bain, MBBS, FRACS, FA(Ortho)A, PhD
Professor
Upper Limb and Research
Department of Orthopedic Surgery
Flinders University and Flinders Medical Centre
Bedford Park, Adelaide, SA, Australia

Videos can also be accessed at
http://link.springer.com/book/10.1007/978-3-319-34226-9

ISBN 978-3-319-34224-5 ISBN 978-3-319-34226-9 (eBook)
DOI 10.1007/978-3-319-34226-9

Library of Congress Control Number: 2016941340

© Springer International Publishing Switzerland 2016
This work is subject to copyright. All rights are reserved by the Publisher, whether the whole or part of the material is concerned, specifically the rights of translation, reprinting, reuse of illustrations, recitation, broadcasting, reproduction on microfilms or in any other physical way, and transmission or information storage and retrieval, electronic adaptation, computer software, or by similar or dissimilar methodology now known or hereafter developed.
The use of general descriptive names, registered names, trademarks, service marks, etc. in this publication does not imply, even in the absence of a specific statement, that such names are exempt from the relevant protective laws and regulations and therefore free for general use.
The publisher, the authors and the editors are safe to assume that the advice and information in this book are believed to be true and accurate at the date of publication. Neither the publisher nor the authors or the editors give a warranty, express or implied, with respect to the material contained herein or for any errors or omissions that may have been made.

Printed on acid-free paper

This Springer imprint is published by Springer Nature
The registered company is Springer International Publishing AG Switzerland

*I dedicate this book to my fellowship director James N. Wilson, MD. Jim introduced me to the mysteries of Kienböck's disease and kick-started my lifelong interest in this fascinating subject.*

David M. Lichtman

*I dedicate this book to my beautiful wife Katherine, and our 3 amazing children; Madeleine, Jack and Annabel. It is our families that inspire us to strive and achieve in life.*

Gregory Ian Bain

# Foreword

Following the initial identification of Kienböck's disease in the early twentieth century, clinical observational reports, imaging and histological studies, and anatomical experiments in human cadavera have concluded uniformly that the essential abnormality is an irreversible osteonecrosis of bone. While the cause of lunate osteonecrosis has been related to a number of factors, including a unique external and internal vascular supply and negative ulnar variance, its occurrence is notable for an absence of those factors associated with osteonecrosis in other anatomical locations (i.e., focal arterial injury, such as that to the medial femoral circumflex artery, ethanol and corticosteroid administration, and gene polymorphisms associated with disorders of lipid metabolism). As a result, advances in the assessment and treatment of lunate osteonecrosis over the past century have been based largely on empirical observational reports from a broad array of clinical disciplines and less on the results of hypothesis-driven experiments in well-validated animal models.

The persistence of fundamental unanswered questions on the nature of Kienböck's disease notwithstanding, scientific advances in recent years have steadily improved clinical assessment and care. Detailed studies of the lunate's macro- and microarchitecture, investigations of the bone's external and internal vascularization, biomechanical studies on the distribution of forces and pressures in affected compared to normal wrists, and improved imaging, including advanced MRI modeling of involved bones, have led to more useful classification systems and to more effective treatment algorithms. Further, recently reported 15- to 20-year cohort studies with validated outcomes measures have provided a more complete understanding of the natural history of the disease and have confirmed the benefit of selected forms of operative treatment.

Drs. Lichtman and Bain, two of the field's foremost authorities on Kienböck's disease, have brought together a remarkable group of international contributors, drawn from academic and private practice settings, for the creation of this very timely and thorough reference. The authors' goals are clear—to improve care by reconciling the diverse body of existing knowledge with the most relevant new scientific data on diagnosis and operative treatment. The result is the most definitive and useful reference on Kienböck's disease to have been compiled, one that effectively couples the scientific underpinnings of the disease with a practical, up-to-date description of traditional and new treatment strategies. The authors conclude with a novel model of the pathologic stages of the disease and a matrix algorithm to assist with assessment and treatment.

While the overarching goal of *Kienböck's Disease: Advances in Diagnosis and Treatment* is to provide a rigorous and comprehensive resource for the clinician scientist and hand surgeon specialist, the practical nature of the book makes it an invaluable addition to the libraries of all those who treat patients who present with this elusive disorder of the wrist.

Richard H. Gelberman
St. Louis, MO, USA

# Preface

## Introduction

For many years it has been popular to introduce articles on Kienböck's disease with some variation of the following statement: "Not much new information has been published on the etiology and natural history of Kienböck's disease since the appearance of the manuscript *On Traumatic Lunatomalacia* by Robert Kienböck in 1910." And, to a degree, this statement is true. No one has yet disproved Professor Kienböck's theory that the disease is caused by a compromised lunate blood supply and that some degree of stress or trauma plays a role in the process of lunate collapse. On the other hand, more recent evidence indicates that the etiology is multifactorial, that the disorder progresses through several distinct stages, that there are sophisticated diagnostic techniques available beyond plane x-rays, and that current treatment options are abundant, effective, and adaptable to the precise needs of the patient.

Realizing that much of this information is widely disseminated throughout the world's literature and that some of the currently popular treatment algorithms are based on incomplete use of this widespread database, we decided that a work collecting and synthesizing all this information would be helpful for most physicians treating osteonecrosis of the lunate. Accordingly, the two of us set out to identify selected individuals who have made significant contributions in recent years and to ask them to contribute to this publication. In almost every instance they have participated enthusiastically and added to its depth and diversity.

The goal of this book, then, has been to dispel the popular notion that we are in a static era with respect to the understanding of this enigmatic disorder. More specifically, the ultimate goal has been to consolidate the most important new information on Kienböck's disease in order to develop a more dynamic and nuanced treatment algorithm. Feeling cautiously optimistic that we have achieved this goal, we also acknowledge that there is much more to be accomplished. The many knowledge gaps that persist will surely stimulate additional basic and clinical research. And the time will eventually come when the material presented here, along with the derivative treatment models, will once again need to be revised and elevated to the next level.

One more observation: Throughout this book we use the traditional title, *Kienböck's* disease, rather than the newly fashionable, *Kienböck* disease. Although an argument can be made for either, we feel that the traditional title is a more appropriate way to honor Professor Robert Kienböck. We hold him in esteem not just for the many professional contributions he made to the fields of radiology and hand surgery but also for the highly honorable way he conducted his personal affairs during the worst turmoil of the twentieth century.

## Organization of the Book

The book commences with a dedication to the life of Robert Kienböck and the many aspects of this fascinating man's remarkable career. It is written by Dr. Martin Chochole, who practices hand surgery in Vienna, Austria, Dr. Kienböck's hometown.

The first section of the book is devoted to the basic sciences such as anatomy, pathology, and biomechanics of the lunate and Kienböck's disease. It also contains an update on the etiology of the disorder.

The next section details the assessment of the patient including radiology, advanced imaging, and arthroscopy. The clinical presentation is integrated with the natural history and radiologic progression of Kienböck's disease in adults, children, and the elderly. This section also introduces important information on classification and natural history based on advances in detection of bone and cartilage viability.

The treatment section is extensive and reviews the roles and methods of traditional and new treatment options. These include nonoperative modalities, minimally invasive techniques, arthroscopy, reconstructive procedures (e.g., various osteotomies, vascularized bone grafts, and limited wrist fusions), and salvage options (e.g., proximal row carpectomy, wrist fusion, and arthroplasty).

In the final chapter, we bring together the concepts provided throughout the book by the multiple authors. We then construct a more inclusive model of the pathologic stages of Kienböck's disease. From this, we present a matrix in table format for the assessment and treatment of the disease. We conclude with recommendations for future research and development.

David M. Lichtman
Fort Worth, TX, USA

Gregory Ian Bain
Adelaide, Australia

# Acknowledgements

Throughout the book there are many fine images and illustrations. However, there are some that the editors consider to be exceptional.

The editors acknowledge the significant contribution of the images provided by Henry V. Crock AO. The osseous arterial and venous studies provide a unique insight into the understanding of vascular components of Kienböck's disease. They are reproduced from *An Atlas of Vascular Anatomy of the Skeleton and Spinal Cord*, published in 1996 by Martin Dunitz. Henry V. Crock AO maintains copyright of these images.

The 3D micro-CT images provide a special insight into the microstructure of the normal and pathological lunate. The lunates have been scanned at Adelaide Microscopy, University of Adelaide, South Australia. We acknowledge the support and imaging skills of Dr. Egon Perilli, School of Computer Science Engineering and Mathematics, Flinders University, Adelaide, South Australia.

David M. Lichtman
Gregory Ian Bain

# Contents

# Contributors

**Brian D. Adams, MD** Department of Orthopedic Surgery, University of Iowa College of Medicine, Iowa City, Iowa, USA

**Ahmadreza Afshar, MD** Department of Orthopedics, Urmia University of Medical Sciences, Imam Khomeini Hospital, Urmia, West Azarbaijan, Iran

**William R. Aibinder, MD** Department of Orthopedic Surgery, Mayo Clinic, Rochester, MN, USA

**Wisam Al-Hakim, MBBS, BSc, PGDip, FRCS (Tr & Orth)** Department of Trauma and Orthopedics, The Royal London Hospital, London, UK

**Andrea Atzei, MD** Sezione di Chirurgia della Mano, Casa di Cura "Giovanni XXIII", Monastier di Treviso, Italy

**Gregory Ian Bain, MBBS, FRACS, FA(Ortho)A, PhD** Professor, Upper Limb and Research, Department of Orthopedic Surgery, Flinders University and Flinders Medical Centre, Bedford Park, Adelaide, SA, Australia

**Richard Blake Barber, BS, MS** University of North Texas Health Science Center–Texas College of Osteopathic Medicine, Fort Worth, TX, USA

**Philippe Bellemère, MD** Institut de la Main Nantes Atlantique, Clinique Jeanne D'Arc, Nantes, France

**Michel E.H. Boeckstyns, MD** Clinic for Hand Surgery, Gentofte Hospital, University of Copenhagen, Hellerup, Denmark

Kloeverbakken, Virum, Denmark

**Heinz K. Bürger, MD** Department of Hand and Microsurgery, Private Clinic Maria Hilf, Klagenfurt, Carinthia, Austria

**Marc A. Caragea, BS** University of North Texas Health Science Center – Texas College of Osteopathic Medicine, Fort Worth, TX, USA

**Kin Ghee Chee, MBBS, MRCS, MMed (Surgery)** Department of Orthopedic Surgery, Tan Tock Seng Hospital, Jalan Tan Tock Seng, Singapore, Singapore

**Harvey Chim, MD** Division of Plastic Surgery, University of Miami Miller School of Medicine, Miami, FL, USA

**Martin Chochole, MD** Department of Orthopedics, Herz Jesu Krankenhaus, Vienna, Austria

**Paul D. Clifford, MD** Department of Diagnostic Radiology, University of Miami Miller School of Medicine, Miami, FL, USA

Miami Beach, FL, USA

**Aude Le Corre, MD** Clinique Jeanne d'Arc, Institut de la Main, Nantes, France

**Ilse Degreef, MD, PhD** Hand Unit, Department of Orthopedic Surgery, University Hospitals Leuven, Pellenberg, Belgium

**Richard H. Gelberman, MD** Department of Orthopedic Surgery, Washington University School of Medicine, St. Louis, MO, USA

**George S. Gluck, MD** Hand and Upper Extremity, Department of Orthopedic Surgery, Wake Forest University Baptist Hospital, Winston Salem, NC, USA

**Benjamin R. Graves, MD** Hand and Upper Extremity, Department of Orthopedic Surgery, Wake Forest University Baptist Hospital, Winston Salem, NC, USA

**Ngoc Buu Ha, MBBS** Department of Orthopedics and Trauma, Royal Adelaide Hospital, Adelaide, Australia

**Bassem Hanalla, BA** University of North Texas Health Science Center–Texas College of Osteopathic Medicine, Fort Worth, TX, USA

Durbridge Trail Dr., Houston, TX, USA

**Guillaume Herzberg, MD, PhD** Department of Orthopedic Surgery, Hopital Edouard Herriot, Pavillon T, Upper Limb Surgery, Lyon, France

**James P. Higgins, MD** Curtis National Hand Center, Union Memorial Hospital, Baltimore, MD, USA

**Hitoshi Hirata, MD, PhD** Department of Hand Surgery, Nagoya University Graduate School of Medicine, Nagoya, Japan

**Pak-cheong Ho, MBBS, FRCS, FHKCOS** Department of Orthopedics and Traumatology, Prince of Wales Hospital, Chinese University of Hong Kong, Shatin, Hong Kong, China

**Carlos Irisarri, MD** Hand Surgery Unit, Hospital Vithas-Fátima, Vigo, Pontevedra, Spain

**Karlheinz Kalb, Dr Med,** Clinic for Hand Surgery, Herz- und Gefaßklinik GmbH der Rhön-Klinikum AG, Bad Neustadt, Germany

**David M. Lichtman, MD** Rear Admiral (Retired), US Navy Adjunct Professor, Department of Surgery, Uniformed Services University of the Health Sciences, Bethesda, MD, USA

Adjunct Professor, Department of Orthopedic Surgery, University of North Texas Health Sciences Center, Fort Worth, TX, USA

**Bo Liu, MD, FRCS** Department of Hand Surgery, Beijing Ji Shui Tan Hospital, Beijing, China

**Steven Marchalleck, BSc, BSc (Med Sci), MBBS** Department of Orthopedics, Princess Alexandra Hospital, Fortitude Valley, QLD, Australia

**Daniel J. Mastella, MD** The Hand Center, University of Connecticut, Glastonbury, CT, USA

**Steven L. Moran, MD** Division of Plastic Surgery, Mayo Clinic, Rochester, MN, USA

**Hisao Moritomo, MD, PhD** Department of Orthopedics, Yukioka Hospital Hand Center, Osaka Yukioka College of Health Science, Osaka-shi, Osaka, Japan

**Levi Morse, BPhty, BMBS (Hons)** Department of Orthopedics and Trauma, Flinders Medical Centre, Bedford Park, SA, Australia

**Fabian Moungondo, MD** Department of Orthopedics and Traumatology, Erasme University Hospital, Université libre de Bruxelles (ULB), Brussels, Belgium

**Ryogo Nakamura, MD, PhD** Department of Orthopedic Surgery, Nagoya Hand Center, Chunichi Hospital, Nagoya, Japan

**Anuj P. Netto, MD, MPH** Department of Orthopedics, Davis Health Care System, University of California, Sacramento, CA, USA

**Timothy Niacaris, MD, PhD** Department of Orthopedic Surgery, University of North Texas Health Science Center, Fort Worth, TX, USA

**Loris Pegoli, MD** Hand and Reconstructive Microsurgery Unit, San Pio X Clinic, Milan, Italy

**Egon Perilli, PhD (Bioeng), MSc (Phys)** Medical Device Research Institute, School of Computer Science, Engineering and Mathematics, Flinders University, Clovelly Park, SA, Australia

**Joideep Phadnis, FRCS (Tr & Orth)** Department of Trauma and Orthopedics, Brighton and Sussex University Hospitals, NHS Trust, Eastern Road, Brighton, East Sussex, UK

**William F. Pientka II, MD** Department of Orthopedic Surgery, John Peter Smith Hospital, Fort Worth, TX, USA

Highwoods Ct., Fort Worth, TX, USA

**Francisco del Piñal, MD DrMed** Department of Hand and Plastic Surgery, Hospital Mutua Montañesa, Santander, Spain

**Gary G. Poehling, MD, PhD** Department of Orthopedic Surgery, Wake Forest University Baptist Hospital, Winston-Salem, NC, USA

**Peter Charles Rhee, DO, MS** Department of Orthopedic Surgery and Rehabilitation, San Antonio Military Medical Center, Fort Sam Houston, TX, USA

Scenic Knoll, San Antonio, TX, USA

**Mark Ross, MBBS, FRACS** Brisbane Hand and Upper Limb Research Institute, Brisbane Private Hospital, Brisbane, QLD, Australia

Department of Orthopedics, Princess Alexandra Hospital, Brisbane, QLD, Australia

School of Medicine, The University of Queensland, Brisbane, QLD, Australia

**Rainer R. Schmitt, MD** Department of Radiology, Herz- und Gefäßklinik GmbH, Bad Neustadt, Germany

**Frédéric A. Schuind, MD, PhD** Department of Orthopedics and Traumatology, Erasme University Hospital, Université libre de Bruxelles (ULB), Brussels, Belgium

**Alexander Y. Shin, MD** Department of Orthopedic Surgery, Mayo Clinic, Rochester, MN, USA

**Meenalochani Shunmugam, MBBS, MSSc** Department Orthopedic Surgery and Trauma, Flinders Medical Centre, North Adelaide, SA, Australia

**Vikas Rajesh Singh, MBBS, MS, DNB** Department Orthopedic Surgery, Lyell Mcewin Hospital, Elizabeth Vale, Australia

**Luc De Smet, MD, PhD** Department of Orthopedics, University Hospitals Leuven, Pellenberg, Belgium

**Robert M. Szabo, MD, MPH** Department of Orthopedics, Davis Health Care System, University of California, Sacramento, CA, USA

**Masahiro Tatebe, MD, PhD** Hand and Microsurgery Center, Anjo Kosei Hospital, Anjo, Japan

**Xiaofeng Teng** Department of Hand Surgery, NingBo Sixth Hospital of Zhejiang, China, Ningbo, Zhejiang, China

**Wing-lim Tse, FRCSEd, FHKCOS** General Office, Department of Orthopedics and Traumatology, Prince of Wales Hospital, Shatin, Hong Kong, SAR China

**Lee Wang, MD** Department of Radiology, University of Miami Miller School of Medicine, Miami, FL, USA

**H. Kirk Watson, MD** The Hand Center, University of Connecticut, Glastonbury, CT, USA

**Terry L. Whipple, MD** Virginia Commonwealth University School of Medicine, Richmond, VA, USA

**Clara Wong Wing-yee, MRCS, FRCSEd, FHKCOS** Department of Orthopedics and Traumatology, Prince of Wales Hospital, Shatin, Hong Kong, China

Sun Tuen Mun Center, Tuen Mun, N.T., Hong Kong, China

**Chong Jin Yeo, MBChB, MRCS, MMed, FAMS** Hand and Microsurgery Section, Department of Orthopedic Surgery, Tan Tock Seng Hospital, Singapore, Singapore

**Michael B. Zlatkin, MD, FRCP (C)** Nationalrad, Commerce Parkway, Weston, FL, USA

Department of Diagnostic Radiology, University of Miami Miller School of Medicine, Miami, FL, USA

# 1 Dedication. Robert Kienböck (January 11, 1871–September 7, 1953): A Life for Radiology and Radiotherapy

Martin Chochole

Robert Kienböck saw the light of day on January 11th 1871 in Vienna as the firstborn of Karl and Adele (née Sandor) Kienböck, a well-respected family. His father, descended from a wealthy farmer in Lower Austria, was a successful lawyer [1, 2]. His mother came from a Hungarian family; her father had been a banker in Budapest [3]. In 1871 the German Empire was restored and Wilhelm, King of Prussia, became Kaiser and König. Robert's younger brother Viktor, after graduating law school, entered his father's office and eventually went into politics. He would later become minister of finance (for two terms) and governor of the National Bank of Austria [4]. Both brothers would later be expelled by the Nazis into insignificance [4, 5]. After World War II the brothers, now in their 70s, returned to their old vocations with much diminished capacity and stature [1, 2, 4–6]. Table 1.1 provides a timeline of his lifetime achievements.

## Early Career

Robert Kienböck, like all male members of the family, attended Schottengymnasium between 1881 and 1889 [1, 2, 6]. He entered medical school in Vienna, passed the winter half-term 1893/1894 in Heidelberg, and graduated on July 25, 1895 [1, 6, 7]. This was the same year Wilhelm Conrad Röntgen discovered X-rays in the laboratory of Würzburg University and took his first radiograph of the hand of his wife, Anna Berta [8]. After graduation Kienböck enrolled at the second military hospital in Vienna and attended until March 1896 [7]. For the next 12 months Robert Kienböck had the opportunity to visit clinics in Paris and London for further studies [1, 7]. While still in London he encountered X-ray beams with the physicist Carlyle, who performed experimental studies in the new field of röntgenology [1].

After returning to Austria, Kienböck attended the Allgemeine Krankenhaus, the leading teaching hospital in Vienna, where he joined the faculty of internal medicine headed by Schrötter [1, 6, 7]. Soon after, he initiated his own studies in radiology, and in 1899 he established a private radiologic institute in the offices of Sanatorium Fürth [5–7]. Although young and having to learn by experience, his ideas were innovative and his advice was sought even by senior colleagues [1]. Throughout the years, the institute would be the base where he would further his research in skeletal radiology [1, 5].

In 1898 he published his first three papers on radio-diagnostics [2] and in 1900 his first paper on radiotherapy. In 1901 he published a paper on the radiologic evaluation of the spine. Experimental studies done by Kienböck at this

M. Chochole, MD (✉)
Department of Orthopedics, Herz Jesu Krankenhaus, Baumgasse 20A, Vienna 1030, Austria
e-mail: martinchochole@hotmail.com

© Springer International Publishing Switzerland 2016

D.M. Lichtman, G.I. Bain (eds.), *Kienböck's Disease*, DOI 10.1007/978-3-319-34226-9_1

**Table 1.1** Timeline of Robert Kienböck

| 1871–1895 | 1896–1905 | 1905–1915 | 1915–1938 | 1938–1953 |
|---|---|---|---|---|
| Born Jan 11, 1871 | Study in London and Paris | Co-founder of German Röntgen Gesellschaft | Co-founder of Vienna Society of Radiology | Quits professional activities 1942 after two strokes |
| Schottengymnasium 1881–1889 | Klinik Schrötter | 1910 Marries Bianka Notburga | Elected first president of the Austrian Society of Radiology | Still working as a scientist |
| Vienna Medical School till 1895 | Publishes first papers on radiodiagnostics and radiotherapy | Skull fracture due to fall from horse | 1933 he has to step down as president of the German Röntgen Congress in Bremen | Stays in contact with his colleagues |
| Second Military Hospital, Vienna | Founds his own radiologic institute | "Über traumatische Malazie des Mondbeines und ihre Folgezustände: Entartungsformen und Kompressionsfrakturen," published in Fortschritte auf dem Gebiet der Röntgenstrahlen | 1934 commences to publish 8 volumes of radiodiagnostics | Elected Honorary President of the Austrian Society of Radiology 1946 |
| | Introduces dosimetry | Perilunate dislocations epiphyseolysis and posttraumatic growth stop | 1938 after the Anschluss Nazis force him to retire | Dies September 7, 1953 |
| | Establishes radiology as distinct discipline in medicine | Appointed extraordinary Professor at Vienna Medical School | Sanatorium Fürth is closed down | • 250 publications |
| | Head of the first radiologic institute within a hospital | | | • 8 volumes on radiodiagnostics<br>• Set basis for safe X-rays |

time were among the first to confirm the deleterious effect of radiation on skin and soft tissues. In 1901 he published a paper on the pathology of skin lesions in humans and beasts caused by X-rays [1]. Kienböck proved the direct effect of radiation on skin and tissue. This ended the erroneous idea that the "electrical side effects" of radiation were therapeutically active agents [1, 2]. These observations on the biologic effects of radiation made him one of the leading experts worldwide [1]. In 1901 the German Society for Nature Science and Medicine appointed Kienböck the head of their study group for radiotherapy [1].

In 1902, while still a "Hilfsarzt" (auxiliary physician) at Kaiser Franz Josef Ambulatorium, Wien X, he published a paper on the topic of traumatic syringomyelia and its differential diagnosis in the traumatic spinal cord lesion [1, 7, 9].

In 1903, together with Guido Holzknecht and Leopold Freund, Kienböck was appointed postdoctoral lecturer in radiology, effectively establishing a new discipline in medicine [1, 6, 10]. His paper, "Die medizinische Radiologie als selbständiger Zweig der medizinischen Wissenschaft," jointly published with Guido Holzknecht, was an important stimulus for the recognition of medical subspecialties [10].

Kienbock was also a pioneer in the safe use of diagnostic and therapeutic X-rays. In 1903 he introduced one of the first dosimeters. Using a so-called Aluminiumtreppe he was able to accurately anticipate the effects of radiation in superficial and deep tissue layers of the body, thus making radiotherapy much safer for use in dermatology and oncology. In 1904 he published an essay on the prophylaxis of professional risks for radiologists: A dramatic call for protection against radiation on behalf of radiologists and their patients [11]. The publication of his handbook on radiotherapy in 1907 was another significant step forward [1, 6] in this area.

In 1904 Kienböck was named head of a new radiologic institute within the prestigious Erste Wiener Allgemeine Poliklinik in Vienna, presumably the first radiologic institute in all of Europe [1, 6, 12]. The Poliklinik was founded in 1872 by faculty members of Vienna's medical school and provided, among other things, free treatment to the poor. In those days the Poliklinik was on the cutting edge of medical science [12] and Kienböck was now on equal terms with other senior colleagues of the faculty (Figs. 1.1, 1.2, 1.3, and 1.4).

Throughout his early career, Kienbock worked with his German and international colleagues to

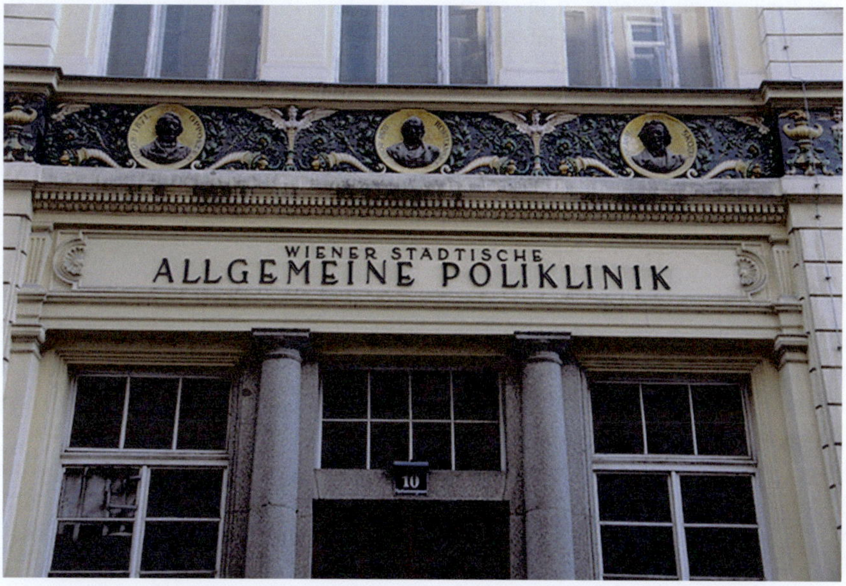


**Fig. 1.1** The portal of Erste Wiener Poliklinik (later: Wiener Städtische Allgemeine Poliklinik)

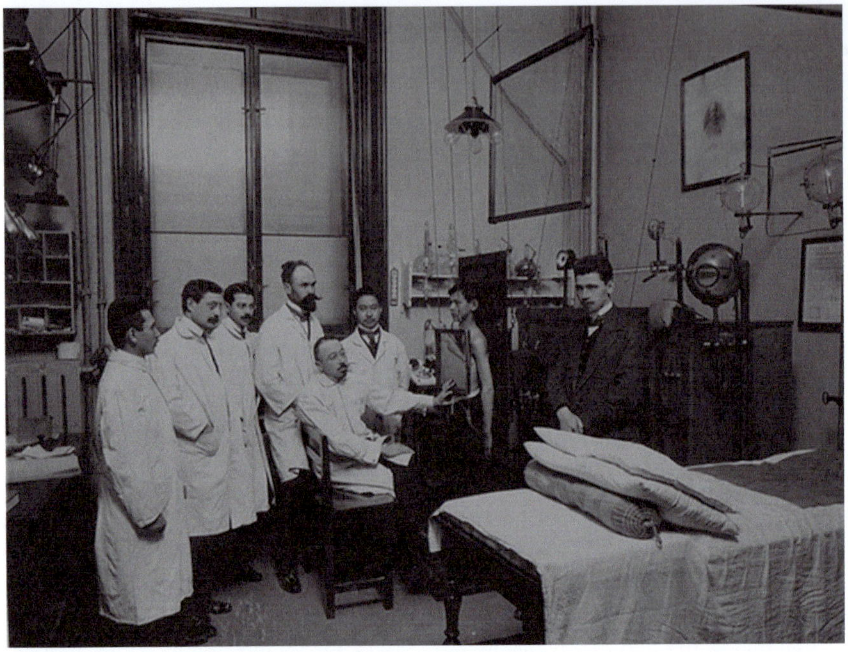

**Fig. 1.2** Robert Kienböck in the radiology department of Poliklinik 1909 (sitting in front of his colleagues). Reprinted with permission from Josephinum, Collection of Pictures, Collections and History of Medicine, MedUni, Vienna, Austria

advance education and research in radiology and radiotherapy. His affable personality and mastery of foreign languages was a great asset for him in that regard. One of his international colleagues was Antoine Béclère, the founder of the French Radiologic Society [1]. In 1905 Kienböck was instrumental in organizing and establishing the Deutsche Röntgen Gesellschaft [1, 2, 8], the national radiologic society of Germany.

The year 1910 was memorable for Robert Kienbock; it was a year with great joy and near disaster. On August 25th he married Bianka Notburga née Schindelmaiser, widowed Barbieri. Later that same year, Kienböck, a passionate horseman, fell from his mount and was hit by a hoof, sustaining a fractured skull. He was brought to the Poliklinik but the case looked desperate. Against all odds Kienböck recovered, although slowly. He would never be the same cheerful man again. He turned out to be a quiet and ponderous laborer. Attendance at meetings was hardly bearable due to a dramatic hyperacusis [1, 2, 6]. He reduced his workload at the Poliklinik and focused more on his private diagnostic center in Sanatorium Fürth. But in 1910 he also published his 90th paper, which made his name unforgotten in the field of hand surgery [1, 2, 13] (Figs. 1.5 and 1.6). In 26 pages he outlined the pattern of lunatomalacia with porosis, sclerosis, and initial fragmentation of the proximal lunate pole. He envisioned the pathogenesis as malnutrition and overuse rather than traumatic causes [13]. Remarkably, the very next publication in the same issue of Fortschritte auf dem Gebiete d. Röntgenstrahlen was a paper by Kienbock on perilunate dislocations [14]. Later the same year he published on epiphyseolysis and posttraumatic inhibition of bone growth [15].

In 1913 he lectured on the radiotherapy of malignant bone tumors in London and on dosimetry in Berlin. In the next few years, he became recognized as a leading authority in the diagnosis of bone diseases and tumors [1, 2, 16]. He contributed to the resolution of the diagnostic dilemma between Mb. Paget and Mb. Recklinghausen (and in 1940 and 1941 he

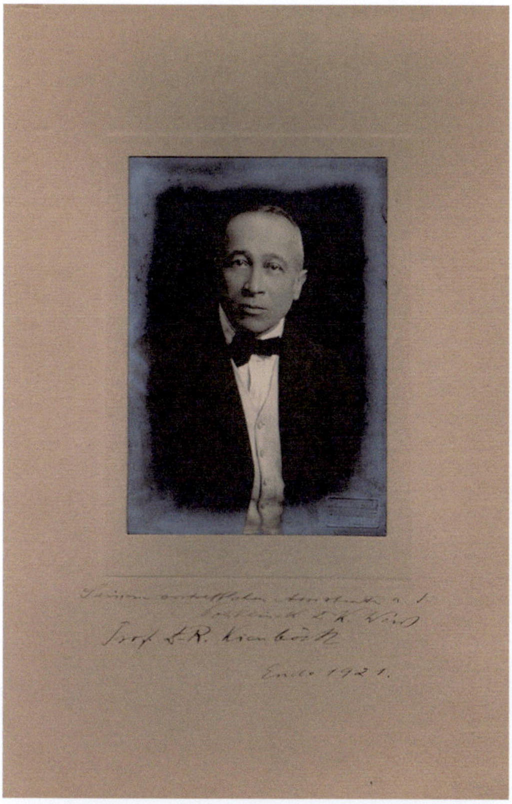

**Fig. 1.3** Portrait of Robert Kienböck, 1921. Reprinted with permission from Josephinum, Collection of Pictures, Collections and History of Medicine, MedUni, Vienna, Austria

published a small booklet on each of these entities, later embedded in the first volume of his Radiology [1]). In 1915 Kienböck was appointed extraordinary Professor at Vienna Medical School [1, 5]. He held this position until 1938, when he was dismissed by the Nazis [5].

## The Nazi Era and WWII

Most of Robert Kienbock's appointments and projects were prematurely terminated during the Nazi's rise to power and especially after the Anschluss, or the Nazi annexation of Austria in 1938. He was persecuted for two reasons: one was because of the political positions held by his brother and the other because Kienbock himself was half Jewish (his mother came from a Jewish family). Nevertheless, in the so-called Reichsärzteregister (the board of medical doctors in the Third Reich), he was considered of "German blood" [5].

In 1923 Kienböck, Holzknecht, and Haudek co-founded the Vienna Society of Radiology (Wiener Gesellschaft für Röntgenkunde). In 1933 Robert Kienböck was told to step down as president of the German Röntgen Congress in Bremen because the political class had decided to accept only speakers of German blood. Kienböck, although being Catholic but half Jewish on his mother's side, was informed of this in a letter by his substitute. Ultimately, none of the Viennese radiologists would attend the congress in Bremen [6]. In 1934, the Austrian Society of Radiology was founded with Kienböck elected as its first president [1, 2, 6]. Both the Viennese and Austrian societies existed separately until annexation of Austria by the Third Reich [6]. In 1934, Robert Kienböck started writing his eight volumes on radiology (Fig. 1.7a, b). Unfortunately, the work was abandoned in 1942 [1, 2].

Not only was the Anschluss the end of Austria and its institutions, above all it was an immense and cruel human tragedy. The Sanatorium Fürth was shut down by the Nazis and the building was confiscated by the Wehrmacht for their own purposes. Most of the former patients, many of them Jewish, never returned. Jewish scholars and physicians were deported or had to flee penniless. Many colleagues chose to commit suicide. Fürth, the owner of the sanatorium, was one of those. He and his wife took their own lives in the operating theatre of the sanatorium [17]. In 1938 the Poliklinik was "aryanized" by the Nazis and lost two-thirds of its outstanding, highly valued faculty [12]. Both Kienböck brothers were forced to retire but were permitted to remain in Vienna [5].

During the war, Kienböck continued his studies and his work on the eight volumes on Radiology. Two of these are still available. Interestingly, volume two was published in 1938 in two parts, and the first volume came out in 1941 (authors' own copies).

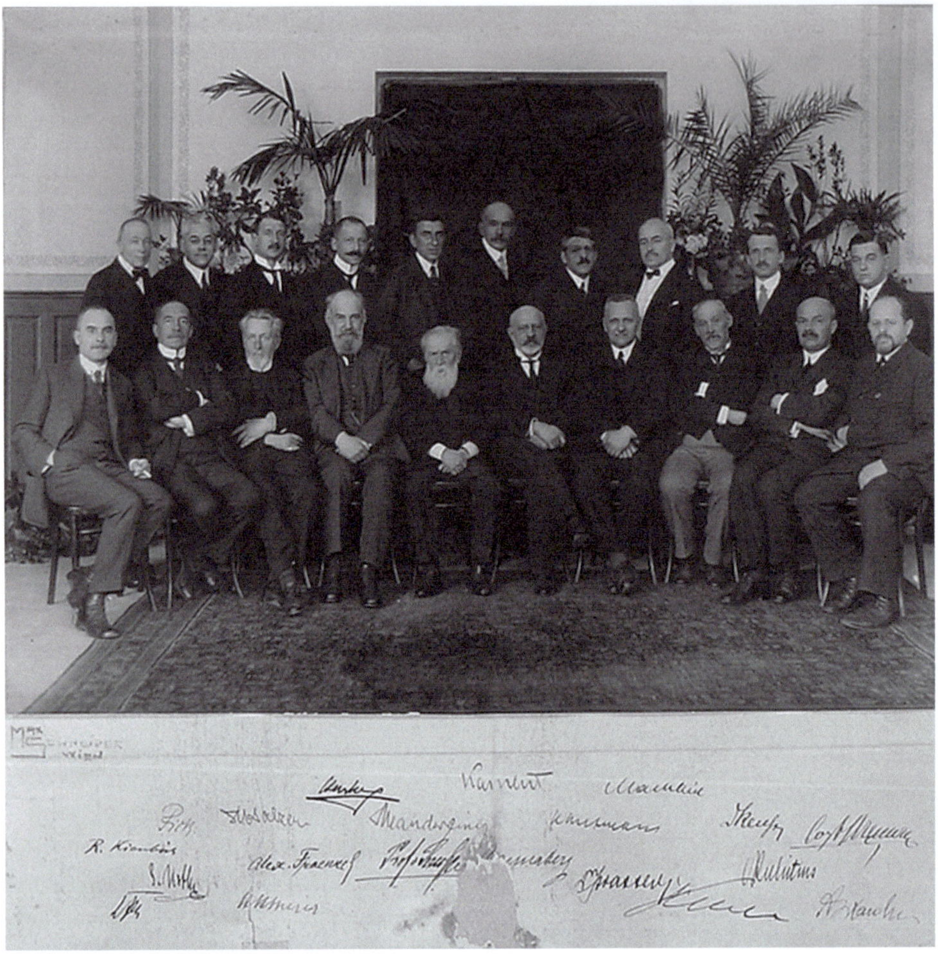

**Fig. 1.4** The faculty of Erste Wiener Poliklinik, 1923. Robert Kienböck is the leftmost in the second row. Reprinted with permission from Josephinum, Collection of Pictures, Collections and History of Medicine, MedUni, Vienna, Austria

## Post-WWII

After World War II the Poliklinik was taken over by the City of Vienna and renamed Wiener Städtische Allgemeine Poliklinik. It was operated as a hospital until 1998, and then as a home for the aged for about 10 years. The Sanatorium Fürth building was recovered by the Austrian Government after the war and was later turned over to the US authorities as part of the US Embassy in Austria [17].

Robert Kienböck never returned to his professional activities as a radiologist [5] but did maintain a strong interest in the activities of the scientific community. Two consecutive strokes at the age of 71 handicapped him and he was further hindered by severe depression [1]. Nevertheless, he was named honorary president of the Austrian Röntgen Society, which was established at the Poliklinik on November 30, 1946 [1, 6] (Fig. 1.8). When Robert Kienböck died on September 7, 1953, he had written 250 publications and completed eight volumes on radiology. He was a pioneer in establishing radiology as a specialty and set the standards for a safer practice of radiotherapy [18]. He never personally suffered the effects of uncritical use of X-ray [1, 2, 6, 19].

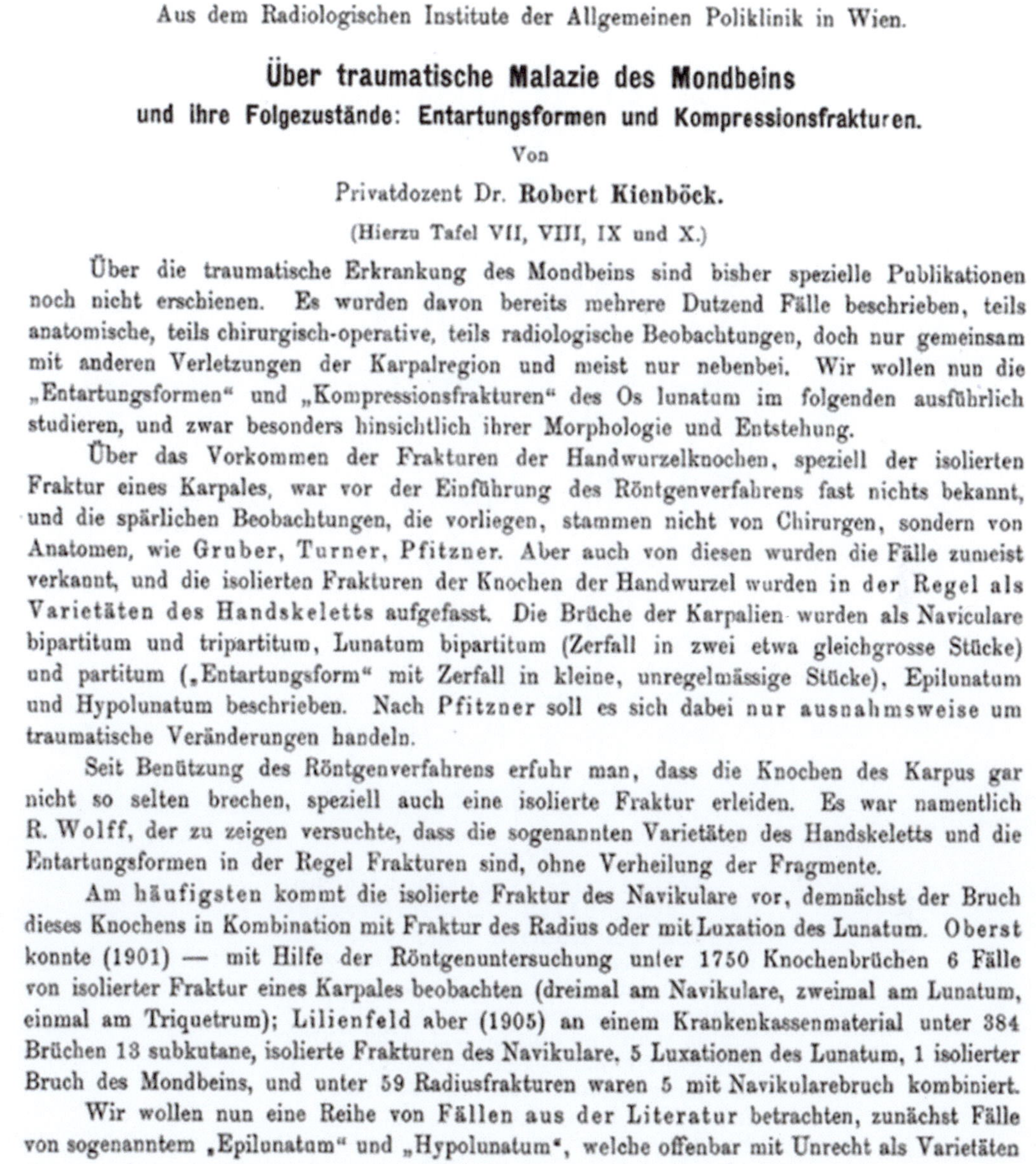

Aus dem Radiologischen Institute der Allgemeinen Poliklinik in Wien.

**Über traumatische Malazie des Mondbeins**
**und ihre Folgezustände: Entartungsformen und Kompressionsfrakturen.**

Von

Privatdozent Dr. **Robert Kienböck.**

(Hierzu Tafel VII, VIII, IX und X.)

Über die traumatische Erkrankung des Mondbeins sind bisher spezielle Publikationen noch nicht erschienen. Es wurden davon bereits mehrere Dutzend Fälle beschrieben, teils anatomische, teils chirurgisch-operative, teils radiologische Beobachtungen, doch nur gemeinsam mit anderen Verletzungen der Karpalregion und meist nur nebenbei. Wir wollen nun die „Entartungsformen" und „Kompressionsfrakturen" des Os lunatum im folgenden ausführlich studieren, und zwar besonders hinsichtlich ihrer Morphologie und Entstehung.

Über das Vorkommen der Frakturen der Handwurzelknochen, speziell der isolierten Fraktur eines Karpales, war vor der Einführung des Röntgenverfahrens fast nichts bekannt, und die spärlichen Beobachtungen, die vorliegen, stammen nicht von Chirurgen, sondern von Anatomen, wie Gruber, Turner, Pfitzner. Aber auch von diesen wurden die Fälle zumeist verkannt, und die isolierten Frakturen der Knochen der Handwurzel wurden in der Regel als Varietäten des Handskeletts aufgefasst. Die Brüche der Karpalien wurden als Naviculare bipartitum und tripartitum, Lunatum bipartitum (Zerfall in zwei etwa gleichgrosse Stücke) und partitum („Entartungsform" mit Zerfall in kleine, unregelmässige Stücke), Epilunatum und Hypolunatum beschrieben. Nach Pfitzner soll es sich dabei nur ausnahmsweise um traumatische Veränderungen handeln.

Seit Benützung des Röntgenverfahrens erfuhr man, dass die Knochen des Karpus gar nicht so selten brechen, speziell auch eine isolierte Fraktur erleiden. Es war namentlich R. Wolff, der zu zeigen versuchte, dass die sogenannten Varietäten des Handskeletts und die Entartungsformen in der Regel Frakturen sind, ohne Verheilung der Fragmente.

Am häufigsten kommt die isolierte Fraktur des Navikulare vor, demnächst der Bruch dieses Knochens in Kombination mit Fraktur des Radius oder mit Luxation des Lunatum. Oberst konnte (1901) — mit Hilfe der Röntgenuntersuchung unter 1750 Knochenbrüchen 6 Fälle von isolierter Fraktur eines Karpales beobachten (dreimal am Navikulare, zweimal am Lunatum, einmal am Triquetrum); Lilienfeld aber (1905) an einem Krankenkassenmaterial unter 384 Brüchen 13 subkutane, isolierte Frakturen des Navikulare, 5 Luxationen des Lunatum, 1 isolierter Bruch des Mondbeins, und unter 59 Radiusfrakturen waren 5 mit Navikularebruch kombiniert.

Wir wollen nun eine Reihe von Fällen aus der Literatur betrachten, zunächst Fälle von sogenanntem „Epilunatum" und „Hypolunatum", welche offenbar mit Unrecht als Varietäten

**Fig. 1.5** Front page of the famous paper on avascular necrosis of the lunate

Ruckensteiner called Kienböck an everlasting star in the firmament of radiology [19]. He established the fundamentals of radiotherapy and he made it a secure and reliable treatment by adding his method of radioquantimetry [20].

For hand surgeons Kienböck's name always will stand for the entity of lunatomalacia [13]. He not only encountered the radiologic phenomenon but described its pathogenesis, as well. He even anticipated histologic changes that decades later have been confirmed [19]. His ideas on therapy are at least partly true today, as are his splendid observations and deductions on perilunate dislocation of the wrist [14].

For young colleagues in radiology the yearly "Kienböck Award" of the Austrian Radiologic

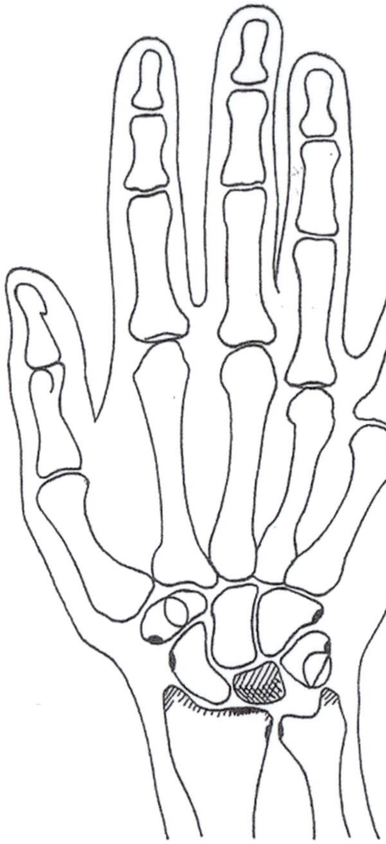

Fig. 23.

Skizze zur Veranschaulichung der sekundären Begleiterscheinungen bei isolierter traumatischer Erkrankung des Lunatum: Ausschleifung und oberflächliche arthritische Veränderung am Radiusende, sowie Formveränderung am Stylus radii und ulnae. Die sechs schwarzen Punkte markieren die Rauhigkeit an den Ansatzstellen von drei Bändern, infolge von Lockerung und Zerrung des Handgelenkes.

13

**Fig. 1.6** The figure in his 1910 paper on avascular necrosis of the lunate. The translation of the figure legend states, "Drawing to visualize the sequelae of isolated post-traumatic lunatomalacia: Sclerosis and apophytes at the distal rim of radius, deformation of radial and ulnar styloid. The blackened patches mark the ligament insertions roughened due to secondary laxity of the carpus"

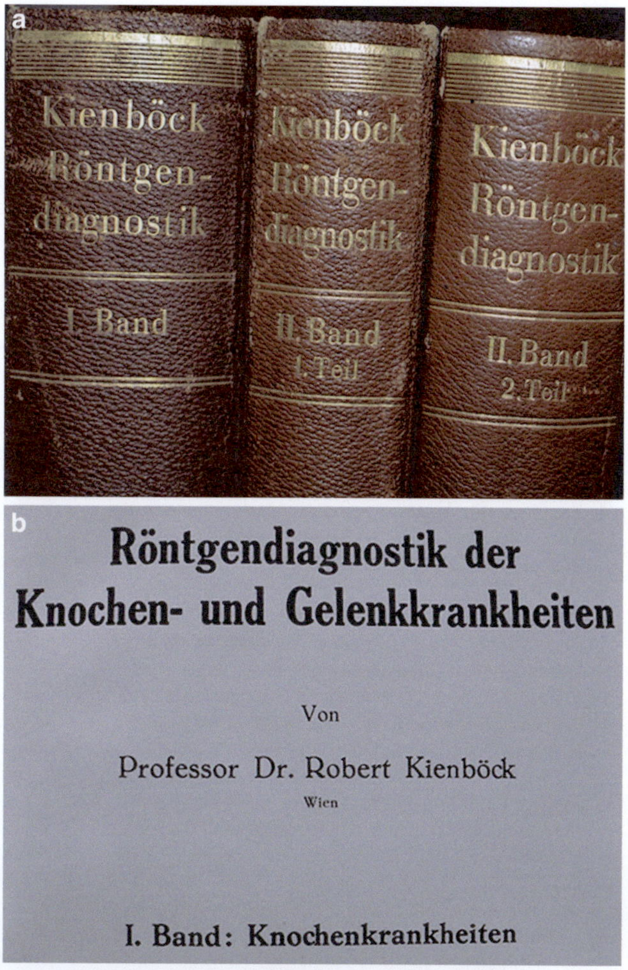


**Fig. 1.7** (**a**) Kienböck, Röntgendiagnostik der Knochen und Gelenkkrankheiten. (**b**) Kienböck, Röntgendiagnostik der Knochen und Gelenkkrankheiten, front page

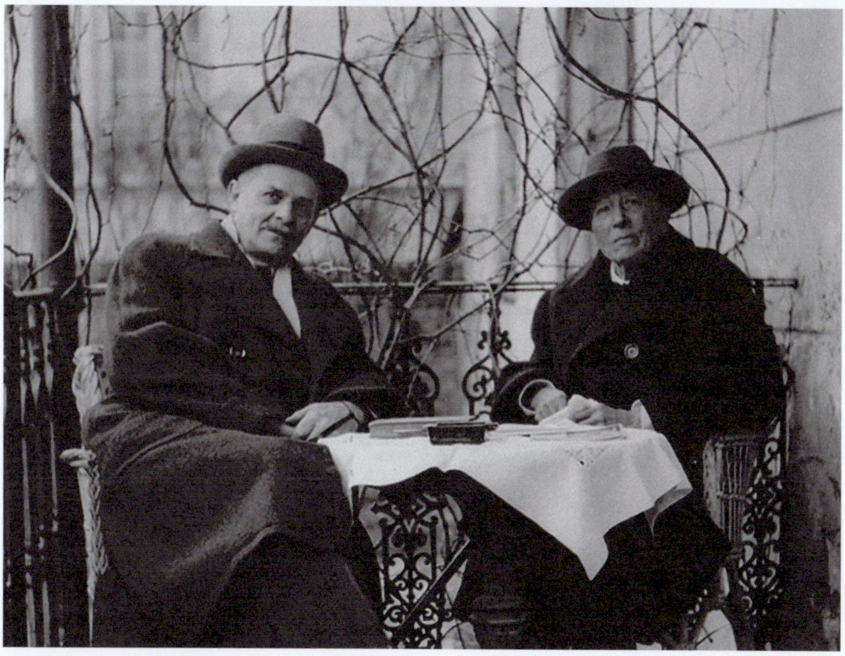

**Fig. 1.8** Robert Kienböck (*right*) at his 80th birthday with Konrad Weiss, First President of the Austrian Society of Radiology, after WW II (thus, successor of R. Kienböck)

Society is the stimulant to submit extraordinary, brilliant publications, quite in the spirit and of the standards set by Robert Kienböck himself [21].

## References


1. Weiss K. In memoriam Robert Kienböck, Eulogy held at the 6th Congress of the Austrian Röntgen Society in Innsbruck. Radiol Austriaca. 1954;VIII(2):109–16.
2. Weiss K. Professor Robert Kienböck. Wien Klin Wochenschr. 1953;65(42):883–4.
3. Opll F. Wiener Stadt- und Landesarchiv, MA 8, personal communication.
4. Kienböck M. Viktor Kienböck. Vierteljahresschrift für Zeitgeschichte, Sozial-, Kultur und Wirtschaftsgeschichte, 12. Jg. Nr.2/95, Wien 1995.
5. Huber A. Robert Kienböck, Gedenkbuch für die Opfer des Nationalsozialismus an der Universität Wien 1938 aktualisiert 2014/06/12. http:// gedenkbuch.univie.ac.at/index.php?id=435&no_cache=1&person_single_id=34.
6. Ellegast HH. Robert Kienböck in Hundert Jahre medizinische Radiologie in Österreich 1995, Hrsg.: Ellegast HH. Kogelnik HD., Strasser E, pp. 51–7.
7. Archiv des Medizinhistorischen Museum Wien IX, Josephinum (Personalakt) Allgemeines Krankenhaus, Verzeichnis der feierlichen Inaugurationen, Fischer I., S. 758.
8. Busch U. Die Gründung der Deutschen Röntgengesellschaft im Jahr 1905. http://www.drg.de/.
9. Kienböck R. Kritik der sogenannten, traumatischen Syringomyelie. Jahrb Psychiatrie Neurol. 1902; 21(4):162.
10. Holzkecht G, Kienböck R. Die medizinische Radiologie als selbständiger Zweig der medizinischen Wissenschaft. Wien Klin Wochenschr 1904; pp. 1–16.
11. Kienböck R. Über Prophylaxe des Radiologen gegen Beschädigung im Beruf. Wien Klin Wochenschr. 1904;51:1382–4.
12. Thurnher B. 1972. Das Röntgeninstitut der Poliklinik. Österreichische Ärztezeitung. 27(11).
13. Kienböck R. Über traumatische Malazie des Mondbeins und ihre Folgezustände: entartungsformen und Kompressionsfrakturen. Fortschritte ad Gebiete d Röntgenstrahlen. 1910;XVI(2):77–103.
14. Kienböck R. Über Luxationen im Bereiche der Handwurzel A. Dorsale Luxation der Hand in der perilunären Gelenkslinie und isolierte volare Luxation des Os lunatum, B. Dorsale Luxation der Mittelhand. Fortschritte ad Gebiete d Röntgenstrahlen. 1910; XVI(2):103–15.
15. Kienböck R. Über traumatische Epiphysenlösung und Wachstumshemmung. Zentralblatt für Röntgenstrahlen, Radium und verwandte Gebiete. 1910;3(4):81–6.
16. Kienböck R. Über Röntgendiagnostik der Geschwülste der Knochen und Gelenke Erstbeschreibung primärer und sekundärer Knochentumoren. Wien Klin Wochenschr. 1921;39:472–3.
17. Walzer T. Vom Böhmerwald aus in die Welt, Einblicke in die Geschichte der Familie Fürth. David, Jüdische Kulturzeitschrift. 2005; (12) 67. http://www.davidkultur.at/ausgabe.php?ausg=67&artikel=592.
18. Kienböck R. Über die Arten der photochemischen Radiometer für Messung des Röntgenlichtes. Strahlentherapie, 1913; (2): 556–67.
19. Ruckensteiner E. Dem Gedenken von Robert Kienböck (1871–1953) und Josef Paluguay (1890–1953). Fortschritte Röntgen Nuklearmedizin. 1954;81(Suppl):20–3.
20. Kienböck R. Das quantimetrische Verfahren. Wien Klin Wochenschr. 1906;14:405–8.
21. Österreichische Röntgengesselschaft Gesselschaft für Medizinische Radiologie und Nuklearmedizin. http://www.oerg.at/index.php/aktuelles.html.

# Part I

# Basic Science

# Osseous Anatomy and Microanatomy of the Lunate

2

Chong Jin Yeo, Gregory Ian Bain, and Egon Perilli

## Introduction

The name of the lunate bone derives from the "crescent-shaped" (Latin: *lunatus*), from Latin *luna* ("moon"), from the bone's resemblance to a crescent moon. The lunate has been described as the keystone of the wrist. It is the "intercalated" segment of the intercalated proximal carpal row.

An understanding of the normal anatomy and variants is of value before delving into the pathological anatomy.

C.J. Yeo, MBChB, MRCS, MMed, FAMS
Hand and Microsurgery Section, Department of Orthopedic Surgery, Tan Tock Seng Hospital, 11 Jalan Tan Tock Seng, Singapore 308433, Singapore

G.I. Bain, MBBS, FRACS, FA(Ortho)A, PhD (✉)
Professor, Upper Limb and Research, Department of Orthopedic Surgery, Flinders University and Flinders Medical Centrer, Bedford Park, Adelaide, SA, Australia
e-mail: greg@gregbain.com.au

E. Perilli, PhD (Bioeng), MSc (Phys)
Medical Device Research Institute, School of Computer Science, Engineering and Mathematics, Flinders University, 1284 South Rd, Clovelly Park, SA 5082, Australia

## Gross Anatomy of the Normal Lunate

Dr. Henry Gray, in 1858, described the lunate in his classic text "Anatomy: Descriptive and Surgical" as follows:

> "The *Semi-lunar* bone may be distinguished by its deep concavity and cresentic outline. It is situated in the centre of the upper range of the carpus, between the scaphoid and cuneiform. Its *superior surface*, convex, smooth and quadrilateral in form, articulates with the radius. Its *inferior surface* is deeply concave, and of greater extent from before backwards, than transversely; it articulates with the head of the os magnum, and by a long narrow facet (separated by a ridge from the general surface) with the unciform bone. Its *anterior* or *palmar* and *posterior* or *dorsal surface* are rough, for the attachment of ligaments, the former being broader, and of somewhat rounded form. The *external surface* presents a narrow, flattened, semilunar facet, for articulation with the scaphoid. The *internal surface* is marked by a smooth, quadrilateral facet, for articulation with the cuneiform (Fig. 2.1).
>
> To ascertain to which hand this bone belongs, hold it with the dorsal surface upwards, and the convex articular surface backwards; the quadrilateral articular facet will then point to the side to which the bone belongs.
>
> *Articulations*. With five bones: the radius above, os magnum and unciform below, scaphoid and cuneiform on either side."

© Springer International Publishing Switzerland 2016
D.M. Lichtman, G.I. Bain (eds.), *Kienböck's Disease*, DOI 10.1007/978-3-319-34226-9_2

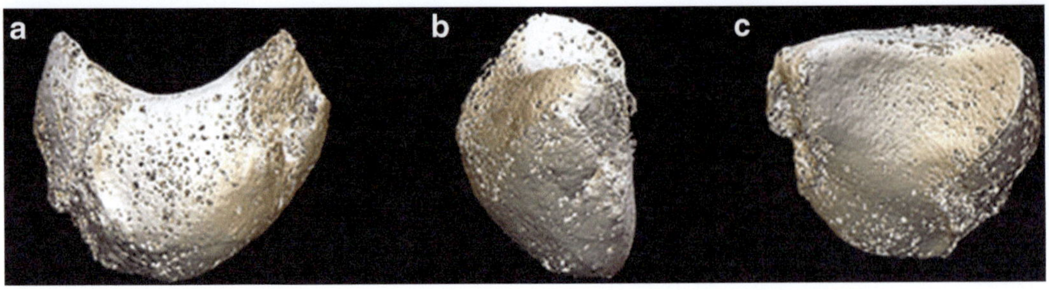


**Fig. 2.1** Micro-CT 3D images of the normal lunate from a (**a**) radial view, (**b**) volar view, and (**c**) distal view. Reproduced with permission from Low S, Bain GI, Findlay DM, Eng K, Perilli E, External and internal bone micro-architecture in normal and Kienböck's lunates: A whole-bone micro-computed tomography study. J Orthop Res 2014; 32 (6): 826–833.© 2014 Orthopedic Research Society. Published by Wiley Periodicals, Inc.

In addition to some changes in nomenclature of the bones, this description is still very much applicable today.

The lunate is cartilaginous at birth and usually has one ossification center that begins to ossify during the fourth year [1]. Ossification has been noted to take place from 1.5 to 7 years of age in boys, and between 1 and 6 years of age in girls. There have also been observations of double-ossification centers in the lunate.

Several accessory bones can be associated with the lunate. Accessory bones, if present, usually are the result of a secondary or an additional ossification center that does not fuse with the associated bone. These have been associated with the lunate: the os epilunatum (os centrale II), the os hypolunatum (os centrale III), the os hypotriquetrum, the os epitriquetrum (epipyramis, os centrale IV), and the os triangulare (os intermedium antebrachii, os triquetrum secundarium) [2]. The os epilunatum is located between the lunate, scaphoid, and capitate, along the distal border of the scaphoid and lunate. The os hypolunatum is located between the lunate and the capitate, just ulnar to the site of the os epilunatum. The os hypotriquetrum is located in the vicinity of the lunate, capitate, proximal pole of the hamate, and the triquetrum. The os epitriquetrum is located between the lunate, hamate, and triquetrum, just ulnar to the site of the os hypotriquetrum. The os triangulare is located between the lunate, triquetrum, and the distal ulna [2].

The lunate is crescentic, concave distally, and convex proximally. It consists of internally cancellous bone, surrounded by a cortical shell. The dorsal and palmar surfaces where the carpal ligaments attach to are rough. The palmar surface is roughly triangular and is larger and wider than the dorsal portion. The smooth, convex proximal articular surface articulates with the lunate fossa of the distal radius and with a portion of the triangular fibrocartilage on its proximal ulnar aspect. The lateral surface is crescent shaped, flat, and narrow, with a relatively narrow surface area with which it contacts the scaphoid. The medial surface is square or rectangular, and fairly flat, and articulates with the triquetrum. The distal surface is deeply concave and articulates with the proximal portion of the capitate. There are variations noted for the distal articulations that will be touched upon later in the chapter.

Of note, there are no muscle origins or insertions on the lunate, but has a volar and dorsal capsule, and the scapholunate and lunotriquetral ligaments.

Five bones articulate with the lunate: the radius, scaphoid, capitate, hamate, and triquetrum. The lunate articulates with the radius on its proximal surface where it lies in the lunate fossa of the radius, located on the ulnar aspect of the distal radius. The lunate articulates with the scaphoid along the lunate's radial surface, with a relatively small, crescent-shaped articular surface area. The lunate articulates with the capitate distally, where the proximal pole of the capitate sits in the distal, crescent-shaped articular surface of the lunate. Between the articular surfaces for the triquetrum and the capitate, there usually is a narrow strip of articular surface for articulation with the proximal portion of the hamate. A curved ridge separates the articular surfaces for the hamate and capitate. Contact with the hamate is maximized with ulnar deviation.

## Normal Lunate Morphology

Viegas et al. described two types of lunate based on the existence of a distal medial facet. Type I lunates (35 %) had no distal medial facet while type II (65 %) lunates had a distal medial facet that articulates with the hamate [3] (Fig. 2.2).

Zapico in 1966 categorized lunate morphology into three types (Fig. 2.3) and also noted a relation-

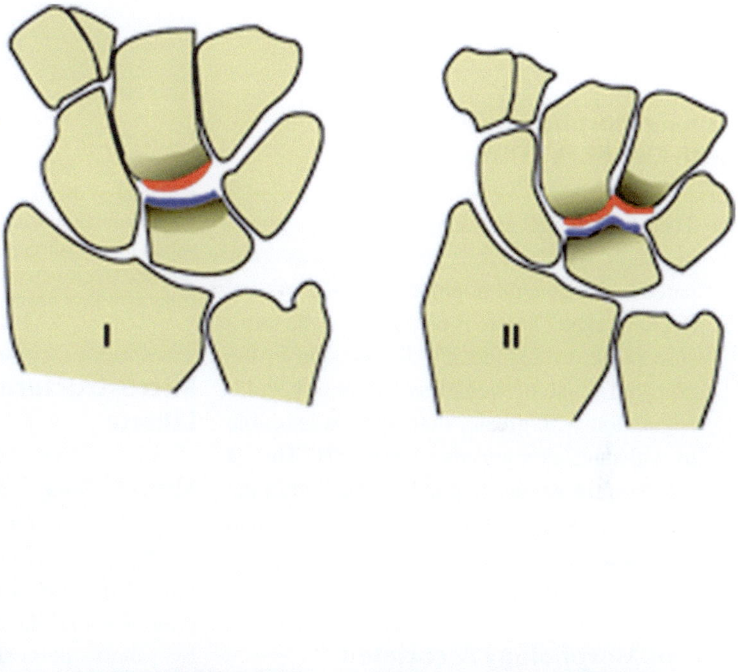


**Fig. 2.2** Lunate morphology as described by Viegas. Type I has an absent medial facet, while type II had a medial facet articulating with the hamate

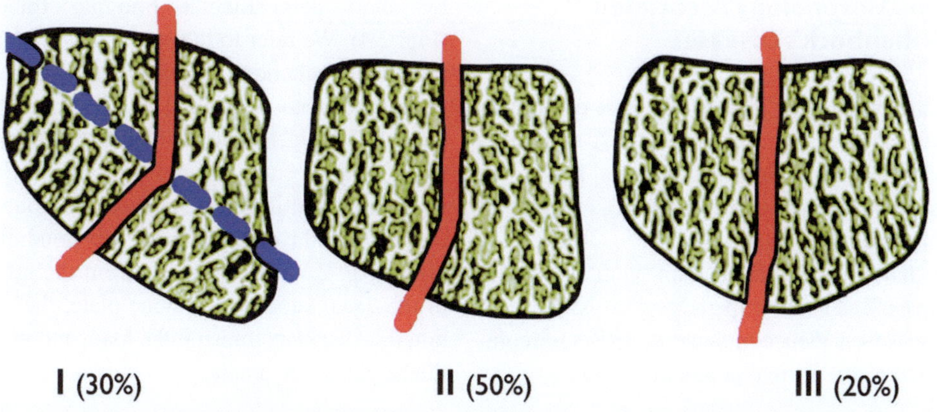


**Fig. 2.3** Lunate morphology as described by Zapico. The Zapico type I lunates have a trabecular angulation of greater than 135°, making it less able to tolerate compressive loads and thus at risk for Kienböck's disease. Modified from [4]

ship between the ulnar variance and type of lunate [4, 5]. Type I lunates are trapezoidal in shape and associated with negative ulnar variance. Type II lunates are more rectangular in shape and associated with ulnar neutral wrists. Type III lunates are pentagonal, with two proximal joint surfaces, and found typically with positive ulnar variance.

## Wrist Morphology Associated with Kienböck's Disease

There are a number of morphological factors of the lunate, radius, and ulnar that are known to be associated with Kienböck's disease.

### Lunate Morphology Associated with Kienböck's Disease

1. There is a higher incidence of Viegas' type I lunates in Kienböck's disease patients as compared to the general population [6–8].
2. Zapico's type I lunate is postulated to be more susceptible to Kienböck's disease due to the potential plane of weakness as the trabecular angulation with greater than 135° is less able to withstand compressive forces [9]. This is based on the studies that trabeculae within the lunate run perpendicular to the proximal and distal articular surfaces [4, 9].

### Radius Morphology Associated with Kienböck's Disease

1. Ulnar variance is one of the most commonly cited factors for lunate loading. A short ulna will increase the load on the radial half of the lunate. There are numerous studies to support this mechanism [10–13].
2. A flatter radial inclination with a smaller lunate was noted in patients with Kienböck's disease on their contralateral wrists as compared to the normal population [14].

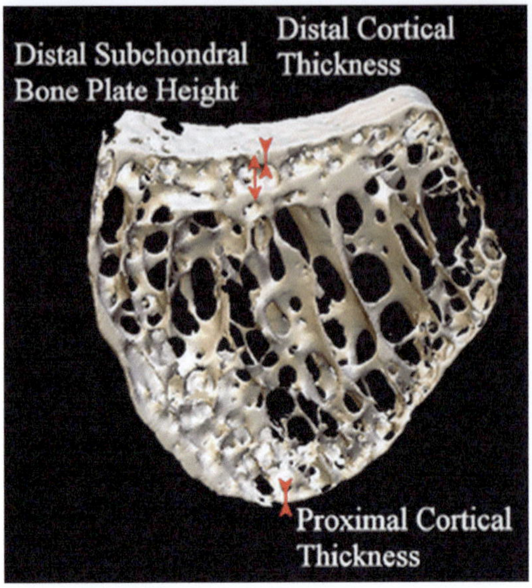


**Fig. 2.4** 3D micro-CT image demonstrating posterior view of left lunate, with trabeculae spanning from the proximal to the distal subchondral bone plate. Note that the proximal subchondral bone plate is a single layer, which may predispose to a stress fracture of the proximal surface, and it is repeatedly loaded in the same location. Copyright Dr. Gregory Bain

## Microstructure of the Normal Lunate

Micro-CT images demonstrate that the lunate has single-layered cortices, except the distal subchondral bone plate that articulates with the capitate [15]. This distal lunate subchondral bone plate was multilayered with each layer separated by short perpendicular bridging trabeculae (Fig. 2.4). We refer to the superficial layer as the primary subchondral bone plate, and then the secondary plate below it [15]. The coronal 3D micro-CT images demonstrated multiple radially arranged trabeculae, spanning from the distally reinforced multilayered subchondral bone plate to the single-layered proximal subchondral bone plate (Fig. 2.5). By spanning from the proximal to the distal subchondral bone plate, they maintain this distance, transmit the load, and maintain the height of the lunate.

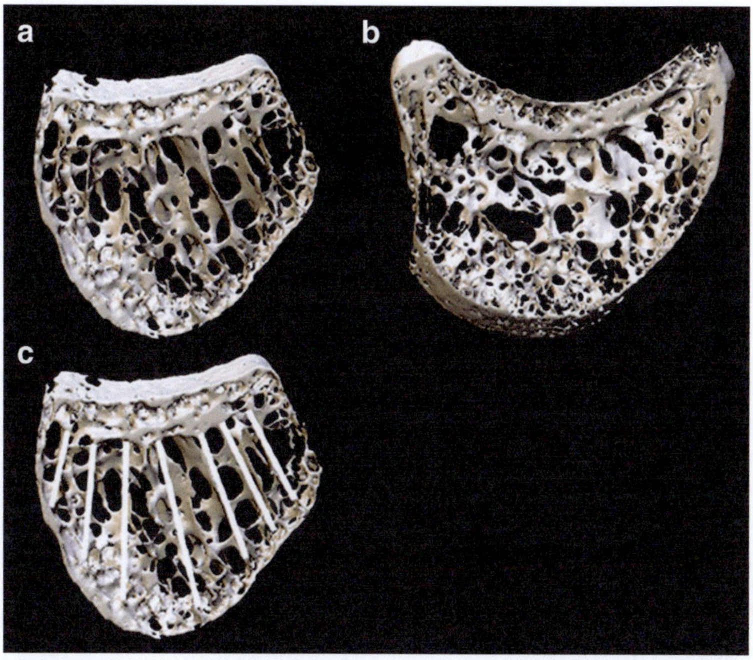


**Fig. 2.5** 3D micro-CT images, 1 mm thick cross sections of the lunate: (**a**) coronal section showing radial pattern of the trabeculae, spanning from distal to the proximal subchondral bone plate, (**b**) sagittal section, and (**c**) coronal section with radial lines highlighted in *white*, evidencing radial spanning trabeculae. Reproduced with permission from Low S, Bain GI, Findlay DM, Eng K, Perilli E, External and internal bone micro-architecture in normal and Kienböck's lunates: A whole-bone micro-computed tomography study. J Orthop Res 2014; 32 (6): 826–833.© 2014 Orthopedic Research Society. Published by Wiley Periodicals, Inc.

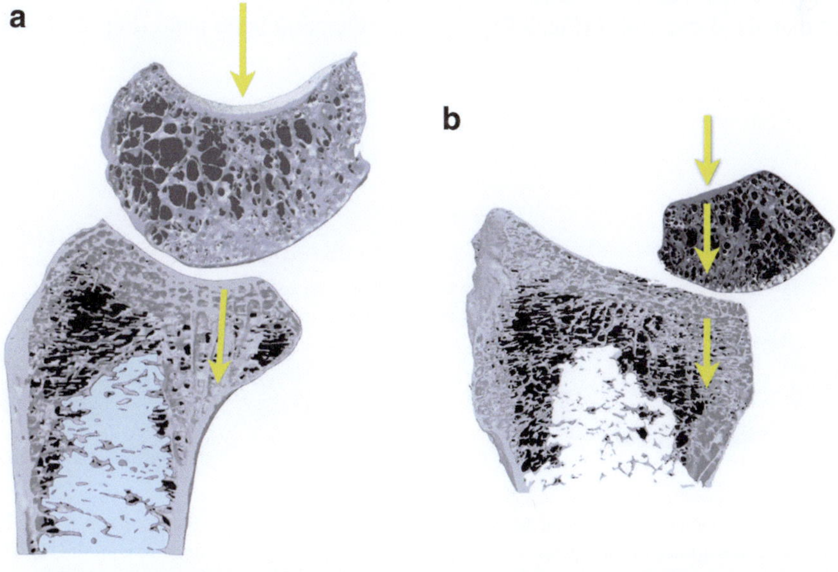


**Fig. 2.6** Micro-CT images showing the internal trabeculae and subchondral structures for the lunate and radius. (**a**) Sagittal view with the *bold arrow* illustrating the loading force from distal, and the *transparent arrows* showing the thickened trabeculae and subchondral bone. (**b**) Coronal view. Copyright Dr. Gregory Bain

The subchondral bone is a shock absorber and can be seen morphologically to distribute the joint stresses (Fig. 2.6). Below it, intermediate spanning trabeculae extend from the proximal to the distal articular surfaces and maintain the lunate height. The proximal articular "condyle" is the common site of Kienböck's disease. It is to be noted that the subchondral bone plate on the convex proximal surface is *only a single layer*, and it is this surface that is prone to the lunate fracture of Kienböck's disease. The distal multilayered cortex is self-reinforcing, and typically has a coronal fracture due to the impinging capitate. The main soft-tissue attachments, which include the vascular pedicles, are on the volar and dorsal aspects. Unlike long bones, there is almost no periosteum on the lunate.

## Microstructure of the Kienböck's Lunate

3D micro-CT images reveal that the lunates in Kienböck's disease had lost the normal crescent shape, and are fractured and fragmented, showing destruction of the bone, with only part of the cortex being present, both proximally and distally. The proximal cortex was more severely fragmented than the distal aspect (Fig. 2.7).

Internal morphology displayed regions of dense trabeculae bone interspersed with regions devoid of bone, with some residual evidence of the distal subchondral bone plate (Fig. 2.8). However, the radially patterned trabeculae that normally span from the distal to the proximal lunate subchondral bone plate were largely absent, due to bone fragmentation and resorption.

The micro-CT demonstrates the sparse pattern of normal lunate, compared to the avascular lunate, in which there are twice as many trabeculae that are thicker (×3). However, the total bone volume of the lunate is reduced, as a consequence of the bone resorption [4] (Fig. 2.9).

The subchondral bone plate is an important morphological structure that transmits the load, and provides a consistent platform for the articular cartilage. The subchondral bone plate can be compromised by fracture, or it can be eroded such that the articular cartilage has no support (Fig. 2.10).

## Histology of the Kienböck's Lunate

Gross examination demonstrates the ulcerated changes of the articular surface, and the necrotic subchondral bone plate (Fig. 2.11). Histological

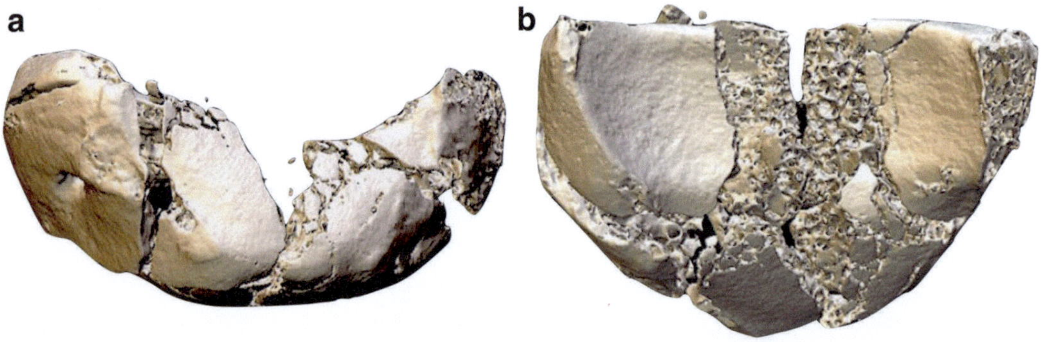


**Fig. 2.7** 3D micro-CT images of fractured Kienböck's lunates in various orientations of (**a**) radial view, with volar and dorsal fragments, (**b**) distal view, with the common coronal fracture. The Kienböck's lunate has lost the crescent shape, and is flattened and wider. The subchondral bone plate has fragmented, producing irregular articular surfaces. Copyright Dr. Gregory Bain

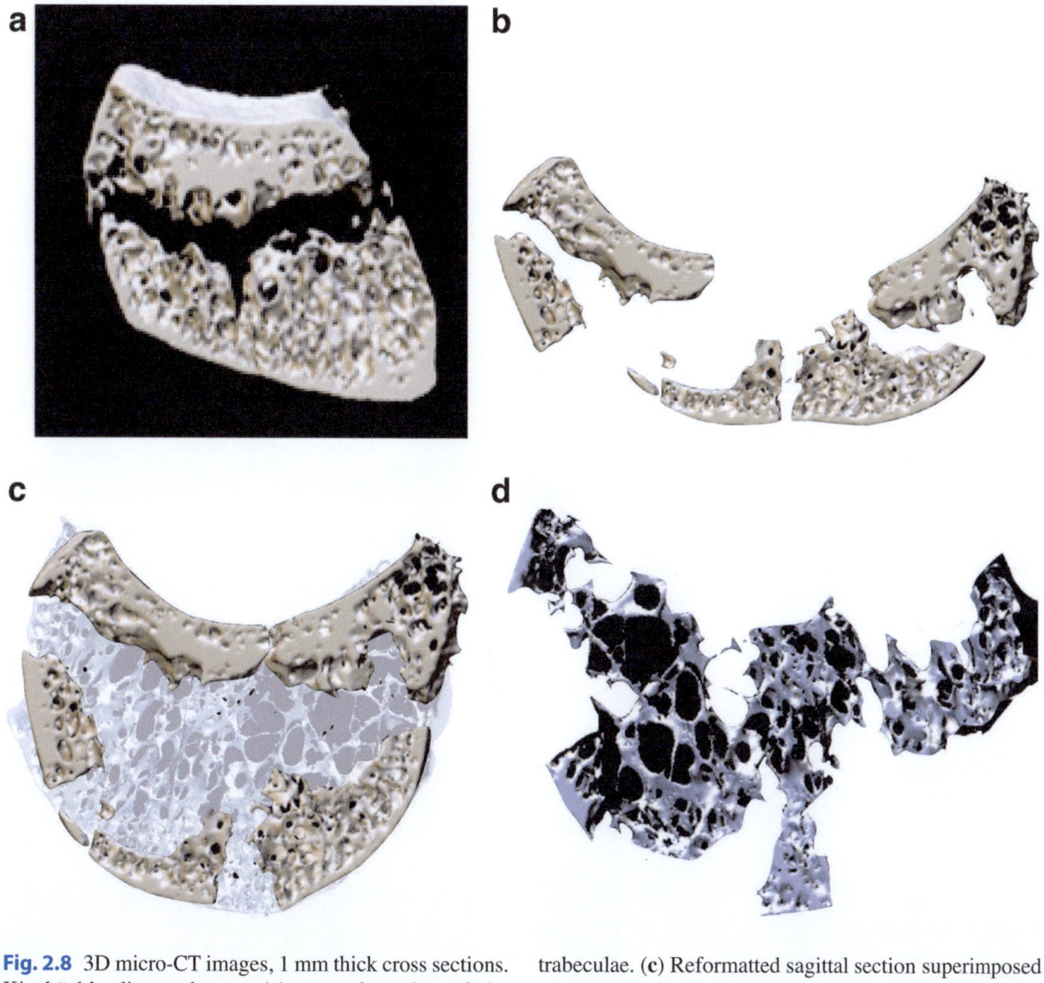

**Fig. 2.8** 3D micro-CT images, 1 mm thick cross sections. Kienböck's disease lunate: (**a**) coronal section of the lunate, consistent with a sheering fracture. (**b**) Sagittal section, with fragmentation of the cortical and subchondral bone plate and resorption of the spanning radial trabeculae. (**c**) Reformatted sagittal section superimposed on a normal lunate. Note the multiple cortical fractures, and extensive loss of trabeculae due to fracture and resorption. (**d**) The proposed area of reabsorption of bone. Copyright Dr. Gregory Bain

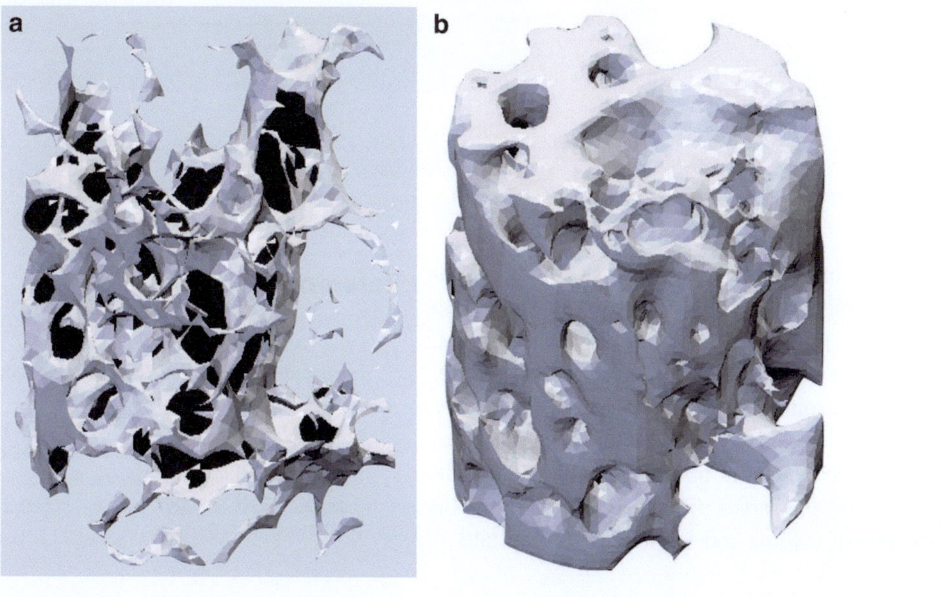

**Fig. 2.9** 3D morphometric analysis of the cylindrical trabecular volume of interest (3 mm diameter, 3 mm length). (**a**) Normal lunate and (**b**) Kienböck's lunate, which has more trabeculae that are thicker. However the total bone volume of the lunate is less than the normal lunate due to bone resorption

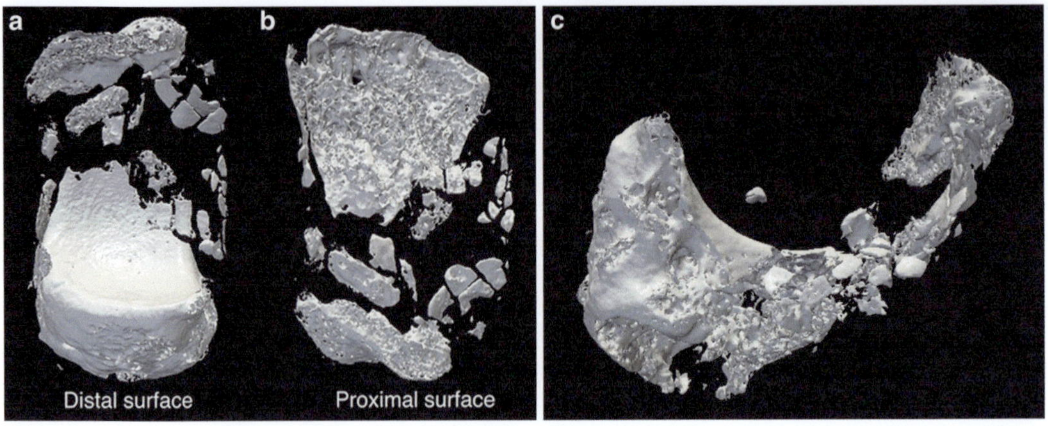


**Fig. 2.10** Micro 3D CT scan images of Kienböck's lunate demonstrating extensive fragmentation and almost complete loss of the proximal subchondral bone plate, which exposes the medullary trabecular bone. This "honeycomb" is not designed to be a load bearing surface and is therefore eroded. Distal and proximal (**a**, **b**) and lateral (**c**) views. Copyright Dr. Gregory Bain

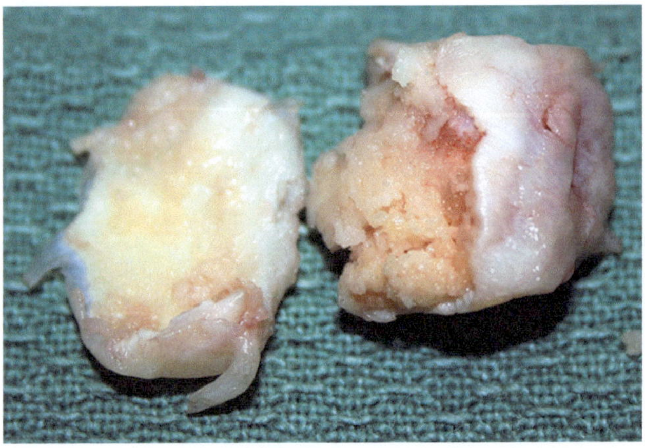

**Fig. 2.11** Excised Kienböck's lunate. Note the ulcerated articular surface, has lost its usual glistening surface. The subchondral bone plate has been replaced with granulation tissue. The medullary bone is fragmented, pale, and avascular. Copyright Dr. Gregory Bain

assessment of the lunate provides another insight into the morphology of the lunate (see Chap. 6 on pathology). Extensive voids can be identified, which are filled with areas of necrotic bone, scarred fibrous tissue, and cysts [16]. There are also areas of reparative tissue including granulation tissue and new bone. The new bone will respond to the forces placed upon it and take on the role of loading and supporting the capitate.

## References

1. Garn SM, Rohmann CG. Variability in the order of ossification of the bony centers of the hand and wrist. Am J Phys Anthropol. 1960;18:219–30.
2. O'Rahilly R. Developmental deviations in the carpus and the tarsus. Clin Orthop. 1957;10:9–18.
3. Viegas SF, Wagner K, Patterson R, Peterson P. Medial (hamate) facet of the lunate. J Hand Surg Am. 1990;15(4):564–71.

4. Zapico J. Enfermedad de Kienbock. Rev Ortop Traumatol. 1993;37 Suppl 1:100–13.
5. Zapico J. Malacia del semilunar. Valladolid: Universidad de Valladolid; 1966.
6. Tatebe M, Imaeda T, Hirata H. The impact of lunate morphology on Kienbock's disease. J Hand Surg Eur Vol. 2015;40:534.
7. Tatebe M, Shinohara T, Okui N, Yamamoto M, Kurimoto S, Hirata H. Arthroscopic lunate morphology and wrist disorders. Surg Radiol Anat. 2013; 35(1):79–83.
8. Rhee PC, Moran SL, Shin AY. Effect of lunate morphology in Kienbock disease. 29th International Wrist Investigators' Workshop; 2013; Moscone West Convention Center, San Francisco, CA.
9. Owers KL, Scougall P, Dabirrahmani D, Wernecke G, Jhamb A, Walsh WR. Lunate trabecular structure: a radiographic cadaver study of risk factors for Kienbock's disease [corrected]. J Hand Surg Eur Vol. 2010;35(2):120–4.
10. Hùlten O. Über anatomische variationen der handgelenkknochen. Acta Radiol. 1928;9:155–68.
11. Stahl S, Reis ND. Traumatic ulnar variance in Kienbock's disease. J Hand Surg Am. 1986;11(1): 95–7.
12. Gelberman RH, Bauman TD, Menon J, Akeson WH. The vascularity of the lunate bone and Kienbock's disease. J Hand Surg Am. 1980;5(3):272–8.
13. Chen WS, Shih CH. Ulnar variance and Kienbock's disease. An investigation in Taiwan. Clin Orthop Relat Res. 1990;255:124–7.
14. Tsuge S, Nakamura R. Anatomical risk factors for Kienbock's disease. J Hand Surg Br. 1993;18(1):70–5.
15. Low S, Bain GI, Findlay DM, Eng K, Perilli E. External and internal bone micro-architecture in normal and Kienböck's lunates: a whole-bone micro-computed tomography study. J Orthop Res. 2014; 32(6):826–33.
16. Bain G, Yeo CJ, Morse LP. Kienböck disease: recent advances in the basic science. Assessment and treatment. Hand Surg. 2015;20(3):352–65.

# 3 Vascularity of the Lunate

Kin Ghee Chee, Chong Jin Yeo, and Gregory Ian Bain

## Introduction

Dr. Robert Kienböck, an Austrian radiologist, first described lunatomalacia in 1910 in his clinical series and felt that the cause of the collapse of the lunate was repetitive trauma to the lunate from work activities [1, 2]. This opinion was backed by the study of Muller in 1920 who coined the term occupational lunatomalacia [3]. The etiology of avascular necrosis of the lunate remains uncertain to this day, but a common theory persists that it is due to disruption of the vascular supply to the lunate. The exact cause of this disruption is still a source of considerable debate.

There are few papers describing in detail the blood supply to the carpal bones. The vascular supply is difficult to delineate as the vessels supplying the carpal bones are small and the capsular tissues and ligaments surrounding the carpal bones are relatively thick. Arterial injection studies with chemical debridement and decalcification were used to identify the arterial anatomy of the carpal bones more accurately in modern days. We review papers that described arterial anatomy of the carpal bones with particular attention being paid to the lunate bone.

K.G. Chee, MBBS, MRCS, MMed (Surgery)
Department of Orthopedic Surgery,
Tan Tock Seng Hospital, Jalan Tan Tock Seng,
Singapore 308433, Singapore

C.J. Yeo, MBChB, MRCS, MMed, FAMS
Hand and Microsurgery Section, Department
of Orthopedic Surgery, Tan Tock Seng Hospital,
11 Jalan Tan Tock Seng, Singapore 308433,
Singapore

G.I. Bain, MBBS, FRACS, FA(Ortho)A, PhD (✉)
Professor, Upper Limb and Research, Department of
Orthopedic Surgery, Flinders University and Flinders
Medical Centre, Bedford Park, Adelaide, SA,
Australia
e-mail: greg@gregbain.com.au

## Extraosseous Blood Supply to the Carpus [4]

There are five named blood vessels that give off direct supply to the carpal bones. There are the radial artery, ulnar artery, anterior interosseous artery, deep palmar arch, and accessory ulnar recurrent artery. These five arteries form a palmar network and a dorsal network that supply the carpal bones. Each network can be divided into three transverse arches which give off branches of nutrient arteries that supply the carpal bones (Figs. 3.1 and 3.2).

© Springer International Publishing Switzerland 2016
D.M. Lichtman, G.I. Bain (eds.), *Kienböck's Disease*, DOI 10.1007/978-3-319-34226-9_3

## Palmar Transverse Arches

Palmarly, the arches formed are the radiocarpal arch, the intercarpal arch and the deep palmar arch. The radiocarpal arch is the most proximal and is found about 5–8 mm proximal to the radiocarpal joint at the level of the metaphysis of the distal radius and ulna. It is encased in the wrist capsule. This arch is constantly supplied by the radial, ulnar, and the anterior interosseous artery in 87 % of the specimens and in 13 % the anterior interosseous artery does not contribute to this arch. The radiocarpal arch gives off branches that supply the palmar surface of the lunate and triquetrum (see Fig. 3.1).

The palmar intercarpal arch receives its supply from radial, ulnar, and anterior interosseous arteries. One-quarter of the specimens do not have any contribution from the anterior interosseous artery. It is present in about half the specimens and it lies in between the proximal and distal arches of the wrist. This arch is not a consistent contributor to the carpal bones and is usually small in diameters.

The deep palmar arch is the most distal in location. It is located at the base of the metacarpals about 5–10 mm distal to the carpometacarpal joints. It presents consistently and gives off the ulnar and radial recurrent arteries, and sends perforating branches to the palmar metacarpal arteries and dorsal basal metacarpal arch.

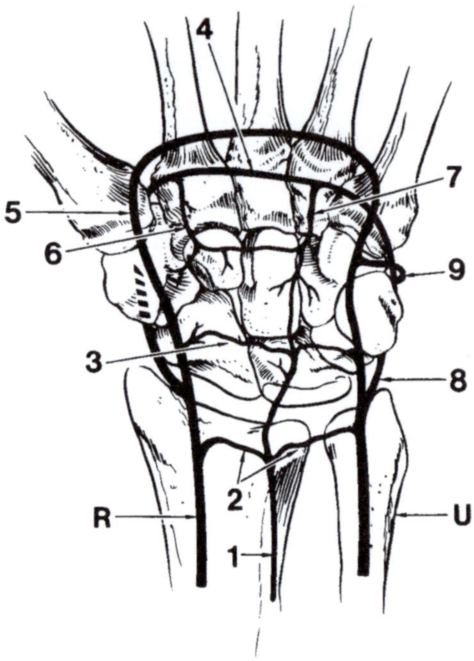


**Fig. 3.1** The palmar carpal arterial supply. *R* radial artery, *U* ulnar artery, *1* palmar branch, anterior interosseous artery, *2* palmar radiocarpal arch, *3* palmar intercarpal arch, *4* deep palmar arch, *5* superficial palmar arch, *6* radial recurrent artery, *7* ulnar recurrent artery, *8* medial branch, ulnar artery, *9* branch off ulnar artery contributing to the dorsal intercarpal arch. Reprinted from The Journal of Hand Surgery, 8(4), Gelberman RH, Panagis JS, Taleisnik J, Baumgaertner M, The arterial anatomy of the human carpus. Part I: The extraosseous vascularity, 367–375, Copyright © 1983 American Society for Surgery of the Hand, Published by Elsevier Inc. All rights reserved

## Dorsal Transverse Arches

On the dorsal aspect of the carpus, the blood supply also comes from three transverse arches. The most proximal of them, the dorsal radiocarpal arch is present in 80 % of the specimens and obtains its supply from the radial, ulnar, and anterior interosseous arteries. The radiocarpal arch is located at the level of the radiocarpal joint and provides main nutrient vessels to the lunate and triquetrum. Occasionally, the anterior interosseous artery or the ulnar artery may not contribute to this arch (see Fig. 3.2).

The dorsal intercarpal arch is the most consistent arch dorsally and is the largest. It receives its supply from radial, ulnar, and anterior interosseous arteries in 53 % of the specimens, radial and ulna arteries alone in 20 % of the specimens, and 7 % from ulnar and anterior interosseous arteries only. It is located in between the proximal and distal carpal rows. It gives off anastomoses to the radiocarpal arch and supplies the lunate and triquetrum (Fig. 3.3).

The basal metacarpal arch is the most distal of the dorsal transverse carpal arch. It is the most inconsistent of the arches and does not play an important roll in the vascularity of the lunate. The basal metacarpal arch is located in between second to fourth metacarpal bases and supplies the distal carpal bones.

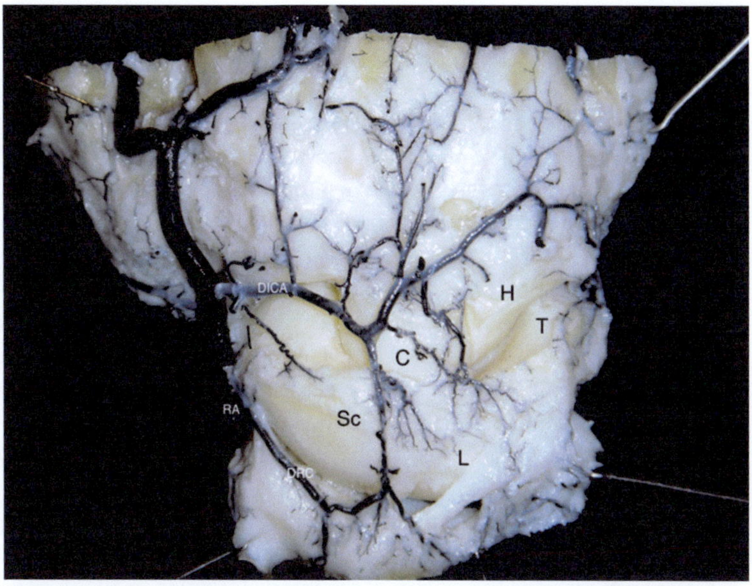


**Fig. 3.2** The dorsal carpal arterial supply. Cadaveric specimen of the arterial anatomy with latex injection and acid submersion, to erode the soft tissues. Radial artery (RA), with the dorsal radiocarpal artery (DRC), dorsal intercarpal artery (DICA), scaphoid (S), lunate (L), hamate (H), capitate (C), and triquetrum (T). Copyright Dr. Carlos Zaidenberg, Argentina

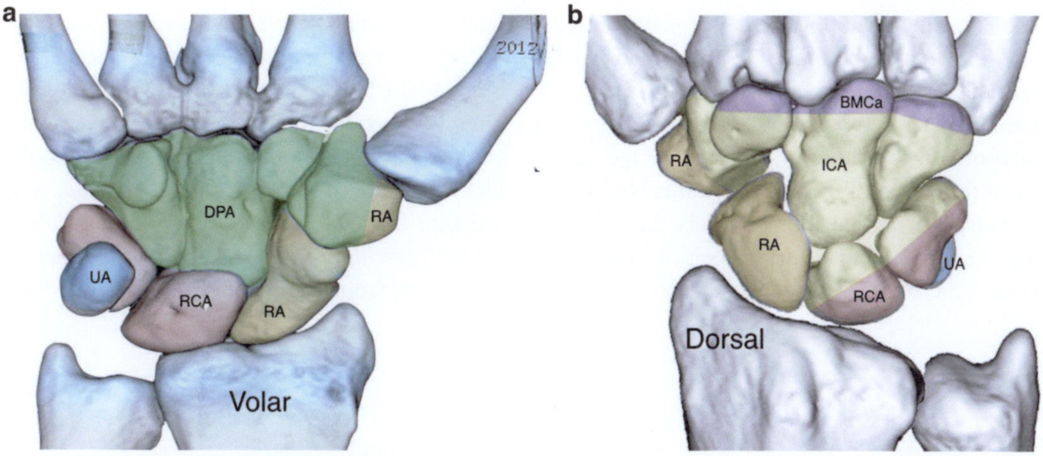


**Fig. 3.3** Contributions of the five named arteries supplying the carpus; radial, ulnar, anterior interosseous, accessory recurrent ulnar artery, and deep palmar arch. Note areas of vascular contribution to each carpal bone. (**a**) Volar. (**b**) Dorsal. Image drawn with information from [4]. Copyright Dr. Gregory Bain

## Extraosseous Blood Supply of the Lunate [4–6]

The lunate receives its blood supply from the palmar and dorsal sources. The main nutrient arteries' supply come palmarly from the radiocarpal and the intercarpal arches. The dorsal radiocarpal and intercarpal arches also give nutrient arteries to the lunate but are usually smaller. Eighty percent of the specimens receive supply from both the dorsal and palmar supplies; 20 % of the specimens only receive their supply from the palmar arches alone. The lunate is covered mostly by articular cartilage and hence no other nutrient arteries enter the bone. After entering the bone these nutrient vessels branch proximally and distally.

## Intraosseous Blood Supply of the Lunate [5, 6]

Lee in 1963 and Gelberman in 1980 have studied the intraosseous vascular anatomy of the lunate. Lee reported that 26 % of the lunates had only a single major blood supply either from the dorsal or the volar arch [5, 6]. These blood vessels enter volarly (15 %) or dorsally (11 %) and traverse obliquely across the lunate to supply the whole lunate (Fig. 3.4). There was a dorsal and volar supply, but with no anastomosis in 7.5 % of the specimens. In 66.5 % of the specimens, there were both vessels entering the lunate bone from either the dorsal or the volar surfaces. About 20 % of them form a ring anastomosis, while the other 80 % form a single anastomosis in the center of the lunate.

Gelberman reported the pattern of the internal vascularity of the lunate. Fifty-nine percent of them form a three-vessel anastomosis (Y pattern), of which half of them have two volar nutrient vessels and the other half have two palmar nutrient vessels. Thirty-one percent of the specimens that anastomosed formed a single-vessel anastomosis (I pattern), and 10 % of the specimens formed the X pattern anastomosis with two vessels entering the lunate volarly and dorsally and formed a single anastomosis in the center (Fig. 3.5a, b). In a subsequent paper his group reported that in 20 % of the specimens, nutrient vessels were seen entering only the palmar surface of the lunate [8]. In these specimens, one or two medium-sized vessels penetrated the palmar surface and gave off numerous branches that supplied the entire lunate [8]. The group at risk of Kienböck's disease is likely to be those with a single arterial supply or those with no anastomosis between the vessels. The development of the vascularity of the lunate can be appreciated from this image provided by Dr. Henry Crock [7]. Note how there is only a volar arterial supply in this lunate from a 4-year-old. It helps explain how some lunates will have a dominant volar or dorsal supply.

Lamas et al. reported that nutrient vessels entered the lunate through the dorsal and volar poles in all the specimens [9]. Dorsal lunate vascularity is supplied by branches originating from the dorsal plexus as well as the radiocarpal, intercarpal, and transverse metacarpal arch. The dorsal intercarpal and radiocarpal arches supply blood to the lunate from plexus of vessels located directly over the lunate's dorsal pole. Vessels entered the dorsal lunate through 1–3 foramina located in the proximal, central, or ulnar, nonarticular aspect of the bone (Fig. 3.5c). Palmar lunate vascularity is supplied by branches originating from a palmar plexus as well as direct

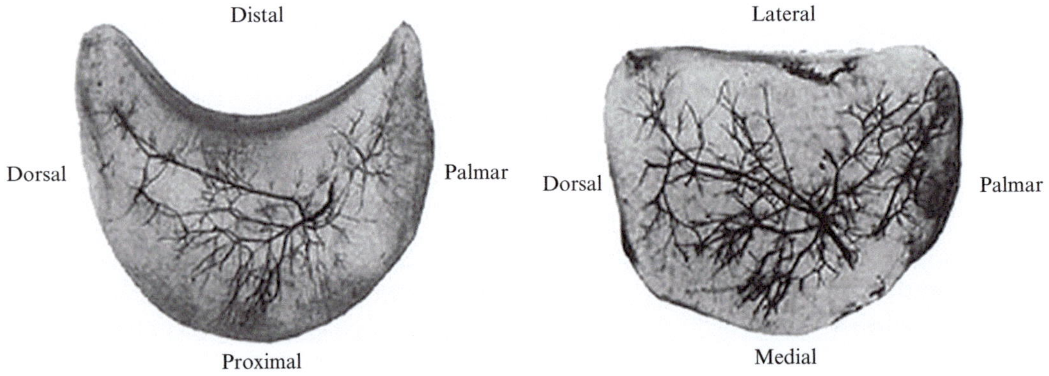


**Fig. 3.4** Lunate with single volar artery as seen from the lateral and distal view. The intraosseus arterial pattern of the carpal lunate bone and its relation to avascular necrosis. Note the single volar vessel. Reproduced with permission from Lee ML. The intraosseus arterial pattern of the carpal lunate bone and its relation to avascular necrosis. Acta Orthop Scand. 1963;33:43–55. Courtesy of Taylor & Francis Ltd., www.tandfonline.com

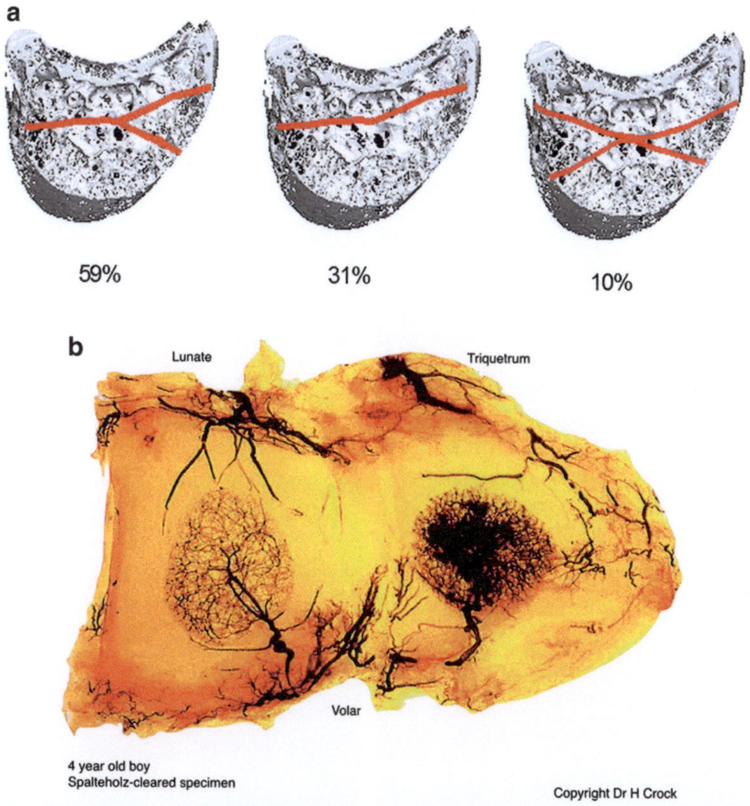


**Fig. 3.5** (**a**) Schematic drawing to illustrate the various lunate blood supply. Image drawn with information from [6]. Copyright Dr. Gregory Bain. (**b**) Left lunate and triquetrum of a 4-year-old boy. Note the single large volar vessel in the lunate and the triquetrum. There are dorsal vessels that now have an established anastomosis with the triquetrum and are just starting with the lunate. Copyright HV Crock AO [7]. (**c**) Dorsal aspect of the lunate with three dorsal foramina and vessels entering the lunate. (**d**) Transverse section of the wrist with Spalteholz technique. Arterial supply of the dorsal and palmar aspect of the wrist. Dorsal nutrient vessels entering the lunate through the dorsal radiocarpal arch. Palmar nutrient vessels entering the lunate through the RSL ligament of Testut-Kuentz, RLT ligament, and ULT ligament. (**e**, **f**) Transverse section with Spalteholz technique. Magnified view of the osseous ligamentous interface, through which the vessels enter the lunate. Parts (**c**), (**d**), (**e**), and (**f**) reproduced from Lamas C, Carrera A, Proubasta I, Llusà M, Majó J, Mir X. The anatomy and vascularity of the lunate: considerations applied to Kienböck's disease. Chirurg Main 2007; 26:13–20. Copyright © 2007 Elsevier Masson SAS. All rights reserved

ulnar, radial, and anterior interosseous artery branches. Palmar radiocarpal arches were present in all specimens, while the intercarpal arch was present in 70 %. The nutrient vessels (1–5) entered the volar pole through various ligament insertions, including the ligament of Testut-Kuentz (RSL ligament) and the radiolunate triquetrum ligament and ulnar lunate triquetral ligament (Fig. 3.5d–f) [9].

## Venous Anatomy of the Lunate [7, 10]

The work of Dr. C. Lamas and Professor M. Llusa provides some insight into the extraosseous venous system of the carpus (Fig. 3.6). The interconnections of the venous drainage system reflect the arterial supply.

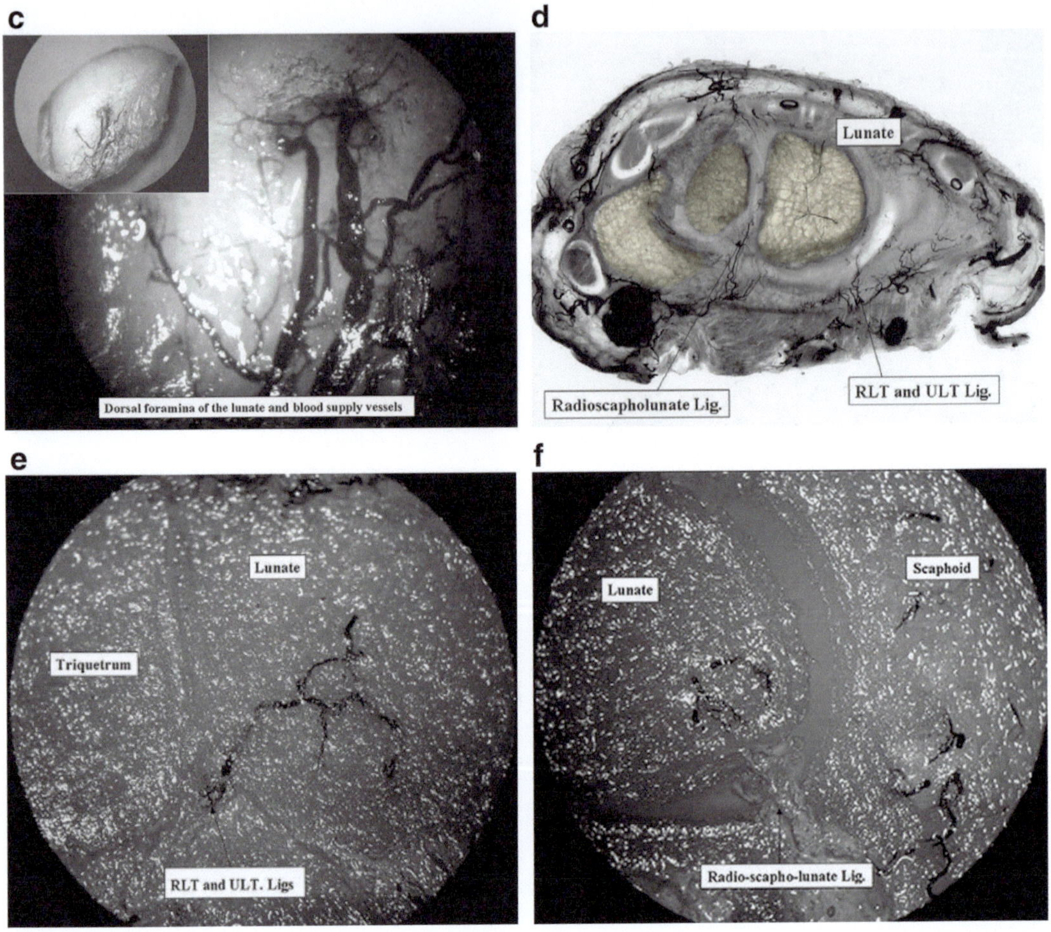


**Fig. 3.5** (continued)

Crock studied the intraosseous lunate venous system of the lunate and the lower limb (Fig. 3.7a–c) [7, 11]. He reports that there is a complex subarticular venous system, collecting blood from the subchondral plate. In the lower femur he states that the veins mirror the arteries, except that they are a wider diameter and are wavy in configuration [11]. The venous limbs of the capillaries perforate the subchondral bone plate, to drain into the subarticular plexus, which lies immediately adjacent to the subchondral bone plate. The plexus is arranged in parallel as a dense subarticular plexus that drains to the margins of the articular surface, into collecting trunks which join the lower radiate veins. In the lunate specimen there is some connections between the dorsal and volar lunate intraosseous veins. The wavy veins are seen to pass to the volar and dorsal margins, and then pass towards the mid-volar and dorsal aspects of the lunate where they coalesce before exiting the osseous lunate [7].

The venous drainage from the lunate then forms a dorsal venous plexus and a palmar venous plexus (Fig. 3.8). Dorsally the venous

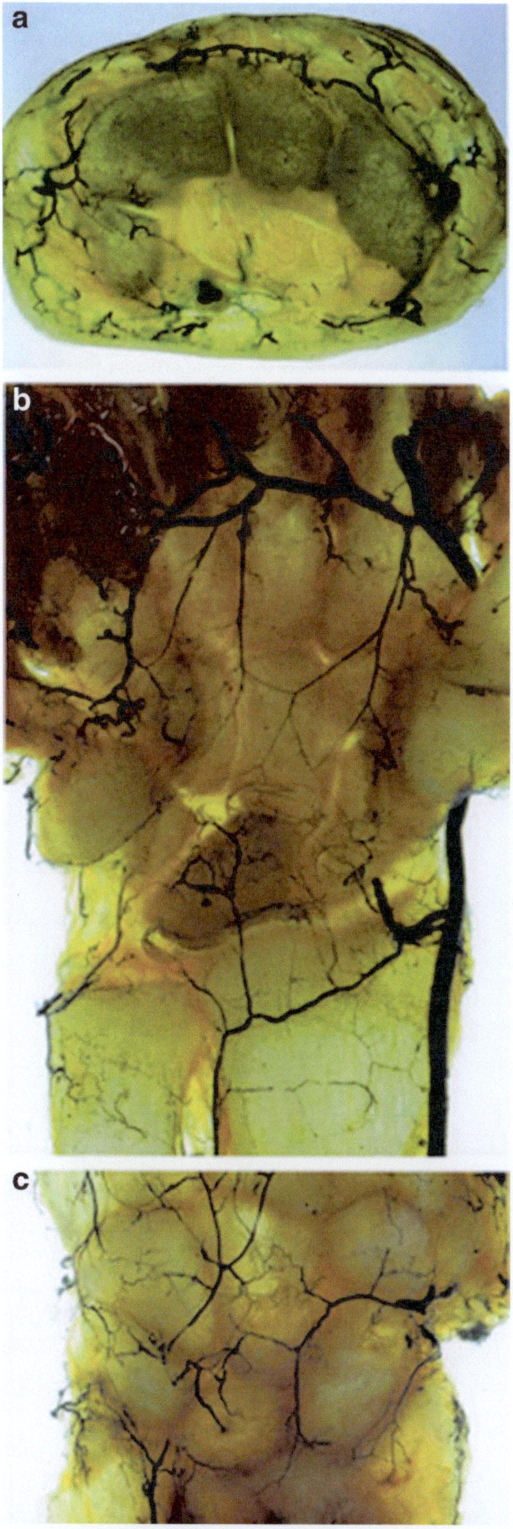

Fig. 3.6 (a–c) Angiogram of the carpus. Note the extensive array of vessels around the carpus. Reprinted with permission from Lluch A, Garcia-Elias M. Etiology of Kienbock's disease. Tech Hand Up Extrem Surg 2011; 15(1): 33–37 [14]

plexus continues into the contiguous capsule of the wrist joint. The system continues radialward via the dorsal intercarpal arch and into the comitant veins of the radial artery. The plexuses also communicate with the subcutaneous veins via small connective vessels which went through the deep dorsal fascia of the hand. A consistent large-caliber vein runs through the two sections of the first dorsal interosseous muscle into the hand after coming between the radial veins and the subcutaneous dorsal venous plexus. Less frequently, one or two veins stretch along the base of the fourth synovial sheath and discharge into the dorsal interosseous veins.

Palmarly, the typical venous plexus merges into the contiguous parts of the palmar capsule 8. Venous blood vessels from surrounding tissues and the palmar venous plexus drain ulnarward along the concavity of the ulnar part of the carpal bones and reach the ulnar comitant veins after leaving the proximal hiatus of Guyon's ulnar canal into the distal forearm (Fig. 3.9). A few parallel vessels within the deep palmar fascia drain radially into the comitant veins of the deep palmar arch.

The palmar venous plexus drains into the radial comitant veins that swerve in the dorsal direction from the ventral distal radius under the long tendons of the thumb muscles (Fig. 3.10).

A single vein runs beneath the pronator quadratus in the proximal direction as the palmar interosseous vein. The topographic attribution of the veins to the complex ligamentous apparatus is difficult because of the narrowness of the carpal ligaments and their close contact with the joint capsule of the carpus. As the vessels leave the lunate the small veins fill the connective tissue intervals of the deep, middle, and superficial carpal ligamentous structures and run in palmar and dorsal directions in the deep fascia of the hand.

## Conclusion

The relationship of the anatomy (vascular, osseous, and cartilaginous) and how it is affected by the pathological processes will be the key to the puzzle of Kienböck's disease [12, 13].

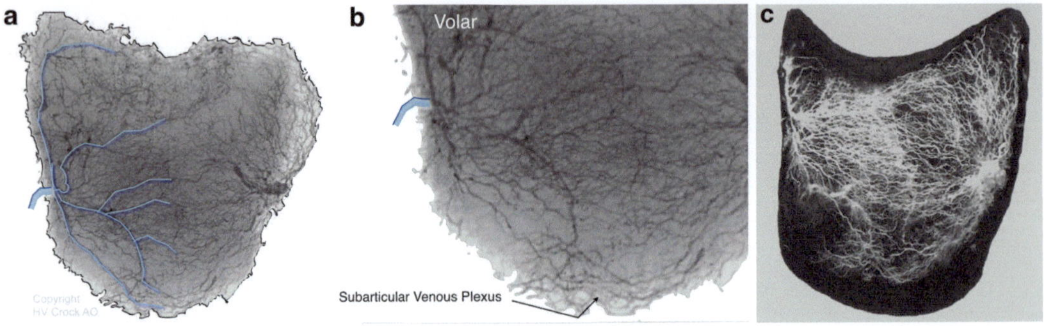


**Fig. 3.7** (**a**) Lateral view of an adult lunate with venous injection. The main veins emerge on the volar and dorsal surfaces in the middle of the lunate. (**b**) Magnified view of specimen from (**a**). Note the volar and dorsal plexus. With the extra magnification the sinusoids (*small black dots*) can be better appreciated. Note that on the inferior surface the parallel venules make up the subarticular plexus, and that there is a single vein exiting the volar lunate. (**c**) This is the same specimen as in (**a**), illuminated with incident light and Spalteholz cleared, showing the complex subarticular collecting veins arranged in parallel wavy lines. Figures copyright HV Crock AO [7]

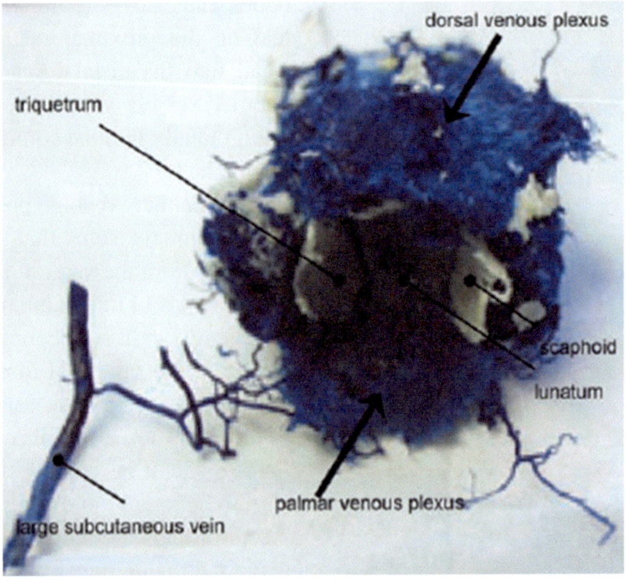


**Fig. 3.8** The venous drainage of the lunate. Used with permission from Springer Science+Business Media: Surg Radiol Anat, 2003, Pichler M, Putz R [24]

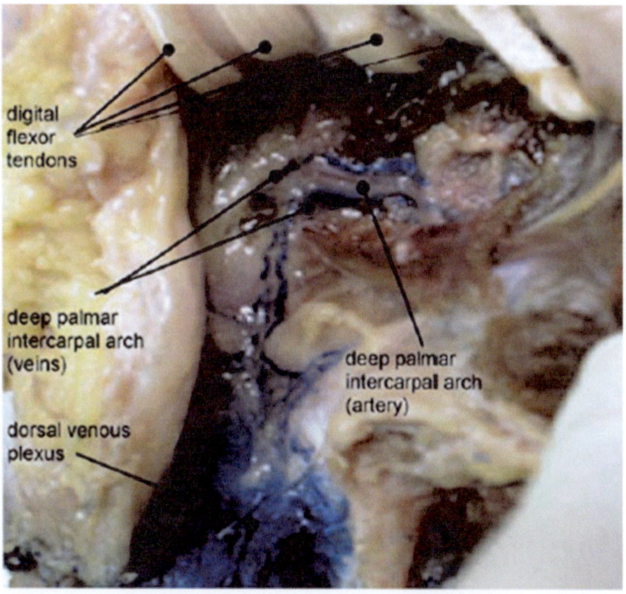


**Fig. 3.9** The deep palmar intercarpal arch with both arteries and veins. With permission from Springer Science+Business Media: Surg Radiol Anat, The venous drainage of the lunate bone, 2003, Pichler M, Putz R

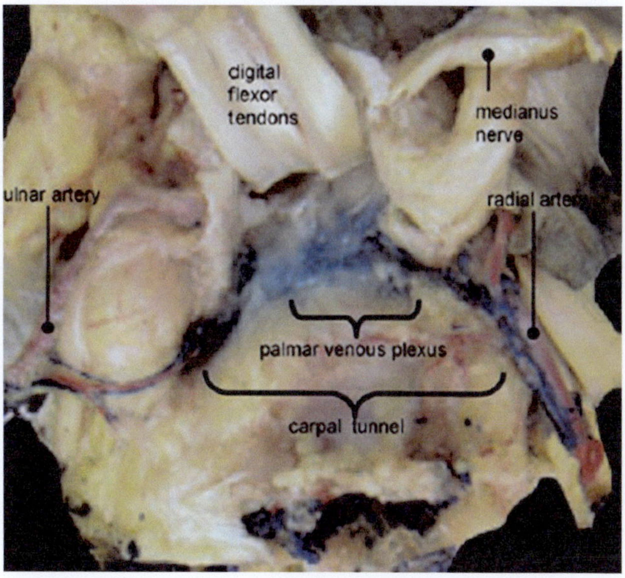


**Fig. 3.10** The palmar venous plexus. With permission from Springer Science+Business Media: Surg Radiol Anat, The venous drainage of the lunate bone, 24, 2003, 372–376, Pichler M, Putz R

## References


1. Kienböck R. Concerning traumatic malacia of the lunate and its consequences: joint degeneration and compression. Fortsch Geb Roentgen. 1910;16: 77–103.
2. Peltier LF. The classic. Concerning traumatic malacia of the lunate and its consequences: degeneration and compression fractures. Privatdozent Dr. Robert Kienbock. Clin Orthop Relat Res. 1980;149:4–8.
3. Müller W. Über die Erweichung und Verdichtung des Os Lunatum, eine Typische Erkrankung des Handgelenks. Beiträge Zur Klinischen Chirurgie. 1920;119:664.
4. Gelberman RH, Panagis JS, Taleisnik J, Baumgaertner M. The arterial anatomy of the human carpus. Part I: The extraosseous vascularity. J Hand Surg Am. 1983;8(4):367–75.
5. Lee ML. The intraosseus arterial pattern of the carpal lunate bone and its relation to avascular necrosis. Acta Orthop Scand. 1963;33:43–55.

6. Gelberman RH, Bauman TD, Menon J, Akeson WH. The vascularity of the lunate bone and Kienbock's disease. J Hand Surg Am. 1980;5(3):272–8.
7. Crock HV. An atlas of vascular anatomy of the skeleton & spinal cord. 1st ed. London: Martin Dunitz; 1996.
8. Panagis JS, Gelberman RH, Taleisnik J, Baumgaertner M. The arterial anatomy of the human carpus. Part II: The intraosseous vascularity. J Hand Surg Am. 1983;8:375–82.
9. Lamas C, Carrera A, Proubasta I, Llusà M, Majó J, Mir X. The anatomy and vascularity of the lunate: considerations applied to Kienböck's disease. Chirurg Main. 2007;26:13–20.
10. Pichler M, Putz R. The venous drainage of the lunate bone. Surg Radiol Anat. 2003;24:372–6.
11. Crock HV. The blood supply of the lower limb bones in man. Philadelphia, PA: Churchill Livingstone; 1967.
12. Low S, Bain GI, Findlay DM, Eng K, Perilli E. External and internal bone micro-architecture in normal and Kienböck's lunates: a whole-bone micro-computed tomography study. J Orthop Res. 2014; 32(6):826–33.
13. Bain G, Yeo CJ, Morse LP. Kienböck disease: recent advances in the basic science, assessment and treatment. Hand Surg. 2015;20(3):352–65.
14. Lluch A, Garcia-Elias M. Etiology of Kienbock's disease. Tech Hand Up Extrem Surg. 2011;15(1):33–7.

# Lunate Bone Morphology and Its Association with Kienböck's Disease

4

Peter Charles Rhee and Steven L. Moran

## Introduction

The etiology for Kienböck's disease has been attributed to many factors including vascular insufficiency, repetitive microtrauma, corticosteroid use, and a hypercoagulability state [1, 2]. Mechanical factors such as decreased radial inclination and negative ulnar variance have also been postulated as risk factors for the development of Kienböck's disease [1, 2]. More recently, variations in lunate morphology have been theorized to play a role in the pathogenesis of avascular necrosis within the lunate [3–9].

The lunate is the keystone of the wrist. The lunate is integral to the central column of the carpus and may be subjected to marked axial loads [10–12]. Variations in lunate shape have been shown to affect carpal kinematics. In addition, lunate shape may predispose to asymmetric loading of the lunate, which in turn could predispose to microtrauma and avascular necrosis [6, 13–17]. This chapter reviews the different classifications of lunate morphology and how they apply to Kienböck's disease.

## The Effect of Lunate Morphology on the Pathogenesis and Management of Kienböck's Disease

Lunate morphology has been described according to several variables including overall size and position [8, 9], dorsal and volar height [4, 18, 19], and proximal [3–5, 20] and distal articular surfaces [15, 17, 21, 22].

### Lunate Size and Position (Coronal Plane Morphology)

Lunate size and the angle of the distal articular facet may affect the lunate's ability to transmit force within the central column and alter the linkage between the proximal and distal rows [9, 10]. Radiographic population-based assessments of lunate size have been reported. Tsuge et al. assessed lunate height (LH), diameter (LD), distal facet width (DF), and tilt (LT) on standard posteroanterior radiographs of 66 normal male controls (mean age 32 years, range 14–67) (Fig. 4.1) [9]. Thienpont et al. performed similar measurements on 126 normal wrists in 68 men and 58 women (mean age 36 years, range 17–69)

P.C. Rhee, DO, MS
Department of Orthopedic Surgery and Rehabilitation, San Antonio Military Medical Center, 3551 Roger Brooke Dr., Fort Sam Houston, TX 78234, USA

1310 Scenic Knoll, San Antonio, TX 78258, USA

S.L. Moran, MD (✉)
Division of Plastic Surgery, Mayo Clinic, 200 First St. SW, Rochester, MN 55905, USA
e-mail: moran.steven@mayo.edu

© Springer International Publishing Switzerland 2016
D.M. Lichtman, G.I. Bain (eds.), *Kienböck's Disease*, DOI 10.1007/978-3-319-34226-9_4

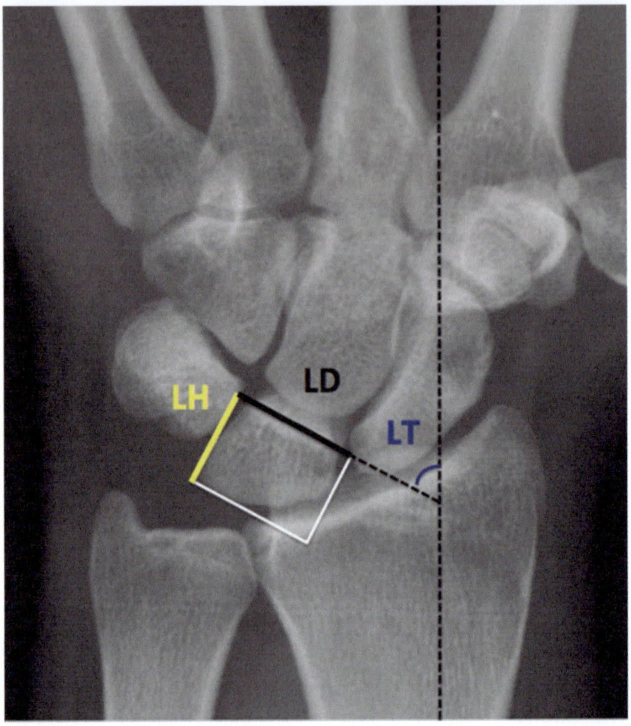


**Fig. 4.1** Measurement of lunate size and tilt (coronal plane morphology). A tangential line connecting the ulnar and radial most distal aspect of the lunate articular surface is drawn from which the width of the lunate body is measured and defines the lunate diameter (LD, *solid black line*). A perpendicular line along the ulnar surface of the lunate defines the lunate height (LH, *yellow line*). The LD line is extended to transect the longitudinal axis of the radius (*dotted black line*) to determine the lunate tilting angle (LT, *blue*)

**Table 4.1** Lunate dimensions and Kienböck's disease[a]

| Author | Sample (*n*) | Lunate height (LH) | Lunate diameter (LD) | Lunate tilt (LT) | Distal facet width (DFW) |
|---|---|---|---|---|---|
| Tsuge et al. | | | | | |
| • Normal | 66 | 11.5 ± 1.1 mm | 16.1 ± 1.6 mm | 18.8° ± 4.4° | 8.9 ± 1.2 mm |
| • Kienböck | 41 | 11.0 ± 1.0 mm | 15.0 ± 2.1 mm | 21.2° ± 3.8° | 8.8 ± 1.5 mm |
| *P*-values | | 0.04 | 0.003 | 0.004 | 0.5 |
| Thienpont et al. | | | | | |
| • Normal | 126 | 11.5 ± 0.7 mm | 15.4 ± 1.6 mm | 17.7° ± 5.4° | N/A |
| • Kienböck | 54 | 10.1 ± 1.2 mm | 14.2 ± 1.0 mm | 20.9° ± 4.6° | N/A |
| *P*-values | | 0.04 | 0.004 | 0.004 | N/A |

• Reported as mean ± standard deviation
[a]Created with data from Thienpont [8] and Tsuge [9]

[8]. The mean values for lunate size and position are noted in Table 4.1. Tsuge then compared his controls to the unaffected contralateral wrists in 41 male Kienböck patients (mean age 34 years, range: 15–58) and Thienpont compared them to the contralateral wrists in 54 patients, 31 men and 23 women (mean age 35 years, range: 17–58) (see Table 4.1) [8, 9]. They observed a significantly smaller lunate, in height and diameter, in the Kienböck group compared to the control group and concluded that a smaller lunate may be subjected to a higher relative load of transmitted force and a greater likelihood of microtrauma and avascular necrosis [20, 23].

A more radially inclined lunate with increased lunate tilt may predispose the lunate to increased intraosseous pressure and/or avascular necrosis (see Fig. 4.1). It is known that the trabeculae

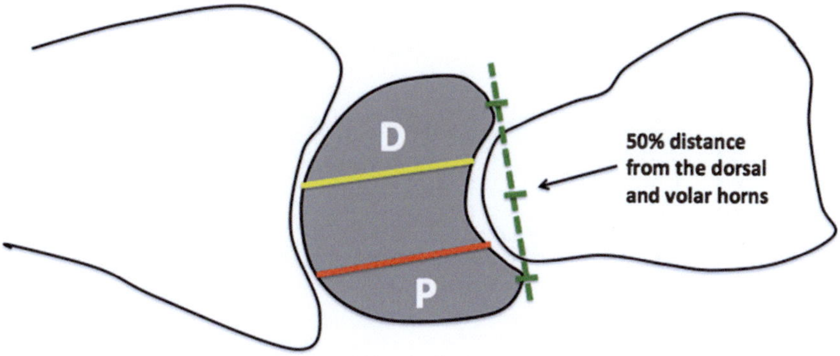


**Fig. 4.2** Lunate volar and dorsal rim height measurement method (lateral plane morphology). A baseline (*dotted green*) is drawn which connects the dorsal and palmar horns of the lunate. On the baseline, the volar and dorsal quarters are marked (at 25 and 75 percentiles between the volar and dorsal horns). Perpendicular lines are drawn from these quarter lines, and the height of the lunate measured. In a wedge-shaped lunate, the dorsal height (*yellow*) will be shorter than the palmar height (*red*)

within the lunate are arranged perpendicular to the articular surface [24]. While it is plausible, Tsuge et al. did not find a correlation between lunate inclination or tilt (LT, Fig. 4.1) and the age of onset of Kienböck's disease [9].

## Dorsal and Volar Height (Sagittal Plane Morphology)

The lunate is predominantly wedge shaped on lateral projection with a propensity to rotate dorsally or extend. Kauer et al. reviewed sagittal sections through cadaveric wrists and observed that the lunate was wedge shaped (greater distance between the volar distal and proximal articular surfaces than the dorsal surfaces) (Fig. 4.2) [18]. Watson et al. evaluated the lateral lunate morphology of 292 normal wrists on standard radiographs and noted shorter dorsal height, or wedge shaped, in 67 % of wrists ($n=196$) [19]. Kato et al. also observed a wedge-shaped lunate in 88 % (21 of 24) of normal wrists [4]. It is postulated that the capitate head will drive a wedge-shaped lunate into extension, whereas the opposite morphology, shorter volar distal to proximal articular distance, would result in a predisposition for lunate flexion [18, 19].

Lateral, or sagittal plane, lunate morphology has not been shown to be a clear risk factor for development of Kienböck's disease. Kato et al. compared the unaffected, contralateral wrists in 23 wrists (mean age 40 years, range: 14–63) diagnosed with Kienböck's disease to 24 control patients (mean age 39 years, range: 12–68 years) with normal wrists [4]. The authors did not observe a significant difference in the incidence of a wedge-shaped lunate between the Kienböck's disease patients (74 %, $n=17$) and the control (88 %, $n=21$) group. Despite a theoretical propensity for wedge-shaped lunates to dorsiflex, there was no significant difference for the mean radiolunate angle (6° and 7°) and the mean radioscaphoid angles (58° and 58°) in the Kienböck and control groups, respectively [4].

## Variation in Proximal Articular Surface

The proximal articular surface of the lunate has been shown to exist in three distinct forms as defined by Antuña-Zapico [3, 20]. In type I, the proximal and radial surfaces of the lunate converged at >130° forming an apex or crest (referred to as AZ-type I). Type II has an angle of approximately 100°–110°, resembling a square or rectangle (AZ-type II). Type III has two discrete facets to articulate with the radius or the triangular fibrocartilage complex (AZ-type III, Fig. 4.3)

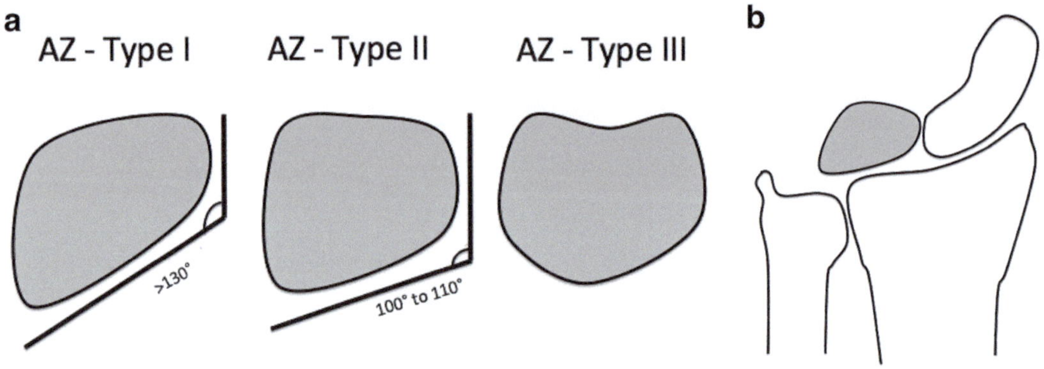


**Fig. 4.3** Lunate morphology based on the proximal articular surface (Antuña-Zapico). AZ-type I, the proximal and radial surfaces of the lunate converged at >130° forming an apex or crest, AZ-type II has an angle of approximately 100°–110°, resembling a square or rectangle, and AZ-type III has two discrete facets to articulate with the radius and the triangular fibrocartilage complex (**a**) [3, 9]. Relationship of the lunate to the distal radius (**b**)

[3, 9]. The existence of a separate proximal ulnar facet (AZ-type III) was also confirmed by Shepherd who anecdotally noted that the size of the facet varied between patients [25]. Llamas et al. evaluated 24 cadaveric specimens and noted the prevalence of lunate shape as 21 % ($n$=5) AZ-type I, 75 % ($n$=18) AZ-type II, and 4 % ($n$=1) AZ-type III [5]. The mean proximal articular surface of AZ-type I and AZ-type II lunates was 237 mm$^2$ and 251 mm$^2$, respectively. There was no significant difference in surface area between the proximal, radial, or ulnar surfaces of the lunate, or in their relationships to lunate morphology [5].

The trabecular structure within an AZ-type I lunate may render it the weakest to resisting compressive stress. As mentioned previously, the trabeculae within the lunate runs perpendicular to the proximal and distal articular surface. Therefore, the external frame of the lunate corresponds to the trabecular structure [2, 24, 26]. Based on this principle, compressive loads through an AZ-type I lunate, with an increased intratrabecular angulation, are most at risk for bone fatigue, stress fractures, and inability to effectively heal fractures or microtrauma (see Fig. 4.3) [2, 3, 20]. Additionally, an AZ-type I lunate has been associated with ulnar negative variance, which is also postulated to be an independent risk factor for the development of Kienböck's disease due to extreme shear stress on the lunate imparted by the capitate and the ulnar articular surface of the distal radius, similar to a "nutcracker" [1–3, 20]. Consequently, lunate fragmentation is more frequently seen in wrists with an AZ-type I lunate and ulnar negative variance [3].

Lunate morphology at the proximal articular surface has not been shown to clearly play a role in the pathogenesis of Kienböck's disease. Lamas et al. evaluated 24 cadaveric wrists and did not observe a correlation between lunate morphology, as described by Antuña-Zapico, and the presence of wrist arthrosis or to the number of vascular foramina within the lunate. Kato et al. did not report any significant difference in the incidence of AZ-type I lunates in the unaffected, contralateral wrists in patients with Kienböck's disease (44 %, 10 of 23) compared to control wrists (38 %, 9 of 24) [5].

## Distal Articular Surface

Two types of lunates have been described by Viegas et al. based on the absence (V-type I) or presence (V-type II) of a distal articular medial facet that articulates with the proximal pole of the hamate (Fig. 4.4) [22]. The authors evaluated 165 cadaveric wrists and observed lunates without a medial (hamate) facet in 35 % (V-type I, $n$=57) and with a medial facet in 66 % (V-type II, $n$=108) (22). When present, the medial facet width ranged from 1 to 6 mm

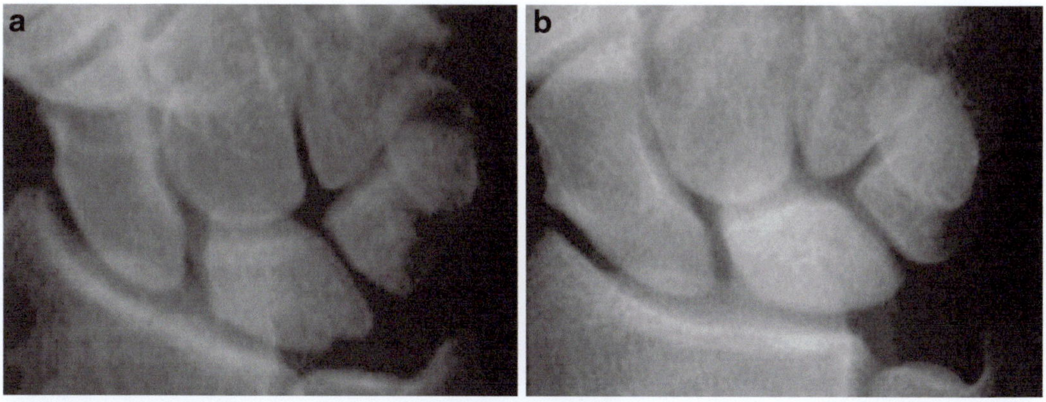

**Fig. 4.4** Lunate morphology based on the absence (**a**) or presence (**b**) of a medial hamate facet (Viegas) [22]

[5, 17, 22]. In a similar cadaveric study, Nakamura et al. noted an incidence of 29 % ($n$=49) V-type I and 71 % ($n$=121) V-type II lunates [17]. A magnetic resonance imaging (MRI) study confirmed that the medial facet articulates with the hamate in ulnar deviation. This articulation may be affected by arthritis and arthrosis at the proximal pole of the hamate has been seen in 44–49 % of wrists with a V-type II lunate in cadaveric specimens [5, 16, 17].

The presence of the medial (hamate) facet can influence the overall kinematics of the carpus [22]. Nakamura et al. noted the existence of a separate ligament originating from the triquetrocapitate ligament and coursing to the proximal pole of the hamate in patients with a type II lunate. In Nakamura's study, this ligament was present in 96 % (47 of 49) of cadaveric specimens. These findings suggest that variations in the intrinsic carpal ligament anatomy are associated with lunate shape; these ligaments may affect carpal kinematics [17]. Further work by Nakamura and colleagues showed a greater total arc of radioulnar deviation in the presence of a type II lunate. V-type II lunates extend later during ulnar deviation and flex earlier in radial deviation when compared to the V-type I lunate in a cadaveric motion analysis study [16]. An in vivo motion analysis study, performed by Galley et al., noted greater scaphoid flexion in wrists with a V-type II lunate and greater scaphoid translation in wrists with a V-type I lunate during radial deviation [14]. Bain et al. performed a three-dimensional kinematic analysis of the carpus in cadaveric specimens and reported more restricted midcarpal motion through a flexion to extension arc in wrists with a V-type II compared to V-type I lunates. Thus type II lunate wrists have more motion through the radiocarpal than the midcarpal joint in flexion and extension [13].

Viegas et al. remarked that the presence of the medial (hamate) facet may alter the vascular pattern and load characteristics of the lunate [22]. Additionally, Nakamura et al. reported greater force distribution between the radius and a V-type II lunate compared to a V-type I lunate, concluding that the presence of the additional facet may be an anatomical risk factor for Kienböck's disease [15]. However, Kato et al. and Tsuge et al. did not observe a significant difference in the incidence of a V-type II lunate in the contralateral, unaffected wrist in patients with Kienböck's disease (26 % V-type II, 6 of 23 and 37 %, 15 of 41) compared to a control group of normal wrists (29 % V-type II, 7 of 24 and 42 %, 28 of 66), respectively, on standard radiographs [4, 9]. In fact, Tatebe et al. noted a significantly higher prevalence of V-type II lunates, confirmed on arthroscopy, in the control group of wrists with non-traumatic diseases (32 %), such as ganglion cysts or monoarthritis, compared to patients who underwent surgery for Kienböck's disease (22 %)

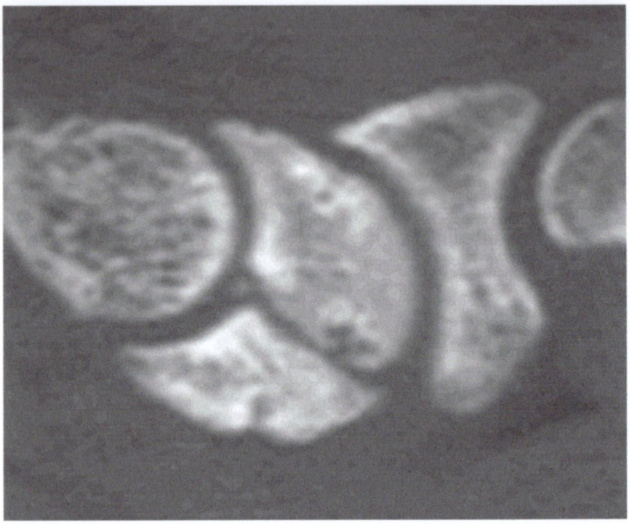

**Fig. 4.5** Coronal fracture of the lunate in Kienböck's disease seen on computed tomography

[7]. Thus, it does not appear that a medial hamate facet within the lunate contributes to the cause of Kienböck's disease.

While not contributing to the cause of Kienböck's disease, the presence of a medial hamate facet (V-type II) may be protective against coronal lunate fractures in established Kienböck's disease [6]. Armistead et al. theorized that during wrist extension, the stout radiolunate and volar lunotriquetral ligaments concentrated stress at their insertion onto the palmar rim of the lunate [27]. In combination with the loads exerted onto the lunate between the distal radius and capitate or "nutcracker effect," mechanical failure of the lunate, such as coronal fractures, can occur (Fig. 4.5) [27]. However, Rhee et al. reviewed 106 wrist radiographs in patients with Kienböck's disease and noted a higher prevalence of coronal fractures in V-type I lunates (77 %, $n=58$ of 75) compared to V-type II lunates (58 %, 18 of 31) [6].

A V-type II lunate can inhibit abnormal scaphoid flexion deformity and may decelerate the progression of Kienböck's disease [6]. The presence of a medial (hamate) facet has been previously shown to protect against dorsal intercalated segment instability (DISI) in cases of scaphoid nonunion and scapholunate dissociation [28, 29]. Rhee et al. noted smaller radioscaphoid angles in intact V-type II (45°, range: 30°–58°) compared to intact V-type I (53°, range: 38°–79°) lunates in patients with Kienböck's disease [6]. However, in the presence of a coronal fracture, the protective effect of the V-type II lunate against scaphoid flexion deformity was lost. Nonetheless, the authors also reported significantly higher stages of Kienböck's disease at the time of initial presentation in wrists with V-type I (stage IIIA–IV = 85 %, 64 of 75) compared to V-type II (stage IIIA–IV = 61 %, 19 of 31) lunates [6]. This may be explained by the fact that excessive scaphoid flexion, as seen in scapholunate advanced collapse, can result in radiocarpal and midcarpal arthritis due to abnormal loading of the carpus [6].

Decreased radioscaphoid angles associated with a V-type II lunate may result in improved clinical outcomes after joint leveling or unloading procedures in early stages of Kienböck's disease (stage II–IIIA) [6]. Condit et al. reviewed 23 patients with Kienböck's disease that underwent radial shortening osteotomy ($n=14$, mean age 28 years) or scaphoid-trapezoid-trapezium (STT) arthrodesis ($n=9$, mean age 32 years) with a mean clinical follow-up of 62 months and 54 months, respectively [30]. The authors observed that the preoperative radioscaphoid angle (smaller values) was the only factor that correlated with improved clinical outcomes (wrist motion, function, and grip strength) [30]. Another study noted no correlation between scaphoid flexion (radioscaphoid angle) and carpal collapse, indicating that these radiographic parameters are independent of each other [31]. Similarly, Goldfarb et al. remarked that scaphoid flexion, as determined by the radioscaphoid angle, is the best predictor of outcome after surgery for Kienböck's disease [31].

Scaphoid-trapezoid-trapezium arthrodesis should be performed with caution in wrists with a V-type II lunate. Wrist kinematic studies have illustrated greater scaphoid flexion in V-type II wrists, as opposed to greater scaphoid translation in V-type I wrists [13, 14, 17]. This is supported by the higher incidence of STT arthritis in wrists with a V-type II (83 %) compared to a V-type I (64 %) lunate [32]. Many authors have recommended against STT arthrodesis in the presence of a V-type II lunate since it could result in a greater loss of motion by eliminating scaphoid flexion [14, 33]. Similarly, Condit et al. recommended radial shortening osteotomy over STT arthrodesis in early stages of Kienböck's disease due to an unacceptable nonunion rate for STT arthrodesis (33 %, 3 of 9), radial styloid impingement, and loss of wrist motion observed in their cohort [30]. The authors recommended STT arthritis only in wrists with ulnar positive variance and a radioscaphoid angle < 60° [30]. Tatebe et al. performed a radial closing wedge osteotomy in 67 patients with V-type I ($n=51$) and V-type II ($n=16$) lunates and noted no significant difference in wrist function (Mayo wrist scores) between the two groups at a mean of 39-month follow-up [7].

## Limitations of the Literature

Evaluating the effect of lunate morphology in the pathogenesis and management of Kienböck's disease is difficult due to the destructive changes within the lunate. Tsuge et al. recognized the challenges in characterizing lunate morphology in the patient with Kienböck's disease [9]. The authors reviewed bilateral wrists in 20 healthy male patients (mean age 33 years, range: 23–44) and confirmed that paired wrists were anatomically equivalent based on a variety of radiographic parameters [9]. As a result, subsequent studies have utilized the unaffected, contralateral wrists to detect any radiographic markers that may serve as a risk factor for the development of Kienböck's disease [4, 8, 9]. However, the reported incidence of bilateral Kienböck's disease is 3–7 %, thus evaluating the unaffected, contralateral wrist may not provide an accurate assessment of the affected wrist [34]. In addition, there is wide variability in classifying lunate morphology on imaging studies [29]. For example, the ability to accurately detect the medial (hamate) facet on the lunate, V-type II, ranges from 64 to 72 %, and a medial facet of less than 3 mm can be mistaken for a V-type I lunate, which is the most common width of the additional facet [5, 17, 35, 36]. As such, erroneous classification of lunate morphology can occur complicating outcome-based studies.

## Conclusion

Variations in lunate morphology may play a role in the pathogenesis and management of Kienböck's disease. Alterations in the structural anatomy of the lunate or the associated influence on carpal kinematics with abnormal transmitted loads may be a risk factor for avascular necrosis. In addition, lunate morphology may influence the clinical outcomes in the surgical treatment of Kienböck's disease. However, further studies are necessary to identify the true influence of lunate morphology in Kienböck's disease.

## References

1. Beredjiklian PK. Kienböck disease. J Hand Surg Am. 2009;34(1):167–75.
2. Lluch A, Garcia-Elias M. Etiology of Kienböck disease. Tech Hand Up Extrem Surg. 2011;15(1):33–7.
3. Antuna-Zapico J. Malacia del semilunar. Tesis doctoral. Valladolid: Universidad de Valladolid; 1966.
4. Kato H, Nakamura R. Lunate morphology of Kienböck disease on x-ray study. Hand Surg. 1999; 4(1):75–9.
5. Lamas C, Carrera A, Proubasta I, Llusa M, Majo J, Mir X. The anatomy and vascularity of the lunate:

considerations applied to Kienböck disease. Chir Main. 2007;26(1):13–20.
6. Rhee PC, Jones DB, Moran SL, Shin AY. The effect of lunate morphology in Kienböck disease. J Hand Surg Am. 2015;40:738.
7. Tatebe M, Imaeda T, Hirata H. The impact of lunate morphology on Kienböck disease. J Hand Surg Eur Vol. 2015;40:534.
8. Thienpont E, Mulier T, Rega F, De Smet L. Radiographic analysis of anatomical risk factors for Kienböck disease. Acta Orthop Belg. 2004;70(5):406–9.
9. Tsuge S, Nakamura R. Anatomical risk factors for Kienböck disease. J Hand Surg Br. 1993;18(1):70–5.
10. Taleisnik J. The ligaments of the wrist. J Hand Surg Am. 1976;1(2):110–8.
11. Navarro A. Luxaciones del carpo. Anal Facult Med. 1921;6:113–41.
12. Craigen MA, Stanley JK. Wrist kinematics. Row, column or both? J Hand Surg Br. 1995;20(2):165–70.
13. Bain GI, Clitherow HD, Millar S, Fraysse F, Costi JJ, Eng K, et al. The effect of lunate morphology on the 3-dimensional kinematics of the carpus. J Hand Surg Am. 2015;40(1):81–9.e1.
14. Galley I, Bain GI, McLean JM. Influence of lunate type on scaphoid kinematics. J Hand Surg Am. 2007;32(6):842–7.
15. Nakamura K, Beppu M, Matsushita K, Arai T, Ide T. Biomechanical analysis of the stress force on midcarpal joint in Kienböck disease. Hand Surg. 1997;2: 101–15.
16. Nakamura K, Beppu M, Patterson RM, Hanson CA, Hume PJ, Viegas SF. Motion analysis in two dimensions of radial-ulnar deviation of type I versus type II lunates. J Hand Surg Am. 2000;25(5):877–88.
17. Nakamura K, Patterson RM, Moritomo H, Viegas SF. Type I versus type II lunates: ligament anatomy and presence of arthrosis. J Hand Surg Am. 2001;26(3): 428–36.
18. Kauer JM. Functional anatomy of the wrist. Clin Orthop Relat Res. 1980;149:9–20.
19. Watson HK, Yasuda M, Guidera PM. Lateral lunate morphology: an x-ray study. J Hand Surg Am. 1996; 21(5):759–63.
20. Taleisnik J. The wrist. New York, NY: Churchill Livingstone; 1985.
21. Viegas SF, Patterson RM, Hokanson JA, Davis J. Wrist anatomy: incidence, distribution, and correlation of anatomic variations, tears, and arthrosis. J Hand Surg Am. 1993;18(3):463–75.
22. Viegas SF, Wagner K, Patterson R, Peterson P. Medial (hamate) facet of the lunate. J Hand Surg Am. 1990;15(4):564–71.
23. Youm Y, McMurthy RY, Flatt AE, Gillespie TE. Kinematics of the wrist. I. An experimental study of radial-ulnar deviation and flexion-extension. J Bone Joint Surg Am. 1978;60(4):423–31.
24. Franck P. Die pathogenese der lunatum necrose. Une ihre bezielung zur funktionellen. Belastung des handgelenks. Beitr Z Klin Chir. 1936;164.
25. Shepherd FJ. Note on the radio-carpal articulation. J Anat Physiol. 1891;25(Pt 3):349–51. PubMed PMID: 17231926, Pubmed Central PMCID: 1328173.
26. Owers KL, Scougall P, Dabirrahmani D, Wernecke G, Jhamb A, Walsh WR. Lunate trabecular structure: a radiographic cadaver study of risk factors for Kienböck disease [corrected]. J Hand Surg Eur Vol. 2010;35(2):120–4.
27. Armistead RB, Linscheid RL, Dobyns JH, Beckenbaugh RD. Ulnar lengthening in the treatment of Kienböck disease. J Bone Joint Surg Am. 1982;64(2):170–8.
28. Haase SC, Berger RA, Shin AY. Association between lunate morphology and carpal collapse patterns in scaphoid nonunions. J Hand Surg Am. 2007; 32(7):1009–12.
29. Rhee PC, Moran SL, Shin AY. Association between lunate morphology and carpal collapse in cases of scapholunate dissociation. J Hand Surg Am. 2009; 34(9):1633–9.
30. Condit DP, Idler RS, Fischer TJ, Hastings 2nd H. Preoperative factors and outcome after lunate decompression for Kienböck disease. J Hand Surg Am. 1993;18(4):691–6.
31. Goldfarb CA, Hsu J, Gelberman RH, Boyer MI. The Lichtman classification for Kienböck disease: an assessment of reliability. J Hand Surg Am. 2003; 28(1):74–80.
32. McLean JM, Turner PC, Bain GI, Rezaian N, Field J, Fogg Q. An association between lunate morphology and scaphoid-trapezium-trapezoid arthritis. J Hand Surg Eur Vol. 2009;34(6):778–82.
33. Nuttall D, Trail IA, Stanley JK. Movement of the scaphoid in the normal wrist. J Hand Surg Br. 1998; 23(6):762–4.
34. Yazaki N, Nakamura R, Nakao E, Iwata Y, Tatebe M, Hattori T. Bilateral Kienböck disease. J Hand Surg Br. 2005;30(2):133–6.
35. Sagerman SD, Hauck RM, Palmer AK. Lunate morphology: can it be predicted with routine x-ray films? J Hand Surg Am. 1995;20(1):38–41.
36. Dyankova S, Marinov G. Comments about "The hamate facet of the lunate: a radiographic study in an Arab population from Bahrain". Surg Radiol Anat. 2007;29(2):181. author reply 3.

# Wrist Biomechanics as Applied to the Lunate and Kienböck's Disease

5

Hisao Moritomo

## Introduction

Normal carpal mechanics depends on a complex interplay between a sophisticated arrangement of carpal ligament and carpal bone geometry [1]. Although the origin and natural history of Kienböck's disease remain unclear, treatment of Kienböck's disease has been designed to decrease compressive loading of the lunate to prevent lunate collapse and to allow lunate revascularization. Information regarding the load transfer characteristics, contact area, and pressures on the lunate has offered a basis to better understand the pathomechanics of Kienböck's disease. It has also served as a means to assess the possible efficacy of different types of surgical decompression procedures. This chapter first reviews the kinetics and kinematics of the normal wrist, followed by the morphological influence on and kinetics of Kienböck's disease, and, finally, the kinetic efficacy of different types of surgical decompression procedures.

H. Moritomo, MD, PhD (✉)
Department of Orthopedics, Yukioka Hospital Hand Center, Osaka Yukioka College of Health Science, 2-2-3, Ukita, Kita-ku, Osaka-shi, Osaka 530-0021, Japan
e-mail: hisao-moritomo@yukioka-u.ac.jp

## Kinetics and Kinematics of Normal Lunate

### Midcarpal Joint

The midcarpal joint consists of the scaphoid–trapezium–trapezoid joint, scaphoid–capitate joint, lunate–capitate joint, and triquetrum–hamate joint. The distal row has been considered as a relatively fixed or constrained group of bones, and the proximal carpal row is, by comparison, much less constrained [1]. The normal load mechanics of the midcarpal joint were studied using pressure-sensitive film, and load distribution through the midcarpal joint was reported to be as follows: scaphoid–trapezium–trapezoid, 23 %; scaphoid–capitate, 28 %; lunate–capitate, 29 %; and triquetrum–hamate, 20 % [1]. When the scaphoid flexes in normal wrists, the flexion moment is constrained by the extension moment of the triquetrum, and stable equilibrium is achieved via the lunate as a bony link [2]. Gupta studied the effect of physiological axial loading on carpal alignment [3]. He concluded that physiological axial loading resulting from the normal tone of the forearm muscles tends to flex the scaphoid and the lunate. This is contrary to the classical description of the lunate as having a tendency to extend under axial loading [4]. If the link is broken (e.g., due to scapholunate dissociation [SLD], scaphoid nonunion, or advanced Kienböck's disease), the scaphoid flexes and the capitate translate proximally, i.e., carpal collapse occurs.

© Springer International Publishing Switzerland 2016

D.M. Lichtman, G.I. Bain (eds.), *Kienböck's Disease*, DOI 10.1007/978-3-319-34226-9_5

In Viegas et al.'s original cadaveric study of 165 wrists, in 35 % of wrists (*N*=57), the lunate articulates only with the capitate (type I lunate); in the other 65 % of wrists (*N*=108), a second distal joint surface is present articulating with the hamate (type II lunate) [5]. When present, the medial facet of the lunate articulates with the hamate during midcarpal motion, which can result in degenerative change at the proximal pole of the hamate in 44 % of type II lunate wrists [5]. Harley et al. cited hamate-lunate impaction as a cause of ulnar wrist pain and found a 91 % correlation between hamate arthritis and lunotriquetral ligament tears [6]; however, De Smet et al. noted that this degenerative change is often asymptomatic [7]. In a magnetic resonance imaging study in six positions of radial-ulnar deviation the wrists with a type I lunate did not have contact between the lunate and hamate in any position; the wrists with a type II lunate did have contact between the hamate and the lunate, but only in ulnar deviation [8]. We investigated contact between the type II lunate and the hamate using computed tomography in nine wrist positions and found that the type II lunate contacts the hamate only in wrist ulnar extension, ulnar deviation, and ulnar flexion (Fig. 5.1). This result suggests that pain at the ulnar midcarpal joint in these positions can be clues for hamate-lunate impaction.

We studied in vivo three-dimensional kinematics of the midcarpal joint during radioulnar deviation and flexion–extension motion in healthy wrists using a markerless bone registration algorithm [9, 10]. These kinematic studies revealed that the direction of capitate motion relative to the scaphoid was rotation in a radial extension–ulnoflexion plane, the so-called dart-throwingers motion, during both radioulnar deviation and flexion–extension of the wrist. By comparison, capitate motion relative to the lunate was rotation in a radial extension–ulnoflexion plane during radioulnar deviation, and rotation in an almost flexion–extension plane during wrist flexion–extension [9]. Substantial intercarpal motion between the scaphoid and the lunate must occur during flexion–extension motion to compensate for this discrepancy. Capitate motion relative to the lunate and triquetrum in the midcarpal joint was essentially similar and synchronous with one another, regardless of the type of wrist motion [9]. The lunate–triquetrum unit always moves along the oval convex surface of the capitate and the hamate in either type I lunate wrist or type II lunate wrist [9]. At the extreme ulnar position of the lunate–triquetrum unit, the concave part of the hamate contacts the triquetrum in both types and the lunate facet of the hamate contacts the lunate in type II lunate wrists (Fig. 5.2).

Several investigators have studied the potential association between lunate morphology and alterations in carpal kinematics. Nakamura et al. have investigated the difference in carpal kinematics between types I and II lunate wrists two-dimensionally, and have reported that the type II lunate articulation, with the shorter radius of curvature of the capitate, would have much more motion than the type I lunate articulation with the more gradual curvature of the capitate [8]. Bain et al. reported the effects of lunate morphology on the three-dimensional kinematics of the carpus [11]. They found that significantly greater motion occurred at the radiocarpal joint during flexion–extension of a type I lunate wrist than a type II lunate wrist. However, we cannot make a definitive statement about wrist kinematics regarding the difference between types I and II lunate wrists at present. Further research is required to increase the database.

## Radiocarpal Joint

The lunate articulates proximally with the radius and with the triangular fibrocartilage. The investigation of force transmission through the normal wrist using discrete element analysis models revealed that, on average, 90.3 % of the total radioulnocarpal force was transmitted to the radius, with 61.0 % through the radioscaphoid joint and 39.0 % through the radiolunate joint [12]. A mean of 9.7 % was dissipated through the triangular fibrocartilage. The proximal pole of the scaphoid was constantly transmitting most of

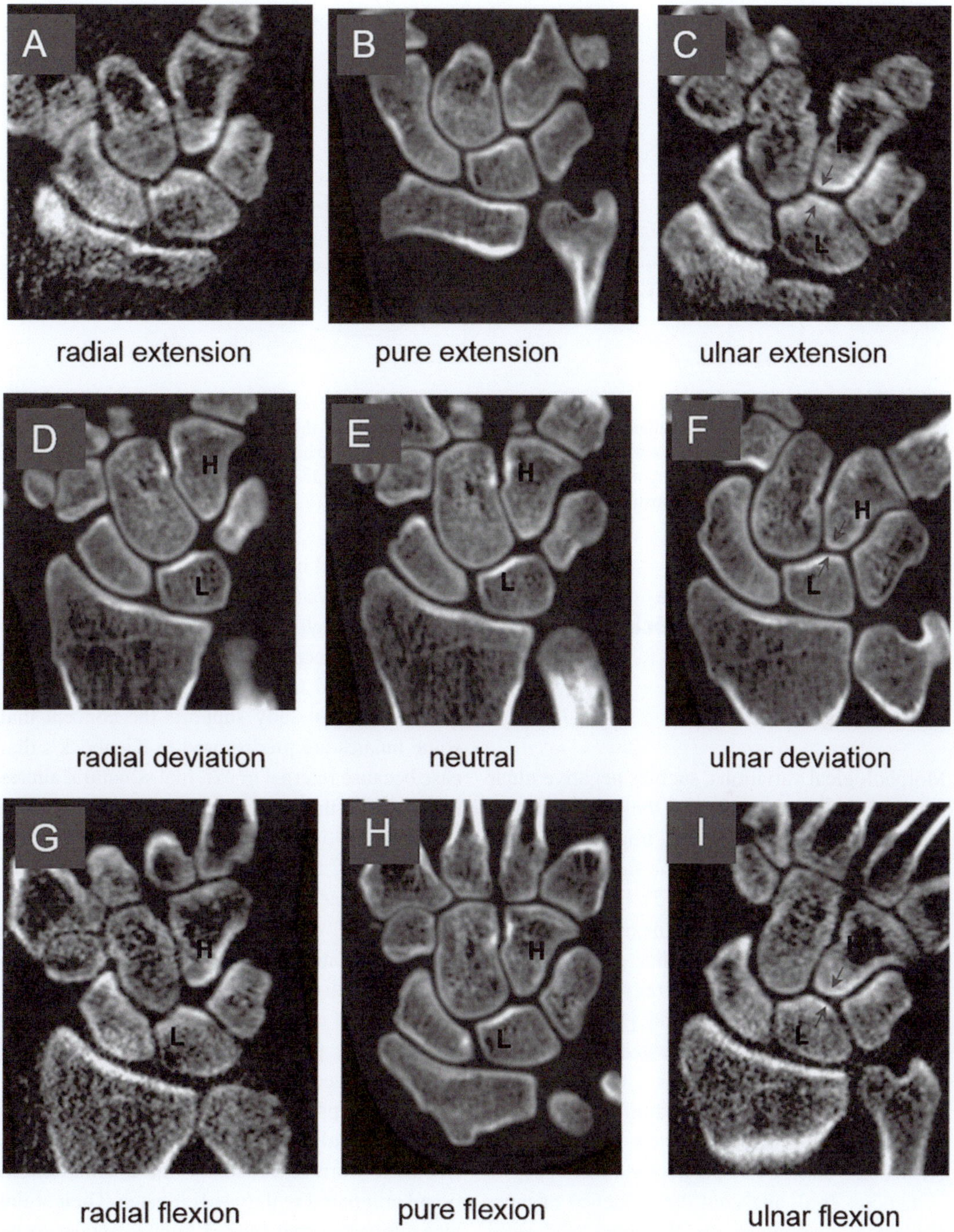


**Fig. 5.1** Computed tomography of the wrist with the type II lunate in nine wrist positions. The type II lunate contacts the hamate at wrist ulnar extension, ulnar deviation, and ulnar flexion (*arrows*), and does not contact at other wrist positions. L, lunate; H, hamate

the scaphoid load, with a radioscaphoid versus radiolunate peak pressure ratio of 1.6, and a radiolunate versus ulnolunate peak pressure ratio of 4.0 [12].

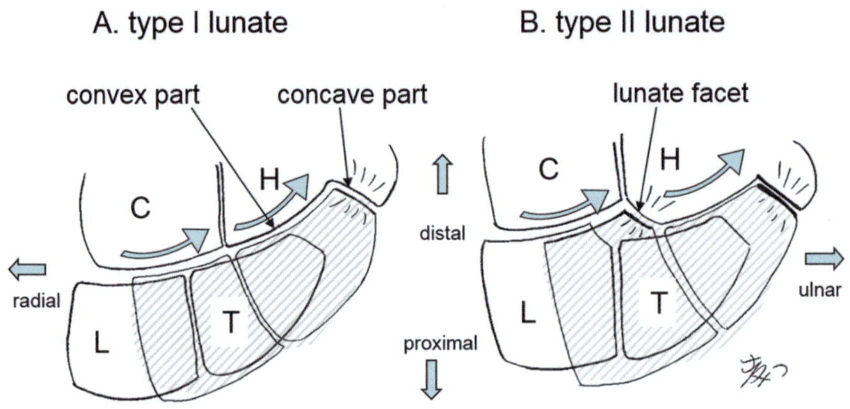


**Fig. 5.2** Motion of the lunate and the triquetrum relative to the capitate and hamate. The lunate–triquetrum unit always moves along the oval convex surface of the capitate and the hamate in either (**a**) type I or (**b**) type II lunate wrist. At the extreme ulnar position of the lunate–triquetrum unit (*shaded area*) the concave part of the hamate contacts the triquetrum in both types and the lunate facet of the hamate contacts the lunate in type II. T, triquetrum; C, capitate

## Morphological Influence on and Kinetics of Kienböck's Disease

### Morphological Influence

Morphological variations, such as negative ulnar variance, high uncovering of the lunate, abnormal radial inclination, and/or a trapezoidal shape of the lunate, and the particular vascular pattern, may be predisposing factors [13]. Hultén noted in 1928 that a short ulna (ulnar negative variance) was present in 78 % of his patients with Kienböck's disease, whereas only 23 % of normal patients had a short ulna [14]. However, D'Hoore et al. found no statistically significant relationship between ulnar variance and Kienböck's disease [15]. In addition, Nakamura et al. noted that most Japanese patients with Kienböck's disease had positive variance [16].

Ledoux et al. analyzed the influence of morphological variations on Kienböck's disease using a finite element analysis model [17]. The ulnar variance had a strong influence on the ratios of radiolunate/ulnolunate total load and peak pressures. The distribution of internal stresses was markedly affected by the lunate uncovering index. The evolution of a simulated incomplete fracture was dramatically influenced by morphological parameters: with positive ulnar variance, the fracture did not progress, but in the presence of three associated conditions—negative ulnar variance, a high lunate uncovering index, and angulated trabeculae of the lunate—the fracture progressed and the proximal part of the lunate collapsed. This study supports the concept that some lunates are predisposed to Kienböck's disease because internal or external structural alterations make them unable to absorb excessive stress, and allows an incomplete fracture to progress resulting in progressive collapse and localized trabecular osteonecrosis.

Rhee et al. studied the incidence of type I and type II lunates in patients presenting with Kienböck's disease [18]. They reported a 29 % prevalence of type II lunates in the affected wrist of Kienböck patients. There was significantly more advanced disease (stage IIIA or greater) upon initial presentation in wrist with a type I compared with a type II lunate. Coronal plane fractures were significantly more common in type I compared with type II lunates. Their study also suggested that type II lunates appear to be protective against scaphoid flexion deformities.

### Kinetics

According to the Lichtman classification scheme, carpal collapse and osteoarthritis gradually develop as Kienböck's disease progresses [19].

Iwasaki et al. [20] studied the effects of lunate collapse and demonstrated that in the early stages of the disease (stages II and IIIa), the normal position of the scaphoid prevented, to some extent, transmission of excessive forces to the lunate. However, as the scaphoid assumed its flexed position (in stage IIIb), the loads across the lunate were increased, thereby accelerating the process of collapse and fragmentation. Ueba et al reported that the proximal articular cartilage facing the radius is generally more affected than the distal articular cartilage facing the capitate [21].

Clinically, however, some patients with advanced Kienböck's disease can be asymptomatic, and the symptoms do not correlate well with the changes in shape of the lunate and the degree of carpal collapse [22]. Taniguchi et al. have reported patients with asymptomatic stage IV Kienböck's disease that was associated with marked carpal collapse, and their radioscaphoid joint (RSJ) space was retained [23]. In contrast, it was revealed that wrists with SLD had RSJ incongruity caused by dorsal subluxation of the scaphoid proximal pole as well as carpal collapse, and the incongruity caused osteoarthritis in RSJ [24, 25]. These facts suggest that the deformity pattern of SLD is different from that of stage IIIb Kienböck's disease. We examined three-dimensional carpal alignment in stage IIIa and IIIb Kienböck's disease to determine whether RSJ incongruity involving dorsal subluxation of the scaphoid proximal pole was present [26]. These results were compared with those for normal wrists and wrists with SLD and RSJ incongruity involving scaphoid rotatory subluxation. We found that normal RSJ congruity of both stage IIIa and IIIb Kienböck's disease was retained (Figs. 5.3a and 5.4a–c). Conversely, in SLD, the scaphoid flexed to the same extent as in stage IIIb Kienböck's disease but also shifted

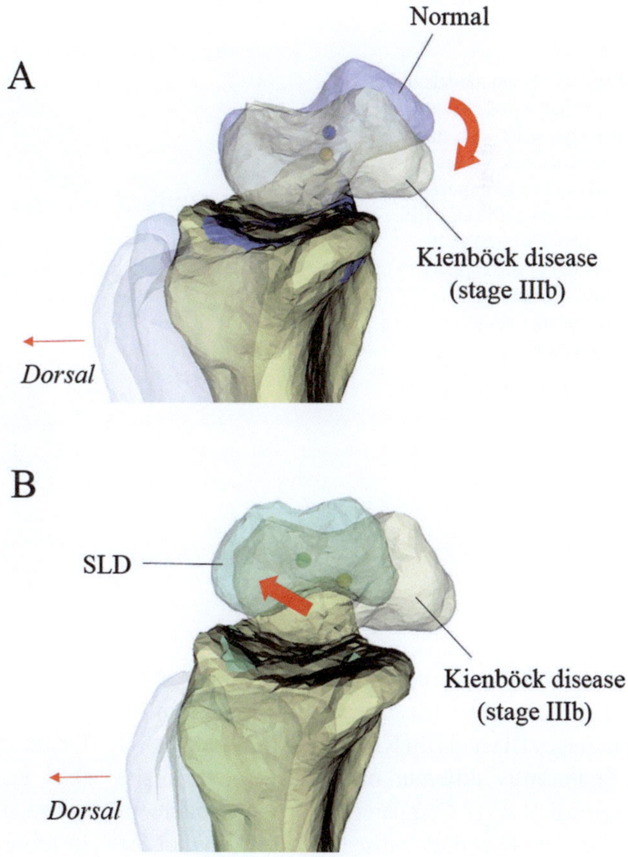


**Fig. 5.3** Models of the scaphoid and radius in the right wrist with normal, stage IIIb Kienböck's disease, and scapholunate dissociation (SLD) superimposed and viewed from the ulnar side. The similar color points represent centroids of each scaphoid. Compared with a normal scaphoid, the scaphoid in stage IIIb Kienböck's disease is flexed, and the centroids are located proximally (**a**). Compared with stage IIIb Kienböck's disease, the centroid and the proximal pole of the scaphoid with SLD show significant translation in the dorsal and distal directions (**b**)

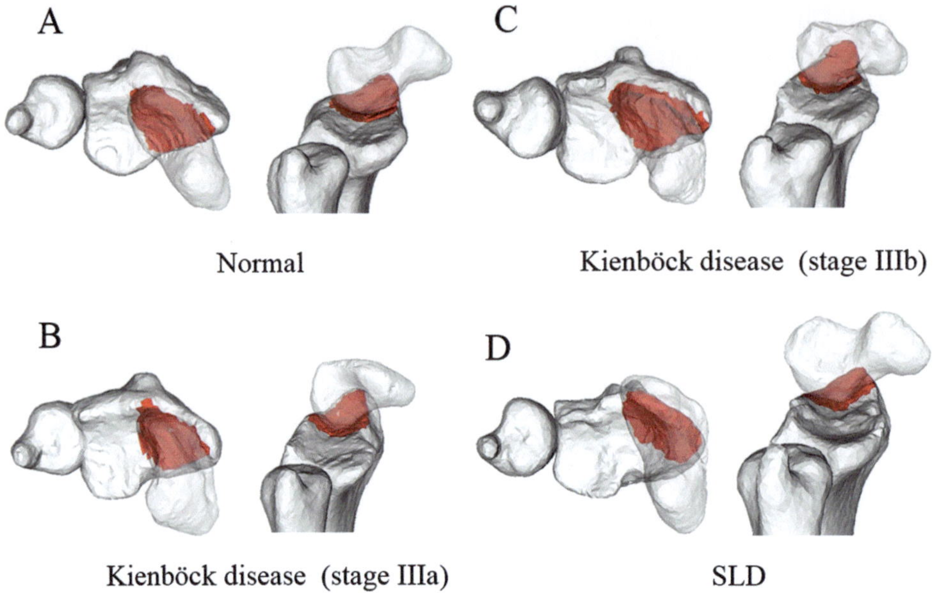


**Fig. 5.4** Inferred contact areas of the articular surface of the radioscaphoid joint (RSJ). A typical example of each joint is shown. The left illustration of each shows a distal view, and the right illustration shows the ulnar view. The contact areas in the RSJ of normal, stage IIIa, and stage IIIb Kienböck's disease wrists are similar, and congruency is retained (**a–c**). In RSJ with scapholunate dissociation (SLD), the contact area is located on the dorsal side and there is a joint incongruity for dorsal subluxation of the scaphoid proximal pole (**d**)

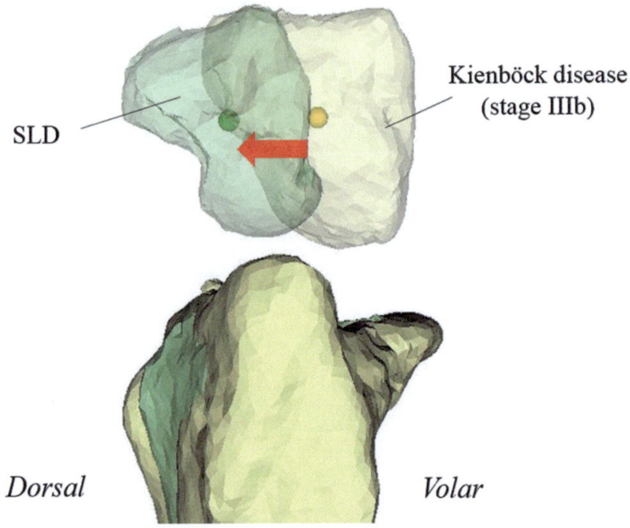


**Fig. 5.5** Bone models of the capitate and radius in the right wrist with stage IIIb Kienböck's disease and SLD superimposed. Compared with stage IIIb Kienböck's disease, the centroid of the capitate with SLD shows significant dorsal translation

dorsodistally, producing RSJ incongruity (Figs. 5.3b and 5.4d). The centroid of the capitate in stages IIIa and IIIb Kienböck's disease was not significantly different from the capitate in the normal wrists. Compared with the capitate in stage IIIb Kienböck's disease, the centroid of the capitate with SLD significantly translated 5.2 mm in the dorsal direction where dorsiflexion of the lunate was associated (Fig. 5.5). We concluded that the patterns of carpal collapse differed between stage IIIb Kienböck's disease and SLD in terms of RSJ congruity. Our results suggest that carpal collapse in Kienböck's disease is not associated with RSJ incongruity, which may explain why there are asymptomatic patients with Kienböck's disease and carpal collapse. This study also explains why excision of the lunate in Kienböck's disease showed favorable clinical results after long-term follow-up [27].

## Kinetic Efficacy of Different Types of Surgical Decompression Procedures

### Radial Shortening Osteotomy

As Kienböck's disease could be the result of excessive bone stress, studies have been conducted to understand how it might be possible to unload the lunate [13]. The most common procedure for unloading the lunate in patients with ulnar negative variance is radial shortening osteotomy [28–30]. Radial shortening or ulnar lengthening appears to redistribute some of the radiolunate load to the radioscaphoid joint and the ulnocarpal joint [31–33]. Werner et al. examined the effect of ulnar lengthening in cadavers and found that the radiolunate pressure was halved with a 2.5 mm ulnar lengthening [33]. On the other hand, radial shortening or ulnar lengthening increases the ulnocarpal pressure [33], which potentially produces postoperative ulnocarpal impaction syndrome, which requires ulnar-shortening osteotomy (Fig. 5.6).

### Radial Wedge Osteotomy

Radial wedge osteotomy, or lateral closing wedge osteotomy, which decreases radial inclination, has been proposed for patients with neutral or positive ulnar variance [34]. Conflicting results have been published regarding the unloading effects of changing the radial inclination [33, 35–37]. It is likely that the lateral closing wedge osteotomy does not actually decrease the total radiolunate load; however, by allowing better covering of the lunate by the distal radius, it enlarges radiolunate joint contact, thereby decreasing its deleterious peak pressures [13, 36].

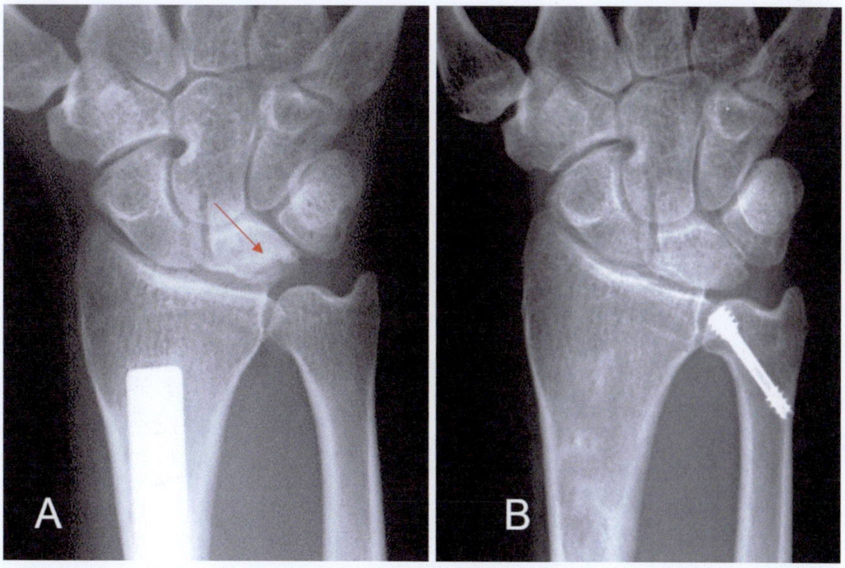


**Fig. 5.6** Ulnocarpal impaction syndrome that occurred 1 year after radial shortening performed for a 19-year-old girl with stage II Kienböck's disease (**a**). Note the cystic changes at the proximal and ulnar aspect of the lunate facing the ulnar head (*arrow*). Pain was resolved by distal metaphyseal ulnar shortening osteotomy (modified Kitano procedure) (**b**)

## Capitate Shortening Osteotomy

Decompression procedures for the treatment of Kienböck's disease include the capitate shortening procedure [41, 42]. In the classical capitate shortening procedure, a transverse osteotomy is located at the capitate waist, and both the lunate and scaphoid facets of the capitate are shortened. Capitate shortening is particularly useful in positive or neutral ulnar variance because its operative indication does not depend on ulnar variance, whereas the radial shortening procedure is only appropriate for negative ulnar variance [41, 42]. Biomechanically, Werber et al. noted that significant load reduction on the lunate was evident in all specimens after capitate shortening [43]. An average decrease of 49 % was observed under a 9.8-N load, and 56 % under a 19.6-N load [43]. Horii et al. verified that among surgical treatment options, the largest reduction of compressive forces on the lunate is obtained by the capitate shortening procedure [32]. The authors noted a 66 % decrease in the radiolunate load and a 26 % increase in the radioscaphoid load. However, they also suggested that this operation causes the scaphoid–trapezium joint to be tremendously overloaded and, under such forces, the scaphoid progressively adopts an abnormal palmar flexed position. Along with this collapse, the distal carpal row migrates proximally until capitate–lunate contact is reestablished (Figs. 5.7 and 5.8).

## Partial Capitate Shortening

To preserve scaphoid–capitate and midcarpal dynamics, in 2001 we developed a modified capitate shortening procedure known as "partial capitate shortening" [44, 45]. Only the lunate facet of the capitate is osteotomized and shortened, leaving the scaphoid–capitate joint intact (Fig. 5.9). In our experience, carpal collapse did not progress postoperatively in most cases, and the lunate-capitate joint space maintained (Fig. 5.10) [45]. Using fresh frozen cadavers, we measured the intra-articular pressure with axial load in the radioscaphoid fossa, radiolunate fossa, and ulnocarpal fossa before and after partial capitate shortening [46]. The radioscaphoid mean pressure significantly increased by an average of 39 %, and the radiolunate mean pressure significantly decreased by an average of 53 %. The ulnocarpal mean pressure did not significantly change. We also investigated whether the effect of lunate decompression is related to the presence or absence of the lunate–hamate articulation (type I or type II lunate) after partial capitate shortening. Despite the presence or absence of the lunate–hamate articulation, the radiolunate mean pressure significantly decreased, and the ulnocarpal mean pressure was unchanged. The early clinical results combined with our biomechanical data demonstrate decreased radiolunate joint loading after partial capitate shortening, and suggest a role for partial capitate shortening in

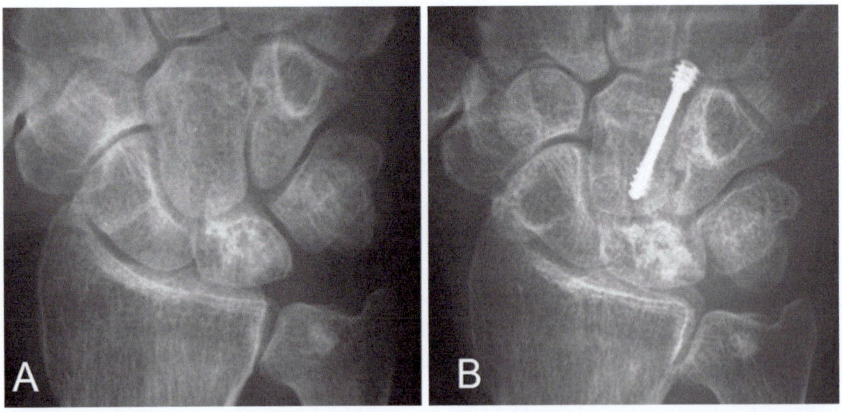


**Fig. 5.7** Preoperative (**a**) and 1.5-year postoperative (**b**) X-rays of classical capitate shortening procedure performed for a 25-year-old man with stage II Kienböck's disease. Note that the scaphoid flexed and carpal collapse progressed postoperatively until capitate–lunate contact is reestablished, decreasing carpal height

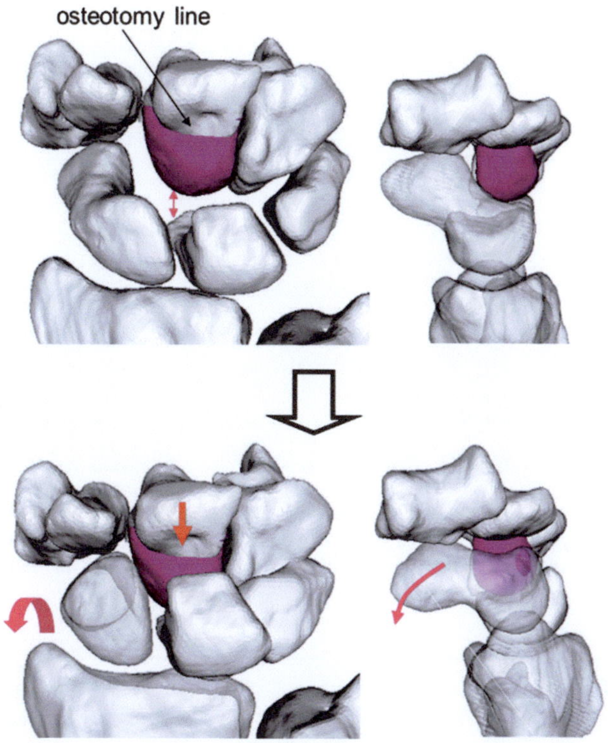


**Fig. 5.8** After classical capitate shortening, the scaphoid progressively adopts an abnormal flexed position. With this collapse, the distal carpal row migrates proximally until capitate–lunate contact is reestablished

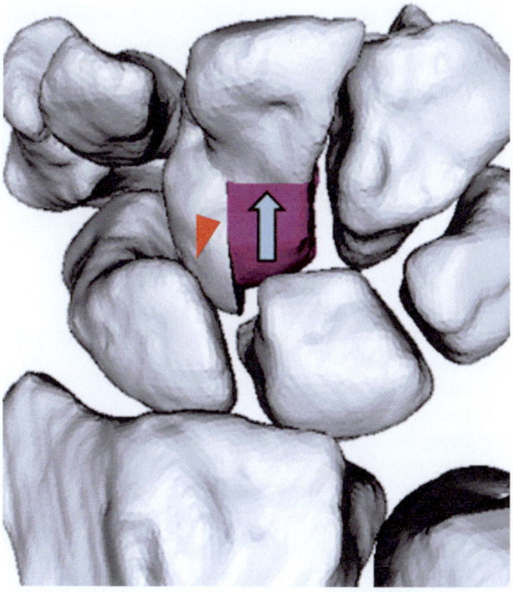

**Fig. 5.9** In partial capitate shortening only the lunate facet of the capitate is osteotomized and shortened, the scaphoid–capitate joint (*arrowhead*) remains intact

the treatment of Kienböck's disease. Clinically, Citlak et al. reported that partial capitate shortening appears to be an effective treatment for Lichtman stage II and IIIA patients [47]. Carpal collapse following the capitate shortening procedure seldom occurred if the articular contact between the capitate and the scaphoid is retained [47]. Additional clinical studies, however, will be necessary to define this role and to determine the long-term results of this procedure.

## Intercarpal Fusions

Some intercarpal fusions also decrease the loading across the radiolunate joint. Two examples are scaphoid–trapezium–trapezoid joint fusion [31, 33, 38, 40] and scaphoid–capitate fusion [32, 39, 40], but Werner et al. did not support the use of capitate–hamate fusion for unloading the radiolunate joint [33, 39].

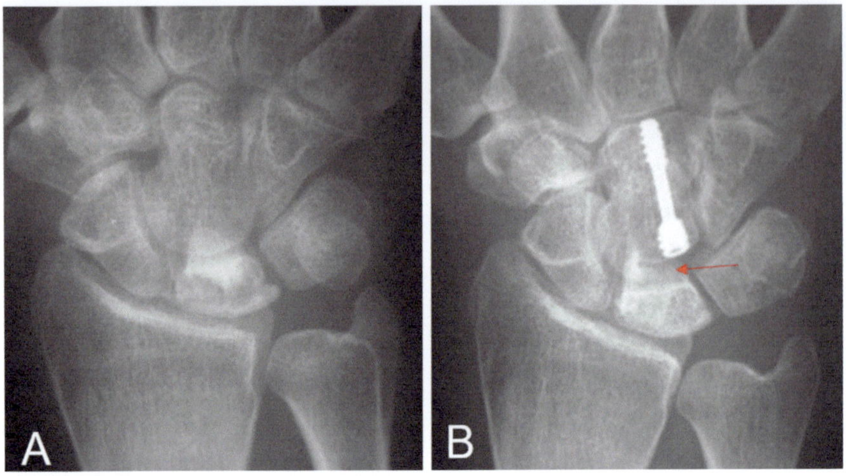


**Fig. 5.10** Preoperative (**a**) and 1-year postoperative (**b**) X-rays of partial capitate shortening procedure performed for a 29-year-old woman with stage IIIA Kienböck's disease. Note that carpal collapse did not progress postoperatively with the lunate-capitate joint space maintained (*arrow*)

## References


1. Viegas SF, Patterson RM, Todd PD, McCarty P. Load mechanics of the midcarpal joint. J Hand Surg Am. 1993;18:14–8.
2. Garcia-Elias M. Kinetic analysis of carpal stability during grip. Hand Clin. 1997;13:151–8.
3. Gupta A. Change of carpal alignment under anaesthesia: role of physiological axial loading on carpus. Clin Biomech. 2002;17:660–5.
4. Kaur JM. The mechanism of the carpal joint. Clin Orthop. 1986;202:16–26.
5. Viegas SF, Wagner K, Patterson R, Peterson P. Medial (hamate) facet of the lunate. J Hand Surg Am. 1990;15:564–71.
6. Harley BJ, Werner FW, Boles SD, Palmer AK. Arthroscopic resection of arthrosis of the proximal hamate: a clinical and biomechanical study. J Hand Surg Am. 2004;29:661–7.
7. De Smet L, Degreef I. Hamate impingement: a rare cause of ulnar wrist pain? In: Del Piñal F, Mathoulin C, Nakamura T, editors. Arthroscopic management of ulnar pain. New York, NY: Springer; 2012. p. 191–7.
8. Nakamura K, Beppu M, Patterson RM, Hanson CA, Hume PJ, Viegas SF. Motion analysis in two-dimensions of radialulnar deviation of type 1 versus type 2 lunates. J Hand Surg Am. 2000;25:877–88.
9. Moritomo H, Goto A, Sato Y, Murase T, Sugamoto K, Yoshikawa H. The triquetrum-hamate joint: an anatomic and in vivo 3-dimensional kinematic study. J Hand Surg Am. 2003;28:797–805.
10. Moritomo H, Murase T, Goto A, Oka K, Sugamoto K, Yoshikawa H. In vivo, 3-dimensional kinematics of the midcarpal joint of the wrist. J Bone Joint Surg Am. 2006;88:611–21.
11. Bain GI, Clitherow HD, Millar S, Fraysse F, Costi JJ, Eng K, McGuire DT, Thewlis D. The effect of lunate morphology on the 3-dimensional kinematics of the carpus. J Hand Surg Am. 2015;40:81–9.e1.
12. Schuind F, Cooney WP, Linscheid RL, An KN, Chao EY. Force and pressure transmission through the normal wrist: a theoretical two-dimensional study in the posteroanterior plane. J Biomech. 1995;28:587–601.
13. Schuind F, Eslami S, Ledoux P. Kienbock's disease. J Bone Joint Surg Br. 2008;90:133–9.
14. Hultén O. Uber die Enstehung und Behandlung der Lunatummalazie (Morbus Kienböck). Acta Chir Scand. 1928;76:121.
15. D'Hoore K, De Smet L, Verellen K, Vral J, Fabry G. Negative ulnar variance is not a risk factor for Kienböck's disease. J Hand Surg Am. 1994;19: 229–31.
16. Nakamura R, Imaeda T, Miura T. Radial shortening for Kienböck's didease: factors affecting the operative result. J Hand Surg Br. 1990;15:40–5.
17. Ledoux P, Lamblin D, Wuilbaut A, Schuind F. A finite-element analysis of Kienbock's disease. J Hand Surg Eur Vol. 2008;33:286–91.
18. Rhee PC, Jones DB, Moran SL, Shin AY. The effect of lunate morphology in Kienböck's disease. J Hand Surg Am. 2015;40:738–44.
19. Lichtman DM, Lesley NE, Simmons SP. The classification and treatment of Kienböck's disease: the state of the art and a look at the future. J Hand Surg Eur Vol. 2010;35(7):549–54.
20. Iwasaki N, Genda E, Minami A, Kaneda K, Chao EY. Force transmission through the wrist joint in

Kienböck's disease: a two-dimensional theoretical study. J Hand Surg Am. 1998;23:415–24.
21. Ueba Y, Kakinoki R, Nakajima Y, Kotoura Y. Morphology and histology of the collapsed lunate in advanced Kienböck's disease. Hand Surg. 2013; 18(2):141–9.
22. Lutsky K, Beredjiklian PK. Kienböck's disease. J Hand Surg Am. 2012;37:1942–52.
23. Taniguchi Y, Tamaki T, Honda T, Yoshida M. Rotatory subluxation of the scaphoid in Kienböck's disease is not a cause of scapholunate advanced collapse (SLAC) in the wrist. J Bone Joint Surg Br. 2002;84: 684–7.
24. Burgess RC. The effect of rotatory subluxation of the scaphoid on radio-scaphoid contact. J Hand Surg Am. 1987;12:771–4.
25. Omori S, Moritomo H, Omokawa S, Murase T, Sugamoto K, Yoshikawa H. In vivo 3-dimensional analysis of dorsal intercalated segment instability deformity secondary to scapholunate dissociation: a preliminary report. J Hand Surg Am. 2013;38: 1346–55.
26. Kawanishi Y, Moritomo H, Murase T, Sugamoto K, Yoshikawa H. In vivo three-dimensional analysis of stage III Kienböck's disease: pattern of carpal deformity and radioscaphoid joint congruity. J Hand Surg Am. 2015;40:74–80.
27. Kawai H, Yamamoto K, Yamamoto T, Tada K, Kaga K. Excision of the lunate in Kienböck's disease. Results after long-term follow-up. J Bone Joint Surg Br. 1988;70:287–92.
28. Quenzer DE, Dobyns JH, Linscheid RL, Trail IA, Vidal MA. Radial recession osteotomy for Kienböck's disease. J Hand Surg Am. 1997;22:386–95.
29. Weiss AP, Weiland AJ, Moore JR, Wilgis F. Radial shortening for Kienböck's disease. J Bone Joint Surg Am. 1991;73:384–91.
30. Almquist EE, Burns Jr JF. Radial shortening for the treatment of Kienböck's disease: a 5- to 10-year follow-up. J Hand Surg Am. 1982;7:348–52.
31. Trumble T, Glisson RR, Seaber AV, Urbaniak JR. A biomechanical comparison of the methods for treating Kienböck's disease. J Hand Surg Am. 1986;11:88–93.
32. Horii E, Garcia-Elias M, Bishop AT, Cooney WP, Linscheid RL, Chao EY. Effect on force transmission across the carpus in procedures used to treat Kienböck's disease. J Hand Surg Am. 1990;15:393–400.
33. Werner FW, Palmer AK. Biomechanical evaluation of operative procedures to treat Kienböck's disease. Hand Clin. 1993;9:431–43.
34. Nakamura R, Tsuge S, Watanabe K, Tsunoda K. Radial wedge osteotomy for Kienböck's disease. J Bone Joint Surg Am. 1991;73:1391–6.
35. Kam B, Topper SM, McLoughlin S, Liu Q. Wedge osteotomies of the radius for Kienböck's disease: a biomechanical analysis. J Hand Surg Am. 2002; 27:37–42.
36. Garcia-Elias M, An KN, Cooney WP, Linscheid RL. Lateral closing wedge osteotomy for treatment of Kienböck's disease. Chir Main. 1998;17:283–90.
37. Watanabe K, Nakamura R, Horii E, Miura T. Biomechanical analysis of radial wedge osteotomy for the treatment of Kienböck's disease. J Hand Surg Am. 1993;18:686–90.
38. Masear VR, Zook EG, Pichora DR, Krishnamurthy M, Russell RC, Lemons J, Bidez MW. Strain-gauge evaluation of lunate unloading procedures. J Hand Surg Am. 1992;17:437–43.
39. Short WH, Werner FW, Fortino MD, Palmer AK. Distribution of pressures and forces on the wrist after simulated intercarpal fusion and Kienböck's disease. J Hand Surg Am. 1992;17:443–9.
40. Viegas SF, Patterson RM, Peterson PD, Pogue DJ, Jenkins DK, Sweo TD, et al. Evaluation of the biomechanical efficacy of limited intercarpal fusions for the treatment of scapho-lunate dissociation. J Hand Surg Am. 1990;15:120–8.
41. Almquist EE. Kienböck's disease. Clin Orthop. 1986;202:68–78.
42. Almquist EE. Capitate shortening in the treatment of Kienböck's disease. Hand Clin. 1993;9:505–12.
43. Werber KD, Schmelz R, Peimer CA, Wagenpfeil S, Machens HG, Lohmeyer JA. Biomechanical effect of isolated capitate shortening in Kienböck's disease: an anatomical study. J Hand Surg Eur Vol. 2013;38(5): 500–7.
44. Moritomo H, Murase T, Yoshikawa H. Operative technique of new decompression procedure for Kienböck's disease: partial capitate shortening. Tech Hand Upper Extrem Surg. 2004;8(2):110–5.
45. Moritomo H, Tsuyoshi M, Shimada K, Yamamoto K, Tada K. Partial capitate shortening for Kienbock's disease. J Jpn Soc Surg Hand. 2005;22:149–54.
46. Kataoka T, Moritomo H, Omokawa S, Iida A, Wada T, Aoki M. Decompression effect of partial capitate shortening for Kienbock's disease: a biomechanical study. Hand Surg. 2012;17(3):299–305.
47. Citlak A, Akgun U, Bulut T, Tahta M, Dirim Mete B, Sener M. Partial capitate shortening for Kienböck's disease. J Hand Surg Eur Vol. 2014;40:957.

# Pathoanatomy of Kienböck's Disease

6

Chong Jin Yeo, Gregory Ian Bain, and Levi Morse

## Introduction

Dr. Robert Kienböck first described lunatomalacia in 1910 in his clinical series, and felt that the cause of collapse of the lunate was repetitive trauma to the lunate from work activities [1, 2]. This opinion was backed up by the study of Muller in 1920 who coined the term occupational lunatomalacia [3]. The etiology of avascular necrosis of the lunate remains uncertain to this day, but a common theory persists that it is due to disruption of vascular supply to the lunate. The exact cause of this disruption is still a source of considerable debate.

There have been many classifications introduced in an attempt to understand the disease process as well as to guide treatment. At present, the most commonly utilized is the radiographical classification proposed by Lichtman in 1977 [4]. This is based upon osseous radiographic changes and orientation of the carpus. Schmidt et al. used magnetic resonance imaging (MRI) with contrast enhancement to identify and classify the vascular changes within the lunate [5]. Bain and Begg developed an articular-based approach via arthroscopy to classify the disease and recommend treatment [6]. However, the pathoanatomical aspects of Kienböck's disease are likely to involve all three components of vascular, osseous, and chondral pathologies (Table 6.1).

Understanding the etiology, anatomy, and pathology will be an important step towards explaining the various aspects of Kienböck's disease. By comprehending the basic science, one can better understand the prognostic and management matrix of Kienböck's disease.

## Normal Bone Healing

Bone is comprised of various components, namely the bone marrow, cancellous bone, subchondral bone plate, cortical bone, and articular cartilage. Healing of the individual components occurs differently. Wolff's law (1892) that bone remodels in response to imposed loads is widely accepted [7]. Strong structural supportive bone is formed where stresses require its presence (Fig. 6.1).

C.J. Yeo, MBChB, MRCS, MMed, FAMS
Hand and Microsurgery Section, Department of Orthopedic Surgery, Tan Tock Seng Hospital, 11 Jalan Tan Tock Seng, Singapore 308433, Singapore

G.I. Bain, MBBS, FRACS, FA(Ortho)A, PhD (✉)
Professor, Upper Limb and Research Department of Orthopedic Surgery, Flinders University and Flinders Medical Centre , Bedford Park, Adelaide, SA 5042, Australia
e-mail: greg@gregbain.com.au

L. Morse, BPhty, BMBS (Hons)
Department of Orthopedics and Trauma, Flinders Medical Centre, Bedford Park, SA 5042, Australia

© Springer International Publishing Switzerland 2016
D.M. Lichtman, G.I. Bain (eds.), *Kienböck's Disease*, DOI 10.1007/978-3-319-34226-9_6

**Table 6.1** Pathoanatomical aspects of Kienböck's disease[a]

| Stage | Pathological staging | Vascular | Bone | Chondral |
|---|---|---|---|---|
| | **Normal** | Perfusion | Structural trabeculae and subchondral bone plate | Glistening, smooth and firm surface |
| 0 | **Predisposition** | Single vessel | Negative ulnar variance | |
| | | Hypercoagulapathy | Lunate shape | |
| | | "Teenbock" protective | | |
| 1 | Physiological response (Reactive) | Hypoperfusion Insult | Edema | Normal |
| | **Challenged** | – Diffuse Reactive hyperemia | | |
| 2 | Acute pathology (reversible) | Ischemia | **Bone healing** | Acute synovitis |
| | **Compensated** | Necrosis of marrow and bone | – Osseous necrosis | Fibrillation |
| | | Neovascularization of necrotic margin | – Laying down of new bone (sclerosis) | |
| | | | – Bone remodeling (soft) | |
| | | | Fracture of sclerotic or soft bone | Cartilage clefts and fracture |
| | | | – Fracture union | |
| 3 | Chronic pathology (irreversible) | Focal hypervascularity | **Failed bone healing** | Chronic synovitis |
| | **Compromised** | – sequestrum and cyst formation | – Nonunion with fibrous tissue formation | Floating cartilage surfaces |
| | | | – Fragmentation | Cartilage degeneration |
| | | | – Subchondral bone resorption | Fibrocartilage/granulation tissue |
| 4 | Lunate failure | Complete necrosis | **Failed lunate** | Lunate OA |
| | | | – Lunate collapse | |
| 5 | Wrist failure | | **Compromised wrist** | Pan carpal OA |
| | | | Carpal collapse | |

[a]Modified from [22]

## Cancellous Bone Healing

Cancellous bone unites very rapidly since it is rich in cells and blood supply. Osteoblastic action is confined to bone surfaces (endosteal or periosteal). Total endosteal surface area is very high in cancellous bone, whereas in cortical bone it is limited to the linings of Haversian canals. The gaps in cancellous bone are filled by the formation of new bone from the points of contact [8, 9]. Cancellous bone comprises 20 % of bone mass, but 80 % of bone turnover, primarily due to its large surface area. Cancellous bone remodels by having osteoblastic deposition of layers of lamellae, followed by osteoclastic absorption.

## Bone Marrow Healing

Interstitial oedema and marrow fat cell swelling occur with detrimental effects on the vascular supply to the rest of the bone. Healing is through formation of granulation tissue, which mainly

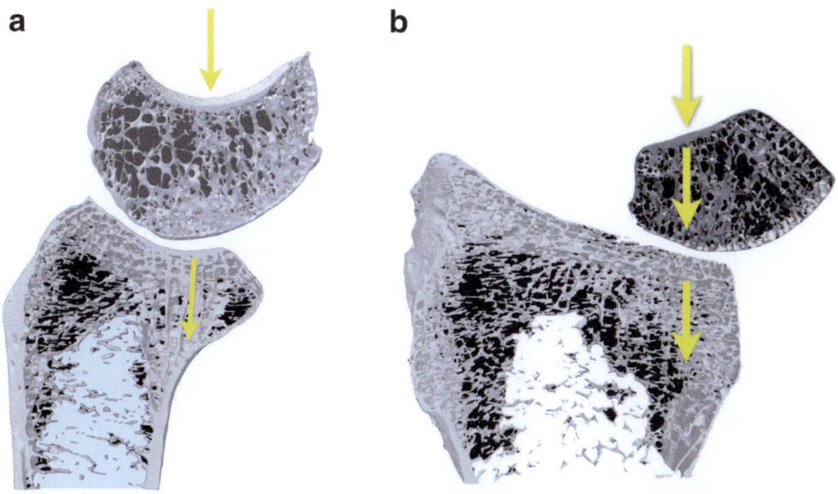


**Fig. 6.1** Micro-CT images showing the internal trabeculae and subchondral structures for the lunate and radius. (**a**) Sagittal view with the *bold arrow* illustrating the loading force from distal, and the transparent *arrows* showing the thickened trabeculae and subchondral bone. (**b**) Coronal view. Copyright Dr. Gregory Bain

consists of new vessel formations and collagen. This progresses to become fibrous tissue that lays a framework for the cancellous bone to heal.

## Cortical Bone/Subchondral Bone Healing

Cortical bone unites by two mechanisms, depending upon the local conditions. When there is exact apposition of cortical bone ends and immobilization is rigid, end-to-end healing takes place from the cortical surfaces with very little external callus (primary bone healing) [10–14]. Where displacement of the fragments occurs, or if immobilization is not rigid, repair occurs by external callus formation (secondary bone healing). This occurs in overlapping phases consisting of the inflammatory phase, the reparative phase (fibrocartilage and bony callus), and the remodeling phase.

In cortical bone, remodeling occurs with osteoclastic tunneling or formation of cutting cones. The osteoclasts make up the head of the cutting cone, followed by capillaries. Capillary loops penetrate this resorptive cavity and eventually establish new Haversian systems, and osteoblasts then lay down the osteoid to fill the cutting cone. Phemister has coined this process "creeping substitution" [15].

## Articular Cartilage Healing

Articular or hyaline cartilage is avascular. The absence of vessels within the cartilage limits the healing potential. Isolated cartilage damage does not mount a vascular response. Chondrocytes in the articular cartilage are capable of cell division and of increasing proteoglycan synthesis; however cartilage regeneration is very slow and the highest potential for growth occurs in the perichondrium, which lies at the periphery of articular cartilage.

The mechanism of repair of the articular cartilage depends on the depth of injury. If the injury extends down to the subchondral bone, capillary injury results in a fibrin clot that will be replaced by granulation tissue and fibrocartilage. If the injury does not penetrate the subchondral bone, healing is reliant on the chondrocytes to synthesize new matrix via diffusion of nutrients from synovial fluid. Therefore healing takes place very slowly and incompletely.

## Osteonecrosis Process

Most of our understanding of osteonecrosis (ON) is based upon research of avascular necrosis (AVN) of the femoral head. The primary mechanism appears to be a circulatory disturbance, though there is still debate upon the location of the occlusion (Fig. 6.2).

## Pathophysiology

Bone is vascularized by small arteries and capillaries, which drain into sinusoids and then exit the bone via veins. ON can be thought of as a type of compartment syndrome, with bone being the rigid compartment. A blood flow blockage at any level can result in significant bone infarct, regardless of the etiology and morphological presentation. Any insult that causes the initial ischemia will cause interstitial oedema. This causes swelling of marrow fat that can lead to capillary or sinusoidal tamponade and intravascular thrombosis. In essence, the blood flow in the bone is inversely proportional to the pressure within the bone marrow. The final common pathway is intravascular coagulation and venous thrombosis, leading to retrograde arterial occlusion and subsequent ischemia. A cycle of recurrent and progressive ischemia can occur leading to eventual bone necrosis (Fig. 6.3).

## Experimental Osteonecrosis

In experimentally induced avascular necrosis, the first histologic changes are in the marrow. Loss of cellular detail occurs in 2–4 days. Necrotic osteocytes may appear normal for weeks under light microscopy, which means that empty lacunae are a late feature of bone death.

Repair begins with the invasion of the necrotic marrow by capillaries and undifferentiated mesenchymal cells. The response is different for each tissue type.

The marrow is resorbed and replaced by hemopoietic and fibrous tissue. With cancellous bone, osteoblasts differentiate to form appositional new bone on the surfaces of necrotic spicules. This explains the increase in radiodensity of cancellous bone during the reparative phase.

With compact bone, including the subchondral bone plate, osteoclasts resorb the compact bone with a net loss of bone mass and a concomitant weakening of the subchondral bone plate and possible fracture. This feature may propagate along the margin of the repair tissue or alternatively along lines of least resistance (Fig. 6.4).

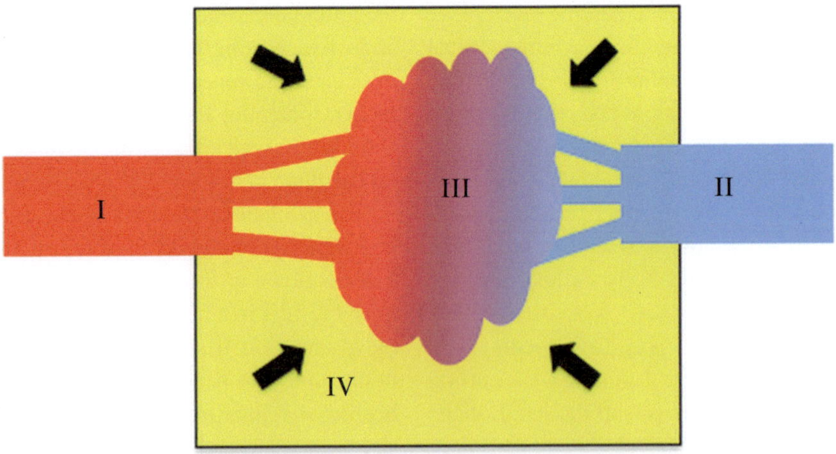


**Fig. 6.2** Diagrammatic representation of possible vascular occlusion in the pathogenesis of osteonecrosis. (I) Arterial insufficiency. (II) Venous occlusion. (III) Intravascular capillary occlusion. (IV) Intraosseous capillary tamponade. Copyright Dr. Gregory Bain

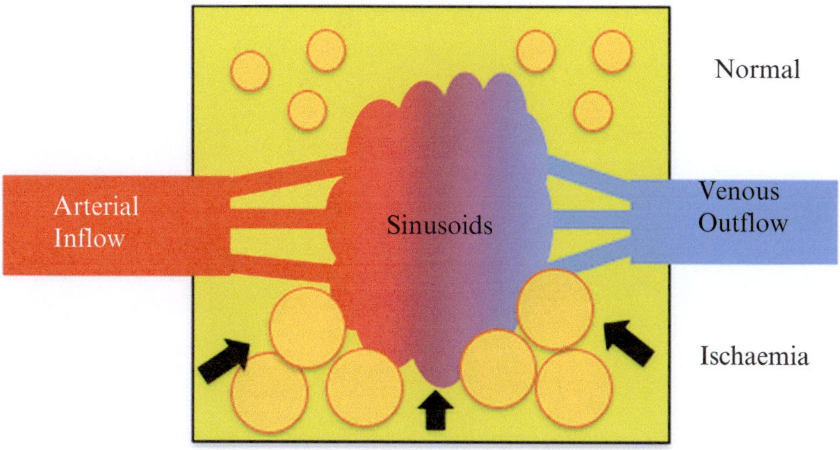


**Fig. 6.3** Diagrammatic representation of the normal process of vascularization of the lunate and with ischemia, the fat cells in the marrow become swollen, and there is interstitial oedema, leading to a tamponade effect on the sinusoids, thus decreasing the venous outflow. This increases the intraosseous pressure, reduced arterial flow and eventually leads to ischemia and necrosis. Copyright Dr. Gregory Bain

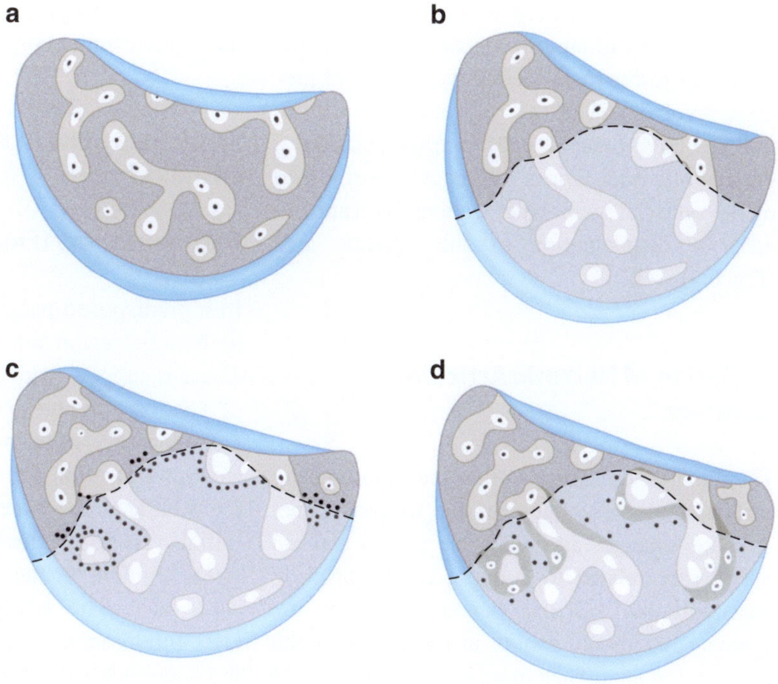


**Fig. 6.4** Evolution of pathological changes in avascular necrosis. (**a**) Normal bone. (**b**) Ischaemic segment with cell death. (**c**) Cellular proliferation and revascularization in the zone between dead bone and live bone. (**d**) Appositional new bone formation upon dead trabeculae. Copyright Dr. Gregory Bain

## Evolution of Necrotic Bone

The evolution of necrotic bone is to either repair or progress to fracture, osteochondral fragment detachment, collapse, fragmentation, and disintegration (resorption).

Fracture occurs through necrotic bone, which is at first difficult to identify on radiographs as it is usually just a thin fracture line. The fracture acts as a secondary stimulus for revascularization. Resorption of compact bone and the subchondral bone plate leads to structural weakening.

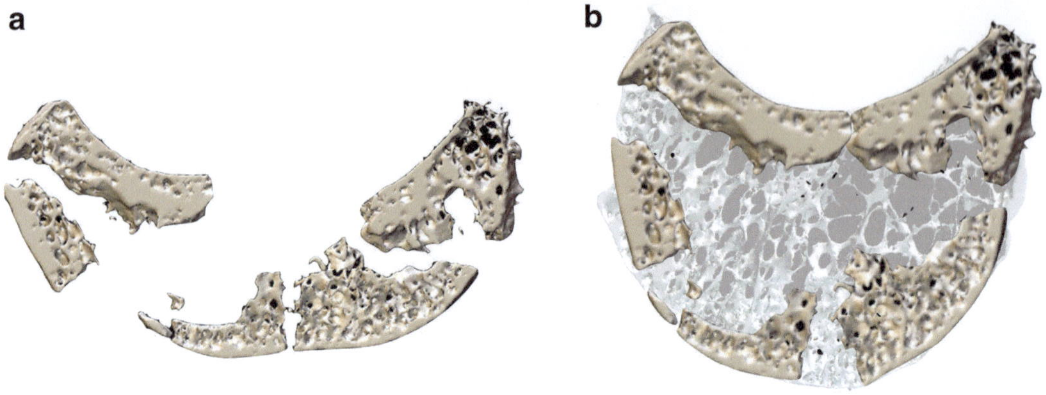


**Fig. 6.5** MicroCT images of the lunate. (**a**) Fragmented lunate in Kienböck's disease. (**b**) Reconstructed fragments superimposed onto a normal lunate, which highlights the fracture path and resorption of the medullary bone. Fractures at the attachment of margins of resorption of cancellous bone, with majority of subchondral bone plate intact. Copyright Dr. Gregory Bain

Normal bone is replaced by fibrous tissue and areas of fibrocartilage. Collapse of the internal structures is due to an ineffective reparative process. Involvement of the resorption pathway in the reparative process leads to fragmentation of the necrotic area. These fragments are resorbed by the synovial membrane, leading to disappearance or disintegration of the necrotic area (Fig. 6.5).

### Evolution of Necrotic Articular Cartilage

The articular cartilage is often preserved during early fracture or collapse of the necrotic bone. Articular changes appear in late phases and are only partly related to collapse of the necrotic area. Initially, vascular penetration from the synovial membrane results in resorption of the subchondral area. Then there is transformation of compact subchondral area to a trabecular structure as vascularization reaches the deep cartilage layers. Vascularization of the normally avascular tissue leads to reduction in matrix content and cell numbers. In the synovial membrane, revascularization occurs through penetration of the cartilage, and the "pannus" formation reduces nutritional supply. All these factors lead to the cartilage developing fibrillations, clefts, fractures, and eventual osteoarthritis.

## What Happens in Kienböck's Disease?

### Pathoanatomy (Fig. 6.6)

In a predisposed patient, repeated insults leads to hypoperfusion and ischemia of the lunate. There is support from literature that impairment of venous drainage plays a critical role in the pathoanatomy of Kienböck's disease [16, 17]. Revascularization and new bone formation is in the middle of the bone, suggesting that there is initial venous occlusion due to compressive stress, evident by the raised intraarticular pressure, leading to arterial blood flow cessation [18]. Intraosseous pressure of the normal versus the Kienböck's disease lunate was also studied. The intraosseous pressure rose significantly on wrist extension, significantly more in the Kienböck's disease lunate as compared to the normal lunate. In some of the Kienböck's disease lunate, the pressure exceeds arterial blood pressure [19].

A vicious cycle of progressive ischemia occurs, with interstitial oedema and marrow fat

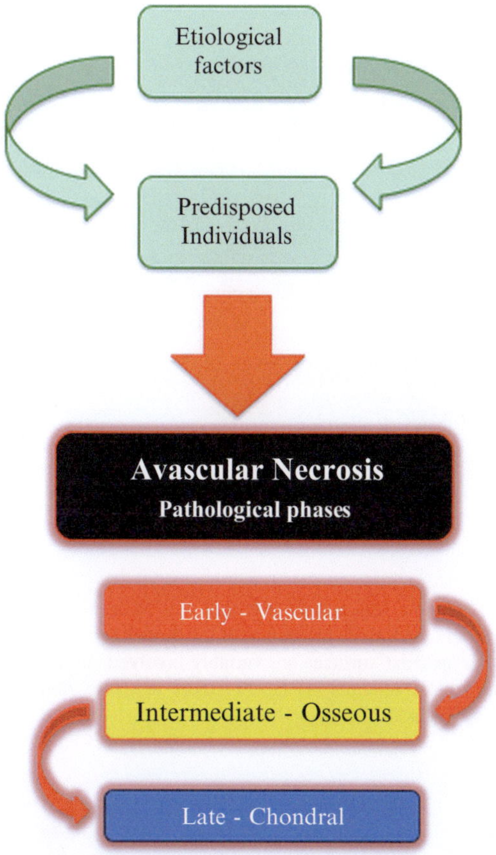


**Fig. 6.6** Flowchart of Kienböck's disease pathoanatomy. Copyright Dr. Gregory Bain

cell swelling. The fat cells lyse and are phagocytosed by macrophages to form foam cells. As the trabeculae, marrow and vascular structures are confined to the osseous compartment, this can produce a tamponade effect on the capillary and sinusoids leading to stasis and intravascular thrombosis that further accentuates oedema. Persistent ischemia eventually produces necrosis of bone and its marrow (Fig. 6.7).

Attempts at healing starts with granulation tissue being laid down that consists of new vessels and collagen. With repeated insults and persistent ischaemic events, the granulation tissue becomes fibrous tissue and fibrocartilage that prevents the new vessels penetrating to supply the necrotic osseous and fibrous tissue (Fig. 6.8).

New bone is laid down on the existing dead trabeculae via osteoblastic activity, creating a thickened trabecular structure that can be seen on plain X-rays and micro-CT (Fig. 6.9) [20, 21].

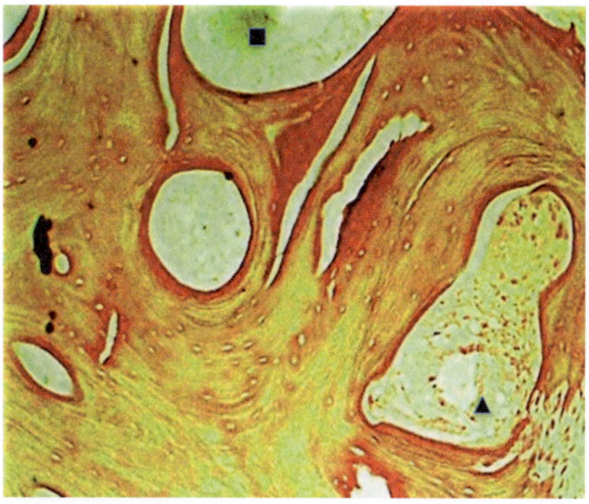

**Fig. 6.7** Histology of a Kienböck's lunate with empty lacunae. ▲ illustrates granulation tissue, ■ fibrous tissue. Copyright Dr. Gregory Bain [20]

Fracture and fragmentation occurs during the remodeling period as the dead bone is resorbed and there is structural weakness. It has been observed that there are a number of fracture types in Kienböck's disease: impaction, oblique, shear, or fragmented (Fig. 6.10).

The sclerosis that is observed on X-rays can be attributed to the following:

1. Fracture, and overlay of fragmented bone
2. Laying down of new bone on necrotic trabeculae
3. Disuse osteopenia of adjacent bone
4. Dystrophic calcification

Fractures of the subchondral bone plate lead to joint irregularity. Resorption of the subchondral bone leads to loss of support for the articular cartilage (Fig. 6.11). Synovitis is a universal finding in Kienböck's disease, which may be due to the necrotic factors of Kienböck's disease or the late degenerative arthritis [6].

Articular cartilage changes include fissuring, fracture and degeneration. Kissing lesions that affect the opposing articular surface then occur (Fig. 6.12). Clinically it has been noted that the proximal surface of the lunate (radiolunate joint) tends to be affected before the midcarpal joint.

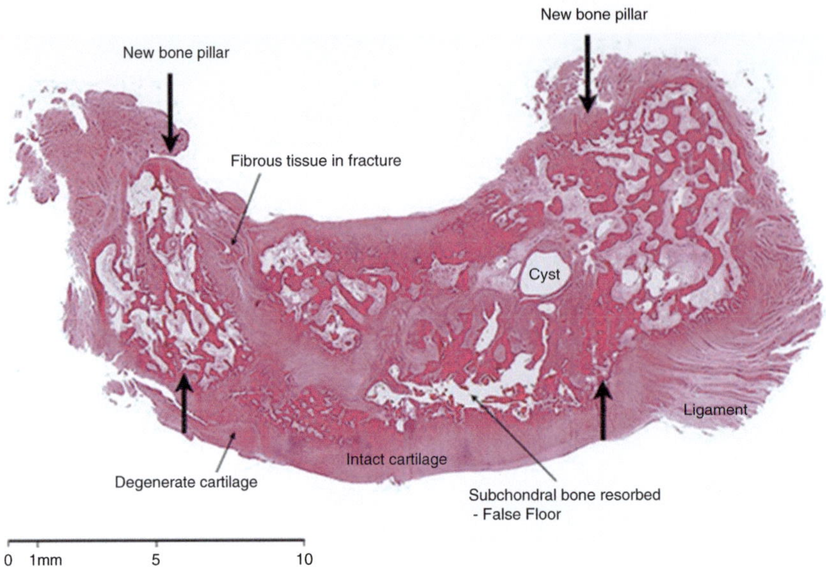


**Fig. 6.8** Histology of Kienböck's lunate. There is extensive osseous necrosis, with intervening fibrous tissue and cysts that fill the osseous voids. The body of the lunate is significantly compromised with reabsorption of the medullary canal of the lunate and the subchondral bone plate. The *arrows* demonstrate pillars of new bone, which transmit the load, since the failure of the medullary trabeculae. The articular surfaces are variably involved. In this case the distal articular surface is more severely involved. Copyright Dr. Gregory Bain

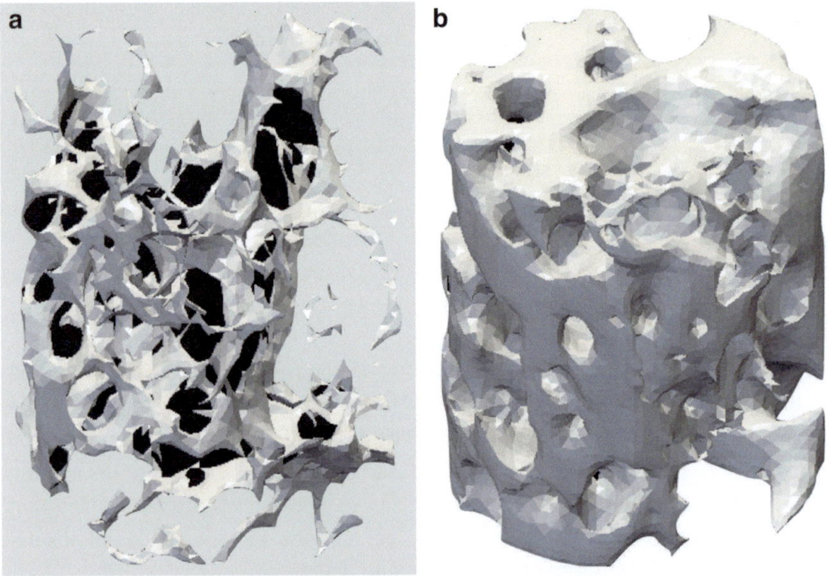


**Fig. 6.9** MicroCT of trabecular structure. (**a**) Trabecular structure in a normal lunate. (**b**) Thickened trabeculae in a Kienböck's lunate. There is up to 3× more trabeculae but a decrease in total bone volume. Reproduced with permission from Low SC, Bain GI, Findlay DM, Eng K, Perilli E. External and internal bone micro-architecture in normal and Kienbock's lunates: a whole-bone micro-computed tomography study. J Orthop Res. Jun 2014;32(6):826–833. © 2014 Orthopedic Research Society. Published by Wiley Periodicals, Inc.

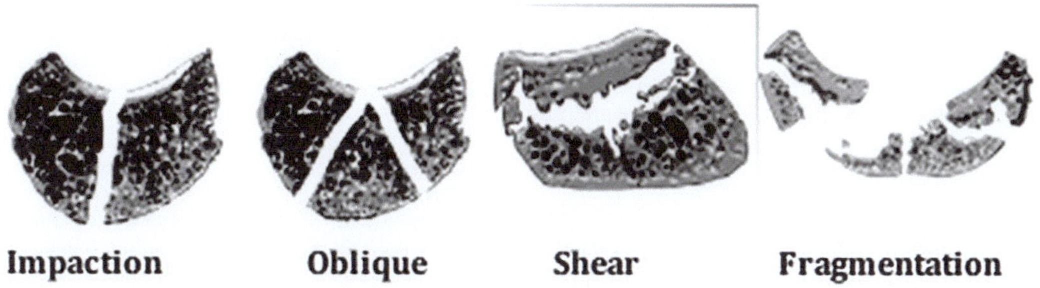


**Fig. 6.10** Fracture types occurring in Kienböck's disease. Copyright Dr. Gregory Bain

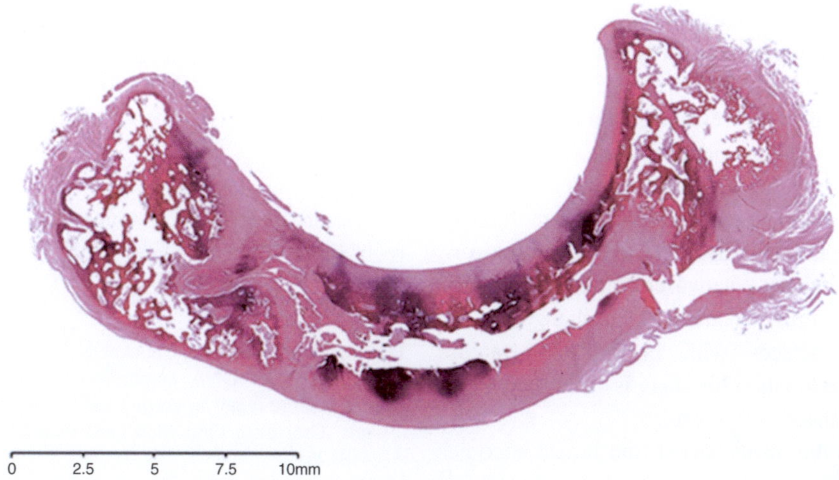


**Fig. 6.11** Histology of the Kienböck's lunate with extensive collapse and disintegration of the internal structures whilst maintaining the cartilage surface. Copyright Dr. Gregory Bain

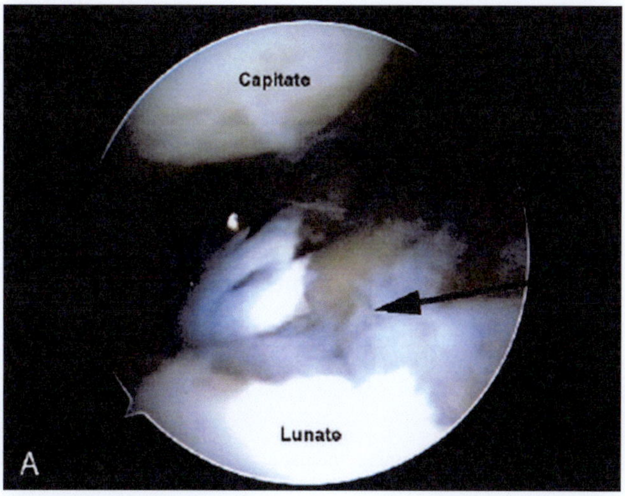


**Fig. 6.12** Arthroscopic image showing the kissing lesions between the distal lunate and the capitate

## Pathoanatomical Staging

Based on our understanding thus far of the pathoanatomy of Kienböck's disease, we are proposing a pathological staging system founded on the vascularity, osseous, and chondral changes of the lunate.

Utilizing a simple analogy, the lunate in Kienböck's disease can be likened to a failing heart. There are certain patients with "risks factors" or predisposing factors for Kienböck's disease that include single vessel in the lunate, hypercoagulopathy, negative ulnar variance, and trapezoidal lunate shape.

When the lunate is initially stressed, there is a physiological response (reactive or challenged stage) to this insult resulting in diffuse reactive hyperemia and bony oedema.

If the insult continues, the lunate progresses to a compensated stage whereby ischemia ensues with resultant necrosis of the bone and marrow, with concurrent neovascularization of the necrotic margins. There will be changes to the cartilage surfaces with or without fracture through the lunate. This stage is still reversible if the initial insult is removed.

Should the insult persist, the lunate becomes compromised. It no longer is able to heal itself and the changes are now irreversible. This is quickly followed by complete failure of the lunate. Since the lunate is the "keystone" to the wrist, the wrist will also start to fail accordingly.

The pathoanatomical staging system presented here, when viewed in combination with the several other staging systems presented elsewhere in this book, can serve as an important component of a highly nuanced treatment algorithm for all phases of Kienböck's disease. This has been done in Chap. 30, where the senior authors (DML and GIB) have intertwined these various systems in order to create a practical, comprehensive, and unified guide to evaluation and treatment.

## References

1. Kienböck R. Concerning traumatic malacia of the lunate and its consequences: joint degeneration and compression. Fortsch Geb Roentgen. 1910;16:77–103.
2. Peltier LF. The classic. Concerning traumatic malacia of the lunate and its consequences: degeneration and compression fractures. Privatdozent Dr. Robert Kienbock. Clin Orthop Relat Res. 1980;149: 4–8.
3. Müller W. Über die Erweichung und Verdichtung des Os Lunatum, eine Typische Erkrankung des Handgelenks. Beitr Klin Chir. 1920;119:664.
4. Lichtman DM, Mack GR, MacDonald RI, Gunther SF, Wilson JN. Kienbock's disease: the role of silicone replacement arthroplasty. J Bone Joint Surg Am. 1977;59(7):899–908.
5. Schmitt R, Heinze A, Fellner F, Obletter N, Struhn R, Bautz W. Imaging and staging of avascular osteonecroses at the wrist and hand. Eur J Radiol. 1997;25(2):92–103.
6. Bain GI, Begg M. Arthroscopic assessment and classification of Kienbock's disease. Tech Hand Up Extrem Surg. 2006;10(1):8–13.
7. Wolff J. The law of bone remodeling. Berlin: Springer; 1986.
8. Charnley J, Baker SL. Compression arthrodesis of the knee; a clinical and histological study. J Bone Joint Surg Br. 1952;34(2):187–99.
9. Charnley J. The closed treatment of common fractures. 3rd ed. Edinburgh: E&S Livingstone; 1968.
10. Müller ME, Allgöwer M, Willenegger H. Technique of internal fixation of fracture. New York, NY: Springer; 1965.
11. Nichols JT, Toto PD, Choukas NC. The proliferative capacity and DNA synthesis of osteoblasts during fracture repair in normal and hypophysectomized rats. Oral Surg Oral Med Oral Pathol. 1968;25(3): 418–26.
12. Pappas AM, Radin E. The effect of delayed manipulation upon the rate of fracture healing. Surg Gynecol Obstet. 1968;126(6):1287–97.
13. Perren SM, Huggler A, Russenberger M, Allgöwer M, Mathys R, Schenk R, et al. The reaction of cortical bone to compression. Acta Orthop Scand Suppl. 1969;125:19–29.
14. Penttinen R. Biochemical studies on fracture healing in the rat, with special reference to the oxygen supply. Acta Chir Scand Suppl. 1972;432:1–32.
15. Phemister DB. Repair of bone in the presence of aseptic necrosis resulting from fractures, transplantations, and vascular obstruction. Clin Orthop Relat Res. 1930;1992(277):4–11.
16. Pichler M, Putz R. The venous drainage of the lunate bone. Surg Radiol Anat. 2003;24(6):372–6.
17. Schiltenwolf M, Martini AK, Eversheim S, Mau H. Significance of intraosseous pressure for pathogenesis of Kienbock disease. Handchir Mikrochir Plast Chir. 1996;28(4):215–9.
18. Ueba Y, Kakinoki R, Nakajima Y, Kotoura Y. Morphology and histology of the collapsed lunate in advanced Kienbock disease. Hand Surg. 2013;18(2): 141–9.
19. Schiltenwolf M, Martini AK, Mau HC, Eversheim S, Brocai DR, Jensen CH. Further investigations of the intraosseous pressure characteristics in necrotic

lunates (Kienbock's disease). J Hand Surg Am. 1996;21(5):754–8.

20. Low SC, Bain GI, Findlay DM, Eng K, Perilli E. External and internal bone micro-architecture in normal and Kienbock's lunates: a whole-bone micro-computed tomography study. J Orthop Res. 2014;32(6):826–33.
21. Han KJ, Kim JY, Chung NS, Lee HR, Lee YS. Trabecular microstructure of the human lunate in Kienbock's disease. J Hand Surg Eur Vol. 2012;37(4):336–41.
22. Bain G, Yeo CJ, Morse LP. Kienböck disease: recent advances in the basic science, assessment and treatment. Hand Surg. 2015;20(3):352–65.

# The Etiology of Kienböck's Disease

# 7

Gregory Ian Bain and Carlos Irisarri

## Introduction

Throughout this book, contributing authors introduce their chapters by referring to the general lack of consensus about the etiology of Kienböck's disease (KD). I am sure, however, that even the most skeptical of them assumed that this chapter, devoted entirely to etiology, would issue a definitive statement on the subject. Well, I am sorry to disappoint them. Instead, we recognize that, in common with osteonecrosis in other parts of the body (our pathologist friends assure us that the histopathology of KD is compatible with osteonecrosis, or cellular death of bone) multiple biological factors can contribute to its pathogenesis. And we also recognize that there are specific mechanical and structural factors for each anatomical region that can have their own unique influence on the development of osteonecrosis in that particular area.

What we really do not know is which of these factors, the mechanical/structural or the biologic, play the most significant role in the development of KD. But each theory has its champions. For this reason we have divided the chapter into two independent (yet complementary) sections, the first by my coeditor, Greg Bain, from Adelaide, Australia, who advocates the mechanical/structural theory of lunate osteonecrosis, and the second by Carlos Irisarri from Vigo, Spain, who favors the biologic model. After reading both sections, it is our hope that you, our readers, will be anxious to decide for themselves which theory is correct!

David M. Lichtman, MD

**Electronic supplementary material:** The online version of this chapter (doi:10.1007/978-3-319-34226-9_7) contains supplementary material, which is available to authorized users. Videos can also be accessed at http://link.springer.com/chapter/[10.1007/978-3-319-34226-9_7].

## Basic Science Theory of Kienböck's Disease

Gregory Ian Bain

The first chapters of this monograph review the osseous, vascular, and pathological aspects of Kienböck's disease. There are many factors associated with Kienböck's disease, such as genetics, anatomy, trauma, vascular. and metabolic disorders [2–13]. The aim of this chapter is to develop further the likely etiologies of Kienböck's disease, based on this basic science platform.

G.I. Bain, MBBS, FRACS, FA(Ortho)A, PhD (✉)
Professor, Upper Limb and Research, Department of Orthopedic Surgery, Flinders University and Flinders Medical Centre, Bedford Park, Adelaide, SA, Australia
e-mail: greg@gregbain.com.au

C. Irisarri, MD (✉)
Hand Surgery Unit, Hospital Vithas-Fátima, Vía Norte, 48, Vigo, Pontevedra 36206, Spain
e-mail: irisarri@iies.es

© Springer International Publishing Switzerland 2016
D.M. Lichtman, G.I. Bain (eds.), *Kienböck's Disease*, DOI 10.1007/978-3-319-34226-9_7

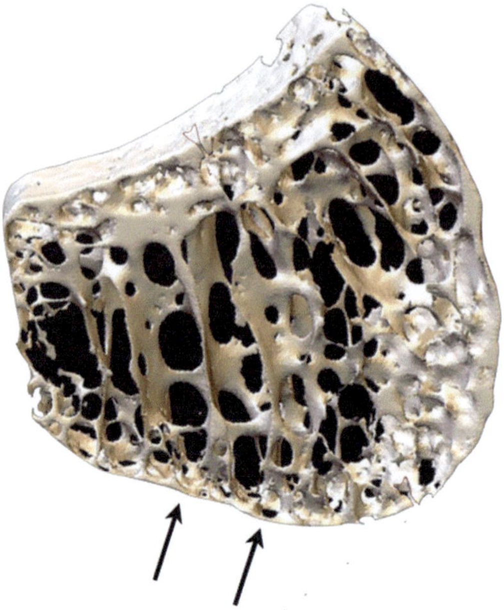

**Fig. 7.1** Micro-anatomy of the lunate. 3D micro-CT scan of the lunate demonstrating the thin proximal single layer of subchondral bone plate, which was measured to be 0.1-mm thick. There are spanning trabeculae principally on the radial aspect [14]. Copyright Dr. Gregory Bain

Avascular necrosis is often considered to be a compartment syndrome of bone [23, 24]. The lunate is the compartment, and the mechanical factors act on the "at risk" fixed osseous lunate. The factors that can change the pressure within the lunate compartment include the (1) arterial inflow, (2) embolization, (3) the compartment contents, and (4) venous outflow.

## The Lunate Compartment

The proximal articular "condyle" is the common site of Kienböck's disease. It is to be noted that the subchondral bone plate on the convex proximal surface is *only a single trabecula layer*, and it is this surface that is prone to the fractures associated with Kienböck's disease [14] (Fig. 7.1). On this specimen we measured the proximal subchondral bone plate in the at risk zone to be 0.1 mm thick. There are multiple trabeculae that span to the distally multilayered subchondral bone plate, that transmit the load and maintain the height of the lunate.

**Table 7.1** "At risk" factors for Kienböck's disease

| | At risk | Effect | Low risk |
|---|---|---|---|
| Lunate | | | |
| Viegas type | I | Radial midcarpal loading | II |
| Zapico type | I | Radial midcarpal loading | II or III |
| Lunate size | Small | Smaller surface area | Large |
| Lunate coverage | Uncovered | Radial radiocarpal loading | Covered |
| Number of vessels | Single | Collateral circulation | Multiple |
| Cortical thickness | Thin | Less fatigue strength | Thick |
| Radius | | | |
| Inclination | Flatter | Increased radiocarpal loading | Inclined |
| Ulnar | | | |
| Variance | Negative | Radial radiocarpal loading | Neutral/ Positive |

## The "At Risk Lunate"

There are a number of morphological factors of the wrist that are know to be associated with Kienböck's disease. These are presented in Table 7.1 and Fig. 7.2 [2–13]. It can be noted that all of these factors increase the loading on the radial aspect of the lunate, although each in a slightly different way.

Briefly reviewing each aspect from distal to proximal:

The Viegas type I lunate positions the capitate in a more radial position, so that it articulates with the radial aspect of the distal lunate [2, 7]. In addition the wrist with a type I lunate will mobilize predominantly through the midcarpal articulation, therefore the radiolunate articulation tends to repeatedly load in the same location (Fig. 7.3) [22].

The Zapico type I lunate loads on the radial aspect of the distal and proximal lunate, therefore creating a shearing force on the lunate [3, 4].

The flatter distal radial inclination causes the loading of the proximal lunate to be greater on the radial half.

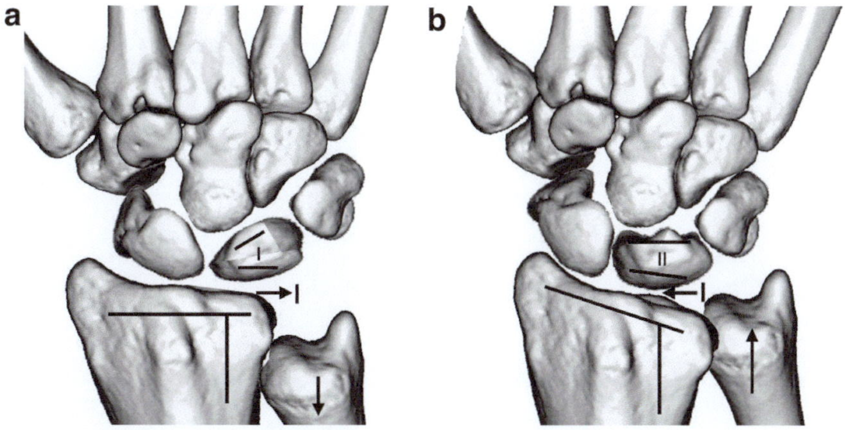


**Fig. 7.2** Morphological factors associated with Kienböck's disease. (**a**) The "at risk" factors increase the load and shear stresses on the radial aspect of the lunate. (**b**) The "low risk" factors lead to a wide distribution of the stresses on the lunate

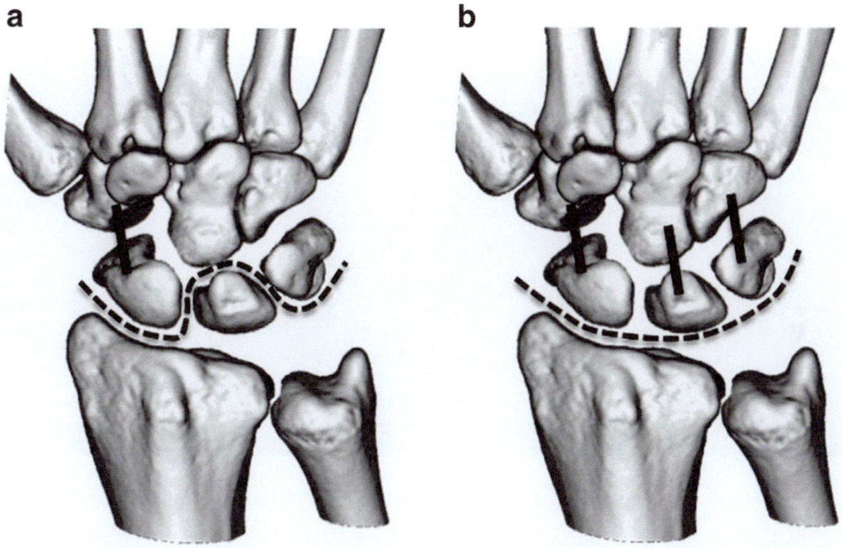


**Fig. 7.3** Kinematics of Viegas type I and II wrist. (**a**) The motion of the central column in the type I lunate is principally through the midcarpal articulation for the flexion/extension and the ulnar/radial deviation planes. (**b**) The type II lunate wrist articulates principally through the radiocarpal joint [22]. Copyright Dr. Gregory Bain

The "uncovered" lunate (i.e., ulnar position of the lunate, so that it hangs off the radius) will only be loaded on that portion of the lunate that articulates with the radius (Fig. 7.4a). In addition, it creates loading on the very radial edge of the distal radius.

A negative ulnar variance causes less of the carpal load to be distributed to the ulna, therefore more of the load is distributed from the radial aspect of the lunate to the radius [9].

All of these anatomical factors cause the loading during power grip to be concentrated on the radial aspect of the lunate.

## Stress Fracture in Progression

To create a stress fracture, there must be a time when the lunate is being loaded, but the fracture had not yet occurred. We refer to this as a "stress

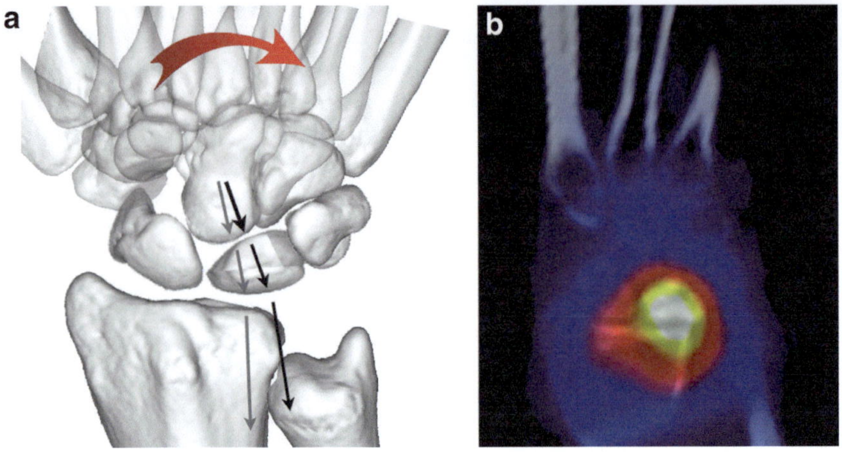

Fig. 7.4 The uncovered type I lunate. (**a**) The uncovered type I lunate is positioned on the radial edge of the lunate, and with power grip in ulnar deviation loads on the radial edge of the radius. (**b**) The SPECT scan demonstrates increased uptake within the lunate due to new bone formation and remodeling within the lunate. There is also increased uptake on the radial aspect of the distal radius due to the abnormal loading

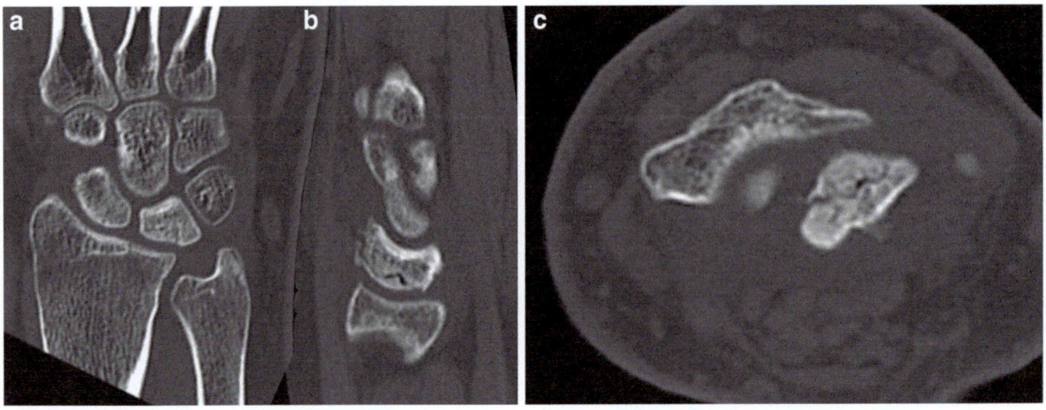

Fig. 7.5 (**a–c**) Early case of Kienböck's disease. The distribution of the fractures corresponds to the shape of the distal radius

fracture in progress." However, this phenomenon creates a reactive physiological response, which can be identified with imaging. This includes edema, hyperemia (gadolinium-enhanced MRI; see Chap. 11) and osteoblastic activity as seen on a SPECT scan (Fig. 7.4b).

Once the micro-fracture has occurred, it is likely to heal spontaneously, if it is not over loaded. With repeated loading the fracture will reoccur, and ultimately propagate through the lunate, and the fracture will be a "die punch" of the shape of the impacting distal radius (Fig. 7.5). The lunate fracture and collapse almost always include the radial half of the lunate, to the level of the ulnar edge of the radius (Fig. 7.6). However, in only the most extensive cases, is the ulnar aspect of the lunate fragmented.

Kienböck's disease is thought not to be due to a major traumatic episode. We performed a systematic review of lunate fracture dislocations, and found only two cases with a volar coronal fracture that developed AVN of the lunate (see Chap. 12). Kienböck's disease is more likely to occur with repeated stresses placed on the lunate and explains the higher incidence in young active male workers [15].

The black arrows demonstrate the areas of loading and the yellow line the zone of propagation.

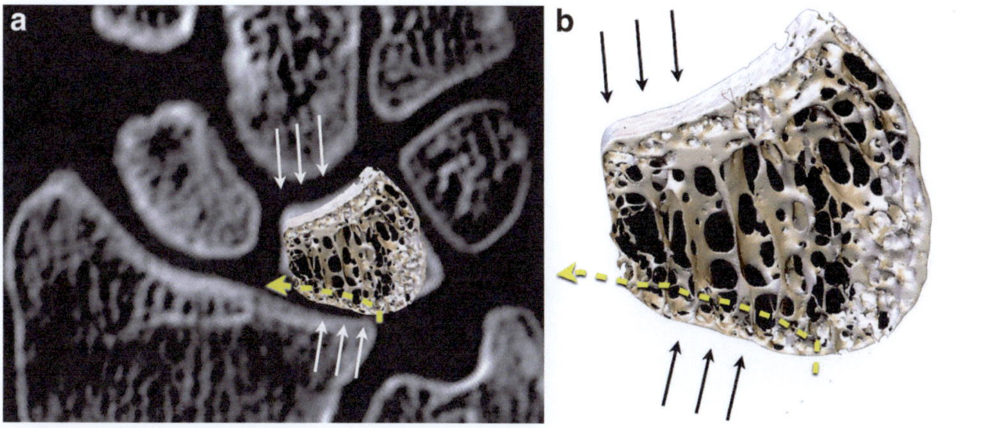


**Fig. 7.6** Kienböck's disease stress fracture concept. (**a**) Micro-CT lunate superimposed on a plane radiograph of Kienböck's wrist, with the areas of load identified with *arrows*. (**b**) In this dry cadaveric bone, a small fracture of the subchondral bone plate can be seen

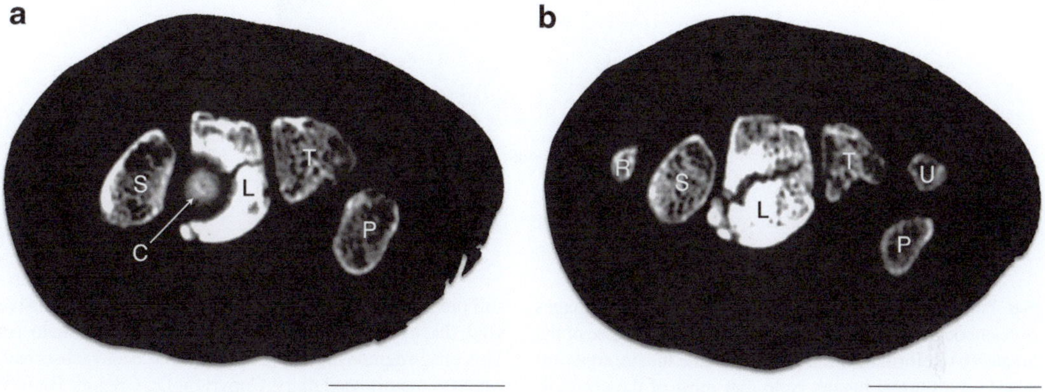


**Fig. 7.7** Capitate nutcracker. (**a**) The capitate is seen at the center of the "target sign" on the radial aspect of the lunate. (**b**) A coronal fracture propagates across the lunate

## Nutcracker Effect of the Capitate

The stress fracture concept can also occur at the distal lunate, due to the loading of the capitate. The distribution of the lunate fracture is dependent upon the type of force applied. In this case the capitate is a nutcracker, which splits the lunate in the coronal plane (Fig. 7.7, Video 7.1).

## Comminution

Once the lunate has fractured at the proximal and distal aspects, it is common for it become comminuted and for the lunate to collapse (Fig. 7.8). However, carpal collapse does not occur until there is significant lunate collapse [15].

## Medullary Abrasion

The medullary bone is designed to span from the proximal to distal cortex. However, once the outer cortices are compromised, the friable medullary bone is exposed. The trabecular bone cannot withstand loading, and therefore the lunate becomes comminuted and the lunate collapses (Fig. 7.9).

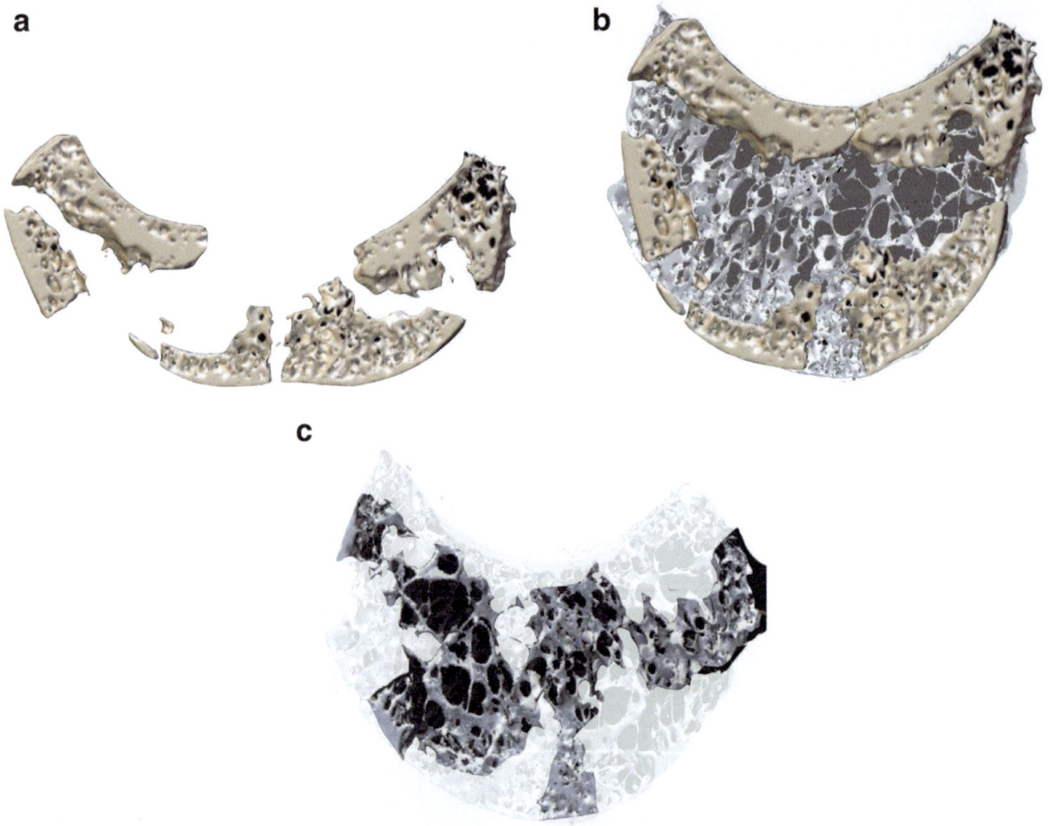


**Fig. 7.8** Lunate fragmentation. Micro-CT sagittal images of Kienböck's lunate: (**a**) Fragmentation and collapse of the lunate. (**b**) Reformatted image of the same lunate, superimposed on a normal lunate. Note that most of the cortex is still present but fragmented. However, there is an extensive void, due to resorption of much of the medullary lunate. (**c**) This image demonstrates the bone that has been reabsorbed, which is mainly medullary. Copyright Dr. Gregory Bain

## Subchondral Bone Plate

The articular cartilage is critical to a normal functioning articular joint. The subchondral bone plate is an important morphological structure that transmits the load and provides a consistent platform for the articular cartilage. Fractures and reabsorption of the subchondral plate will undermine the articular cartilage and affects its function.

## Compartment Syndrome of Bone

The above covered the lunate osseous compartment. The remainder of the chapter will cover the other components of the compartment syndrome model (Fig. 7.10).

## Arterial

There has been much attention to the arterial supply of the lunate in Kienböck's disease of the lunate (Fig. 7.11) [11, 19]. Arterial obstruction can cause avascular necrosis of the lunate, however it is really very uncommon for AVN to occur as a consequence of even complex injuries of the lunate. For example, AVN rarely occurs with perilunate dislocations of the lunate. In a review of the trans-lunate carpal injuries we identified that it was only in two cases where there was a

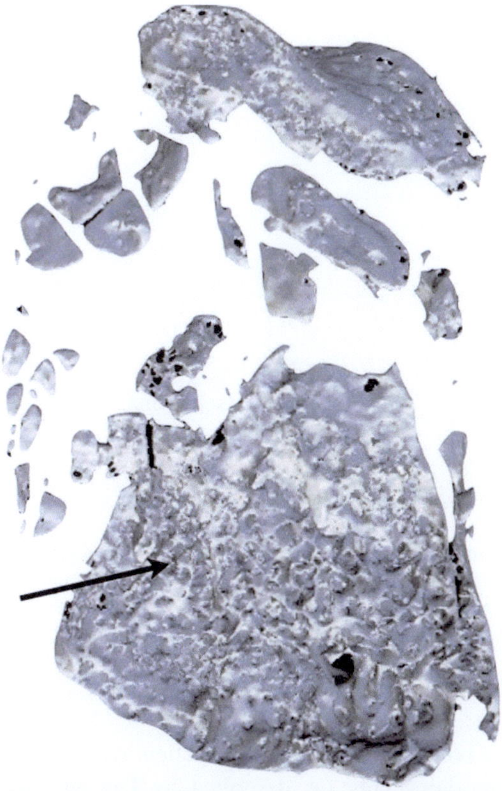

**Fig. 7.9** Medullary erosion. Micro-CT of Kienböck's lunate with extensive fragmentation and almost complete loss of the proximal subchondral bone plate. This exposes the friable medullary bone that is unable to withstand load, and therefore crumbles and is reabsorbed. Copyright Dr. Gregory Bain

volar oblique fracture that AVN of the lunate occurred.

## Emboli

Embolization of the arteries can cause localized necrosis, but it is really uncommon to have AVN be a complication of atrial fibrillation or other embolic diseases [23, 24].

## Compartment Contents

The main contents of the lunate are the bone marrow and its fat. There are conditions that can increase these components, such as Gaucher's disease, which is a rare cause of AVN. However, alcohol abuse also increases the fat content, and is a common cause of AVN of the femoral head [23, 24]. Fortunately it is rarely associated with Kienböck's disease, demonstrating that the factors associated with AVN are multifactorial. The factors associated with AVN are different depending upon the patients' age, sex, race, comorbidities, activities and are also anatomically specific.

However, the intra-osseous fat is very sensitive to ischemia and once necrosis occurs there is significant edema, and this can have a real impact of local vascularity of the lunate. Therefore, the contents of the lunate are unlikely to initiate the AVN, but are likely to potentiate the condition.

## Venous

Hungerford demonstrated that the intraosseous pressure is significantly raised in femoral head AVN [24]. Jensen demonstrated that the intraosseous pressure in Kienböck's lunate was significantly increased compared to the normal population [16, 17]. The intraosseous pressure rose significantly on wrist extension, significantly more in the Kienböck's disease lunate as compared to the normal lunate. In some cases the Kienböck's lunate intraosseous pressure exceeds arterial blood pressure. He postulated that the compromised venous outflow, and the increased intraosseous pressure, was a factor in the development of Kienböck's disease.

Crock studied the venous osseous drainage of the lunate, and described the extra-osseous veins followed the corresponding arteries. He also described the subarticular venous plexus, just below the subchondral bone plate (Fig. 7.12) [18]. He noted that these veins are parallel, and therefore do not communicate as a network as other venous systems do.

In a predisposed patient, repeated insults leads to hypoperfusion and ischemia of the lunate. There is support from the literature that impairment of venous drainage plays a critical role in the pathoanatomy of AVN of the lunate and femoral head [20, 21, 23, 24]. Revascularization and new bone formation is evident throughout the lunate, suggesting that there is initial venous occlusion, that produces ischemia.

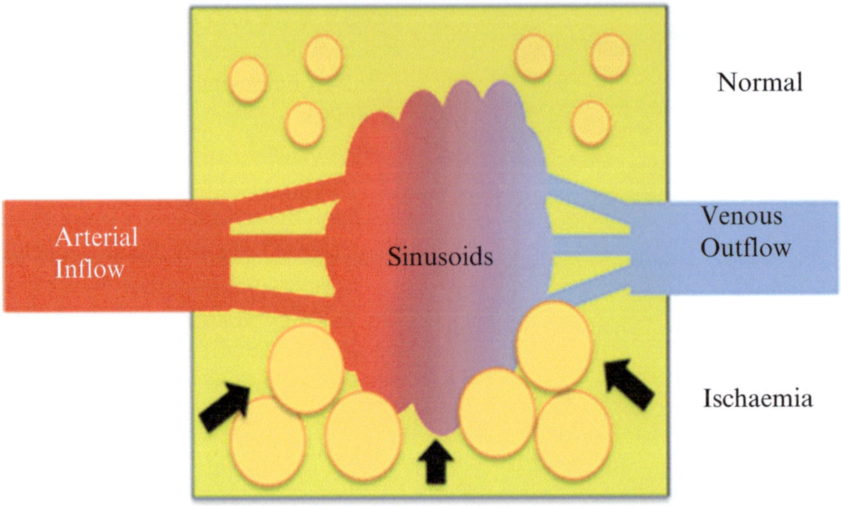


**Fig. 7.10** Compartment syndrome of bone. Diagrammatic representation of the normal vascularization of the lunate (superior half) with the normal fat cell and venous drainage. With ischemia (inferior half), there is interstitial edema and the marrow fat cells become swollen. This leads to tamponade of the sinusoids, thus decreasing the venous outflow. This further increases the intraosseous pressure, reduces arterial inflow, and produces necrosis. Copyright Dr. Gregory Bain

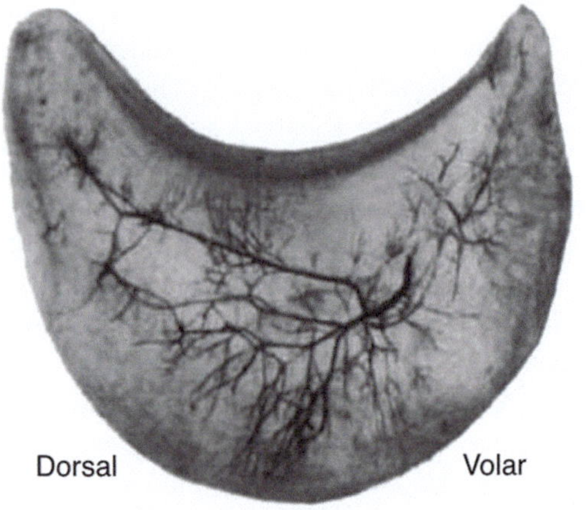


**Fig. 7.11** Lunate arterial supply. Lunate with single volar artery as seen from the lateral and distal view. Reproduced with permission from Lee ML. The intraosseus arterial pattern of the carpal lunate bone and its relation to avascular necrosis. Acta Orthop Scand. 1963;33:43–55. Courtesy of Taylor & Francis Ltd., www.tandfonline.com

Based on this and other works we propose that there are **two** potential models of venous obstruction that can produce AVN. These can be considered as global or localized aspects of the lunate (Fig. 7.13). Crock advised that the extra-osseous venous supply of bone mirrors the arterial supply of bone [18]. Therefore, the patient with a single arterial supply (as described by Lee and also Gelberman [11, 19]) will have a single venous drainage. An obstruction at the osseous vascular foramen or external to the lunate will produce a *global* venous hypertension of the entire lunate.

Localized obstruction can be caused by a stress fracture and lead to *localized* venous hypertension. Once the stress fracture occurs, the adjacent subarticular plexus must be violated, and lead to a localized venous obstruction (Fig. 7.14). This can cause local edema and fat necrosis, which in turn potentiates the entire cycle.

These concepts then invite the question as to whether there are one or two types of avascular necrosis of the lunate. We postulate that the common type of AVN is a stress fracture, as described in the initial section of this chapter. The stress fracture begins at the proximal lunate, in the "at risk" lunate, in the "at risk individual." The stress fracture also disrupts the delicate subarticular plexus, producing local venous hypertension and ischemia. This leads to local edema and fat necrosis. There may be a capitate nutcracker coronal fracture of the lunate; medullary abrasion and reabsorption, comminution, and subsequent collapse of the lunate.

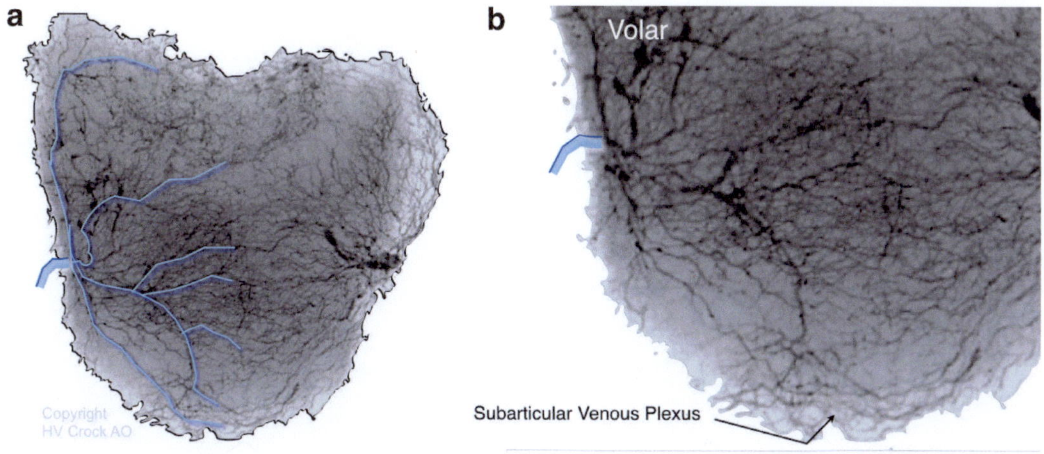


**Fig. 7.12** Venous drainage of the lunate. The majority of the lunate venous system has multiple interconnections. However, the subarticular plexus is made up of small parallel vessels, just below the subchondral bone plate. The venous system exits the lunate via large volar and dorsal veins (**a**) Venogram of lunate. (**b**) Magnified view. Copyright HV Crock AO [18]

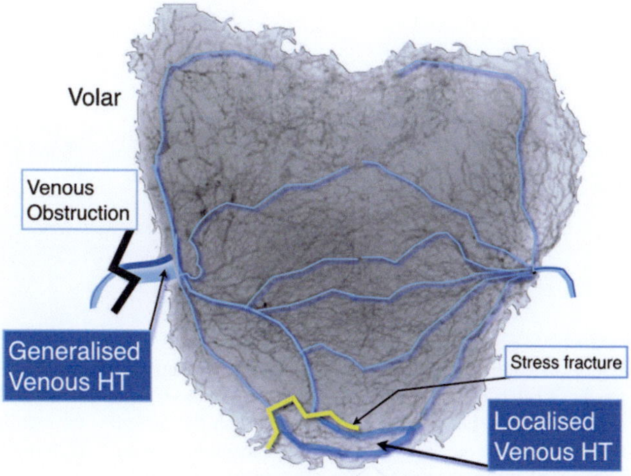


**Fig. 7.13** Venous obstruction models. Generalized venous hypertension can occur with extra-osseous obstruction. Localized venous obstruction can occur with a stress fracture of the subchondral bone plate, which interrupts the parallel venules of the subarticular plexus. This local venous hypertension can cause swelling of the adjacent fat cells and further increases local venous hypertension

The second type is the global AVN of the lunate, which has the entire sclerotic lunate, but usually not associated with collapse (Fig. 7.15). This corresponds to the Lichtman grade 1 [1]. Schmitt reported on the role of gadolinium enhancement MRI, and has demonstrated examples that correspond to this global type of AVN [20]. In their examples they report that this type has a positive enhancement, and a good prognosis (see Chap. 11).

Venous ischemia is not a new concept. There are examples of both acute and chronic venous engorgement that can lead to necrosis. Acute venous obstructing will lead to a free flap failure within hours, if the venous drainage is not restored. Chronic venous engorgement due to failure of the valves of the saphenous vein produces venous hypertension, which ultimately leads to peri-venous fibrosis, local ischemia and subsequent ulceration of the cutaneous tissues. Acute or chronic venous obstruction will cause devastating effects.

## Healing

Although the Kienböck's lunate is considered to be avascular and necrotic, there are often areas of

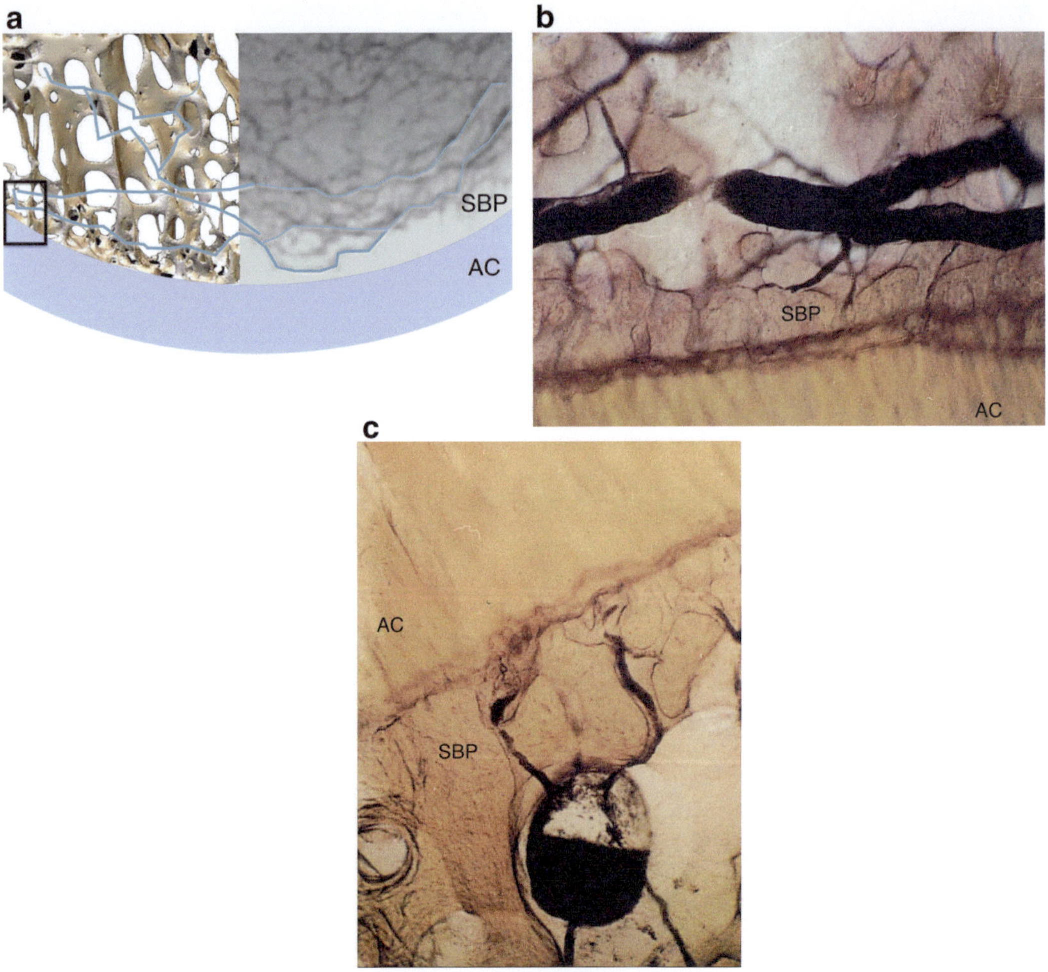


**Fig. 7.14** Subarticular venous plexus. (**a**) A composite image of subarticular venous plexus and 3D micro-CT of the subchondral bone plate. The *small box* on the *left* of image depicts the area demonstrated in the magnified views show in (**b**), where the venule within the subarticular plexus seen in profile. The subarticular venous plexus is directly adjacent, making it particularly at risk, even with a stress fracture. The calcified zone of the articular cartilage (AC), and subchondral bone plate (SBP) are well seen. (**c**) This cross-sectional image graphically shows the venous limb of the capillaries perforating the subchondral bone plate, and then draining into a subarticular collecting vein. The fluid line within the vein demonstrates the position of the specimen at time of preparation. These magnified views are from the knee, which has a similar pattern of venous drainage as the proximal lunate. Copyright HV Crock AO [18]

hyperemia and new bone formation adjacent to the necrotic area. The majority of the bone is alive and reactive, attempting to compensate for the ischemic insult. The SPECT scan will often have extensive increased uptake due to the osteoblastic activity (see Fig. 7.4b). There is laying down of new bone, which then can remodel, based on the stresses placed upon it, as described with Wolfe's law (Fig. 7.16).

## Conclusion

In this chapter we review the conceptual aspects of the etiology of Kienböck's disease. The stress fracture model would account for many of the cases we see in clinical practice with the "at risk" lunate. The fracture commences on the proximal radial aspect of the lunate and corresponds to the shape of the distal radius. There can be a coronal fracture of the

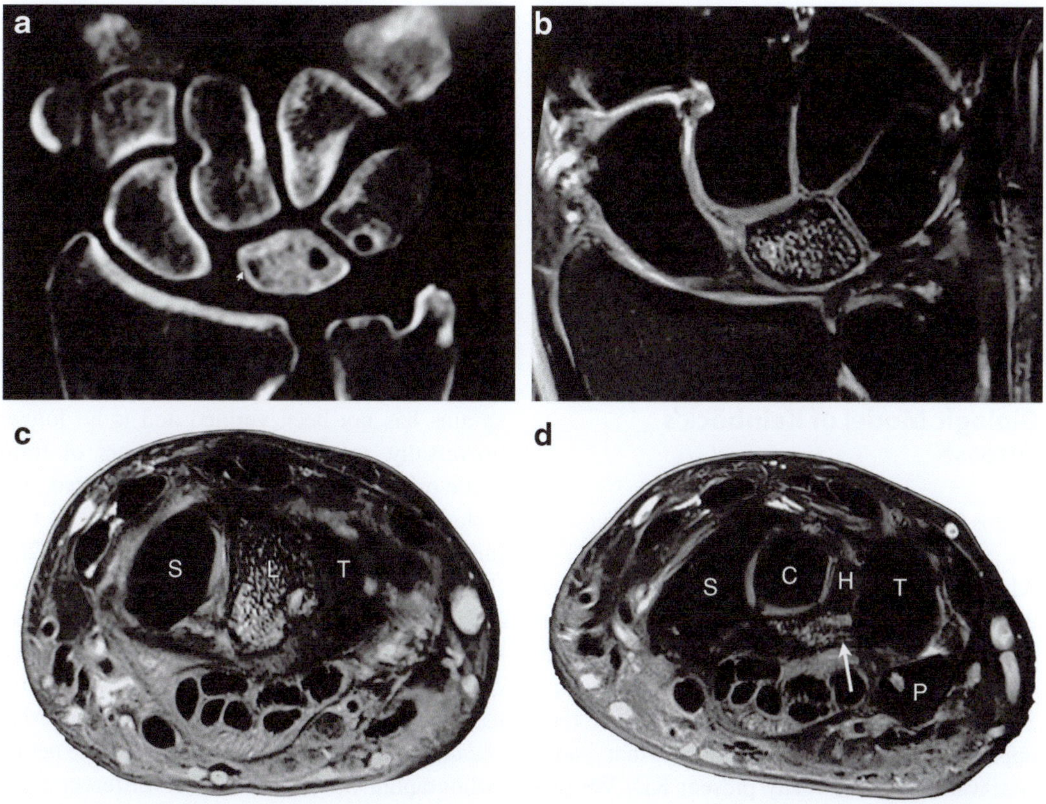


**Fig. 7.15** Global AVN of the lunate. (**a**, **b**) Global sclerosis of the lunate, with large volar perforations of the lunate and triquetrum. We believe this is in part related to the venous hypertension. There is also some localized sclerosis around the venous perforation of the triquetrum. (**c**, **d**) Note the changes on the MRI, including the edema of the volar ligaments at the lunotriquetral articulation (*white arrow*)

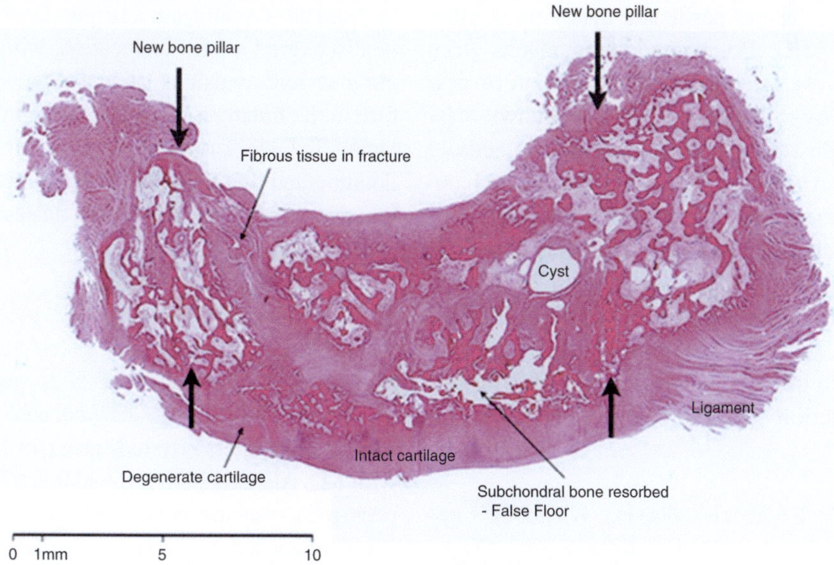


**Fig. 7.16** Histology of the healing lunate. There is extensive osteonecrosis, with intervening fibrous tissue and cysts that fill the osseous voids. There is significant reabsorption of the medullary bone and the subchondral plate. The *arrows* mark pillars of new bone, which transmit the load, since the failure of the medullary trabeculae. The articular surfaces are variably involved. The proximal articular surface has viable articular cartilage, but the subchondral bone has reabsorbed, to leave a false floor. The distal articular surface is more severely involved, with ulceration and fracture. Copyright Dr. Gregory Bain

lunate due to the nutcracker effect. Abrasion and reabsorption of the medullary bone can lead to comminution and collapse of the lunate.

Finally, there is a small group of patients who have a global ischemia, with sclerosis of the entire lunate, and often have a reactive enhancement of the lunate with gadolinium. These patients have a better prognosis.

## Biologic Model of Keinböck's Disease

Carlos Irisarri

**Abstract** A definite genesis for Kienböck's disease (KD) has not yet been identified. In our clinical experience, anatomical or mechanical factors such as repetitive minor trauma do not seem to be the primary cause. Instead, they appear to act more like catalysts that cause aggravation of an already present KD. We feel that more effort should be spent searching for a biological cause rather than a mechanical one. The most likely first step is an avascular non-traumatic process with minor infarction, starting in the proximal subchondral area. Even at this early stage, severe perilunate synovitis is often noted on MRI. Bone remodeling results from resorption by osteoclasts and formation of new bone by osteoblasts. It is still unknown why osteoclastic action exceeds osteoblastic activity in the repair process. We know that lunatomalacia can be present in children and adolescents but the disorder behaves differently than in adults. Fortunately, the so-called infantile and juvenile forms have a better prognosis. Genetic research to date has been inconclusive. Research in the field of reactive arthritis with polymerase chain reaction is a promising new tool to be explored.

**Keywords** Kienböck's disease, Kienböck's etiology, Lunatomalacia, Lunate necrosis, Carpal avascular necrosis, Infantile lunatomalacia, Juvenile lunatomalacia, Lunate osteochondrosis, Kienböck's risk factors, Kienböck genetic research

### Literature Review

#### Trauma

Many hypotheses have been proposed during the century following Robert Kienböck's 1910 report [25] on lunatomalacia, but at this time the genesis of the disease remains speculative. Kienböck's concept that the condition ("*traumatische Malazie*") was due to a disturbance in the nutrition of the lunate following repeated wrist sprains has not been verified and is no longer universally accepted. Ligament tears of traumatic origin have never been demonstrated, and dislocation of the lunate is not followed by true lunatomalacia. The case reported by Cave [26], frequently mentioned as Kienböck's disease following a dorsal perilunate dislocation, was in fact only increased density of the lunate. Cave considered the 6-month follow-up radiographs as "*suggestive of aseptic necrosis, beginning sequestration, comparable to KD*," but the actual radiographic findings are quite different from those of true KD.

Some authors quote Peste [27] in support of a traumatic genesis for KD. In fact, Peste only presented a short report at *Société Anatomique* (Paris, 1843) on a patient who died from a skull fracture after a fall from a height. During autopsy he discovered a wrist dislocation, with radial and ulnar styloid avulsions, as well as a double fracture in the lunate, a condition far from lunatomalacia. To my knowledge, there are no other documented reports of a traumatic lunate fracture that developed into Kienböck's disease.

#### Occupational Lunatomalacia

Walther Müller [28] pointed out "*minor repeated trauma cause the lunate to be affected by a morbid process*." This concept was later supported by Therkelsen and Andersen [29] because they found 98 manual workers in a study group of 107 patients with KD. Also, Stahl [30] found that 97 % of cases occurred in manual workers. However, these studies were carried out in hospitals dedicated to the care of manual workers, and contradict the results of series collected in general hospitals. The possibility that young, active patients experiencing wrist pain after strenuous use are more likely to seek medical attention than older, more sedentary patients, may have introduced a selection bias into the statistical analyses.

## Lunate Overload due to a Short Ulna

The possible relationship between ulnar variance and KD remains controversial. In 1928, Hultén [9] studied 23 Swedish patients with KD and found that 78 % had ulnar negative variance. This observation raised the possibility that a short ulna increased the shear forces acting on the lunate. Hultén pointed out that "*no wrist in which the ulna was longer than the radius developed Kienböck's disease*"; an uncertain assertion, as indicated by ulnar plus variance in four patients in our own series (Fig. 7.17). In addition, Antuña [31] reviewed 100 cases, with clear ulnar plus variance in five patients. Nakamura et al. [32] reported that more than half of their 70 patients with KD had zero or positive ulnar variance. And finally, Afshar et al. [33], reported six cases (10 %) with ulnar positive variance in their 60-patient series.

Causal relationships with other anatomical factors have been proposed, such as uncovering of the lunate by the distal radius, the presence of a midcarpal facet on the lunate in articulation with the hamate, an Antuña type I lunate shape, and a smaller than usual size of the lunate (Tsuge and Nakamura [13]). Mirabello et al. [34] stated that a flat distal radius might be a risk factor. Analyzing our own cases, we found so many differences in distal radius and carpal anatomy among KD patients that we now disregard the so-called "*anatomical risk factors*." It is interesting to note that Giunta et al. [35], using CT osteoabsorptiometry, failed to find excessive loads on the lunate in KD patients, casting doubt on the theory that anatomical variants increase physiologic stress load.

## Vascular Disturbance

As the affected bone in KD appears both macroscopically and microscopically avascular, the term *avascular necrosis* has been widely used. The radiological pattern in all AVN cases is similar. Kenzora and Glimcher [36] described the "*crescent sign*" or presence of the "*crescent line*" in the subchondral area, and termed it the "*the ubiquitous sign*" because it appears in all forms of bone AVN.

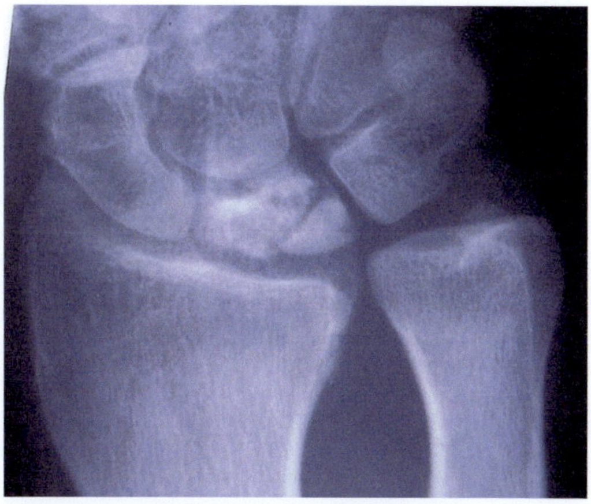

**Fig. 7.17** KD with ulnar plus variance. Lunate's fragmentation simulates a fracture

We should also keep in mind the difference between true early KD and "*lunate bruising*" (for some authors a "*stress fracture*") a condition seen frequently in sports related injuries, which fits better within the so-called "*bone marrow edema syndrome*."

Considering lunatomalacia as a type of osteonecrosis, reduction or disruption of the blood supply to the bone has been implicated in its pathogenesis. Studies of the lunate vascular anatomy by Lee [19] and Gelberman [11] suggested that lunates with only one volar and dorsal vessel are predisposed to avascular necrosis. However, there was evidence of anastomoses between the vessels in all three patterns and all lunates in the study were well vascularized. In addition, there have not been any studies on the vascular anatomy of diseased lunates. Thus, the true influence of variation among individuals has not been determined and it is still unknown whether patients with KD possess a unique lunate vascularity. Schiltenwolf et al. [20] and Jensen et al. [21] reported that the intraosseous pressure in necrotic lunates was increased significantly, hypothesizing that compromise to venous outflow, and the resulting increase in intraosseous pressure, was a factor in the genesis AVN of the lunate. But we really do not know if these changes are related to the disease's genesis or simply a consequence of preexisting pathology.

In keeping with the analogous designation of "*Stage 0*" in the international classification

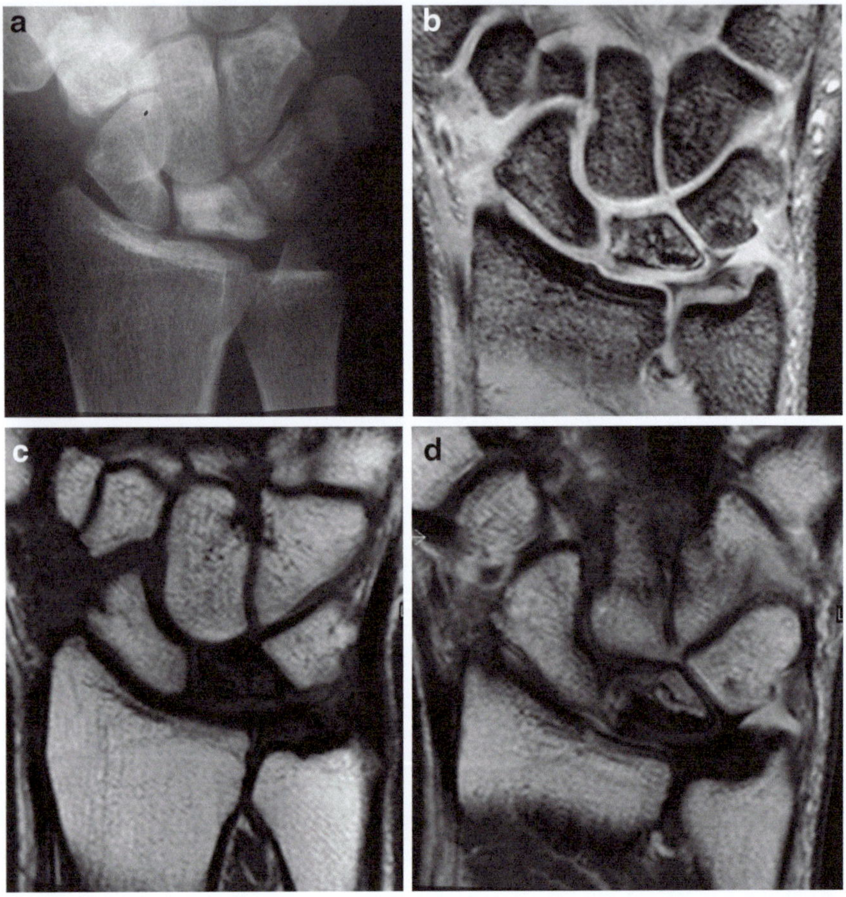


**Fig. 7.18** (**a**) Plain radiograph. (**b**) MRI: T2 sequence. (**c**) MRI: T1 sequence. (**d**) T1 after GDi: positive stage III

system of AVN of the hip, Lichtman et al. [37] proposed consideration of a new "*Stage 0*" *KD*, representing the earliest onset of lunate ischemia. In his point of view this stage represents a transient lunate ischemia, brought on by activities stressful to the wrist. Watson and Weinzweig [38] also described a "*pre-Kienböck* '*stage*'" as the earliest onset of KD. In so-called Stage 0, the unaffected architecture and density of the lunate would result in normal radiographs and MRI studies. Whether contrast-enhanced MRI could identify a lunate suffering intermittent stress ischemia (Stage 0), as suggested by Lichtman, is a controversial topic.

It has been useful [39] to subdivide Lichtman's stage III KD into stage IIIA in the absence of carpal alignment changes, and IIIB if carpal collapse is present, but this subclassification represents a strict biomechanical point of view. Perhaps it would be useful to also establish a biological subdivision, since stage II, and particularly stage III, demonstrate areas of bone necrosis, without vascularity, and areas of bone repair, with active vessel ingrowth. Although a standard MRI does not distinguish between these areas, an MRI taken after intravenous gadolinium infusion clearly identifies areas of perfusion from areas of necrosis. We can thus designate a *positive stage II or III* if signal intensity improves after GDi (Fig. 7.18a–d), and a *negative stage II or III*, if it does not. This information would be most helpful before attempting a lunate revascularization; a *positive* stage II or III clearly having a better prognosis.

Different pathways have been suggested for vascular disorders:

- The role of a vascular disease in KD was first postulated in 1929 by Santozki and Kopeiman [40]. They described an inflammatory vascular process resembling an "*obliterating endarteritis*." Bilz [41] considered the problem a "*traumatic endarteritis*," but this concept never gained widespread acceptance.
- Schwarz [42] pioneered the concept of "*vascular infarction*" in AVN caused by the vascular channels in bone becoming blocked. In the femoral head, as well as the proximal area of the lunate, nutrient channels are essentially end-arteries with limited anastomosis. Impairment of circulation, due to vascular obstruction from any cause, is followed by degenerative changes in these areas of bone.
- In decompression disease, AVN could be the final stage of an intraosseous compartment syndrome, caused by nitrogen bubbles forming during decompression due to supersaturation of nitrogen in fatty marrow cells. In our series, only a 41-year-old professional diver was registered.
- Regulation of thrombosis and hemostasis in endothelium is a complex topic, far from completely understood. A thrombogenic process related to an inflammatory disorder has been suggested in AVN disorders ("*osteochondroses*"). Vasculitis due to microvascular obstruction occurs in immunological diseases (i.e., systemic lupus erythematosus). KD has also been reported in sickle cell disease. Lanzer [43] in 1984 reported a case of KD in a black 18-year-old male with concomitant sickle-cell anemia. There had been no antecedent trauma, and radiographs taken 4 years earlier were normal.
- Culp et al. [44] reported the relationship between AVN and long-term steroid treatment in a patient with Crohn's disease and simultaneous KD and osteonecrosis of the femoral head. Budoff [45] reported a case of avascular necrosis of the scaphoid and lunate 11 years after steroid use. In our series, only one patient, a 45-year-old man with asthma, reported long-term steroid use.
- The relationship between a coagulation disorder and AVN was suggested by Glueck et al. [46]. He found an inherited hypo-fibrinolysis and thrombophilia in patients with Legg–Calvé–Perthes disease (LCPD), with osteonecrosis due to a sequence of venous thrombosis, increased intra-osseous venous pressure, and reduced arterial blood flow and hypoxia. In turn (Siegfried [47]) did not confirm this disorder in association with LCPD.

## Kienböck's Disease and Cerebral Palsy

Patients with cerebral palsy and an abnormally flexed wrist have a higher incidence of KD than the general population. Rooker and Goodfellow [48] found five cases in a group of 53 adults with cerebral palsy. His case no. 1 was a 17-year-old male with athetoid quadriplegia who developed KD in his left nondominant wrist. Case no. 3 was a 17-year-old female who developed the disorder in her left dominant hand.

Joji et al. [49] examined a population of 110 patients with cerebral palsy, and made the radiological diagnosis of KD in six wrists of five patients. Paradoxically, these authors reported that their patients did not necessarily assume a resting posture of wrist flexion except in one case, and their conclusion was "*it is not possible to attribute KD in cerebral palsy to this position*." They favored the influence of negative ulnar variance, although curiously not present in their case no. 1, a 13-year-old girl, who was asymptomatic despite increased radiographic opacity of the lunate.

In reviewing papers from Rooker and Goodfellow [48], Joji et al. [49], and Senda et al. [50], the radiologic images rarely resembles typical evolution and changes in KD, with absence of the "crescent line." Global increased density of the lunate is usually present. An MRI scan has not been performed in any case with cerebral palsy, due to inability of the patients to cooperate.

One pseudo-fracture case (dorsal and volar fragments) was reported from Leclercq and Xarchas [51] in a 25-year-old man with right spastic hemiplegia due to cerebral palsy. The

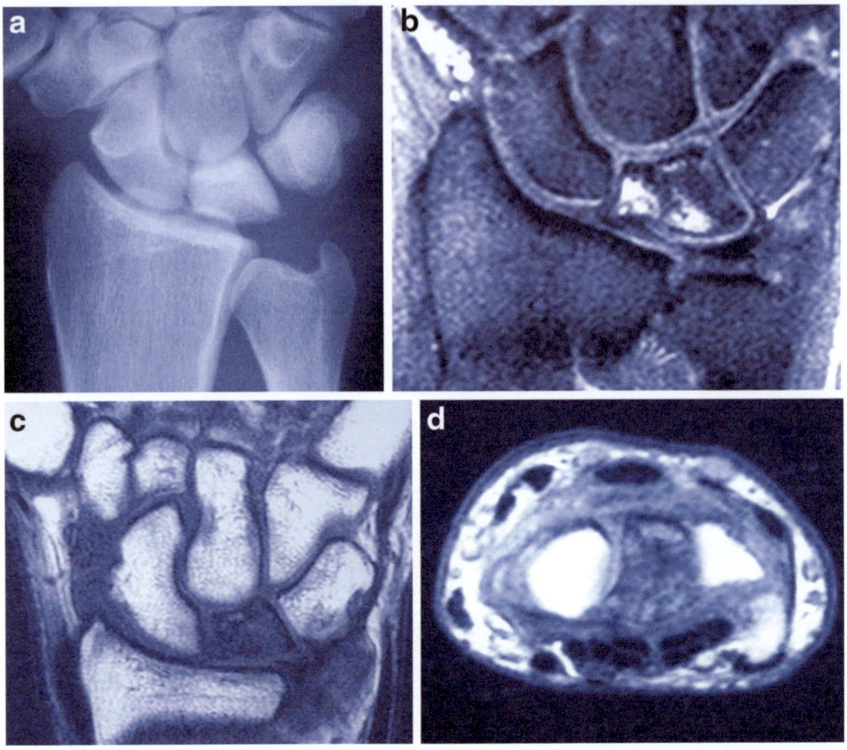

**Fig. 7.19** (**a**) A relatively well-preserved lunate. (**b**) T2 sequence: variable signal intensity throughout the lunate. (**c**) T1 sequence: Loss of lunate signal and severe synovitis is noted. (**d**) Carpal synovitis on axial view

right, affected wrist was used only to assist the left one on gross movements of prehension. The resting position of the wrist had been restored to neutral following a FCU tenotomy carried out 10 years previously.

Greene [52] reported KD in a 10-year-old girl with cerebral palsy. Cast immobilization of the wrist was maintained for 15 weeks. At follow-up exam, age 17, the patient reported no pain and radiographs showed a normal contour of the lunate.

## Miscellaneous Considerations

Clinical symptoms in KD are not uniform. In most cases the onset includes a swollen, painful and stiff wrist. Many experts agree that the first stage in AVN is a "*synovitic stage*," as Ficat [53] pointed out. However, the genesis of the wrist synovitis remains unknown. In several cases in our series, severe synovitis was detected on MRI in the early stages (Fig. 7.19a–d). Synovitis in these cases was considered "*primary*," and not the result of degenerative disease.

Bilateral KD appears in a low percentage of cases statistically, but its presence is very interesting in light of the concept that KD is generally located in the dominant hand. Bilateral KD has been linked to Raynaud's phenomenon and scleroderma (Rennie et al. [54]). The youngest patient with bilateral KD was a 14-year-old girl, with no history of trauma (Blachier et al. [55]). Especially intriguing has been the discovery of cases in which the date of onset of the KD differed many years between both hands. We have seen a 12-year interval in a male who was first affected in the non-dominant hand at age 24. Giunta [35] reported a patient with the onset of acute KD in one wrist and a history of contralateral radial shortening for KD in the other 9 years earlier.

For most of the nineteenth century, physicians thought AVN had a septic origin, including tuberculosis and syphilis. However, the term was later changed to aseptic necrosis because of the failure to culture bacteria from specimens. Later, Phemister [56] considered the possibility of a microbial embolic process as streptococci grew in cultures of two biopsied specimens with KD. In actuality, the positive cultures were most likely due to casual contamination. In several cases we cultured the synovial liquid, synovial tissue, and cancellous bone of the affected lunate, but never found any bacteria.

Mollo [57] suggested the role of genetic predisposition to the disease when considering the presence of "*osteochondritis*" of the lunate in early childhood. Therkelsen and Andersen [29] hypothesized "*perhaps a genetic brittleness of bones may be a contributory factor*." A few familial cases of KD have been reported. In 1932 Ringsted [58] published a report of bilateral KD in two brothers. Unilateral KD in a mother and her daughter was reported by Templeman and Engber [59]. Unilateral KD in two sisters was published by Lichtman et al. [1] as well as in two brothers by Simmons [60].

The possible influence of environmental risk factors in genetically predisposed persons has been introduced in several reports: Giannestras [61] reported LCPD in twins. Kenniston et al. [62] published a case of AVN of the capitellum in fraternal twins, and Tsirikos et al. [63] described bilateral Köhler's disease in identical twins.

## Author's Personal Experience

We retrospectively reviewed the clinical records of 100 patients (104 wrists) seen from October 1992 to December 2014. Radiographs were available in all patients, as well as computed tomography (CT) imaging in 14 cases and MRI in 62 cases.

- Age: The classical assertion "*KD usually affects adults between 20 and 40 years of age, who are predominantly male manual workers*," is not supported by our series, which contains members of the general population as well as manual workers. In our series, we registered four cases with infantile lunatomalacia (IL), nine cases with juvenile lunatomalacia (JL) and eight patients older than 55 years. In this last group all were women but one. The large number of patients with IL and JL may have been attributable to increased referrals following our two publications on this topic (Irisarri [64, 65]). Mean patient age was 35.4 years (range, 9–66).
- Gender: The generally accepted preference of KD for young males was not supported by this series collected from general hospitals. We found a more equal distribution of cases between males (54 cases) and females (46 cases).
- Clinical Symptoms: Radiographic findings of KD have occasionally been reported in films obtained for other reasons, usually after a recent traumatic injury. In our series, completely asymptomatic, incidental KD has been a very rare occurrence. Some patients recall a prior injury, but this was somewhat questionable because of frequent ongoing litigation. A causal association between KD and a previous traumatic event was discounted in the great majority of cases. KD with associated scapholunate dissociation was present in only one patient (Fig. 7.20a, b).
- Ulnar Variance: There was a preponderance of negative ulnar variance in our series. We found 58 patients with ulnar minus (including both wrists in two bilateral cases), 38 patients with ulnar neutral (including both wrists in two bilateral cases) and only four patients with positive ulnar variance.
- Coagulation Disorder: An exhaustive search for coagulation disorders was carried out in ten patients without positive findings.
- Lunate Vascularity: In two female stage III patients an angio-CT was obtained. There were no findings of abnormalities in the extraosseous lunate vascularity. Small intraosseous vessels were not adequately appreciated in these images.
- Bilateral KD: Four cases were recorded in our series, three men and one woman.
- Familial Cases: We have registered four cases in two families. In our first familial case, KD was diagnosed in two brothers. One brother, age 24 was treated for Stage IIIA KD in his

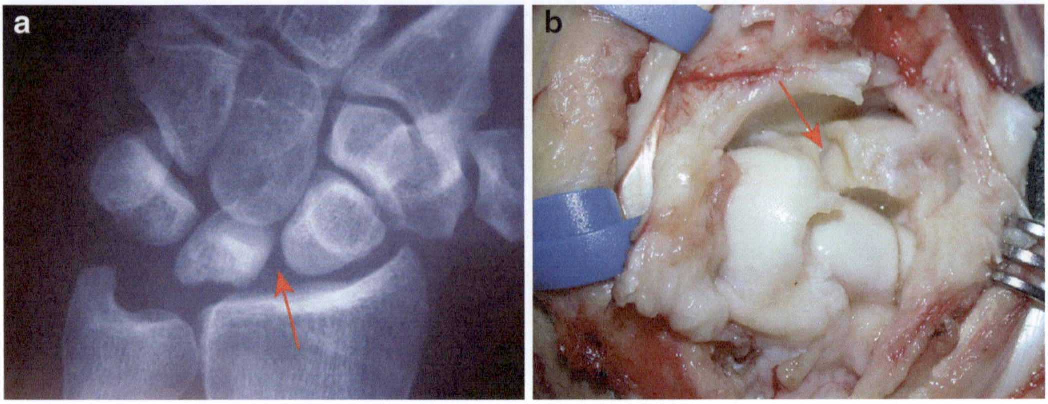


**Fig. 7.20** (**a**) Concomitant KD and scapholunate dissociation (*arrow*). (**b**) Aspect at surgery (*arrow*)

right dominant wrist. No risk factors were identified. One year later, the second brother, age 27, was treated, also with unilateral KD (stage IIIB) in his right dominant hand. He had a history of hepatitis C several years previously.

- Our second familial case was a 37-year-old female with unilateral stage IIIB KD in her right dominant hand. The onset of clinical symptoms was 10 years earlier. No risk factors were found. Several years later we attended her brother, aged 45, with unilateral stage IV KD (IV stage) in his right dominant hand. Again, no risk factors were found.

In an attempt to determine the role of heredity in the genesis of KD, genetic screening was performed on our famililial cases by the Clinical Genetics Department of the University Hospital Santiago. Using current techniques, no genetic anomalies were detected. However, in the future more sophisticated may identify specific genes linked to KD.

## Discussion and Conclusions

The proper treatment of any medical condition requires an understanding of its etiology and natural history. This is not possible in KD because the pathogenesis remains uncertain. Concerns about whether surgical procedures actually improve the natural course of the disease are therefore appropriate. As Stahl [30] pointed out many years ago, the postoperative immobilization, rather than the procedure itself, may be the most important factor in lunate healing—especially following indirect revascularization procedures and in younger patients who have a greater potential for "spontaneous" recovery. As Dias and Lunn pointed out [66] "*there is danger in proceeding to invasive and radical procedures, whereas a more scientific approach would be to 'stand back' and get a more objective view of the condition before advising surgical treatment.*"

Bone cells may be killed in a variety of ways, but the term "*osteonecrosis*" is traditionally associated with ischemia. It is tempting to search for a universal cause of AVN, but in my opinion, we need to revisit the statement that all types of lunatomalacia represent different manifestations of a single disorder, and recognize the possibility of different patterns of KD under different circumstances. Unfortunately, right up until the present, it has rarely been possible to identify the actual causative factor. It may be wishful thinking, but I believe a "*biological cause*" will eventually be identified for most "idiopathic" cases of AVN, in all bones, ages, and circumstances.

In our series, several cases demonstrated severe synovitis in stage II and III on MRI. The role of perilunar synovitis in the genesis of KD is still far from clear, but I believe it is a pathway to be explored. It should be noted that the skeletal behavior in AVN is different from other inflammatory arthropathies, like rheumatoid arthritis, so it seems clear that different patterns and causes for the synovitis of KD are possible.

I also believe "*minor repeated trauma*," including vibration exposure, is probably not the primary cause of KD, but a factor that causes symptomatic aggravation of an underlying disorder. In young, heavy manual laborers, the affected wrist is likely to become painful after strenuous use, whereas less active patients may never seek medical treatment because they only experience mild clinical symptoms. Taniguchi and Tamaki [67] examined 133 patients. There were 47 women, five of whom had bilateral disease. The age at onset for women was significantly higher than that for men. Based on their data, they suggested that the genesis of KD in women might be different from that in men, with biologic factors playing a more important role than mechanical or anatomical ones.

Mennen [68] recently published an interesting study, reviewing radiographs of 1287 South African patients, finding 23 cases (1.9 %) with asymptomatic Lichtman stage II–IV KD. Taniguchi [69] also reported 14 patients with KD diagnosed with wrist radiographs taken for other wrist or hand problems. In my experience, however, patients suffering KD describe at least an initial period of intermittent wrist pain with exertional activities.

My first bilateral KD patient, a self-employed bricklayer, is illustrative. He worked for several years prior to retirement with moderate pain in both wrists but never sought medical advice. My second bilateral KD patient was a 38-year-old miner. He required surgery for both wrists because of severe pain, followed by only partial improvement. He never returned to work. Clearly, one's threshold for pain as well as other personal and social factors influence patients' tolerance of the disease, as well as their outcome after surgery.

Regarding the association of KD and ulnar negative variance (UNV), several authors have reported contradictory findings. Its presence is statistically significant in many series (including ours), but I disagree that this condition influences KD genesis in any patient. Antuña [70] pointed out a possible relationship between lunate morphology and KD evolution. His findings indicate that the presence UNV implies a poor prognosis in an established KD, but I believe that no study has demonstrated that UNV is the true causal factor.

It is surprising that there are so many articles linking the genesis of KD with local anatomical variations, yet there are few reports of capitate AVN—a rare disease, but one similar and proximate enough to stimulate serious research on common etiologic factors.

In AVN, vascular deprivation and minor bone marrow infarctions appear to be the initiating mechanism of bone weakening, but something more than a simple embolus cutting off the circulation must occur. Bone fragmentation and collapse is the result of unbalanced bone remodeling, with increased osteoclastic resorption not being sufficiently counteracted by osteoblastic new bone formation. It is intriguing to note that in contradistinction to the notable resistance of the lunate to collapse in the presence of space occupying lesions (e.g., benign tumor, enchondroma, and intraosseous cyst), the typical progression of collapse of the lunate in KD is relatively rapid.

It is unknown why osteoclastic action surpasses osteoblastic regeneration in KD. Since cellular activity requires a blood supply, the lunate must at least be partially vascularized in order to collapse, thus excluding complete extraosseous arterial deprivation. Endothelial cells play a role in the process of new bone formation, as suggested by Trueta [71, 72], but the mechanism that drives regional vascular endothelial dysfunction is also unknown.

After "*crescent line*" appearance, a dysvascular lunate will collapse starting on the radial side. Only in rare cases is the ulnar side involved first. Later, the entire proximal surface appears collapsed. Resorption of bone leads to weakness and the appearance of a "*pseudo-fracture*." I do not favor the terms "*linear, shear or compressive fracture*" or "*stress fracture*" in KD, because I do not believe it is a true fracture. Perhaps the term "*fault*" (Watson and Guidera [73]) is less equivocal, and adequate even for a complete coronal split of the necrotic lunate, typical in the new

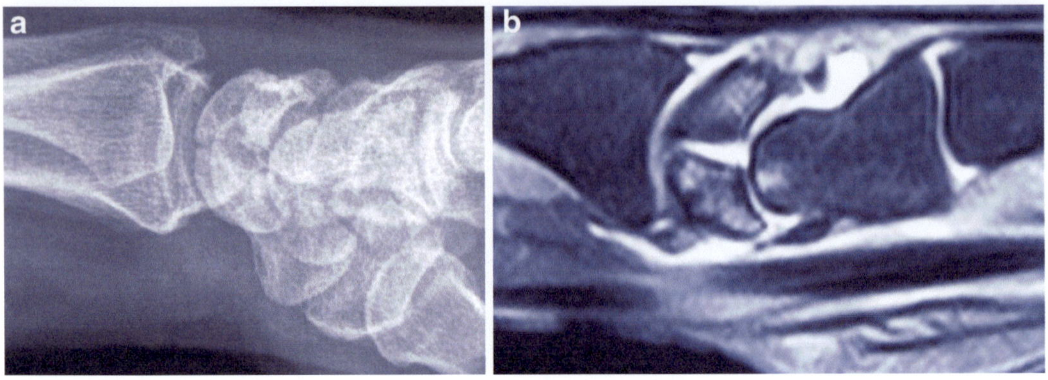


**Fig. 7.21** (**a**) Midcoronal split (Lichtman stage IIIC). (**b**) Sagittal MRI aspect

Lichtman [11] stage III C (Fig. 7.21a, b). He wisely noted that these patients have a poor prognosis, because the lunate does not heal, even after direct or indirect revascularization procedures.

In a 52-year-old male patient of ours, with a doubtful differential diagnosis between KD and traumatic midcoronal lunate fracture, fixation with a screw was followed by rapid post-operative evolution to fragmentation and collapse. In contrast, two of our cases with confirmed traumatic fractures of the lunate obtained union following simple cast immobilization and a third achieved union after screw fixation.

Aspenberg [74] attributes lunate collapse to spontaneous revascularization, and points out that "*stress risers at interfaces between resorbed and sclerotic areas lead to microfractures and collapse.*" It seems that bone destruction in KD results from the attempt of the living cancellous bone to repair the necrotic areas with an unbalanced process of osteogenesis and osteoclasis.

Once a crescent line appears the prognosis is poor in adults. We have only one case that has shown radiological improvement: the patient, a 21-year-old baker, experienced progressive pain for 2 years in his right dominant hand, without a previous acute traumatic event. Once diagnosed at a hospital elsewhere, despite an ulnar plus variance (Fig. 7.22a) a radial shortening was carried with a dorsal plate and a cast for 8 weeks. One year later, the patient arrived in my office complaining of pain in the radio-distal ulnar joint. A clear ulnar impaction syndrome was noted, as well as apparent healing of the radial aspect of the lunate (see Fig. 7.24b).

In several cases that we have treated with proximal row carpectomy, gross examination of the sectioned lunate revealed less avascularity of the distal-ulnar corner, with the presence of "bleeding points" (Fig. 7.23a) in that area. Differences in residual vascularity are also evident in the MRI (see Fig. 7.23b). In more advanced cases, proximal subchondral resorption is clearly noted (Fig. 7.24).

The prognosis for spontaneous healing in children appears to be much greater than in adults, even before mechanical disorders (Greene [52]). In children, the lunate articular cartilage is thicker, and as Therkelsen and Andersen [29] pointed out, its increased plasticity allows considerable deformity without sustaining an actual cortical break. Because of the potentially increased reversibility, I believe that conservative treatment with a period of immobilization is always indicated in young patients. This is similar to the experience noted in Legg–Calvé–Perthes disease and other forms of AVN.

We do not have a definitive answer about whether KD is always an *aseptic* condition or whether it can be triggered by bacterial or viral infection. This is only speculation, but an "*articular inflammation-related synovitis*" could explain AVN in all bones (local or regional) and in all ages. Failure to prove the presence of bacteria does not rule out the presence of a reactive arthritis (ARe), an inflammatory process with

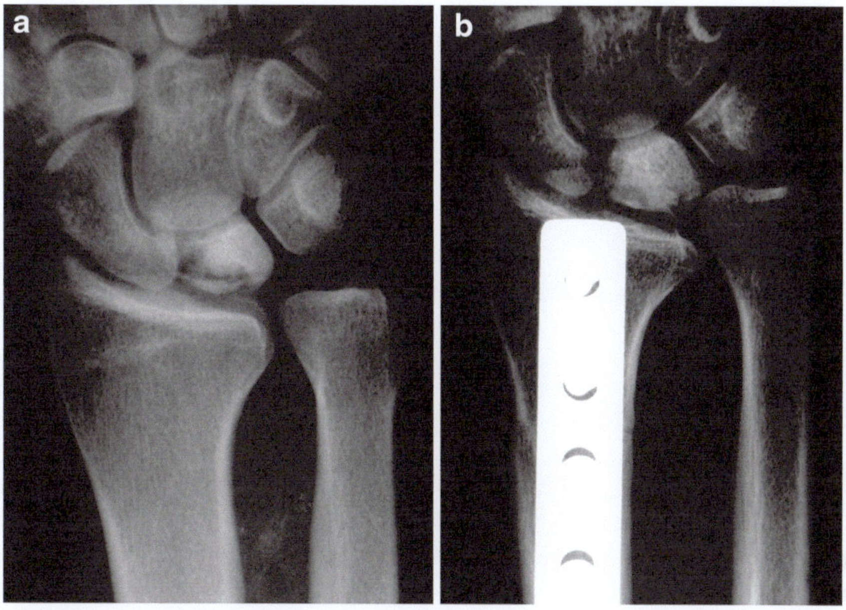


**Fig. 7.22** (**a**) KD with ulnar positive variance. (**b**) Radiological lunate improvement, but now also with and ulnar impaction syndrome since radial shortening

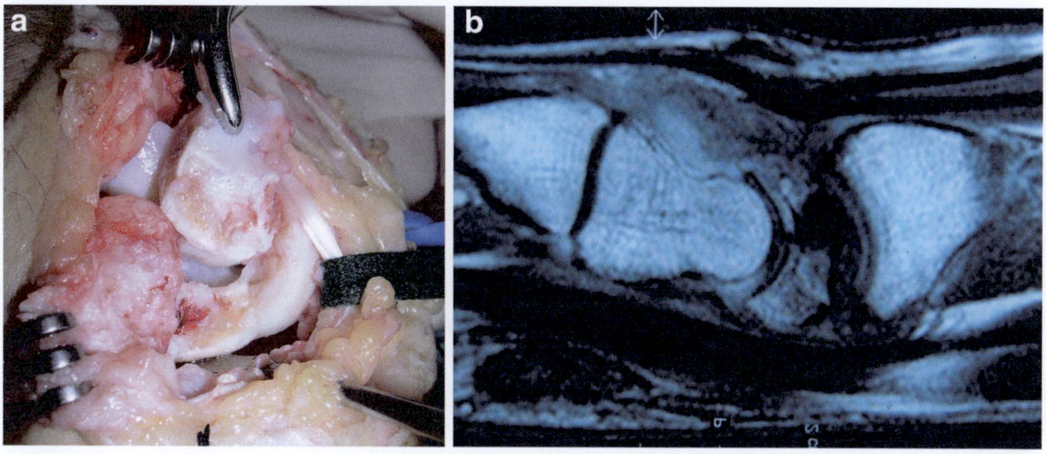


**Fig. 7.23** (**a**) Once the lunate is divided in dorsal (D) and volar (V) fragments, "bleeding points" appear only in the distal-ulnar corner (*arrow*). (**b**) Differences in residual vascularity reflected in MRI

presence of intraarticular bacteria. Polymerase chain reaction is a more sensitive technique than conventional cultures to detect ARe. The relationship of AVN to viral infection must also be considered. Hepatitis C virus has been associated with minor joint disorders, including KD. In our series, we registered two cases of patients with Hepatitis C, both young men. Another patient in our series, a 35-year-old man, was diagnosed with AIDS.

We must remember that the immune system is closely linked to the coagulation cascade and that inflammation and coagulation are also tightly linked. In immune-mediated inflammatory diseases vasculitis can appear. The hypothesis that some subpopulations may be more susceptible to

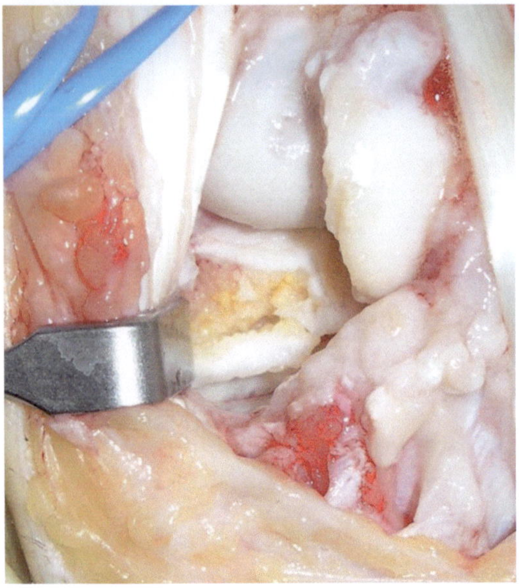

**Fig. 7.24** In a more advanced stage case, scarcely "bleeding point" appears in the distal-ulnar corner. Proximal subchondral resorption is noted

KD than others is worth consideration, but it seems clear that AVN is not a straightforward genetic condition with a predictable mode of inheritance. The possibility that the genetic background of the host can influence the intensity of the reaction after infection and/or immune reaction is another unanswered, yet intriguing, question.

The presence of infantile and juvenile lunatomalacia has caused us to refocus our thinking on "*biological*" as well as "*mechanical*" factors [64, 65] in the genesis of KD. The same is true of bilateral cases and cases involving simultaneous disease in the scaphoid and lunate, as reported by Antuña [70], Watson and Weinzweig [38], and Bhardwaj [75]. In other situations AVN occurs not only bilaterally (LCP disease) but is found in multiple bones, as in Freiberg's disease involving several metatarsal heads of both feet. On the other hand, I have some concerns with reports of "*regional*" AVN of multiple carpal bones, such as the ones by De Smet [76], Budoff [45], and Wollstein [77]. MRI changes are certainly present in all of their cases, but they are not the typical ones of KD. We must therefore question if these cases represent simultaneous KD and Preiser's disease or perhaps completely different disorders.

In summary, the definitive etiology of KD has not been established, but the preponderance of evidence suggests that a vascular nontraumatic process is closest to the truth, starting as a minor infarction pattern in the proximal subchondral area. KD is so widespread in all countries that ethnic differences do not seem to be highly relevant. Concepts of anatomic variations of the radius and ulna, and their effect on ulnar shear stress, as well as the role of arterial and venous anomalies and their potential contribution to lunate AVN, all need to be revisited. Morphology and vascularity of the affected lunate can play a role in the natural history of the disease, but are probably not the factors that initiate AVN.

It is my hope that the next major focus will be on biological research (microbiology and virology studies, polymerase chain reaction [PCR] arrays, etc.). Karyotype genetic screening should be kept in mind, but at present is still an expensive and uncertain tool. To overcome the challenge of KD genesis, as well as the challenge of AVN itself, cooperative efforts are necessary between basic researchers, medical clinicians, and operating surgeons, with an open mind to innovative and diverse viewpoints.

## References


1. Lichtman DM, Mack GR, MacDonald RI, Gunther SF, Wilson JN. Kienböck's disease: the role of silicone replacement arthroplasty. J Bone Joint Surg Am. 1977;59(7):899–908.
2. Viegas SF, Wagner K, Patterson R, Peterson P. Medial (hamate) facet of the lunate. J Hand Surg Am. 1990;15(4):564–71.
3. Zapico J. Enfermedad de Kienböck. Rev Ortop Trauma. 1993;37 Suppl 1:100–13.
4. Zapico J. Malacia del semilunar. Valladolid: Universidad de Valladolid; 1966.
5. Tatebe M, Imaeda T, Hirata H. The impact of lunate morphology on Kienböck's disease. J Hand Surg Eur Vol. 2015;40:534.
6. Tatebe M, Shinohara T, Okui N, Yamamoto M, Kurimoto S, Hirata H. Arthroscopic lunate morphology and wrist disorders. Surg Radiol Anat. 2013;35(1):79–83.

7. Rhee PC, Moran SL, Shin AY. Effect of lunate morphology in Kienböck disease. J Hand Surg Am. 2015;40(4):738–44.
8. Owers KL, Scougall P, Dabirrahmani D, Wernecke G, Jhamb A, Walsh WR. Lunate trabecular structure: a radiographic cadaver study of risk factors for Kienböck's disease [corrected]. J Hand Surg Eur Vol. 2010;35(2):120–4.
9. Hùlten O. Über anatomische variationen der handgelenkknochen. Acta Radiol Scand. 1928;9:155–68.
10. Stahl S, Reis ND. Traumatic ulnar variance in Kienböck's disease. J Hand Surg Am. 1986;11(1): 95–7.
11. Gelberman RH, Bauman TD, Menon J, Akeson WH. The vascularity of the lunate bone and Kienböck's disease. J Hand Surg Am. 1980;5(3): 272–8.
12. Chen WS, Shih CH. Ulnar variance and Kienböck's disease. An investigation in Taiwan. Clin Orthop Relat Res. 1990;255:124–7.
13. Tsuge S, Nakamura R. Anatomical risk factors for Kienböck's disease. J Hand Surg Br. 1993;18(1): 70–5.
14. Low S, Bain GI, Findlay DM, Eng K, Perilli E. External and internal bone micro-architecture in normal and Kienböck's lunates: a whole-bone micro-computed tomography study. J Orthop Res. 2014; 32(6):826–33.
15. Quenzer DE, Dobyns JH, Linscheid RL, Trail IA, Vidal MA. Radial recession osteotomy for Kienböck's disease. J Hand Surg Am. 1997;22(3):386–95.
16. Bain GI, Begg M. Arthroscopic assessment and classification of Kienböck's disease. Tech Hand Up Extrem Surg. 2006;10(1):8–13.
17. Bain G, Yeo CJ, Morse LP. Kienböck disease: recent advances in the basic science, assessment and treatment. Hand Surg. 2015;20(3):352–65.
18. Crock HV. An atlas of vascular anatomy of the skeleton & spinal cord. 1st ed. London: Martin Dunitz; 1996.
19. Lee ML. The intraosseus arterial pattern of the carpal lunate bone and its relation to avascular necrosis. Acta Orthop Scand. 1963;33:43–55.
20. Schiltenwolf M, Martini AK, Mau HC, Eversheim S, Brocai DRC, Jensen CH. Further investigations of the intraosseous pressure characteristics in necrotic lunates (Kienböck's disease). J Hand Surg Am. 1996;21(5):754–8.
21. Jensen CH. Intraosseous pressure in Kienböck's disease. J Hand Surg Am. 1993;18(2):355–9.
22. Bain GI, Clitherow HDS, Millar S, Frayssee F. The effect of lunate morphology on 3-dimensional kinematics of the carpus. J Hand Surg Am. 2015;40(1): 81–9.e1.
23. Solomon L. Idiopathic avascular necrosis of the femoral head; pathogenesis and treatment. Can J Surg. 1981;24:573.
24. Hungerford DS. Bone marrow pressure, venography and core decompression in ischemic necrosis of the femoral head. In the Hip Proceedings, 7th Open Scientific Meeting of the Hip Society. St Louis, MO: CV Mosby Co.; 1979.
25. Kienböck R. Über traumatische Malazie des Mondbeins und ihre Folgezustände Entartungsformen und Kompressions Frakturen. Fortsch Geb Röntgnstr. 1910;16:77–103.
26. Cave EF. Kienböck's disease of the lunate. J Bone Joint Surg Am. 1939;21:858–66.
27. Peste. Société Anatomique, Bulletin no 6, Août 1843, 169–170, Paris.
28. Müller W. Über die Erweichung und Verditchung des os lunatum, eine typische Erkrankung des Handgelenkes. Beitr Klin Chir. 1920;119:664.
29. Therkelsen F, Andersen K. Lunatomalacia. Acta Chir Scand. 1949;97:503–26.
30. Stahl F. On lunatomalacia (Kienböck's disease): clinical and roentgenological study, especially on its pathogenesis and late results of immobilization treatment. Acta Chir Scand. 1947;95 Suppl 126: 1–133.
31. Antuña Zapico JM. Malacia del Semilunar. Doctoral Thesis, Editorial Sever Cuesta. Valladolid University, Spain, 1966.
32. Nakamura T, Tsuge S, Watanabe K, Tsunoda K. Radial wedge osteotomy for Kienböck's disease. J Bone Joint Surg Am. 1991;73:1391–6.
33. Afshar A, Aminzadeh-Gohari A, Yekta Z. The association of Kienböck's disease and ulnar variance in the Iranian population. J Hand Surg Eur Vol. 2012;38:496–9.
34. Mirabello S, Rosenthal D, Smith R. Correlation of clinical and radiographic findings in Kienböck's disease. J Hand Surg Am. 1987;12:1049–54.
35. Giunta R, Löwer N, Wilhem K, Keirse R, Rock C, Müller-Gerbl M. Altered patterns of subchondral bone mineralization in Kienböck's disease. J Hand Surg Br. 1997;22(1):16–20.
36. Kenzora J, Glimcher M. Pathogenesis of idiopathic osteonecrosis: the ubiquitous crescent sign. Orthop Clin North Am. 1985;16:681–96.
37. Lichtman D, Lesley N, Simmons S. The classification and treatment of Kienböck's: the state of the art and a look at the future. J Hand Surg Eur Vol. 2010;35: 549–54.
38. Watson HK, Weinzweig J. Theory and etiology of Kienböck's disease. In: Watson HK, Weinzweig J, editors. The wrist. Philadelphia, PA: Lippincott, William & Wilkins; 2001. p. 411–7.
39. Lichtman D, Alexander A, Mack G, Gunther S. Kienböck's disease- update on silicone replacement arthroplasty. J Hand Surg Am. 1982;7:343–7.
40. Santozki M, Kopeiman S. Ein Beitrag zur sogenannten Malacia ossis Lunati. Fortsch Geb Röntgnstr. 1929;39:1060.
41. Bilz L. Die Lunatumnekrose. Würzburg, 1934. Roll, University of California.
42. Schwarz E. Eine typische Erkrankung der oberen Femurepihyse. Beitr Klin Chir 1914; 93:1 (A typical disease of the upper femoral epiphysis, reprinted in Clin Orthop Relat Res, 1986; 209: 5–12.)

43. Lanzer W, Szabo R, Gelberman R. Avascular necrosis of the lunate and sickle cell anemia: a case report. Clin Orthop Relat Res. 1984;187:168–71.
44. Culp R, Schaffer J, Osterman A, Bora F. Kienböck's disease in a patient with Crohn's enteritis treated with corticosteroids. J Hand Surg Am. 1989;14(2 Pt 1): 294–6.
45. Budoff J. Concomitant Kienböck's and Preiser's diseases: a case report. J Hand Surg Am. 2006;31: 1149–53.
46. Glueck C, Freiberg R, Fontaine R, Tracy T, Wang P. Hypofibrinolysis, thrombophilia, osteonecrosis. Clin Orthop Relat Res. 2001;386:19–33.
47. Sigfried G. The role of inherited thrombotic disorders in the etiology of Legg-Calvé -Perthes disease. J Pediatr Orthop. 1999;19:82–3.
48. Rooker G, Goodfellow J. Kienböck's disease in cerebral palsy. J Bone Joint Surg Br. 1977;59:363–5.
49. Joji S, Mizuseki T, Katayama S, Tsuge K, Ikuta Y. Etiology of Kienböck's disease based on a study of the condition among patients with cerebral palsy. J Hand Surg Br. 1993;18:294–8.
50. Senda H, Terada S, Okamoto H. Radial wedge osteotomy for IIIB Kienböck's disease in cerebral palsy: a case report. J Hand Surg Eur Vol. 2010;35:588–9.
51. Leclercq C, Xarchas C. Kienböck's disease in cerebral palsy. J Hand Surg Br. 1998;23(6):746–8.
52. Greene W. Kienböck disease in a child who has cerebral palsy. J Bone Joint Surg Am. 1996;78(10):568–73.
53. Ficat R, Arlet J. Ischemia and necrosis of bone. In: Hungerford DS, editor. Bone and circulation. Baltimore, MD: Williams & Wilkins; 1980.
54. Rennie C, Britton J, Prouse P. Bilateral avascular necrosis of the lunate in a patient with severe Raynaud's phenomenon and scleroderma. J Clin Rheumatol. 1999;5:165.
55. Blachier D, Renaux P, Forestier A, Moutad G. Maladie de Kienböck bilaterale chez l' adolescent. Rev Chir Orthop. 1992;78:408–10.
56. Phemister D. Repair of bone in the presence of aseptic necrosis resulting from fractures. Transplantations, and vascular obstructions. J Bone Joint Surg Am. 1930;12:679.
57. Mollo L. La necrosi dell'osso semilunare del carpo. Chir Org Mov. 1934;19:343.
58. Ringsted A, Doppelseitiger M. Kienböck bei 2 Brüdern. Acta Chir Scand. 1932;LXIX:185–96.
59. Templeman D, Engber W. Kienböck's disease—Case report of familial occurrence. Iowa Orthop J. 1985;5: 107–9.
60. Simmons E. Kienböck's disease. Orthop Consult. 1981;2:111.
61. Giannestras N. Legg-Perthes disease in twins. J Bone Joint Surg Am. 1954;36:149.
62. Kenniston J, Beredjiklian P, Bozentka D. Osteochondritis dissecans of the capitellum in fraternal twins; case report. J Hand Surg Am. 2008;33: 1380–3.
63. Tsirikos A, Riddle E, Kruse R. Bilateral Köhler in identical twins. Clin Orthop Relat Res. 2003; 409:195–6.
64. Irisarri C. Aetiology of Kienböck's disease. J Hand Surg Br. 2004;3:281–7.
65. Irisarri C, Kalb K, Ribak S. Infantile and juvenile lunatomalacia. J Hand Surg Eur Vol. 2010;35: 544–8.
66. Dias J, Lunn P. Ten questions on Kienböck's disease of the lunate. J Hand Surg Eur Vol. 2010;35(7): 538–43.
67. Taniguchi Y, Tamaki T. Kienböck's disease in women. J Hand Surg Br. 1999;24(5):596–7.
68. Mennen U, Sithebe H. The incidence of asymptomatic Kienböck's disease. J Hand Surg Eur Vol. 2009;34(3):348–50.
69. Taniguchi Y, Nakao S, Tamaki T. Incidentally diagnosed Kienböck's disease. Clin Orthop Relat Res. 2002;395:121–7.
70. Antuña Zapico JM. Enfermedad de Kienböck. Rev Orthop Trauma. 1993;37IB(Suppl I):100–13.
71. Trueta J, Morgan J. The vascular contributions to osteogenesis. J Bone Joint Surg Br. 1960;42(1): 97–109.
72. Trueta J. Papel de los vasos en la osteogenesis. In: La estructura del cuerpo humano. Barcelona: Editorial Labor; 1975.
73. Watson HK, Guidera P. Aetiology of Kienböck's disease. J Hand Surg Br. 1997;22:5–7.
74. Aspenberg P, Wang J, Jonsson K, Hagert C. Experimental osteonecrosis of the lunate: revascularisation may cause collapse. J Hand Surg Br. 1994; 19:565–9.
75. Bhardwaj P, Sharma C, Sabapathy S. Concomitant avascular necrosis of the scaphoid and lunate. Hand Surg. 2012;17(2):239–41.
76. De Smet L. Avascular necrosis of multiple carpal bones. A case report. Chir Main. 1999;18:202–4.
77. Wollstein A, Tantawi D, Wollstein R. Bilateral Kienböck disease concomitant with bilateral Legg-Calvé-Perthes disease: a case report. Hand. 2013;8(1): 120–2.

# Part II

# Clinical Assessment

# Radiological Risk Factors for Kienböck's Disease

**8**

Luc De Smet and Ilse Degreef

## Introduction

The blood supply of the lunate is probably the key factor in the pathogenesis of Kienböck's disease. Extrinsic factors such as fractures or repetitive minor trauma can damage the intra-osseous blood supply leading to osteonecrosis. However, rather than causing the necrosis the fracture may also be a consequence of the necrosis. In 1928 Hulten [1] noted an association between Kienböck's disease and ulnar minus variance. Since then, several other variations in the morphology of the lunate and distal radius have been shown to play a role in the pathogenesis of the disorder.

## Ulnar Variance

The relation between ulnar variance and Kienböck's disease is not yet entirely clear. Since Hulten [1] first described the association between Kienböck's disease and ulnar minus variance, other authors [2–8] have also noted these findings (Table 8.1). Biomechanical concepts such as the "nutcracker theory" [9] are based on this association. As a consequence, levelling procedures have become popular (e.g., radial shortening and ulna lengthening). Numerous studies have reported favorable outcomes for these procedures (Tables 8.2 and 8.3) [2, 7, 10–31]. The basic concept is to unload the lunate and prevent further collapse. Most classical papers and handbooks still recommend an osteotomy for Lichtman stages one and two, provided that there is an ulna minus variance.

Some authors believe that rather than joint levelling the regional hyperemia provided by the surgical insult is responsible for the pain relief. Based on this, Illarramendi et al. [32] proposed performing fenestration of the distal radius and ulna rather than changing the length or orientation.

Several authors, however, have found that measurements of ulnar variance are affected by age, sex, and position of the wrist as well as degenerative arthritis secondary to the effects of Kienböck's disease [20, 21, 23] (Fig. 8.1). Due to the arthritic process there is bone apposition on the distal radius in front of the (collapsed) lunate. This phenomenon is called "pseudo-lengthening of the radius" [20] (see Fig. 8.1). Recently, several authors have demonstrated that there is no significant difference between the ulnar variance in Kienböck's patients and sex- and age-matched control groups [33–39].

L. De Smet, MD, PhD (✉)
Department of Orthopedics, University Hospitals Leuven, Weligerveld 1, Pellenberg 3210, Belgium
e-mail: luc.desmet@uzleuven.be

I. Degreef, MD, PhD
Hand Unit, Department of Orthopedic Surgery, University Hospitals Leuven, Belgium, Weligerveld 1, Pellenberg 3212, Belgium

© Springer International Publishing Switzerland 2016
D.M. Lichtman, G.I. Bain (eds.), *Kienböck's Disease*, DOI 10.1007/978-3-319-34226-9_8

**Table 8.1** Ulnar variance and Kienböck's disease

| Author | Year | UV |
|---|---|---|
| Hulten | 1928 | −2.04 |
| Gelberman | 1975 | −1.40 |
| Armistead | 1982 | −3.01 |
| Sundberg | 1983 | −2.04 |
| Kristensen | 1986 | −1.42 |
| Kristensen | 1987 | −1.04 |
| Mirabello | 1987 | −1.10 |
| Wun | 1990 | −1.22 |
| Nakamura | 1991 | −0.37 |

**Table 8.2** Radial shortening

| Author | Year | *N* | % Good |
|---|---|---|---|
| Calandriello | 1966 | 10 | 90 |
| Axelson | 1973 | 19 | 100 |
| Rosemeyer | 1976 | 19 | 69 |
| Eiken | 0980 | 8 | 87 |
| Oversen | 1981 | 8 | 87 |
| Almquist | 1982 | 12 | 91 |
| Schattenkerk | 1987 | 20 | 70 |
| Nakamuro | 1990 | 23 | 83 |
| Weiss | 1991 | 29 | 87 |
| Gomis | 1994 | 28 | 85 |
| Garbuio | 1996 | 13 | 84 |
| Siala | 2000 | 31 | 80 |

**Table 8.3** Ulnar lengthening

| Author | Year | *N* | % Good |
|---|---|---|---|
| Tillberg | 1968 | 10 | 100 |
| Armistead | 1982 | 20 | 90 |
| Sundberg | 1983 | 19 | 95 |
| Schattenkerk | 1987 | 15 | 70 |
| Quenzer | 1993 | 64 | 90 |
| Ducarmois | 1999 | 9 | 100 |

The source of the discrepancy in variance among apparently well-conducted surveys remains a matter of discussion. A lack of standardized radiographic technique and positioning has been shown to materially affect comparisons of ulnar variance [21, 23, 40–42]. However, since 1983, the technique introduced by Epner et al. [42] and Palmer et al. [42] has been the gold standard for determination of variance.

Another reason for the discrepancy in results is the difference in ulnar variance among various populations (Table 8.4) [43–47]. A crucial feature is the control group. For example, since ulnar variance can be affected by age, a proper

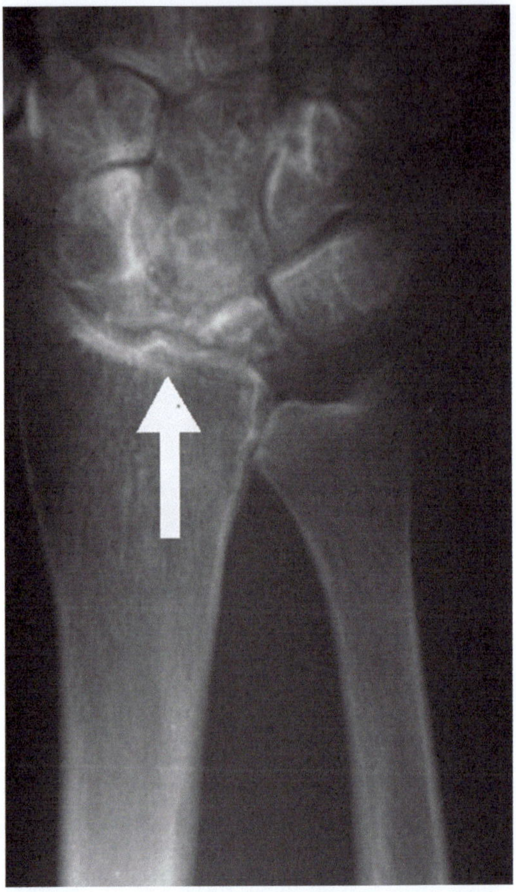

**Fig. 8.1** Pseudolengthening of the radius in a longstanding Kienböck's disease

**Table 8.4** Ulnar variance in different populations

| Author | Year | *N* | UV |
|---|---|---|---|
| Hulten | 1928 | 400 | −0.7 mm |
| Gelberman (Caucasians, USA) | 1975 | 419 | 0.7 |
| Gelberman (Blacks, USA) | 1975 | idem | 0.3 |
| Chan (China) | 1980 | 400 | 0.8 |
| Kristensen (Denmark) | 1986 | 100 | −0.8 |
| Czintrom (USA) | 1987 | 65 | −0.4 |
| Mandelbaum (USA) | 1989 | 25 | −0.5 |
| Nakamura (Japan) | 1991 | 325 | 0.2 |
| Schuind (USA) | 1992 | 120 | −0.9 |
| Hollevoet (Belgium) | 2000 | 50 | −0.4 |
| D'Hoore (Belgium) | 1994 | 125 | −0.4 |

age-matched control group is required before a significant difference in ulnar variance can be established.

Although there may be no proven etiological link between a shorter ulna and the occurrence of Kienböck's disease, the shorter ulna may contribute to progression of an already established disease, including fragmentation and collapse of the lunate. A finite element analysis reported in 2008 by Ledoux et al. [47] pointed in this direction. In 2010, Goeminne et al. reviewed the radiographic files of 70 patients with Kienböck's disease. Ulnar variance and Kienböck stage were determined. A significant difference in ulnar variance was seen between early and late stages of the disease. In later stages there is a marked negative ulnar variance, not caused by bone apposition on the radius. The authors hypothesize that negative ulnar variance encourages further progression of the collapse of the lunate, while neutral or positive ulnar variance seems to protect the lunate against deformation and with revascularization the shape of the lunate remained intact [48].

Two meta-analyses have been reported on this topic [33, 49]. Chung et al. [33] could not find a significant correlation between negative ulnar variance and lunatomalacia. Stahl et al. [49] did find a correlation by adding additional series reported after Chung's paper [36, 49, 50]. They explained this by the selection bias in the control groups. Further statistical methods (i.e., Bradford Hill criteria) did not support a causal relationship between negative ulnar variance and Kienböck's disease.

## Morphology of the Lunate and Distal Radius

In addition to the ulna, morphological (or radiological) features of the distal radius and the lunate itself have been investigated to study the pathogenesis and treatment of Kienböck's disease. Razemon in 1982 [51] studied the lunate coverage ratio and reported that in Kienböck's disease ($n=36$), the lunate was less covered by the radius than in a control population ($n=97$). The study of Thienpondt et al. [37], however, could not confirm this finding. Mirabello et al. [52] reported that a flat distal radius may predispose to Kienböck's disease and that there is a correlation between the slope of the radial distal articular surface and the age of onset. Thienpondt et al. [37] also found a flatter distal radius. Tsuge and Nakamura [4] found a positive correlation with a smaller lunate diameter and height, a flatter radial inclination, and a radially more inclined lunate-tilting angle. These findings were confirmed by Thienpondt [37] (Table 8.5 and Fig. 8.2). In theory, a smaller lunate will concentrate a greater proportion of the axial load per unit area. According to the studies of Frank [53] and Zapico [54], a lunate with a more radially inclined tilting angle is less able to resist axial loading because of its trabecular pattern. It therefore undergoes more shear forces than simple compression forces.

**Table 8.5** Lunate and radial morphology in Kienböck's disease

| | Kienböck group Mean ± SD | Control group Mean ± SD | *P* |
|---|---|---|---|
| Lunate diameter (mm) | 14.23 ± 1.02 | 15.43 ± 1.60 | 0.0037* |
| Lunate height (mm) | 10.08 ± 1.20 | 11.50 ± 0.70 | 0.04* |
| Lunate tilting angle (°) | 20.94 ± 4.6 | 17.68 ± 5.4 | 0.0036* |
| Radial inclination (°) | 23.72 ± 4.3 | 25.42 ± 4.8 | 0.018* |
| Ulnar variance (mm) | −0.89 ± 0.9 | −0.42 ± 1.4 | 0.51 |
| Lunate fossa inclination (°) | 13.81 ± 4.1 | 13.61 ± 4.4 | 0.88 |
| Lunate uncovering index (%) | 33.65 ± 10.5 | 39.32 ± 9.3 | 0.17 |

*$p<0.05$ Statistical significance for Student's *t*-test
From Thienpont E, Mulier T, De Smet L. Radiographic analysis of anatomic risk factors for scapholunate dissociation. Acta Orthop Belg 2003; 69: 246–251 [37]

Lunate morphology may also affect the severity of Kienböck's disease at the time of initial presentation. Patients with Viegas type 1 lunates present with more advanced Kienböck's disease compared with those with type II lunates [55, 56]. In type 1 lunates, there is a greater likelihood of lunate coronal fracture; and, in the absence of

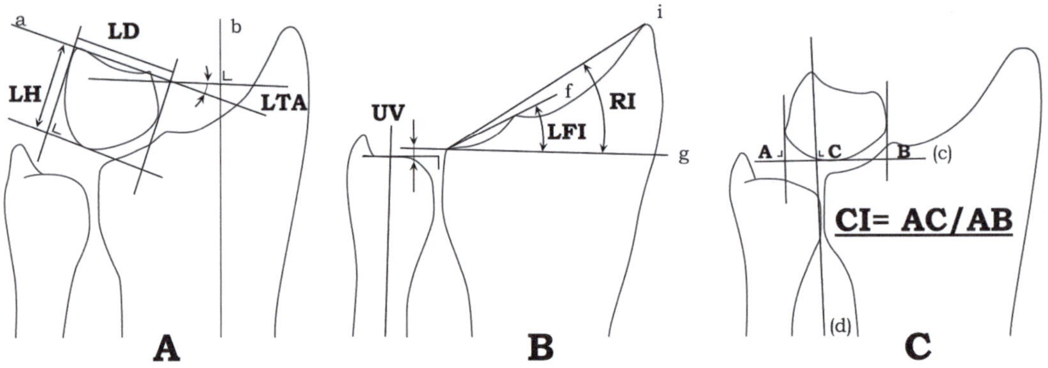


**Fig. 8.2** (a) Measurement of lunate diameter (LD) and height (LH) from the baseline of the lunate (a). Measurement of the lunate-tilting angle (LTA) which is the angle between a perpendicular line drawn to the base of the lunate (a) and the axis of the radius (c). (b) Measurement of the ulnar variance (UV) which is the distance between the most distal part of the ulnar cortical rim and a line drawn from the ulnar side of the articular surface of the distal radius towards the ulna (11). Measurement of the lunate fossa inclination (LFI) which is the angle between the sclerotic line of the lunate fossa of the radius (f) and a line perpendicular (g) to the long axis of the distal ulna (h). Measurement of the radial inclination (RI) which is the angle between a line from the ulnar side of the carpal surface of the radius to the tip of the radial styloid (i) and a line perpendicular (j) to the axis of the ulna (h). (c) Measurement of the lunate uncovering index (LCI) which is the index between the uncovered portion of the lunate (AC) on a line perpendicular (d) to the longitudinal axis of the radial side of the DRUJ (e) and the projection of the entire lunate on the same line (AB) (LCI = AC/AB)

a coronal fracture, the radioscaphoid angles are greater. Type II lunates, therefore, appear to be protective against coronal fractures and scaphoid flexion deformities.

## Conclusion

Since 1928, when Hulten reported an association between Kienböck's disease and ulnar minus variance there has been considerable interest in the morphological features of Kienböck's disease. Finite element modelling suggests that ulnar minus variance is important for progression of the lunate collapse, and that ulnar minus variance is probably not the cause of Kienböck's disease, but contributes to the progression of the collapse.

Other factors that are associated with the pathogenesis or progression of Kienböck's disease include a smaller lunate diameter and height, a more radially inclined lunate-tilting angle, and a flatter radial inclination. The Viegas type 1 lunate wrists have significantly more advanced disease compared with those with type 2 lunates. If there is a type 1 lunate, then there is a greater chance that there will be a coronal fracture; and in the absence of a coronal fracture, radioscaphoid angles are greater. These anatomic factors may result in a greater load transmission across the lunate. Alternatively the type II lunates appear to be protective against coronal fractures and scaphoid flexion deformities.

## References

1. Hulten O. Uber anatomische variationene der Handgelenckknochen. Acta Radiol. 1928;9:155–69.
2. Armistead R, Linscheid R, Dobyns J, Beckenbauch J. Ulnar lengthening in the treatment of Kienbock's disease. J Hand Surg Am. 1982;64:170–8.
3. Gelberman RH, Salamon PB, Jurist JM, Posh JL. Ulnar variance in Kienböck's disease. J Bone Joint Surg Am. 1975;57:674–6.
4. Mirabello SC, Rosenthal DI, Smith RJ. Correlation of clinical and radiographic findings in Kienböck's disease. J Hand Surg Am. 1987;12:1049–54.
5. Nathan PA, Meadows KD. Ulna-minus variance and Kienböck's disease. J Hand Surg Am. 1987;12:777–8.
6. Stahl F. A lunatomalacia. Acta Chir Scand. 1947; 95(Suppl):126.
7. Sundberg S, Lincheid R. Kienbock's disease: results of treatment with ulnar lengthening. Clin Orthop. 1984;187:43–51.

8. Wun-Schen C, Chun-Hsiung S. Ulnar variance and Kienbock's disease. Clin Orthop. 1990;225:124–7.
9. Rossak K. Drukverhaltnisse am andgelenk unter besonderer beruchsichtigung von frakturmechanismen. Verh Dtsch Orthop Ges. 1966;53:296–9.
10. Amillo S, Martinez-Peric R, Barrios RH. Radial shortening for the treatment of Kienböck's disease. Int Orthop. 1993;17:23–6.
11. Almquist EE, Burns Jr JF. Radial shortening for the treatment of Kienböck's disease--a 5- to 10-year follow-up. J Hand Surg Am. 1982;7:348–52.
12. Axelson R. Niveau Operationen bei Mondbein nekrose. Handchir. 1973;5:187–96.
13. Calandriello B, Palandie C. Die Behandlunge der Lunatum-Malacie durch Speichenverkurtzung. Z Orthop. 1966;101:531–4.
14. Ducarmois P, Van Innis F. Long-term results of 9 cases of elongation of the ulna in treatment of Kienböck's disease. Ann Chir Main Memb Super. 1997;16:16–24.
15. Eiken O, Niechajev I. Radius shortening in malacia of the lunate. J Plast Reconstr Surg. 1980;14:191–4.
16. Garbuio P, Obert L, Tropet Y, Vichard P. Kienböck's disease treated by shortening osteotomy of the radius. Analysis of the results apropos of 13 cases. Ann Chir Main Memb Super. 1996;15:226–37.
17. Gomis R, Martin B, Idoux O, Chammas M, Allieu Y. Kienboeck disease: treatment by shortening osteotomy of the radius. Rev Chir Orthop Reparatrice Appar Mot. 1994;80:196–204.
18. Iwasaki N, Minami A, Oizumi N, Suenaga N, Kato H, Minami M. Radial osteotomy for late-stage Kienböck's disease. Wedge osteotomy versus radial shortening. J Bone Joint Surg Br. 2002;84:673–7.
19. Koh S, Nakamura R, Horii E, Nakao E, Inagaki H, Yajima H. Surgical outcome of radial osteotomy for Kienböck's disease-minimum 10 years of follow-up. J Hand Surg Am. 2003;28:910–6.
20. Kristensen S, Soballe K. The influence of arthrosis on UV measurements. J Hand Surg Br. 1987;12:301–5.
21. Kristensen SS, Thomassen E, Christensen F. Ulnar variance determination. J Hand Surg Br. 1986;11:255–7.
22. Nakamura R, Imaeda T, Miura T. Radial shortening for Kienböck's disease: factors affecting the operative result. J Hand Surg Br. 1990;15:40–5.
23. Nakamura R, Tanaka Y, Umaeda T, Miura T. The influence of age and sex on ulnar variance. J Hand Surg Br. 1991;16:84–8.
24. Ovesen J. Shortening of the radius in the treatment of lunatomalacia. J Bone Joint Surg Br. 1981;63:231–2.
25. Quenzer DE, Dobyns JH, Linscheid RL, Trail IA, Vidal MA. Radial recession osteotomy for Kienböck's disease. J Hand Surg Am. 1997;22:386–95.
26. Rosemeyer B, Artmann M, Viernstein K. Lunatomalacie: nachuntersuchungsgebenisse und therapeutische Erwagungen. Arch Orthop Unfallchir. 1976;85:119–27.
27. Schattenkerk M, Nollen A, Van Hussen F. The treatment of lunatomalacia: radial shortening or ulnar lengthening? Act Orthop Scand. 1987;58:652–4.
28. Siala A, Ben Ayeche ML, Frikha R, Ghannouchi G, Moula T. Results of diaphyseal shortening of the radius in the treatment of Kienböck's disease: a series of 31 cases. Rev Chir Orthop Reparatrice Appar Mot. 2000;86:151–7.
29. Tilberg B. Kienbock's disease treated with osteotomy of to lengthen the ulna. Act Orthop Scand. 1968; 39:359–68.
30. Weiss AP. Radial shortening. Hand Clin. 1993;9: 475–82.
31. Chan KP, Huang P. Anatomic variations in radial and ulnar lengths in the wrists of Chinese. Clin Orthop. 1971;80:17–20.
32. Illarramendi AA, Schulz C, De Carli P. The surgical treatment of Kienböck's disease by radius and ulna metaphyseal core decompression. J Hand Surg Am. 2001;26:252–60.
33. Chung KC, Spilson MS, Kim MH. Is negative ulnar variance a risk factor for Kienböck's disease? A meta-analysis. Ann Plast Surg. 2001;47:494–9.
34. D'Hoore K, De Smet L, Verellen K, Vral J, Fabry G. Negative ulnar variance is not a risk factor for Kienböck's disease. J Hand Surg Am. 1994;19: 229–31.
35. Kristensen SS, Thomassen E, Chistensen F. Ulnar variance in Kienböck's disease. J Hand Surg Br. 1986; 11:258–60.
36. Muramatsu K, Ihara K, Kawai S, Doi K. Ulnar variance and the role of joint leveling procedure for Kienböck's disease. Int Orthop. 2003;27:240–3.
37. Thienpont E, Mulier T, De Smet L. Radiographic analysis of anatomic risk factors for scapholunate dissociation. Acta Orthop Belg. 2003;69:246–51.
38. Tsuge S, Nakamura R. Anatomical risk factors for Kienböck's disease. J Hand Surg Br. 1993;18:70–5.
39. Weiss AP. Negative ulnar variance is not a risk factor for Kienböck's disease. J Hand Surg Am. 1994;19: 1057–8.
40. Palmer AK, Glisson RR, Werner FW. Ulnar variance determination. J Hand Surg Am. 1982;7:376–9.
41. Steyers C, Blair W. Measuring ulnar variance: a comparison of techniques. J Hand Surg Am. 1989;14: 607–12.
42. Epner R, Bowers W, Guilford W. Ulnar variance the effect of positioning on roentgen filming technique. J Hand Surg Am. 1982;7:298–305.
43. Czitrom A, Dobyns J, Linscheid R. Ulnar variance in carpal instability. J Hand Surg Am. 1987;12: 205–12.
44. Mandelbaum B, Bortolozzi A, Dary C, Teurlings L, Bragonier B. Wrist pain syndrome in gymnasts. Am J Sports Med. 1989;17:305–17.
45. Schuind F, Linscheid R, An K, Chao E. A normal data base of posteroanterior roentgenographic measurements of the wrist. J Bone Joint Surg Am. 1992;74:1418–29.
46. Hollevoet N, Van Maele G, Van Seymortier P, Verdonk R. Comparison of palmar tilt, radial inclination and ulnar variance in left and right wrists. J Hand Surg Br. 2000;25:431–3.

47. Ledoux P, Lamblin D, Wuilbaut A, Schuind F. A finite-element analysis of Kienbock's disease. J Hand Surg Eur Vol. 2008;33:286–9.
48. Goeminne S, Degreef I, De Smet L. Negative ulnar variance has prognostic value in progression of Kienböck's disease. Acta Orthop Belg. 2010;76:38–41.
49. Stahl S, Stahl AS, Meisner C, Hentschel PJ, Valina S, Luz O, Schaller HE, Lotter O. Critical analysis of causality between negative ulnar variance and Kienböck disease. Plast Reconstr Surg. 2013;132:899–909.
50. Afshar A, Aminzadeh-Gohari A, Yekta Z. The association of Kienbock's disease and ulnar variance in the Iranian population. J Hand Surg Eur Vol. 2013;38:496–9.
51. Razemon JP. Pathological study of Kienböck's disease. Ann Chir Main. 1982;1:240–2.
52. Thienpont E, Mulier T, Rega F, De Smet L. Radiographic analysis of anatomical risk factors for Kienböck's disease. Acta Orthop Belg. 2004;70: 406–9.
53. Frank P. Die pathogenese der lunatumnekrose und ihre Beziehung zur funktionellen belastung des handgelenks. Bruns Beitr Klin Chir. 1936;164:2002–225.
54. Antuna Zapico JM. Malacia del semilunar. Doctoral thesis, Valladolid, 1966.
55. Rhee PC, Jones DB, Moran SL, Shin AY. The effect of lunate morphology in kienböck disease. J Hand Surg Am. 2015;40:738–44.
56. Viegas SF, Patterson RM, Hokanson JA, Davis J. Wrist anatomy: incidence, distribution, and correlation of anatomic variations, tears, and arthrosis. J Hand Surg Am. 1993;18:463–75.

# Clinical Presentation, Natural History, and Classification of Kienböck's Disease

9

William F. Pientka II, Bassem Hanalla, Richard Blake Barber, Timothy Niacaris, and David M. Lichtman

## Introduction

Kienböck's disease is most prevalent in young adults; however, the natural history in this age group is based primarily on empirical observations on patients who were treated shortly after the diagnosis was confirmed. The true natural history of untreated adult Kienböck's patients is therefore somewhat speculative. Nevertheless, in an attempt to select an appropriate treatment plan based on the severity (or stage) of the disease at presentation, several classification systems have been developed based upon these empiric observations [1–4].

Despite the prevalence of this disorder in young adults, Kienböck's disease can also occur in the pediatric and geriatric populations. Since the clinical findings, prognosis, and response to treatment appear to be distinct for the three age groups, they will be discussed individually in separate sections of this chapter.

## Clinical Diagnosis, Classification, and Natural History in Adults

Kienböck's disease usually presents in patients 20–40 years of age with a 2:1 male-to-female predominance. Hand dominance has not been shown to contribute its development [5]. The incidence of bilateral disease in adults is extremely low [6, 7]. The typical presentation is intermittent dorsal wrist pain aggravated by stressful wrist activities, especially extension. Patients may or may not report a history of wrist trauma [8]. With disease

W.F. Pientka II, MD (✉)
Department of Orthopedic Surgery, John Peter Smith Hospital, 1500 S. Main St., Fort Worth, TX 76104, USA

6155 Highwoods Ct., Fort Worth, TX 76112, USA
e-mail: wpientka@jpshealth.org

B. Hanalla, BA
University of North Texas Health Science Center–Texas College of Osteopathic Medicine, 3500 Camp Bowie, Fort Worth, TX 76107, USA

13306 Durbridge Trail Dr., Houston, TX 77065, USA

R.B. Barber, BS, MS
University of North Texas Health Science Center–Texas College of Osteopathic Medicine, 4901 Bryce Ave., Apt B, Fort Worth, TX 76107, USA

T. Niacaris, MD, PhD
Department of Orthopedic Surgery, University of North Texas Health Science Center, 800 5th Avenue, Suite 400, Fort Worth, TX 76104, USA

D.M. Lichtman, MD
Rear Admiral (Retired), US Navy Adjunct Professor, Department of Surgery, Uniformed Services University of the Health Sciences, Bethesda, MD, USA

Adjunct Professor, Department of Orthopedic Surgery, University of North Texas Health Sciences Center, Fort Worth, TX, USA

© Springer International Publishing Switzerland 2016
D.M. Lichtman, G.I. Bain (eds.), *Kienböck's Disease*, DOI 10.1007/978-3-319-34226-9_9

progression, localized swelling, tenderness, and pain compatible with perilunate synovitis appear. These findings are most prominent in the perilunate area and can be present along the ulnar aspect of the carpus as well. Wrist range of motion and grip strength decrease [9] in proportion to the pain and swelling, while forearm rotation is generally preserved [10]. Later in the course of the disease, signs and symptoms of acute synovitis are replaced by findings of carpal instability and degenerative arthritis (i.e., clicking, crepitus, and restricted motion). After several years, the acute symptoms tend to abate and the patient typically notices mild to moderate residual wrist stiffness with occasional flares of pain associated with stressful activities. These residual findings can last indefinitely. Given that the signs and symptoms are relatively non-specific throughout the course of the disease, a diagnosis of Kienböck's disease should be considered in any adult presenting with lingering, undiagnosed wrist pain.

In 1977, the senior author developed a classification system based on personal observations of X-ray changes during the natural course of Kienböck's disease in adult patients (Table 9.1) [1, 2]. Although this classification has also been applied to children and the elderly, the associated treatment algorithm should be used with caution in these populations because of age related variations in the revascularization potential and response to treatment.

In stage I Kienböck's disease, X-rays are normal (Fig. 9.1a, b). The diagnosis of stage I was initially made in retrospect, after lunate density changes appeared on standard X-rays. With MRI, however, low intensity signal on T1-weighted images can confirm the diagnosis (see Fig. 9.1b) prior to X-ray changes. The symptoms and signs at this stage are predominantly those of intermittent perilunate synovitis, and are often initiated by stressful wrist activities.

In stage II disease, the lunate becomes sclerotic on plain X-ray; however, the external architecture is preserved (Fig. 9.2a, b). Measurements of lunate height and carpal height are normal. In stages II and IIIA, the findings of wrist synovitis are more constant and are accompanied by a decrease in wrist motion and grip strength.

**Table 9.1** Lichtman classification of Kienböck's disease

| Disease stage | X-ray findings | MRI findings |
|---|---|---|
| I | Normal | T1 signal: decreased |
| | | T2 signal: variable |
| II | Lunate sclerosis | T1 signal: decreased |
| | | T2 signal: variable |
| IIIA | Lunate collapse | T1 Signal: decreased |
| | | T2 signal: variable |
| IIIB | Lunate and carpal collapse | T1 signal: decreased |
| | Scaphoid rotation (RS angle > 60) | T2 signal: usually decreased |
| IV | Pan carpal arthritis | T1 signal: decreased |
| | KDAC | T2 signal: decreased |

In stage III, there is collapse of the lunate in the frontal plane, with lunate widening in the sagittal plane (Fig. 9.3a, b). Lunate fragmentation is a frequent accompaniment. As the lunate collapses further, the capitate migrates proximally, the proximal carpal row widens, and the scaphoid flexes giving the characteristic ring sign on anteroposterior radiographs (see Fig. 9.4). Stage III is differentiated into stages IIIA (Fig. 9.3a, b) and IIIB (Fig. 9.4), with the determining factor being the absence (IIIA) or presence (IIIB) of fixed scaphoid flexion (radioscaphoid angle greater than 60° [11]). Fixed scaphoid flexion can be due to scapholunate dissociation, flexion deformity of the proximal row and/or fragmentation of the lunate. Symptoms in stage IIIA are similar to those in stage II with increasing pain, stiffness and more constant swelling due to synovitis. In stage IIIB, the predominant findings are those of carpal instability (clicking, grinding, and crepitus) along with gradually increasing wrist stiffness. In most cases the symptoms abate gradually as the inflammation (synovitis) surrounding the necrotic lunate resolves.

Lunate collapse and fragmentation along with radiocarpal and midcarpal degenerative changes denote stage IV (Fig. 9.5). In this stage, symptoms and signs are frequently diminished with intermittent flares following stressful activities.

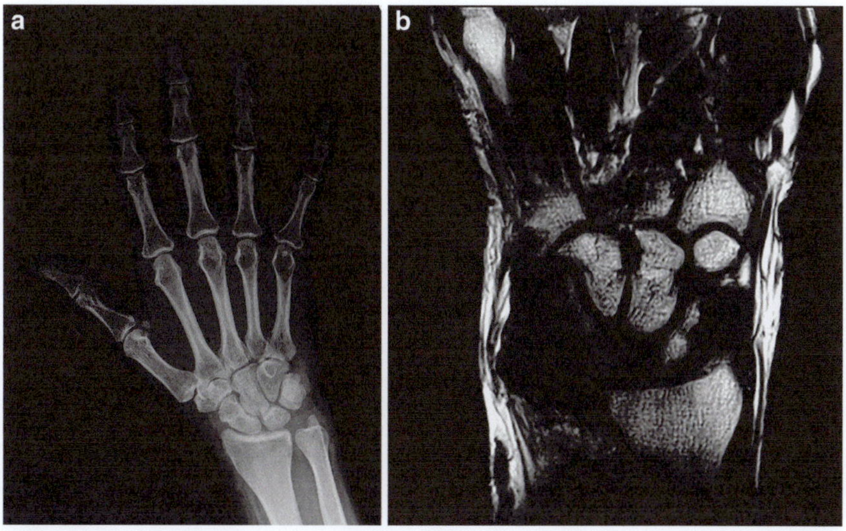


**Fig. 9.1** (a) Anteroposterior view of a wrist of a 46-year-old female with known stage I disease, showing no acute changes. (b) Coronal T1-weighted MRI sequence of the same patient showing decreased signal intensity throughout the entirety of the lunate. With normal radiographs, this is consistent with stage I Kienböck's disease

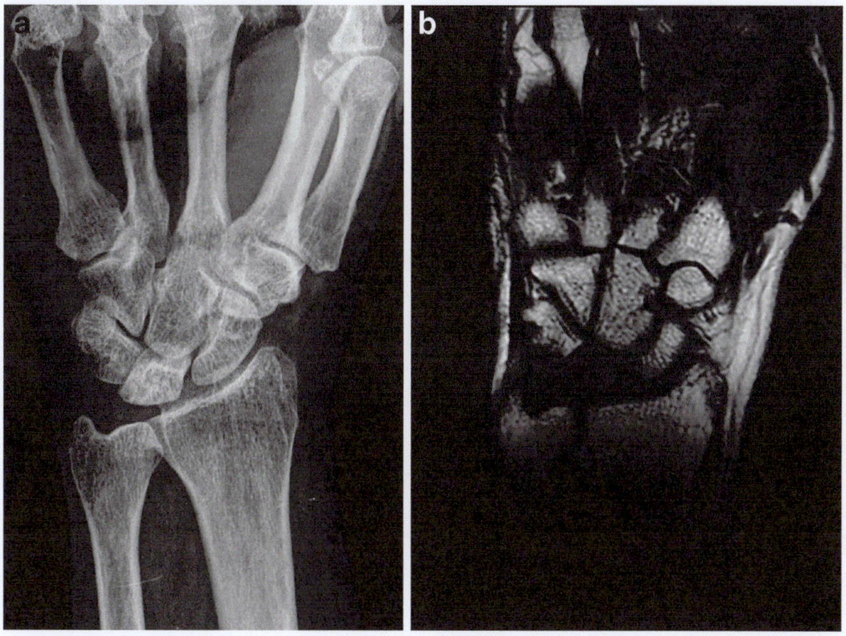


**Fig. 9.2** (a) Anteroposterior radiograph of a 56-year-old female showing sclerosis and cystic changes with the lunate. There is no apparent disruption in the normal architecture of the lunate. These findings are consistent with stage II Kienböck's disease. (b) T1 coronal MRI of the same patient showing decreased signal throughout the lunate

The typical findings of clinical and radiographic degenerative arthritis closely resemble those caused by chronic scaphoid non-union (SNAC) or scapholunate dissociation (SLAC); hence our nickname for this stage, "KDAC" (Kienböck's Disease Advanced Collapse).

Throughout all four stages the T1 MRI signal, which represents healthy bone marrow, remains

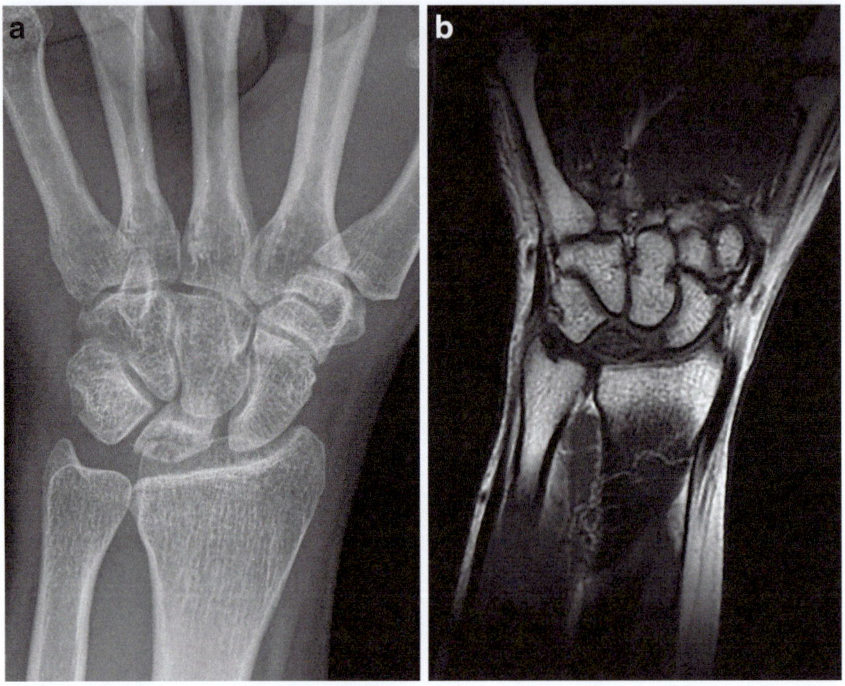


**Fig. 9.3** (**a**) Anteroposterior radiograph of a 34-year-old female showing a sclerotic lunate which has collapsed. The patient did not have fixed scaphoid hyperflexion, consistent with stage IIIA Kienböck's disease. (**b**) T1-weighted coronal MRI of the same patient with decreased signal intensity throughout the lunate

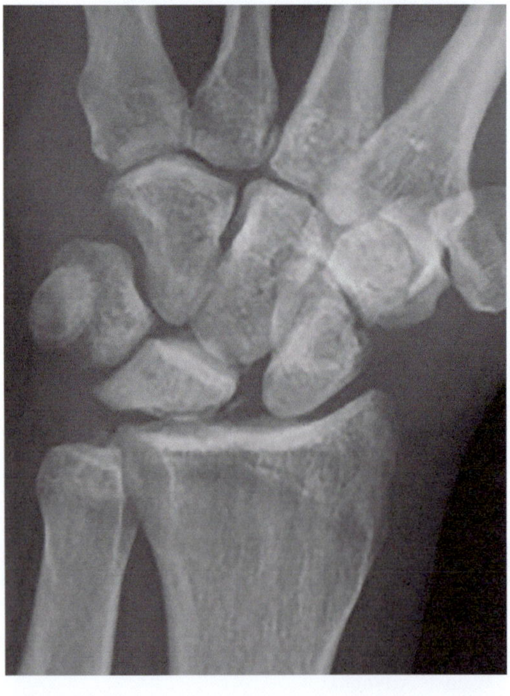

**Fig. 9.4** Anteroposterior radiograph showing lunate sclerosis and collapse, with a prominent ring sign with the scaphoid suggesting scaphoid hyperflexion. This flexion was fixed, consistent with stage IIIB Kienböck's disease

low unless there is spontaneous revascularization of the lunate. On the other hand, the T2 signal, which reflects either lunate edema or revascularization, is variable depending on the amount of fluid in the bone. In general, however, lower signal on T2 sequences correlates with a poorer prognosis for spontaneous revascularization of the lunate. In recent years, investigators have studied the four traditional stages of Kienböck's using advanced imaging [12] and arthroscopic [13] techniques and discovered that the stages can be further divided to add additional nuance to the derived treatment algorithm. The correlation of these findings and their clinical significance will be presented in greater detail elsewhere in this text.

In 2010, the osseous classification system was expanded to include a hypothetical stage 0 and a well-represented stage IIIC disease [14]. Stage 0 disease is analogous to stage 0 of the ARCO International classification [15] of hip osteonecrosis where patients present with intermittent pain but standard radiographs and MR images are normal. The advantage of diagnosis at this stage would be the potential to abort true

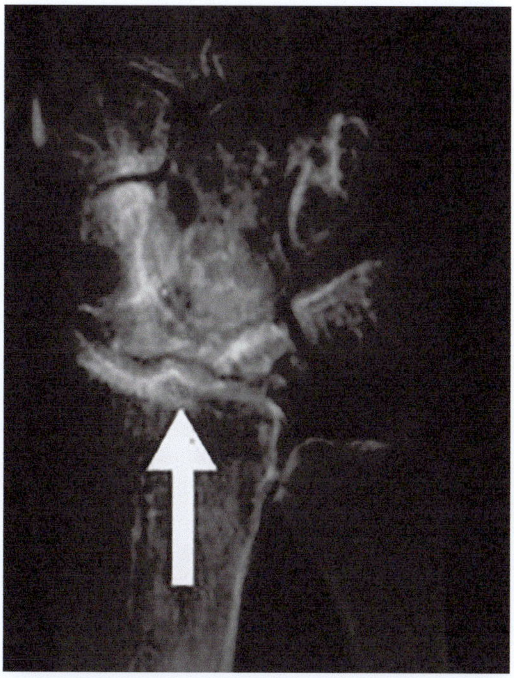

**Fig. 9.5** Anteroposterior image of a wrist with a sclerotic, collapsed lunate with associated diffuse degenerative changes within the radiocarpal and midcarpal joints. This is consistent with stage IV Kienböck's disease. Image courtesy of Luc De Smet

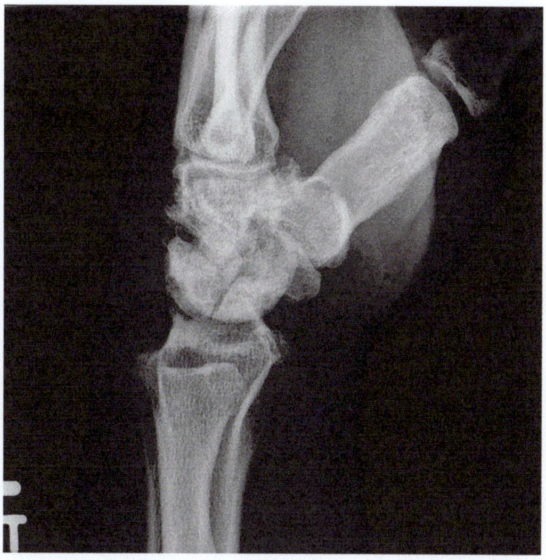

**Fig. 9.6** Lateral radiograph showing a clear coronal fracture of a sclerotic lunate, consistent with stage IIIC Kienböck's disease

osteonecrosis onset by correction of etiologic factors associated with later stages of the disease. In stage IIIC disease, there is a coronal fracture or fragmentation of the lunate (Fig. 9.6). In our experience, when this occurs the prognosis for lunate revascularization is poor. Treatment recommendations for this stage include lunate excision with prosthetic replacement, proximal row carpectomy, or intercarpal arthrodesis.

There are few additional studies that fully confirm the natural history of untreated Kienböck's disease in adults. Keith et al. [16] reported a cohort of 33 wrists with Kienböck's disease treated nonoperatively, and noted that wrist range of motion decreases with increasing disease stage. They also noted a similar deterioration in grip strength in the affected extremity with disease progression. Keith et al. determined that changes in pain, wrist flexion, and DASH scores correlate with disease progression, and that the radioscaphoid angle is the best parameter to evaluate for radiographic progression of the disease.

Reports have shown varying rates of disease progression, with some patients progressing to stage IIIB rapidly [16, 17] while others have followed patients that never progress beyond stage IIIA disease [10]. In 1980, Beckenbaugh et al. [18] reported a retrospective review of 46 patients with Kienböck's disease, and noted that radiographic progression of the disease does not necessarily correlate with worsening symptoms.

In 1986, in a retrospective review by Kristensen [19], 49 wrists with Kienböck's disease were reviewed 8–33 years after diagnosis (mean follow-up 20.5 years). Though intending to compare temporary immobilization with no treatment, their findings are a fair representation of the natural history of the disease. The lunate appeared to progress to fragmentation with a coronal fracture, and they note "without treatment osteoarthritis in the radiocarpal joint supervenes after a number of years." In no patient did the lunate improve in stage at final follow-up. Thirty-three percent of patients ($n=16$) developed a lunate fracture and 66 % ($n=33$) developed radiocarpal arthritis. This relatively large retrospective review with long-term follow-up shows convincing evidence of disease progression when treated nonoperatively.

In 1995 Fujisawa et al. [20] reported on 17 patients with unilateral Kienböck's disease treated nonoperatively and evaluated retrospectively. At minimum 10-year follow-up, five patients remained in the same Lichtman disease stage as presentation, all of which had advanced (stage III or IV) disease. Eight of their nineteen patients progressed in stage, and four patients improved from stage III to stage II. Fujisawa's observation shows a potential for radiographic improvement in early stages of disease, but a trend towards progression to advanced disease with time.

Stahl [21] retrospectively reviewed three cases of nonoperatively treated Kienböck's disease, and noted an expeditious progression from intact lunate architecture (stage II) to stage IIIA in as little as 6 months. This observation is contrary to the more prolonged progression noted previously [20].

In 2015 Vijakka [22] reiterated the fairly predictable disease progression with nonoperative management in a retrospective review of nine wrists with Kienböck's disease (seven patients were stage IIIA, two were stage IIIB). Five patients who presented at stage IIIA did not progress at a mean follow-up of 27.3 years. Two patients who were stage IIIA and both patients who presented at stage IIIB advanced to stage IV at final follow-up. All patients had statistically significant improvement in grip strength from presentation. No significant changes in range of motion in any plane were noted between presentation and final follow-up. The authors conclude that observation alone is not an appropriate treatment recommendation for stage III Kienböck's disease.

Despite a lack of full understanding of the natural history of Kienböck's disease, the structural classification system provides rationale for a generally accepted treatment algorithm for adult patients (Table 9.2). Further details regarding these and many other treatment options are provided elsewhere in this book. Modifications of the algorithm based on recent advances in arthroscopy and advanced imaging will also be presented and discussed in later chapters.

**Table 9.2** Treatment algorithm based on Lichtman classification of Kienböck's disease

| Disease stage | Authors' preferred treatment (alternate in parenthesis) |
|---|---|
| 0, I | Immobilization |
| II or IIIA with ulnar-negative variance | Radial-shortening osteotomy |
| II or IIIA with ulnar-neutral or -positive variance | Capitate shortening with CH fusion (revascularization procedure) |
| IIIB | STT or scaphocapitate fusion (proximal row carpectomy, radial shortening) |
| IIIC, IV | Proximal row carpectomy, wrist fusion, active patient |

## Kienböck's Disease in Pediatric Patients

While the majority of patients diagnosed with Kienböck's disease range in age from 20 to 40 years, there have been various reports of Kienböck's disease in patients as young as 6 years old [5]. As in adults, the etiology of the disease in children is largely unknown, yet it has been recognized that a large proportion of reported patients have a negative ulnar variance.

Disease presentation in pediatric patients is similar to that in adults, with decreased wrist range of motion, decreased grip strength, tenderness, and swelling of the wrist [5, 14, 23–27]. T1-weighted MRI sequences reveal decreased signal within the lunate, while T2-weighted MRI imaging may show either decreased or increased signal intensity. Progressive collapse of the lunate may occur with time, though this is not as frequently observed as in adults [14].

Irisarri [23] categorized Kienböck's disease in children into infantile lunatomalacia (patients 12 or younger) and juvenile lunatomalacia (patients 13 years to skeletal maturity). They treated 13 pediatric patients with Kienböck's disease; four classified as infantile and nine as juvenile. All patients with infantile lunatomalacia were treated with immobilization and were asymptomatic with revascularization noted on MRI at the conclusion of their treatment. Among those with juvenile lunatomalacia, three boys, all 16 years old, failed treatment with immobilization and later underwent successful radial shortening osteotomy. Irisarri concluded that patients under 15 years of age tend to have successful outcomes with immobilization alone. On the other hand, patients older than 15 years tend to show disease progression with nonoperative treatment.

In addition to age, the revascularization potential of the lunate as determined by MRI should be taken into account when considering prognosis and treatment in children. We currently rely on the T2-weighted MRI sequences to detect evidence of possible lunate revascularization [14]. As an example, our group was recently asked to provide a second opinion for a 16-year-old female diagnosed with stage I Kienböck's disease (Fig. 9.7a, b) following 6 months of increasing wrist pain. Based on the significant ulnar minus variance (see Fig. 9.7a), a radial shortening osteotomy had been recommended. Further imaging, however, revealed decreased signal intensity in the lunate on T1-weighted MRI sequences (Fig. 9.8a) but intense signal on T2-weighted sequences (see Fig. 9.8b), suggesting possible early revascularization. We therefore recommended a 3-month trial of immobilization in lieu of surgery. Follow-up MRI at 3 months (Fig. 9.9a, b) and at 7 months (Fig. 9.10a–c) showed a progressive normalization of signal on both T1 and T2 sequences. At 7 months, the patient was asymptomatic and was cleared to resume normal activities.

In 2003, Ferlic et al. [24] reviewed 32 patients with Kienböck's disease ranging from 6 to 19 years old. The review highlighted the case of a 10-year-old girl with cerebral palsy who was treated with 15 weeks of cast immobilization, followed by 15 weeks in a removable wrist splint. At 7-year follow-up, the appearance of the lunate on radiographic images had normalized. In addition, the carpal height ratio increased from 0.48 to 0.56.

Other reports in the literature have shown an improvement in lunate architecture, although the radial aspect of the lunate continued to show some loss of height.

Kim et al. [25] reported three patients under age 12 treated with immobilization, showing improved lunate height with time. Four children older than 12 years did not respond to immobilization and required operative intervention, which provided successful clinical outcomes but did not result in lunate architecture restoration. Kim concluded that the prognosis of patients under 12 years old is good, and often results in remodeling of the lunate. The findings reinforce the concept that adolescent patients tend to respond favorably to nonsurgical treatments.

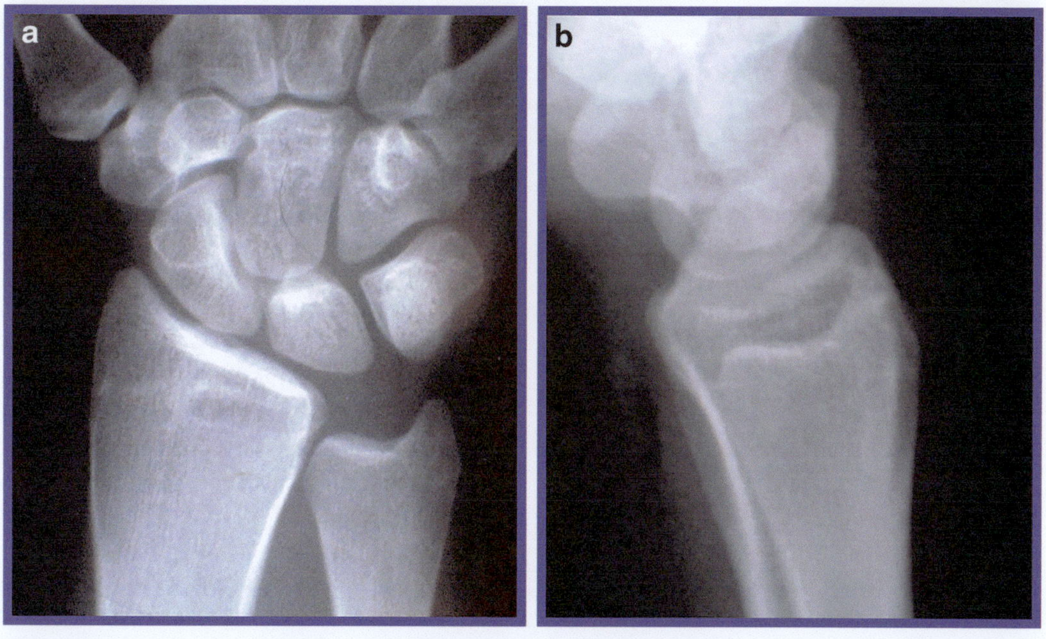


**Fig. 9.7** Plain X-rays before treatment. (**a**) Posteroanterior view reveals a normal appearance of the lunate and a negative ulnar variance. (**b**) Lateral view demonstrates a normal-appearing lunate

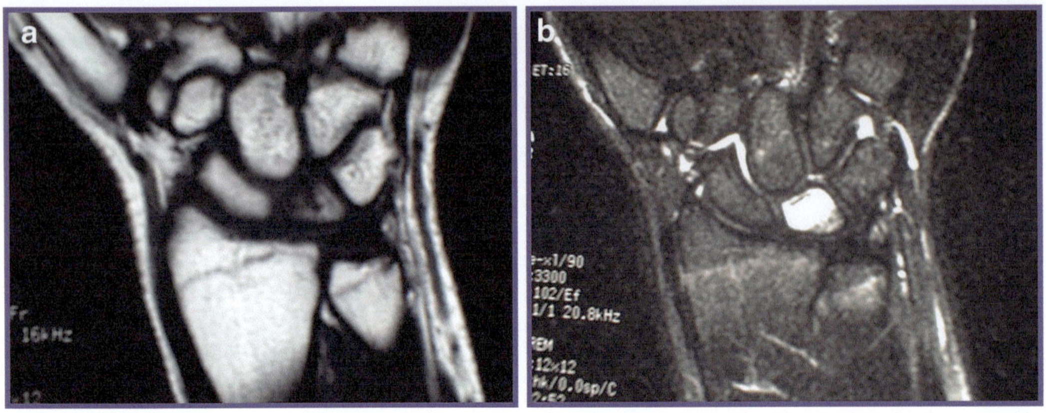


**Fig. 9.8** MRI sequences before immobilization. (**a**) T1-weighted sequence shows decreased signal intensity within the lunate, centered on the radial aspect. (**b**) Markedly increased signal in the lunate on T2

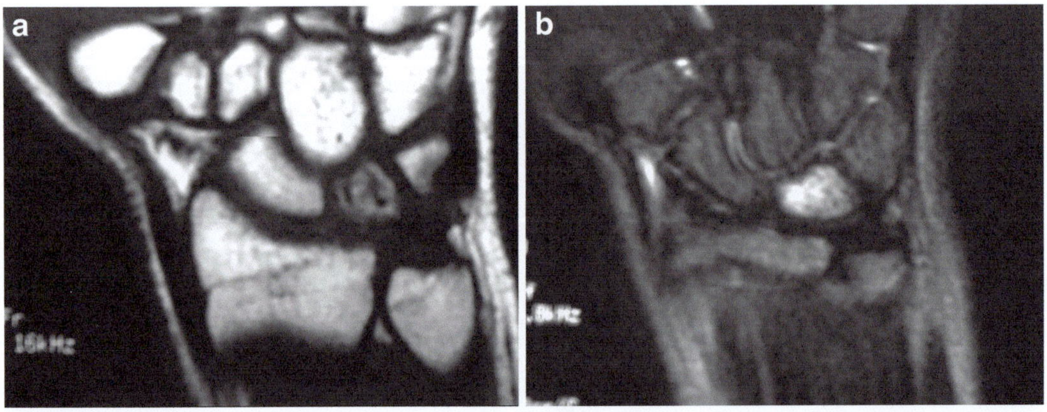


**Fig. 9.9** MRI sequences at 3-month follow-up. (**a**) The T1-weighted sequence shows increased intensity of the lunate compared to the original. (**b**) T2-weighted image shows a slight decrease in intensity from the original

Kim also concluded that, unlike in adults, the lunate in pediatric patients may restore its normal architecture following successful nonoperative treatment.

Since the majority of patients presenting with Kienböck's disease have negative ulnar variance, a popular operative procedure in both children and adults is radial shortening osteotomy. However, in skeletally immature patients, radial shortening increases the risk of postoperative radial overgrowth [27–30]. Matsuhashi [27] reported that overgrowth occurred in four of eight patients treated with radial shortening, but that this did not significantly affect clinical outcome. Nevertheless, it remains a concern in patients with open physes.

A less invasive treatment that does not pose the same risk of overgrowth is temporary fixation of the scaphotrapeziotrapezoidal (STT) joint. Shigematsu et al. [30] and Yasuda et al. [31] both performed this procedure on adolescents with Kienböck's disease and reported favorable results. Kazuki et al. [26] also performed temporary STT pinning on a 15-year-old girl following failure of immobilization alone. At the time of STT pinning, the patient had stage IIIA Kienböck's disease. They used three Kirschner (K) wires, which were removed 6 months postoperative when the signal intensity on T1-weighted MRI normalized. At 2-year follow-up, the patient was pain-free, wrist range of motion increased by 60° and grip strength increased from 20.3 to

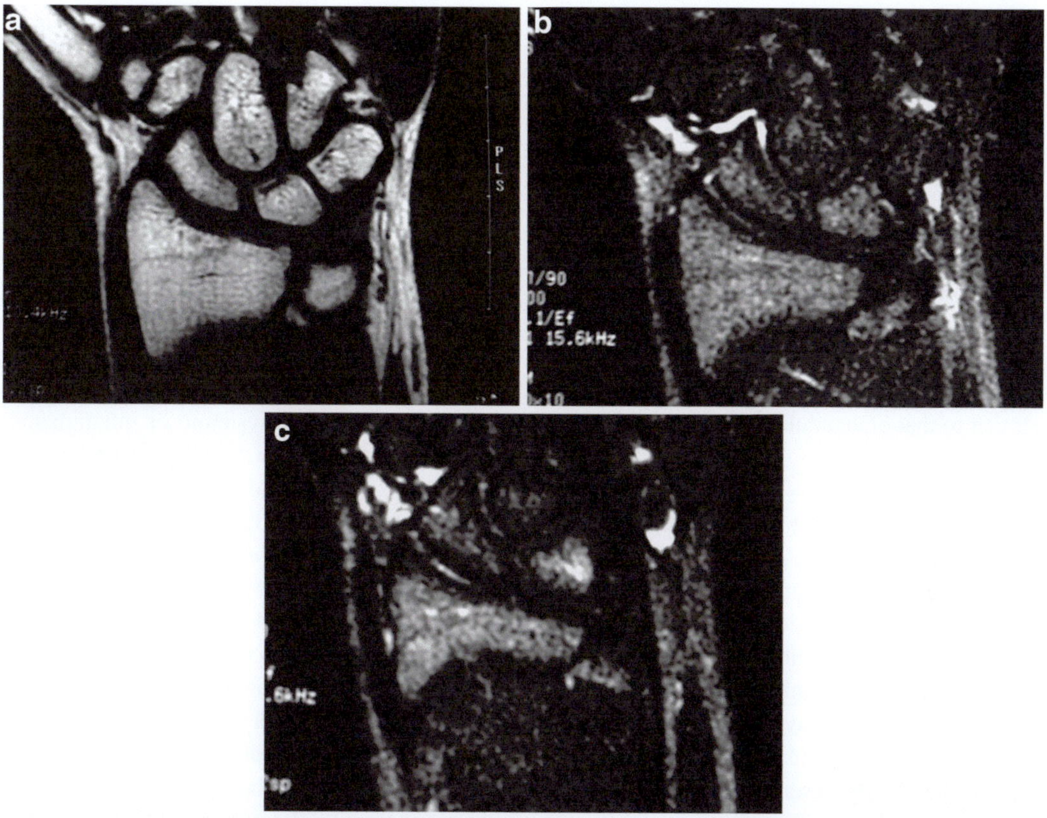

**Fig. 9.10** MRI sequences taken at 7-month follow-up. (**a**) The lunate T1 signal is normalized (except for the very distal aspect). (**b**) The T2 signal is almost normalized in the dorsal aspect of the lunate. (**c**) The T2 continues to show areas of increased signal in the volar lunate, but much improved over earlier sequences

22.9 kg. Despite the clinical improvement, lunate architecture was not restored.

Ando et al. [28] used the same approach in six adolescents (9–17 years old) with type IIIA or IIIB Kienböck's disease. All patients were reported to be pain-free with improved grip strength, increased range of motion, and normalization of MRI changes at final follow-up. STT temporary fixation is therefore an appropriate option for pediatric patients who fail non-operative treatment. It is less invasive than joint leveling procedures, and can be applied regardless of ulnar variance. In addition, this technique avoids the risk of overgrowth associated with radial shortening osteotomy.

Jorge-Mora et al. [29] proposed epiphysiodesis as a new, less invasive alternative to radial shortening for younger patients who do not respond to cast immobilization. Four patients (ages 12–14) were treated with definitive distal radius epiphysiodesis after previous failed attempts at non-operative treatments. This resulted in similar decompression of the radiolunate joint and similar biomechanical effects as a radial shortening osteotomy. The four patients were pain-free and had significantly improved range of motion in the wrist at an average of 4.25 months of follow-up. The authors found several advantages to this procedure: It reduces negative ulnar variance without the risk of radial overgrowth, it is a familiar procedure to pediatric orthopedic surgeons and it has a short recovery time compared to other surgical options. There is, however, limited outcome data for the technique used in this context and further investigation is warranted before advocating its unrestricted use as a treatment for adolescent Kienböck's disease.

Due to the positive prognosis for spontaneous revascularization of the lunate in children, we advise immobilization as the initial treatment for pediatric patients with Kienböck's disease. If there is no clinical or radiologic evidence of healing after 3 months, then surgical options should be considered. Temporary STT joint fixation is recommended for younger patients and for those who show increased signal on T2-weighted MRI sequences. For those 15 years old and over, especially when the MRI indicates minimal revascularization potential, we favor a treatment protocol similar to that of an adult.

## Kienböck's Disease in the Elderly

There are only a few reports of Kienböck's disease in the elderly patient population [32–36]. Despite this paucity of literature, it is evident that Kienböck's disease manifests itself differently in seniors than it does in juveniles or younger adults. Therefore, the natural history of Kienböck's disease in the elderly deserves consideration separate than that of younger patients.

Taniguchi et al. [33] reported the largest series of elderly patients with Kienböck's disease. He observed 14 patients with an average age of disease onset of 65 years. Their series consisted of ten women and four men, as opposed to the male predominance of Kienböck's disease observed in younger populations. Three patients in the study were over 70 years of age, all women. Eleven of the 15 affected wrists involved the dominant hand. One patient had bilateral involvement, and was also diagnosed with lupoid hepatitis. This patient had been treated with corticosteroid therapy for 7 years prior to the onset of wrist symptoms. Two patients presented with a history of wrist trauma; however, ten others reported that their occupation involved manual labor. Negative ulnar variance was present in only 2 of the 14 patients.

Taniguchi used standard radiographic techniques to diagnose and follow disease progression. He recorded the Lichtman disease stage, the carpal height ratio (CHR) as described by Youm [37], and ulnar variance as described by Gelberman [38]. Three wrists were diagnosed at stage II, six wrists were stage IIIA, and six wrists were stage IIIB. At a mean final follow-up of 5.6 years (2.2–9.1) all 15 wrists had progressed to stage IV disease. CHR measurements demonstrated loss of lunate height between the first visit and final follow-up. Despite the progressive carpal collapse and degenerative changes, all patients had either good or excellent clinical outcome scores. Based on his case series, the following observations are pertinent to the natural history of Kienböck's disease in the elderly: It is more common in women, it is not commonly associated with ulnar minus variance, it may be associated with other systemic or inflammatory disorders and despite a predictable progression through the four clinical stages patients respond favorably to nonoperative treatment.

According to separate reviews by Yoshida et al. [34] and Giunta et al. [35], Kienböck's disease in patients over 50 years is causally related to the presence of osteoporosis. They theorize that osteoporosis, a known risk factor for microfracture, could well be a catalyst for the development of osteonecrosis of the lunate. The higher incidence of both Kienböck's disease and osteoporosis in women also suggested to Tanaguchi a possible relationship between the two disorders.

In 2004 Thomas et al. [36] presented a case report of Kienböck's disease in the non-dominant hand of a 70-year-old female patient. The patient's radiographs revealed severe osteopenia and multiple cysts within the carpus of the left hand. X-rays also revealed progressive sclerosis and collapse of the lunate without scaphoid rotation, consistent with stage IIIA Kienböck's disease. Because of the patient's age and rapid progression of disease, proximal row carpectomy (PRC) was performed. They noted that the diagnosis of Kienböck's disease in elderly patients is frequently overlooked because of the many other potential diagnoses, including inflammatory arthritis, carpal tunnel syndrome, infection, or fracture.

A characteristic example of Kienböck's disease in the elderly is represented by a 68-year-old woman who presented to our clinic with intermittent wrist pain of 1-year duration in her dominant right wrist. All relevant laboratory studies were normal. The plain X-rays (Fig. 9.11 a, b) are compatible with diffuse carpal inflammatory arthritis, but the T1- and

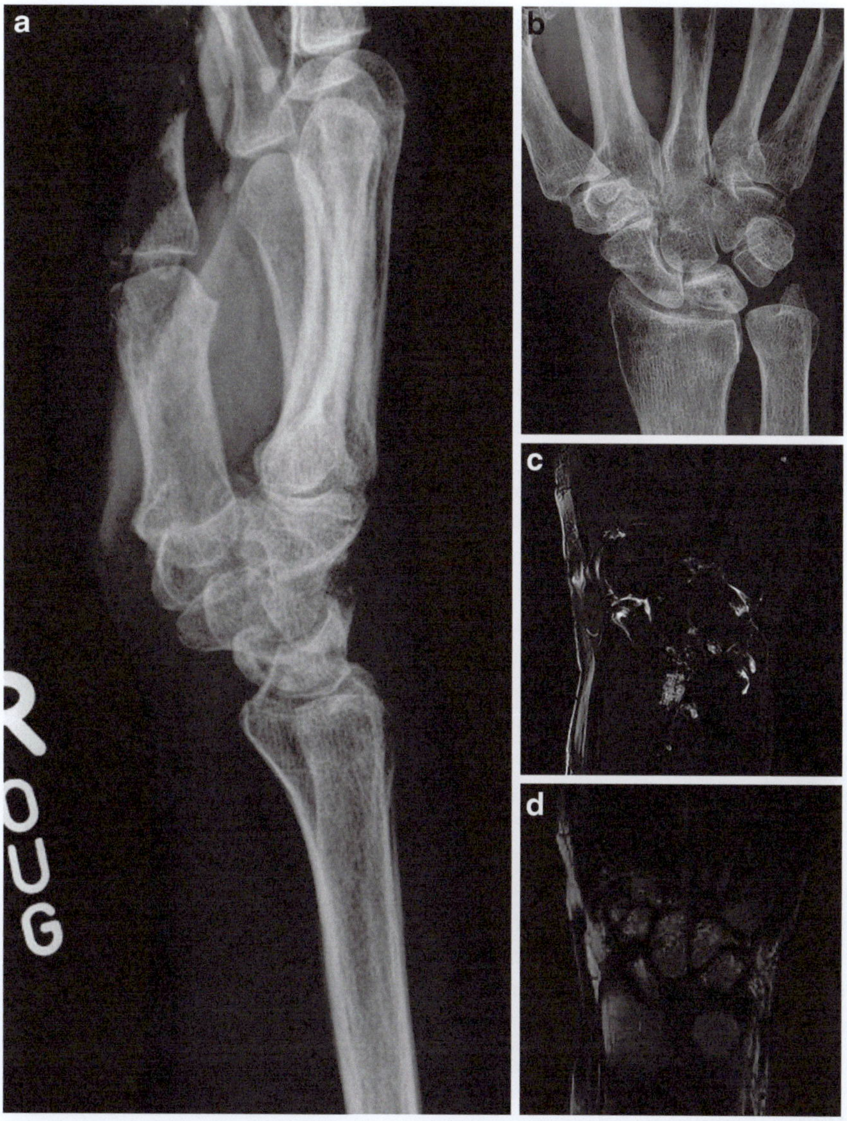

**Fig. 9.11** (**a**) Lateral radiograph of a 68-year-old female with Kienböck's disease, showing sclerosis with cystic changes of the lunate. (**b**) This PA wrist radiograph of the same patient shows evidence of pancarpal arthritis, with lunate sclerosis and collapse consistent with Kienböck's disease. There are cystic changes at the distal radius as well. (**c**) T2-weighted MRI of the same patient showing synovitis, as well as a large cyst in the ulnar aspect of the distal radius and distinct fracture line within the lunate. (**d**) T1-weighted MRI of the same patient showing decreased signal in the lunate, as well as decreased signal in the ulnar distal radius, correlating with the subchondral cyst noted on other imaging studies

T2-weighted MRI sequences (see Fig. 9.11c, d) suggest stage IIIA Kienböck's disease. After the likely course of the disease was explained, the patient elected to continue nonoperative treatment.

The natural history of Kienböck's disease in the elderly differs in many ways from that of younger adults and juveniles. As part of the initial evaluation of Kienböck's disease in the elderly, it is worth exploring the possibility of other causal conditions, such as inflammatory arthritis, autoimmune disorders, and/or osteoporosis. Since most elderly patients do well despite progression to stage IV disease, nonoperative treatment is usually sufficient. For unresponsive patients, radial shortening osteotomy, proximal row carpectomy, synovectomy or wrist arthrodesis may be considered, depending on the extent of joint destruction and pain.

## Conclusion

Kienböck's disease is an uncommon but important cause of wrist pain in children, adults, and the elderly. The natural history of the disorder, as determined by progressive structural changes seen on standard X-rays, is the basis of the classification system commonly used for selecting individualized treatment protocols. Unfortunately, major gaps still exist in our understanding of the natural history the disorder. These gaps in our knowledge relate to the pathogenesis, non-osseous structural changes, pathokinematics, and revascularization potential of the avascular lunate. Fortunately, there is much research ongoing in all of these areas. Hopefully, the findings will lead to a better understanding of the disorder in all age groups and will enable surgeons to create evidence-based treatment algorithms that are attuned to every patient's needs. Other chapters in this book delineate some of the most important ongoing research. The concluding chapter attempts to show how the latest information can be used to create a more nuanced and dependable algorithm.

## References


1. Lichtman DM, Mack GR, MacDonald RI, Gunther SF, Wilson JN. Kienböck's disease: the role of silicone replacement arthroplasty. J Bone Joint Surg Am. 1977;59(7):899–908.
2. Lichtman DM, Degnan GG. Staging and its use in the determination of treatment modalities for Kienböck's disease. Hand Clin. 1993;9(3):409–16.
3. Ståhl F. On lunatomalacia (Kienböck's disease): a clinical and roentgenological study, especially on its pathogenesis and late results of immobilization treatment. Acta Chir Scand. 1947;126(Suppl):1–133.
4. Decoulx P, Marchand M, Minet P, Razemon JP. La maladie de Kienböck chez le mineur: etude clinique et pathogenique avec analyse de 1330 radios du poignet. Lille Chir. 1957;12:65–81.
5. Fontaine C. Kienböck's disease. Chir Main. 2015;34(1):4–17.
6. Morgan RF, McCue 3rd FC. Bilateral Kienböck's disease. J Hand Surg Am. 1983;8(6):928–32.
7. Seah KT, McEachan J, Davidson D. Bilateral Kienböck's disease in association with type 1 diabetes. J Hand Surg Eur Vol. 2012;37(7):697–8.
8. Cross D, Matullo KS. Kienböck disease. Orthop Clin North Am. 2014;45(1):141–52.
9. Lichtman D. The wrist and its disorders. 1st ed. Philadelphia, PA: Saunders; 1997.
10. Lutsky K, Beredjiklian PK. Kienböck disease. J Hand Surg Am. 2012;37(9):1942–52.
11. Goldfarb CA, Hsu J, Gelberman RH, Boyer MI. The Lichtman classification for Kienböck's disease: an assessment of reliability. J Hand Surg Am. 2003;28(1): 74–80.
12. Schmitt R, Krimmer H. Osteonecrosis of the hand skeleton. In: Schmitt R, Lanz U, editors. Diagnostic imaging of the hand. 1st ed. Stuttgart, NY: Georg Thieme Verlag; 2007. p. 351–64.
13. Bain GI, Begg M. Arthroscopic assessment and classification of Kienböck's disease. Tech Hand Up Extrem Surg. 2006;10:8–13.
14. Lichtman DM, Lesley NE, Simmons SP. The classification and treatment of Kienböck's disease: the state of the art and a look at the future. J Hand Surg Eur Vol. 2010;35(7):549–54.
15. Arco News. Association research circulation osseous (ARCO): committee on terminology and classification. ARCO News. 1992;4:41–6.
16. Keith PP, Nuttall D, Trail I. Long-term outcome of nonsurgically managed Kienböck's disease. J Hand Surg Am. 2004;29(1):63–7.
17. Salmon J, Stanley JK, Trail IA. Kienböck's disease: conservative management versus radial shortening. J Bone Joint Surg Br. 2000;82(6):820–3.
18. Beckenbaugh RD, Shives TC, Dobyns JH, Linscheid RL. Kienböck's disease: the natural history of Kienböck's disease and consideration of lunate fractures. Clin Orthop Relat Res. 1980;(149): 98–106.
19. Kristensen SS, Thomassen E, Christensen F. Kienböck's disease--late results by non-surgical treatment. A follow-up study. J Hand Surg Br. 1986;11(3):422–5.
20. Fujisawa K, Hirata H, Tomita Y, Higuchi Y, Morita A, Matsumoto M. Long-term follow up of patients with conservatively treated Kienböck's disease. J Orthop Sci. 1996;1(3):182–6.
21. Stahl S, Hentschel PJ, Held M, Manoli T, Meisner C, Schaller HE, et al. Characteristic features and natural evolution of Kienböck's disease: five years' results of a prospective case series and retrospective case series of 106 patients. J Plast Reconstr Aesthet Surg. 2014;67(10):1415–26.
22. Viljakka T, Tallroth K, Vastamäki M. Long-term natural outcome (7-26 years) of Lichtman stage III Kienböck's lunatomalacia. Scand J Surg. 2016;105:125.
23. Irisarri C, Kalb K, Ribak S. Infantile and juvenile lunatomalacia. J Hand Surg Eur Vol. 2010;35(7):544–8.

24. Ferlic RJ, Lee DH, Lopez-Ben RR. Pediatric Kienböck's disease: case report and review of the literature. Clin Orthop Relat Res. 2003;(408): 237–44.
25. Kim T, Culp R, Osterman A, Bednar J. Kienböck's disease in children. Jefferson Orthopedic J. 1997;25: 53–7.
26. Kazuki K, Uemura T, Okada M, Egi T. Time course of magnetic resonance images in an adolescent patient with Kienböck's disease treated by temporary scapho-trapezoidal joint fixation: a case report. J Hand Surg Am. 2006;31(1):63–7.
27. Matsuhashi T, Iwasaki N, Oizumi N, Kato H, Minami M, Minami A. Radial overgrowth after radial shortening osteotomies for skeletally immature patients with Kienböck's disease. J Hand Surg Am. 2009;34(7): 1242–7.
28. Ando Y, Yasuda M, Kazuki K, Hidaka N, Yoshinaka Y. Temporary scaphotrapezoidal joint fixation for adolescent Kienböck's disease. J Hand Surg Am. 2009;34(1):14–9.
29. Jorge-Mora A, Pretell-Mazzini J, Marti-Ciruelos R, Andres-Esteban EM, Curto de la Mano A. Distal radius definitive epiphysiodesis for management of Kienböck's disease in skeletally immature patients. Int Orthop. 2012;36(10):2101–5.
30. Shigematsu K, Yajima H, Kobata Y, Kawamura K, Nakanishi Y, Takakura Y. Treatment of Kienböck disease in an 11-year-old girl with temporary fixation of the scaphotrapeziotrapezoidal joint. Scand J Plast Reconstr Surg Hand Surg. 2005;39(1):60–3.
31. Yasuda M, Okuda H, Egi T, Guidera PM. Temporary scapho-trapezoidal joint fixation for Kienböck's disease in a 12-year-old girl: a case report. J Hand Surg Am. 1998;23(3):411–4.
32. Geutjens GG. Kienböck's disease in an elderly patient. J Hand Surg Am. 1995;20(1):42–3.
33. Taniguchi Y, Yoshida M, Iwasaki H, Otakara H, Iwata S. Kienböck's disease in elderly patients. J Hand Surg Am. 2003;28(5):779–83.
34. Yoshida T, Tada K, Yamamoto K, Shibata T, Shimada K, Kawai H. Aged-onset Kienböck's disease. Arch Orthop Trauma Surg. 1990;109(5):241–6.
35. Giunta R, Lower N, Wilhelm K, Keirse R, Rock C, Muller-Gerbl M. Altered patterns of subchondral bone mineralization in Kienböck's disease. J Hand Surg Br. 1997;22(1):16–20.
36. Thomas AA, Rodriguez E, Segalman K. Kienböck's disease in an elderly patient treated with proximal row carpectomy. J Hand Surg Am. 2004;29(4): 685–8.
37. Youm Y, McMurthy RY, Flatt AE, Gillespie TE. Kinematics of the wrist. I. An experimental study of radial-ulnar deviation and flexion-extension. J Bone Joint Surg Am. 1978;60(4):423–31.
38. Gelberman RH, Salamon PB, Jurist JM, Posch JL. Ulnar variance in Kienböck's disease. J Bone Joint Surg Am. 1975;57(5):674–6.

# 10 Basic Imaging and Differential Diagnosis of Kienböck's Disease

Lee Wang, Michael B. Zlatkin, and Paul D. Clifford

Robert Kienböck's 1910 publication "Concerning traumatic malacia of the lunate and its consequences" represents one of the earliest applications of radiography to clinical diagnosis [1, 2]. While others before him reported similar anatomic findings in cadaveric specimens, Robert Kienböck was the first to relate imaging findings to clinical symptomatology. He described the radiographic findings of sclerosis and collapse of the lunate with relative sparing of the other bones of the hand in patients presenting with chronic wrist pain [2].

L. Wang, MD
Department of Radiology, University of Miami Miller School of Medicine, 1611 NW 12th Avenue, WW-279, Miami, FL 33136, USA

M.B. Zlatkin, MD, FRCP(C) (✉)
Nationalrad, 1930 N. Commerce Parkway, Suite 5, Weston, FL 33326, USA

Department of Diagnostic Radiology, University of Miami Miller School of Medicine, 1611 NW 12th Avenue, WW-279, Miami, FL 33136-1005, USA
e-mail: mzlatkin@nationalrad.com

P.D. Clifford, MD
Department of Diagnostic Radiology, University of Miami Miller School of Medicine, 1611 NW 12th Avenue, WW-279, Miami, FL 33136-1005, USA

6767 Collins Avenue, Apt. 1802, Miami Beach, FL 33141, USA

Diagnosis has often been delayed in this disease, and the average duration of symptoms prior to diagnosis has been stated to be 1–2 years [3, 4]. Predisposing factors include a vulnerable blood supply, a fixed position of the lunate within the wrist, and the presence of a short ulna.

Even with the passage of time, imaging remains central to the evaluation of Kienböck's disease. With the advent of advanced imaging modalities, including MRI, a more detailed assessment can be made, including diagnosis and staging of Kienböck's disease, While our understanding of the disease process is incomplete, various staging classifications have been created which reflect the natural progression of the disease. The most widely used is a four-stage classification system proposed by Lichtman et al. in 1977 [5]. This system is a modified version of one proposed by Stahl in 1947 [6] and was tailored to guide the selection of treatment options. A number of studies have shown the Lichtman classification to have high inter-observer reliability and reproducibility [3, 7, 8]. It is important to recognize that the Lichtman classification is an assessment of the osseous morphological characteristics of the disease based on imaging examination. Other factors such as vascularity, cartilage integrity, and the morphology of the remainder of the wrist are also important. Patient factors such as functionality, age of the patient, and occupation often must be considered when weighing potential interventions.

© Springer International Publishing Switzerland 2016

D.M. Lichtman, G.I. Bain (eds.), *Kienböck's Disease*, DOI 10.1007/978-3-319-34226-9_10

## Imaging Modalities

### Radiography

The radiological evaluation of a patient with potential Kienböck's disease typically begins with plain radiography. At minimum, three views of the wrist should be obtained in the lateral, 45° oblique, and posteroanterior projection. A standardized set of radiographs will provide a more reproducible image and assessment of ulnar variance. The patient's arm should be in the neutral position—the shoulder abducted at 90°, elbow flexed at 90° with the forearm in neutral rotation. Pronation and supination will increase or decrease ulnar variance, respectively [9, 10]. The axis of the long finger is aligned with the axis of the forearm as radial and ulnar deviation can alter the radiolunocapitate alignment. Well-positioned radiographs are often sufficient to detect lunate fractures, sclerosis, or collapse and may be the only imaging needed for osseous staging of Kienböck's disease.

### Computed Tomography

Computed tomography (CT) is best suited for evaluating the extent of osseous necrosis and trabecular disruption. CT will also demonstrate coronal fractures through the lunate and fragmentation, which may not be seen with radiography. Quenzer reported that the plain radiographs often underscored the severity of the osseous involvement, and that it was common for the wrist to be reclassified after performing a CT scan [11].

### Nuclear Scintigraphy

Prior to the advent of MRI, nuclear scintigraphy frequently followed radiographic evaluation of early Kienböck's disease. Technetium scans applied in this manner are challenging to interpret, in many cases appearing as nonspecific increased radio-isotope uptake. MRI has proven more valuable than scintigraphy for the evaluation of Kienböck's disease as MRI provides better anatomic correlation and higher specificity.

### Magnetic Resonance Imaging

Magnetic resonance imaging (MRI) is most beneficial for the evaluation of early Kienböck's disease at a stage when plain film and CT can be unrevealing. The ability of MRI to detect early disease is valuable as revascularization is often possible [12]. For patients in which revascularization is achieved, a restoration of normal MRI findings can be identified [13, 14]. In established Kienböck's disease, MRI is helpful to detect subchondral collapse and the integrity of the cartilage over the proximal and mid-carpal rows, which may alter surgical management. The Bain and Begg articular cartilage classification was developed from wrist arthroscopy, but MRI can be utilized for grading of the Kienböck's disease [15].

MRI is also suited for the exclusion of other etiologies of patients' chronic wrist pain. Furthermore, MRI may evaluate response to treatment in this disease, and T2-weighted images may be helpful in determining revascularization. Favorable prognostic signs on T2-weighted MR images for revascularization include a focal area of increased signal within bone that manifests diffuse decreased signal and a return to normal or increased marrow signal on T2-weighted images [16, 17].

Studies have shown that functional evaluation may be performed with contrast-enhanced MRI and is complementary to morphologic evaluation, helping to guide treatment in some stages. Further discussion of contrast-enhanced MRI is the subject of a later chapter.

## Wrist Measurements

There are particular measurements, which are important when evaluating radiographs of the wrist. It is important to note the presence or

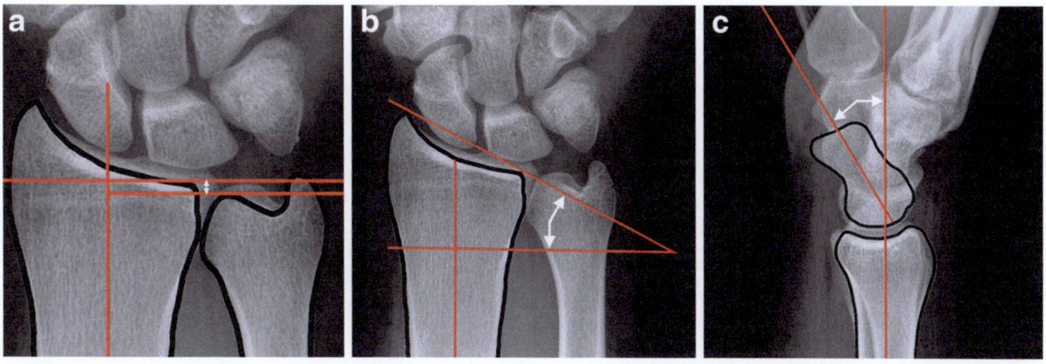


**Fig. 10.1** Wrist measurements. (**a**) Ulnar variance is the distance between two lines which are perpendicular to the long axis of the radius, one drawn through the distal ulnar cortex and the second through the ulnar aspect of the distal radius. Normal ulnar variance is less than or equal to 2 mm. (**b**) Radial inclination is the angle between a line connecting the radial styloid tip to the ulnar aspect of the radius and a line perpendicular to the long axis of the radius. Normal radial inclination is 16–28°. (**c**) Radioscaphoid angle is the angle formed between the long axis of the radius and the long axis of the scaphoid on lateral view. Normal radioscaphoid angle is 30–60°

absence of particular anatomic variants as these may predispose patients to the development of Kienböck's disease. In some cases, the presence of these anatomic variants themselves may prove the basis for or the target of subsequent therapeutic intervention.

Ulnar variance is the distance between two lines which are perpendicular to the long axis of the radius, one passing through the ulnar aspect of the distal radius and a second passing through the distal ulnar cortex (Fig. 10.1a). Negative ulnar variance has been shown to be present in 78% of cases of Kienböck's disease [18]. The term negative ulnar variance denotes an abnormally shortened ulna in comparison to the radius with the variance greater than 2 mm. A number of studies have investigated procedures that normalize ulnar variance with the goal of unloading excessive forces from the lunate [19–24].

A smaller lunate size has been associated with Kienböck's disease [25]. Radiographic measurement of lunate size is usually performed on the posteroanterior view. The relevant measurements are lunate diameter and lunate height with the baseline being the line extending from the ulnar tip to the radial tip of the distal facet. We believe that this measurement has limited clinical value, however, as there are no reference ranges available.

Radial inclination is defined as the angle between a line from the radial styloid to the ulnar aspect of the carpal surface of the radius and a line perpendicular to the long axis of the radius (see Fig. 10.1b). Normal radial inclination is between 16 and 28°. A steeper angle of radial inclinations has been associated with Kienböck's disease [25]. There have been studies that report favorable outcomes with decreasing radial inclination through radial wedge osteotomies [26–28].

The radioscaphoid angle was selected as the key parameter for assessing carpal alignment in Kienböck's disease due to the fact that measurement of the angle does not involve the diseased lunate which may otherwise affect interobserver reliability [3]. The radioscaphoid angle is defined as the angle between the axis of the radius and the axis of the scaphoid on a lateral radiograph (see Fig. 10.1c) with normal range of 30–60° [29]. In addition to the standard radiographs, stress films can prove useful for identification of carpal instability.

## Diagnosis and Classification

A defined set of criteria for the radiological diagnosis of Kienböck's disease is not easily described. The diagnostic features of Kienböck's

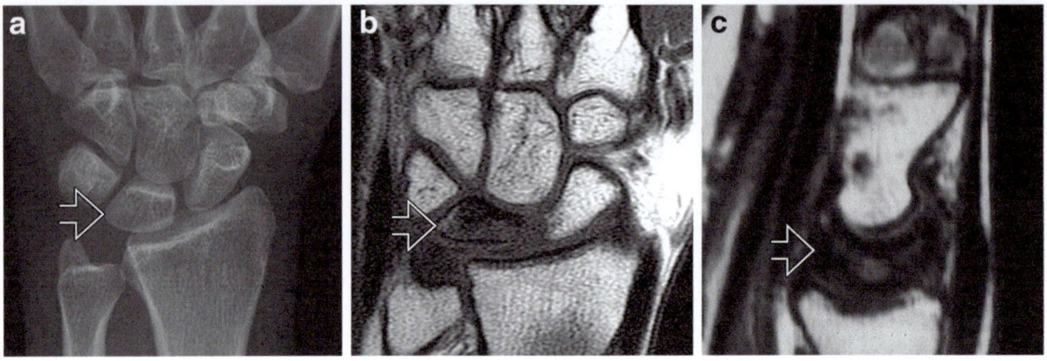

**Fig. 10.2** Stage I Kienböck's disease. (**a**) Radiograph shows normal appearance of the lunate (*arrow*). There is an ulnar-negative variancce. Coronal (**b**) and sagittal (**c**) (separate patient) T1-weighted MR images show decreased signal intensity throughout the lunate (*arrows*)

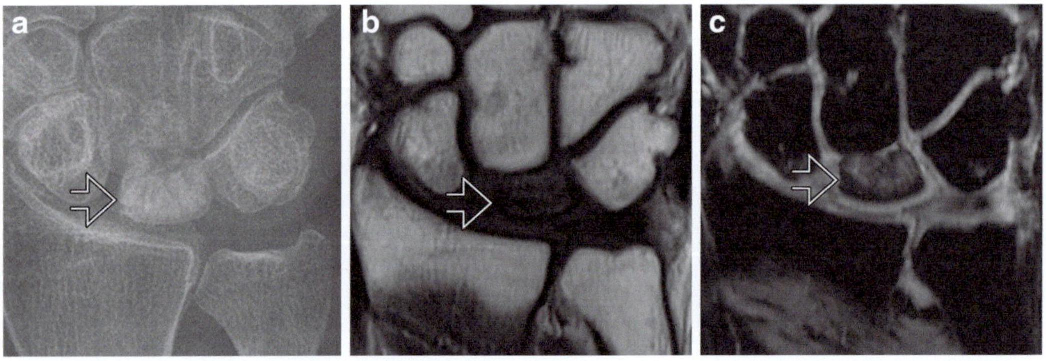

**Fig. 10.3** Stage II Kienböck's disease. (**a**) Radiograph shows increase in density of the lunate (*arrow*). (**b**) Coronal T1-weighted MR image shows decreased signal intensity throughout the lunate (*arrow*). Size and shape of the lunate are preserved. (**c**) Coronal T2-weighted fat-suppressed MR image shows increased signal intensity in the lunate (*arrow*)

disease however are better stratified based on their sequential appearance in the course of the disease. In this manner, the four-stage classification system proposed by Lichtman et al. [5] can serve as a framework for both the diagnosis and classification of Kienböck's disease.

In stage I of Kienböck's disease, radiography and CT demonstrate normal morphology and density of the lunate (Fig. 10.2a). In some cases, a linear or compressive fracture may be appreciated. MRI, however, will be positive at this stage of disease, and typically demonstrates uniformly decreased signal on T1- and T2-weighted sequences [30] (see Fig. 10.2b, c). Less commonly, marrow edema results in increased signal on T2-weighted sequences accompanied by decreased signal on T1-weighted sequences [31]. Relative increased signal on T2-weighted images may indicate residual vascularity and a better prognosis [32].

In stage II, the lunate appears sclerotic with increased density on both radiographs and CT while the morphology of the lunate is largely preserved (Fig. 10.3a). When compared to radiography, CT better demonstrates sclerosis as well as the pseudocystic inclusions which are commonly present at this stage [33]. On MRI, the lunate will exhibit low signal on T1-weighted sequences and variable signal on T2-weighted sequences with areas of low signal on T2-weighted sequences denoting areas of sclerosis (see Fig. 10.3b, c). Signal changes are often greatest at the radial

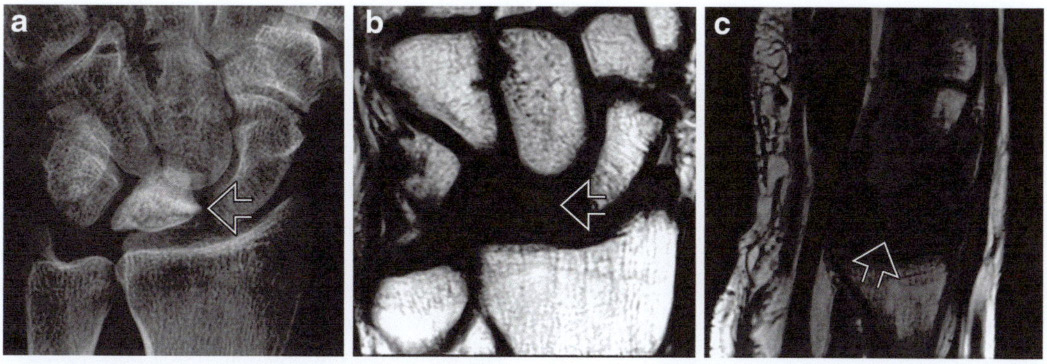


**Fig. 10.4** Stage III Kienböck's disease. (**a**) Radiograph shows lunate sclerosis and collapse (*arrow*). (**b**) Coronal T1-weighted MR image shows decreased signal intensity, flattening, and loss of height of the lunate (*arrow*). (**c**) Sagittal proton density-weighted MR image shows a coronal fracture of the lunate, along with flattening and loss of height (*arrow*)

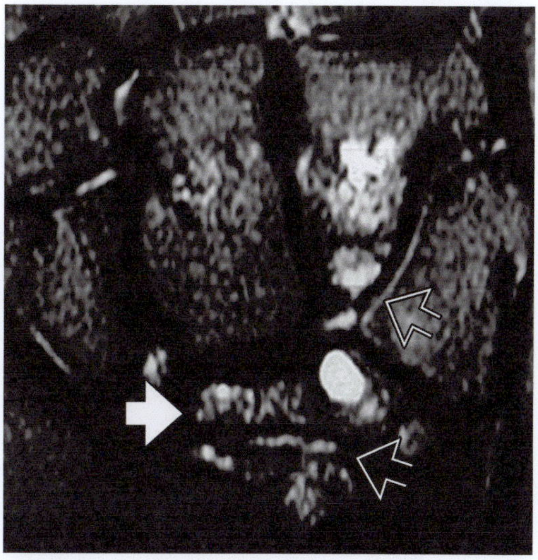

**Fig. 10.5** Stage IV Kienböck's disease. Coronal T2-weighted MRI image revealing lunate collapse (*solid arrow*), with secondary degenerative arthrosis in the radiocarpal and midcarpal joint compartments (*open arrow*)

aspect of lunate, reflecting the propensity of the disease to manifest earliest at this location. Rarely, subtle articular radial surface collapse of the lunate may be seen.

Lunate collapse signifies progression to stage III disease, which is subdivided into stage IIIA and stage IIIB depending on carpal alignment. In stage IIIA, there is lunate sclerosis and collapse with normal carpal alignment (Fig. 10.4a). Under these conditions, the continuity of the proximal row carpals allows for redirection of forces through the scaphoid, thereby alleviating transmission of forces through the lunate [34]. In stage IIIB, there is carpal collapse with abnormal carpal alignment, specifically a radioscaphoid angle of greater than 60° as seen on sagittal projections. Whereas stage I, II, and IIIA may be treated with techniques aimed at revascularization, treatment of stage IIIB must address the carpal instability as its persistence results in accelerated lunate collapse and progression to stage IV disease. Other imaging findings associated with carpal instability include proximal migration of the capitate and ulnar deviation of the triquetrum. A dorsal intercalated segmental instability pattern may also be seen.

MRI of stage III disease demonstrates low signal on T1-weighted sequences and variable signal on T2- and proton density-weighted sequences with high signal usually representing revascularization or granulation tissue (see Fig. 10.4b, c). In stage IIIB, scapholunate dissociation is sometimes seen, and, if so, derangement of the scapholunate ligament can be directly visualized on MRI exam.

Stage IV is characterized by lunate collapse with intra-articular degenerative changes at the midcarpal joint, radiocarpal joint, or both. MRI demonstrates chondral loss, articular collapse, and reactive changes in the midcarpal and radiocarpal articulations (Fig. 10.5). There may be adjacent reactive synovitis and joint effusion. The findings are similar to those seen with scapholunate dissociation advanced collapse (SLAC) and scaphoid nonunion advanced collapse (SNAC). To highlight these similarities, Lichtman et al. coined the term Kienböck's disease advanced collapse (KDAC) [31].

## Differential Diagnosis

Many of the features of Kienböck's disease may overlap with other pathological entities. The most common considerations will be discussed here. In some cases, only a fraction of the lunate may be involved, representing a diagnostic challenge as some other disease processes such as intraosseous ganglia and osteochondral injuries may exhibit a similar appearance. Sagittal sequences usually provide the best evaluation in these cases. Typically, Kienböck's disease may be suggested if abnormal signal changes are present in at least half the lunate. It should be noted however that the extent of involvement can be overestimated since abnormal marrow signal can also be due to reactive granulation tissue and marrow edema. This can be accentuated on fat-saturated T2-weighted images and STIR images.

## Intraosseous Ganglion Cyst

While cysts of the carpal bones are common, an isolated intraosseous ganglion cyst of the lunate presenting with pain is a relatively rare occurrence [35]. Ganglion cysts may occur at any age but most frequently are seen in the second through fourth decades of life. It is thought that these benign lesions occur due to mucoid degeneration of intraosseous connective tissue or synovial herniation into the underlying bone [36, 37]. On radiographs, the lesions appear as round lucencies at the radial aspect or distal ulnar aspect of the lunate, communicating with the scapholunate or lunotriquetral joint space, respectively. MRI demonstrates a round lesion with low signal on T1-weighted sequences and high signal on T2-weighted sequences (Fig. 10.6). There may be surrounding marrow edema, which appears hyper-intense on T2-weighted sequences as well.

## Ulnar Carpal Impaction Syndrome

Ulnar carpal impaction syndrome is a degenerative condition caused by impaction of the ulnar head with the ulnar-sided carpal bones. The abnormal biomechanical forces result in

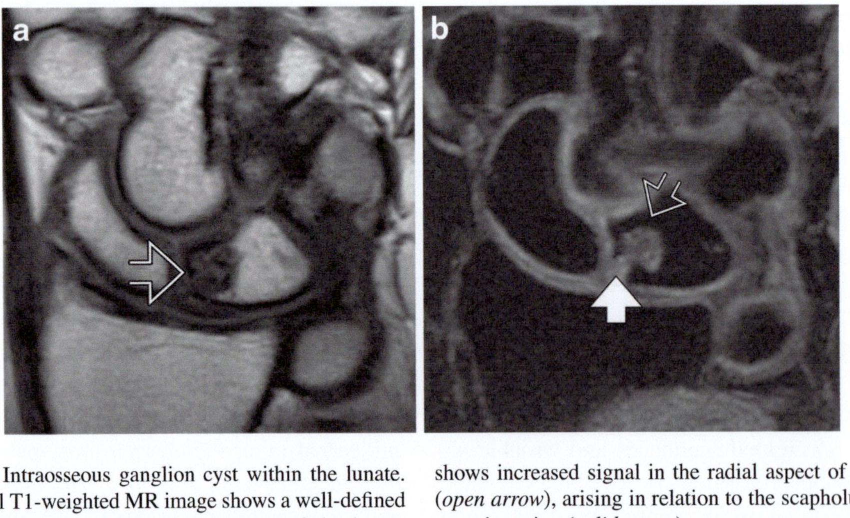


**Fig. 10.6** Intraosseous ganglion cyst within the lunate. (**a**) Coronal T1-weighted MR image shows a well-defined area of hypointensity in the radial aspect of the lunate (*arrow*). (**b**) Coronal T2-weighted fat-suppressed image shows increased signal in the radial aspect of the lunate (*open arrow*), arising in relation to the scapholunate ligament insertion (*solid arrow*)

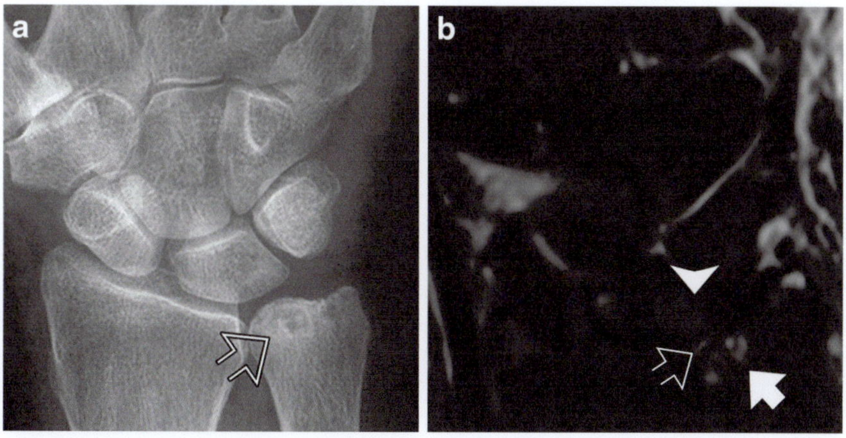


**Fig. 10.7** Ulnar-carpal impaction syndrome, advanced stage (**a**) Radiograph shows positive ulnar variance with cystic changes in the distal ulna (*arrow*). (**b**) Coronal STIR MR image reveals cystic change in the distal ulna (*solid arrow*) as well as chondral loss. There is a large central defect of the TFCC (*open arrow*), and edema along the inferior medial aspect of the lunate bone (*arrowhead*). There is cystic change in the triquetrum and ulnar styloid as well. There is a positive ulnar variance

degeneration of the triangular fibrocartilage disc and chondromalacia overlying the involved osseous structures [38]. The major predisposing factor for ulnar carpal impaction syndrome is positive ulnar variance. In contrast, Kienböck's disease is more commonly associated with ulnar-negative variance. Positive ulnar variance causes abnormal rotational forces and impaction, which leads to attrition and thinning of the TFCC [39]. Radiography demonstrates subchondral sclerosis and cystic changes in the ulnar head (Fig. 10.7a). Similar degenerative changes in the ulnar aspect of the lunate and triquetrum can be seen with advanced disease (see Fig. 10.7b). On MRI, the TFC disc is thinned and often torn, and there is chondromalacia along the ulnar head, lunate, and triquetrum. The key features which distinguish this entity from Kienböck's disease are the association with positive ulnar variance, involvement of the ulnar head, and the predilection for the more inferior ulnar aspect of the lunate rather than its entirety [40].

## Acute Fracture or Contusion

Acute fracture or contusion of the lunate can appear identical to stage I Kienböck's disease on initial imaging. Traumatic lunate fractures are rare, comprising approximately 0.5–1 % of all carpal bone fractures [41]. An acute fracture may appear as a lucent line on radiography and as a hypointense line on T1-weighted MRI sequences. T2-weighted sequences can demonstrate diffuse hyperintensity of the lunate. Marrow contusions are a more common occurrence than fracture and a pattern of diffuse hyperintensity reflective of marrow edema will be seen (Fig. 10.8). In some contusions the typical low signal that may be seen in Kienböck's disease, which is usually the result of fibrosis and/or sclerosis may not be present, and this can at times be a helpful differentiating feature.

Clinical history is important. Fracture or contusion is identified in the setting of acute trauma, and can be associated with carpal dislocation, as a translunate perilunate dislocation [42]. On the other hand, Kienböck's disease is thought to potentially arise from repetitive or chronic forces in anatomically susceptible wrists [31]. Moreover, the signal abnormality on T2-weighted sequences usually resolves with proper immobilization and healing after trauma.

## Arthritis

Arthritides such as rheumatoid arthritis, gout, and posttraumatic arthritis can result in signal changes in the osseous structures of the wrist,

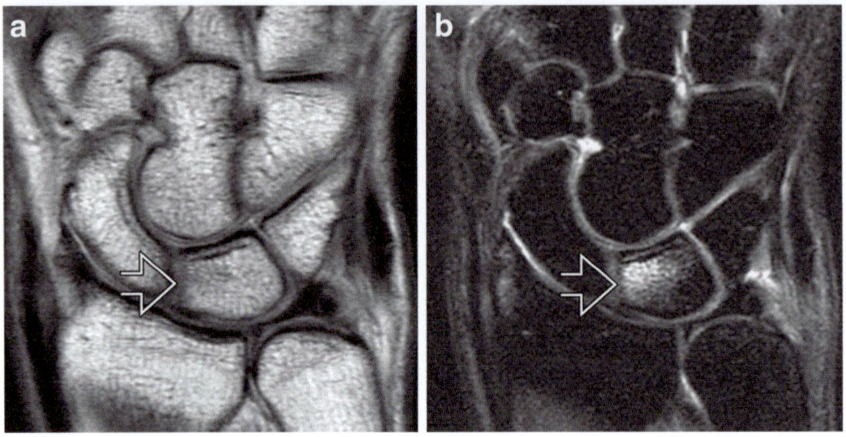


**Fig. 10.8** Lunate contusion. (**a**) Coronal T1-weighted MR image shows only subtle hypointensity in the lunate (*arrow*). (**b**) Coronal T2-weighted fat-suppressed MR image shows relatively diffuse increased signal in the lunate (*arrow*)

mimicking Kienböck's disease. In contrast to Kienböck's disease, these disorders often involve multiple carpal bones and other joints and are associated with a different patient population. However, there can be overlap between the two disease entities as secondary degenerative arthritis is a late-stage manifestation of Kienböck's disease.

## Osteoid Osteoma

Osteoid osteomas are benign osteoblastic neoplasms which typically occur in children and young adults with male-to-female ratio of 2:1 [43, 44]. While the majority of osteoid osteomas occur in the long bones, carpal bone involvement is rare with most published literature on the subject being in the form of isolated case reports [45–49]. Patients with carpal bone involvement present with wrist pain that is usually worse at night and is relieved by aspirin or nonsteroidal anti-inflammatory medications. Unfortunately, the nonspecific nature of the symptoms and low index of suspicion can lead to delayed or incorrect diagnoses. Radiographs demonstrate dense sclerosis and cortical thickening of the affected bone. In some cases, a radiolucent nidus can be seen on radiographs with or without a central sclerotic dot. On MRI, reactive sclerosis and marrow edema are dominant features whereas the nidus is often imperceptible, resulting in an appearance that could potentially be mistaken for Kienböck's disease when the lunate is affected. CT is best suited for demonstrating the radiolucent nidus and central sclerotic dot and is the modality of choice for distinguishing between Kienböck's disease and osteoid osteoma.

## Enchondroma

Enchondromas are benign medullary cartilaginous neoplasms usually found in small tubular bones [50]. In the hand, enchondromas are most common in the phalanges and metacarpals but can rarely appear in the carpal bones [50]. Enchondromas are typically easy to distinguish from Kienböck's disease on radiography and CT, but may sometimes be challenging on MRI. These lesions appear as radiolucent areas in the lunate, which are often well demarcated. They are associated with mild bony expansion, endosteal resorption, and cortical thinning. While uncommon, sclerosis can be seen in cases of pathological fracture. On MRI, the lesions are hypointense on T1-weighted sequences and may have a more lobulated hyperintensity on T2-weighted sequences with low-signal chondroid calcification within.

## Conclusion

Imaging is of significant benefit for the diagnosis, staging, and treatment planning of Kienböck's disease. The imaging-based classification system developed by Lichtman et al. serves as a reliable, reproducible framework for both the diagnosis and characterization of Kienböck's disease. While radiography remains the most common imaging modality for diagnosis, supplemental imaging findings from computed tomography and magnetic resonance imaging have been incorporated into the classification system to allow more accurate staging and comprehensive treatment planning. MRI examination is also of significant benefit in early diagnosis, determining the presence of revascularization, and for following patients after treatment.

## References

1. Chochole M. Robert Kienbock: the man and his work. J Hand Surg Eur Vol. 2010;35(7):534–7.
2. Peltier LF. The classic. Concerning traumatic malacia of the lunate and its consequences: degeneration and compression fractures. Privatdozent Dr. Robert Kienbock. Clin Orthop Relat Res 1980; (149):4–8.
3. Goldfarb CA, Hsu J, Gelberman RH, Boyer MI. The Lichtman classification for Kienbock's disease: an assessment of reliability. J Hand Surg Am. 2003; 28(1):74–80.
4. Amadio PC, Hanssen AD, Berquist TH. The genesis of Kienbock's disease: evaluation of a case by magnetic resonance imaging. J Hand Surg Am. 1987; 12(6):1044–9.
5. Lichtman DM, Mack GR, MacDonald RI, Gunther SF, Wilson JN. Kienbock's disease: the role of silicone replacement arthroplasty. J Bone Joint Surg Am. 1977;59(7):899–908.
6. Stahl F. On lunatomalacia (Kienbock's disease). A clinical and roentgenological study, especially on its pathogenesis and the late results of immobilization treatment. Acta Chir Scand. 1947;95(126):120–33.
7. Goeminne S, Degreef I, De Smet L. Reliability and reproducibility of Kienbock's disease staging. J Hand Surg Eur Vol. 2010;35(7):555–7.
8. Jafarnia K, Collins ED, Kohl 3rd HW, Bennett JB, Ilahi OA. Reliability of the Lichtman classification of Kienbock's disease. J Hand Surg Am. 2000;25(3): 529–34.
9. Yeh GL, Beredjiklian PK, Katz MA, Steinberg DR, Bozentka DJ. Effects of forearm rotation on the clinical evaluation of ulnar variance. J Hand Surg Am. 2001;26(6):1042–6.
10. Quigley RJ, Robicheaux GW, Lee TQ. The proximal and distal position of the radius relative to the ulna through a full range of elbow flexion and forearm rotation. J Hand Surg Eur Vol. 2013;39(5):535–40.
11. Quenzer DE, Linscheid, RL, Vidal MA, Dobyns JH, Beckenbaugh, RD, Cooney WP. Trispiral Tomographic Staging of Kienbock's Disease. J Hand Surg Am. 1997;22(3):396–403.
12. Schuind F, Eslami S, Ledoux P. Kienbock's disease. J Bone Joint Surg Br. 2008;90(2):133–9.
13. Afshar A. Lunate revascularization after capitate shortening osteotomy in Kienbock's disease. J Hand Surg Am. 2010;35(12):1943–6.
14. Nakamura R, Watanabe K, Tsunoda K, Miura T. Radial osteotomy for Kienbock's disease evaluated by magnetic resonance imaging. 24 cases followed for 1-3 years. Acta Orthop Scand. 1993;64(2):207–11.
15. Bain GI, Durrant A. An Articular-based Approach to Kienbock Avascular Necrosis of the Lunate. Techniques in Hand & Upper Extremity Surgery. 2011;15(1):41–7.
16. Imaeda T, Nakamura R, Miura T, Makino N. Magnetic resonance imaging in Kienbock's disease. J Hand Surg Br. 1992;17(1):12–9.
17. Viegas SF, Amparo E. Magnetic resonance imaging in the assessment of revascularization in Kienbock's disease. A preliminary report. Orthop Rev. 1989; 18(12):1285–8.
18. Hn O. Uber anatomische variationen der handgelenkknochen. Acta Radiol Scand. 1928;9:155–68.
19. Horii E, Garcia-Elias M, Bishop AT, Cooney WP, Linscheid RL, Chao EY. Effect on force transmission across the carpus in procedures used to treat Kienböck's disease. J Hand Surg Am. 1990;15(3):393–400.
20. Trumble T, Glisson R, Seaber AV, Urbaniak JR. A biomechanical comparison of the methods for treating Kienböck's disease. J Hand Surg Am. 1986;11(1): 88–93.
21. Masear VR, Zook EG, Pichora DR, Krishnamurthy M, Russell RC, Lemons J, et al. Strain-gauge evaluation of lunate unloading procedures. J Hand Surg Am. 1992;17(3):437–43.
22. Werner FW, Palmer AK. Biomechanical evaluation of operative procedures to treat Kienböck's disease. Hand Clin. 1993;9(3):431–43.
23. Werner FW, Palmer A, Fortino MD, Short WH. Force transmission through the distal ulna: effect of ulnar variance, lunate fossa angulation, and radial and palmar tilt of the distal radius. J Hand Surg Am. 1992;17(3):423–8.
24. Matsui Y, Funakoshi T, Motomiya M, Urita A, Minami M, Iwasaki N. Radial shortening osteotomy for Kienbock disease: minimum 10-year follow-up. J Hand Surg Am. 2014;39(4):679–85.
25. Tsuge S, Nakamura R. Anatomical risk factors for Kienbock's disease. J Hand Surg Br. 1993;18(1):70–5.
26. Iwasaki N, Minami A, Oizumi N, Suenaga N, Kato H, Minami M. Radial osteotomy for late-stage Kienbock's disease. Wedge osteotomy versus radial shortening. J Bone Joint Surg Br. 2002;84(5):673–7.

27. Nakamura R, Tsuge S, Watanabe K, Tsunoda K. Radial wedge osteotomy for Kienböck's disease. J Bone Joint Surg Am. 1991;73-A:1391–6.
28. Watanabe K, Nakamura R, Horii E, Miura T. Biomechanical analysis of radial wedge osteotomy for the treatment of Kienböck's disease. J Hand Surg Am. 1993;18:686–90.
29. Freyschmidt J, Brossmann J, Wiens J, Sternberg A. Koehler/Zimmer's borderlands of normal and early pathological findings in skeletal radiography. 5th ed. New York, NY: Thieme; 2003.
30. Luo J, Diao E. Kienbock's disease: an approach to treatment. Hand Clin. 2006;22(4):465–73. abstract vi.
31. Lichtman DM, Lesley NE, Simmons SP. The classification and treatment of Kienbock's disease: the state of the art and a look at the future. J Hand Surg Eur Vol. 2010;35(7):549–54.
32. Sowa DT, Holder LE, Patt PG, Weiland AJ. Application of magnetic resonance imaging to ischemic necrosis of the lunate. J Hand Surg Am. 1989;14(6):1008–16.
33. Schmitt R, Heinze A, Fellner F, Obletter N, Struhn R, Bautz W. Imaging and staging of avascular osteonecroses at the wrist and hand. Eur J Radiol. 1997;25(2):92–103.
34. Iwasaki N, Genda E, Minami A, Kaneda K, Chao EY. Force transmission through the wrist joint in Kienböck's disease: a two-dimensional theoretical study. J Hand Surg Am. 1998;23:415–24.
35. Tuzuner T, Subasi M, Alper M, Kara H, Orhan Z. Penetrating type intraosseous ganglion cyst of the lunate bone. West Indian Med J. 2005;54(6):384–6.
36. Schajowicz F, Clavel Sainz M, Slullitel JA. Juxta-articular bone cysts (intra-osseous ganglia). J Bone Joint Surg Br. 1979;61:107–16.
37. Uriburu IJ, Levy VD. Intraosseous ganglia of the scaphoid and lunate bones: report of 15 cases in 13 patients. J Hand Surg Am. 1999;24:508–15.
38. Katz DI, Seiler 3rd JG, Bond TC. The treatment of ulnar impaction syndrome: a systematic review of the literature. J Surg Orthop Adv. 2010;19(4):218–22.
39. Sammer DM, Rizzo M. Ulnar impaction. Hand Clin. 2010;26:549–57.
40. Cerezal L, del Piñal F, Abascal F, García-Valtuille R, Pereda T, Canga A. Imaging findings in ulnar-sided wrist impaction syndromes. Radiographics. 2002;22:105–21.
41. Suh N, Ek ET, Wolfe SW. Carpal fractures. J Hand Surg Am. 2014;39(4):785–91. quiz 791.
42. Bain GI, McLean JM, Turner PC, Sood A, Pourgiezis N. Translunate fracture with associated perilunate: Three case reports with introduction of the "Intralunate Arc" concept. J Hand Surg Am. 2008;33(10):1770–6.
43. Mirra J, Picci P, Gold R. Bone tumors: clinical, radiologic, and pathologic correlations. Philadelphia, PA: Lea & Febiger; 1989.
44. Freiberger RH, Loitman BS, Helpern M, Thompson TC. Osteoid osteoma; a report on 80 cases. Am J Roentgenol Radium Ther Nucl Med. 1959;82(2):194–205.
45. Güner MD, Kamburoğlu HO, Bektaş U, Ay Ş. Osteoid osteoma of the lunatum mimicking Kienböck's disease. Case Reports Plast Surg Hand Surg. 2015;2(1):19–21.
46. Arora J, McLauchlan J, Munro N. Recurrent osteoid osteoma of the lunate: a case report and review of the literature. Hand Surg. 2003;8(2):239–42.
47. Ayekoloye C, Lang DM. Osteoid osteoma of the lunate--a case report. Hand Surg. 2000;5(2):185–7.
48. Helbig B. Osteoid osteoma of the lunate. J Hand Surg Am. 1987;12(6):1125.
49. Jackson RP, Reckling FW, Mants FA. Osteoid osteoma and osteoblastoma. Similar histologic lesions with different natural histories. Clin Orthop Relat Res 1977;(128):303–13.
50. Gaulke R. The distribution of solitary enchondromata at the hand. J Hand Surg Br. 2002;27:444–5.

# Advanced Imaging of Kienböck's Disease

# 11

Rainer R. Schmitt and Karlheinz Kalb

## Pathoanatomic Fundamentals of Imaging

To enhance the basic understanding of the imaging findings, we have briefly summarized the multifactorial etiology and underlying mechanisms of pathology in Kienböck's disease [1].

## Etiology

The etiology of Kienböck's disease remains controversial, and there remains no evidence-based explanation. The pathogenesis of Kienböck's disease can't be attributed to a single cause. It seems more likely that a combination of at-risk factors, trigger mechanisms, and modulating factors are required for the initiation and development of the disease [2, 3]. Many hypotheses have been suggested, with vascular, mechanical (extrinsic and intrinsic), and metabolic factors being the most probable factors:

R.R. Schmitt, MD (✉)
Department of Radiology, Herz- und Gefäßklinik GmbH, Campus Bad Neustadt, Salzburger Leite 1, Bad Neustadt 97616, Germany
e-mail: radiodiagnostics@outlook.com

K. Kalb, Dr Med
Clinic for Hand Surgery, Herz- und Gefaßklinik GmbH der Rhön-Klinikum AG, Campus Bad Neustadt, Salzburger Leite 1, Bad Neustadt 97616, Germany

- Anatomically, there is a unique vascularization pattern of the lunate, characterized by a retrograde intraosseous vascularization [4]. Vessels branching from the radial and anterior interosseous arteries enter the lunate via the dorsal pole. Branches of the radial, ulnar, and anterior interosseous arteries, as well as branches from the recurrent deep palmar arch reach the palmar pole of the lunate. The normal nutrient intraosseous vessels are in different configurations, including a Y-shaped (59 %), I-shaped (31 %), or X-shaped (10 %). The vessel density is continuously decreasing from their distal entry sites, to the proximal lunate, which is supplied by only the terminal vessels. The proximal lunate subchondral bone is supplied by only the terminal vessels and is considered the "terminal zone of vascularization" with an increased risk of ischemia if small intraosseous arteries are interrupted by trauma or thromboembolism [4, 5]. A single palmar vessel exists in 7 % of lunates, which theoretically carries a greater risk for avascular necrosis in a traumatic event [6]. Pathoanatomically, the lunate "at risk" is defined either by either a single vessel or by a limited intraosseous collateral network of vessels [3].
- Obviously, carpal injuries play an important role in the onset of Kienböck's disease [7]. Sprains, contusions, and subluxations may lead not only to ligamentous lesions, but also to occlusions of the nutrient vessels to the

© Springer International Publishing Switzerland 2016

D.M. Lichtman, G.I. Bain (eds.), *Kienböck's Disease*, DOI 10.1007/978-3-319-34226-9_11

lunate. Since the dominant hand of males in manual jobs is predominantly affected, chronic repetitive traumas have been thought to be responsible for vascular occlusions, mainly by thrombosis of the intraosseous arteries. Acute injuries of the lunate—mainly impaction or avulsion fractures—can also trigger Kienböck's disease; however, the fracture theory is controversial, as lunate fractures often appear secondarily in the natural course of osteonecrosis. Finally, compromised venous drainage should be mentioned as a possible cause of Kienböck's disease, because increased intra-osseous pressure has been documented, particularly in extended wrists [8].

- Among mechanical risk factors, the short ulna is thought to be the most important contributing for the development of osteonecrosis of the lunate [9]. In negative ulnar variance, which is observed in about 78 % of patients suffering from Kienböck's disease, axial force transmission along the radius-lunate-capitate column is focused onto the radial portion of the lunate, creating an uneven high internal load, whereas the ulnolunate compartment is unloaded. These focal intraosseous strains are considered as the main reason for the preferential manifestation of Kienböck's disease on the radial aspect of the lunate [10]. Furthermore, negative ulnar variance may be associated with a triangular shape of the lunate [11]. However, the causative factor of negative ulnar variance in Kienböck's disease is questioned nowadays [12, 13]. Other mechanical features predisposing to osteonecrosis include decreased radial inclination, a reduced radiolunate contact area [14], the spherical shape of the lunate characterized by large proximal and small distal surfaces, the triangular or square geometry of the lunate [11], and finally the particular architecture of the trabeculae which make the lunate susceptible to fractures under axial load [11, 15].
- In addition, Kienböck's disease has been reported as an infrequent association with neural, metabolic, and endocrine conditions.

## Pathology

Pathoanatomically, Kienböck's disease is not merely a nonreactive, nonviable tissue ("dead bone"), but a dynamic, viable remodeling process of the bone and bone marrow, as has been confirmed in animal experiments [16–18]:

Following the influence of traumatic triggers and modulators on the lunate, cellular repair, and revascularization mechanisms immediately arise from the maintained viable bone marrow [17–20]. As necrotic areas appear, small vessels invade from the periphery of the adjacent living bone. New vessels as well as fibrovascular tissue develop within a hyperemic repair zone, which is interposed between the proximal necrotic (nonviable) tissue and the normal (viable) bone marrow on its distal aspect. This new angiogenetic activity leads to osteoclastic resorption of necrotic bone and laying down of osteoblastic new bone.

The osteonecrotic history of Kienböck's disease can be subdivided into four pathoanatomical phases [19, 20]:

- *Phase of edema*: Any form of ischemia within the lunate induces intercellular edema of the bone marrow with their cells being compromised by an increased water content. Medullary fat cells survive ischemia for only 2–5 days.
- *Phase of cellular necrosis*: After this period, the medullary cells within the lunate die.
- *Phase of repair*: The regenerative processes are initiated already in the phases of edema and necrosis. The first repair mechanism is neogenesis of fibrous and vascular tissues with the presence of fibroblasts and the formation of new vessels. The lunate must be at least partially vascularized for initializing the repair and revascularization processes. Then, the remaining vessels vasodilate and viable bone becomes hyperperfused.
- *Phase of bone remodeling*: Finally, the remaining bone, as well as the rebuilt fibrovascular tissue undergo a remodeling processes. During this phase the osteoblasts and osteoclasts are

intensively activated. On histology, areas of osteonecrosis alternate with areas of new bone formation.

By definition, potentially reversible ischemia must be differentiated from irreversible necrosis of the bone marrow. *Ischemia* is a hypoxic condition of the tissues caused by problems with blood vessels, and characterized by insufficient oxygen and nutrition supply needed for cellular metabolism. Dysfunction of tissue and damage can be the consequences. Ischemic tissue can develop in a reversible manner, if restricted perfusion is eliminated by the onset of repairing mechanisms. *Necrosis* is characterized by severe cell injury and cell death after vascular and tissue repairing has failed [21]. Without intervention, external ischemia may progress to necrosis of the bone marrow and bone substance. In contrast to ischemia, necrotic tissue is definitely irreversible with regard to "ad integrum" healing.

Three different zones can be differentiated in histopathology as well as in contrast-enhanced MRI [19, 22, 23]:

- *Zone of necrosis*: The site of the most intense and frequent osteonecrosis is at the proximal-radial circumference of the lunate. Pathoanatomically, this area is the terminal zone of vascular supply. When reparative vascularization has failed, bone conversion leads to dense osteosclerosis due to an imbalance of osteoblasts with residual activity and insufficient osteoclasts. Osteonecrotic tissue is identified by vacuoles free of osteocytes, sparse osteoid, removal of debris leading to osseous cavities, and comminuted fractures. The articular cartilage of the lunate remains intact for a long time, but is usually damaged in advanced Kienböck's stages [24].
- *Zone of repair*: Microscopic analysis of specimens reveals fibroconnective tissue and shards of bone trabeculae both being suggestive of an ischemic condition. Fibrovascular reparation tissue is found in the middle layer of the lunate, which is characterized by hyperemia, cellular infiltration, granulation tissue, and also by phagocytosis, removal processes, decalcification, and pathologic fractures. In the zone of repair, which resembles a space of osseous nonunion, osteonecrotic foci are alternating with areas of viable bone and new bone formation. There is an attempt to balance the resorption of necrotic bone and the formation of new bone.
- *Zone of viability*: The distal aspects of the lunate, particularly the palmar and dorsal poles, preserve viable bone marrow and bone tissue the longest. Specimens of viable bone have abundant osteoid and osteocytes. The distal aspect of the lunate becomes necrotic in only the advanced stages of Kienböck's disease.

On principle, the new developed repair tissue can take quite different courses with respect to bone viability:

- At its best, the fibrovascular repair tissue is subsequently transformed into fibrous bone tissue, and later into normal lamellar bone. This positive outcome results in a "restitution ad integrum" recovery of Kienböck's disease, and is most often seen in children and adolescents [25, 26], but also in adults under best treatment conditions.
- For reasons not really understood, fibrovascular repair tissue is often not transformed into fibrous and lamellar bone. This progressive event follows a unidirectional course with a "point of no return" pattern that is not clearly determinable in development of osteonecrosis. The final stage is characterized by necrotic (nonviable) bone, osteosclerosis, and formation of sequestra. It is assumed that an increase in vascularization (hyperemia) produces a focal demineralization in the repair zone [27], and this focal osteopenia induces a pathologic fracture of the lunate. The fracture is usually on the proximal aspect or alternatively can be a coronal fracture. Theoretically, a fracture can be the primary event, although this in not thought to be common.
- Fractures of the necrotic lunate lead to a loss of height of the lunate, and a synchronous proximal migration of the capitate and

consequently a loss of height of the proximal carpal row. The final stage is characterized by progressive radiocarpal and midcarpal osteoarthritis (Kienböck's disease advanced collapse), which usually occurs within 5 years, if the wrist is left untreated. Reactive synovitis may be associated.

## Imaging in Kienböck's Disease

The treatment decision in Kienböck's disease is mainly based on four parameters: (1) the stage of the disease, (2) the ulnar variance, (3) the presence of carpal osteoarthritis, and (4) the patient's age. By defining the first three parameters, imaging basically constitutes the main decisive components in the therapeutic concepts of Kienböck's disease. The diagnostic capabilities of CT and MR imaging are emphasized in this text, whereas conventional radiography is only briefly mentioned, because it is covered in another chapter of this book (see Chapter 10).

### Conventional Radiography

True dorso-palmar and true lateral X-ray views are basic imaging tools for assessment of wrist pathology. In most cases of Kienböck's disease (particularly the advanced stages), the diagnosis is made on plain X-rays [7, 28]. But, early in the course of the disease, radiographs may actually be normal. Although being inferior to CT and MRI, X-rays are useful for grading Kienböck's disease and for distinguishing it from other pathologic conditions of the lunate, i.e. the ulnolunate impaction syndrome, intra-osseous ganglion cysts, post-traumatic conditions, lunotriquetral coalitions, and others.

The position of the distal ulna in relation to the distal radial surface changes with varying degrees of forearm rotation. Therefore, it is essential that the dorso-palmar is obtained with the true neutral position, to allow for an exact measurement of the degree of ulnar variance [10, 29].

### Computed Tomography (CT)

The introduction of multi-slice (multidetector) spiral CT has fundamentally improved the capabilities of imaging the osseous anatomy. High-resolution CT is a very powerful tool in evaluating the osseous microstructure of the lunate and the perilunar joints in Kienböck's disease [22, 30].

#### Acquisition and Post-processing Techniques in CT Imaging

High-resolution techniques of both acquisition and reconstruction are recommended for CT imaging of the lunate (Fig. 11.1):

- First, a volumetric data-set is acquired (voltage 120 kV, current 100 mA, field of view 60 mm, slice thickness 0.5 or 0.6 mm, pitch factor 0.9).

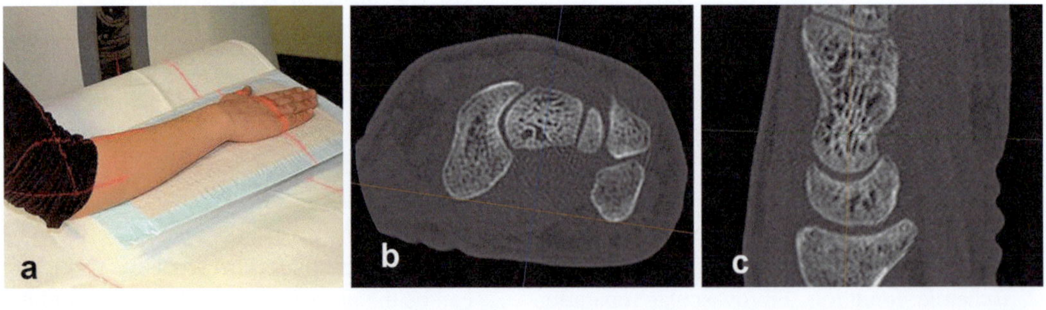


**Fig. 11.1** Acquisition technique of carpal computed tomography (CT). (**a**) Positioning for transaxial CT imaging. The patient is standing beside the CT gantry, and the pronated forearm and hand are placed flat and in longitudinal direction on the gantry table. (**b**) Planning of coronal and sagittal MPR (multiplanar reconstruction) on this transaxial image. The coronal MPR images are planned on the transaxial image with a tangent drawn on the palmar aspect of the scaphoid and pisiform (*yellow line*). Sagittal MPR images (*blue line*) are then perpendicular to the *yellow line*. (**c**) The coronal MPR plane is parallel to the colinear radius-lunate-capitate axis (*yellow line*)

- In the post-processing procedure, transaxial, overlapping source images are reconstructed (slice thickness 0.5 or 0.6 mm, increment 70 %, high-resolution bone kernel)

Sagittal and coronal images are reconstructed (slice thickness 0.5 or 0.6 mm, increment 100 %, high-resolution bone kernel). It must be emphasized that thin slices (0.5–1.0 mm) and overlapping increment are important prerequisites for multiplanar reconstructed (MPR) images. For these reasons CT imaging is superior to X-rays in assessing the fine osseous morphology [23, 30].

## Findings in CT Imaging

Sagittal and coronal MPR images are best for assessing the proximal circumference of the lunate. These MPR images are high-resolution and without any out-of-field and streaking artifacts (these artifacts are often seen in images which have been acquired with primary scans in the sagittal or coronal plane).

- *Evidence of stage II*: Due to the better resolution, CT imaging is able to display mild osteosclerosis of the cancellous bone and pseudo-cystoid inclusions better than plain radiographs (Fig. 11.2). Therefore, stage II of

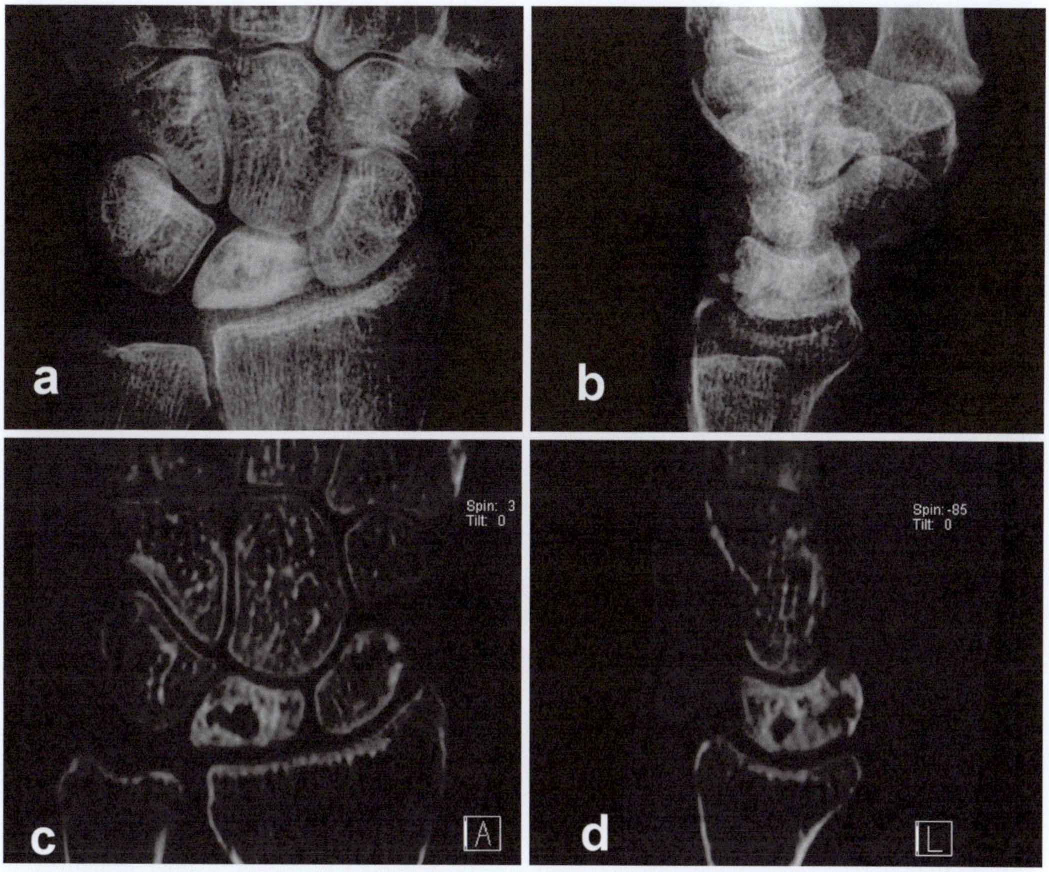


**Fig. 11.2** Plain radiology and CT scan of a 49-year-old female with wrist pain for 3 months. (**a**, **b**) Dorsopalmar and lateral radiographs demonstrate osteosclerosis and flattening of the proximal lunate. This would be defined as a Lichtman stage II. (**c**, **d**) Coronal and sagittal MPR (1-mm slices) demonstrate cystic inclusions, and osteosclerosis is better visualized due to the superior resolution. Additionally, an impacted fracture of the proximal lunate is identified, which would re-define to a Lichtman's stage IIIa

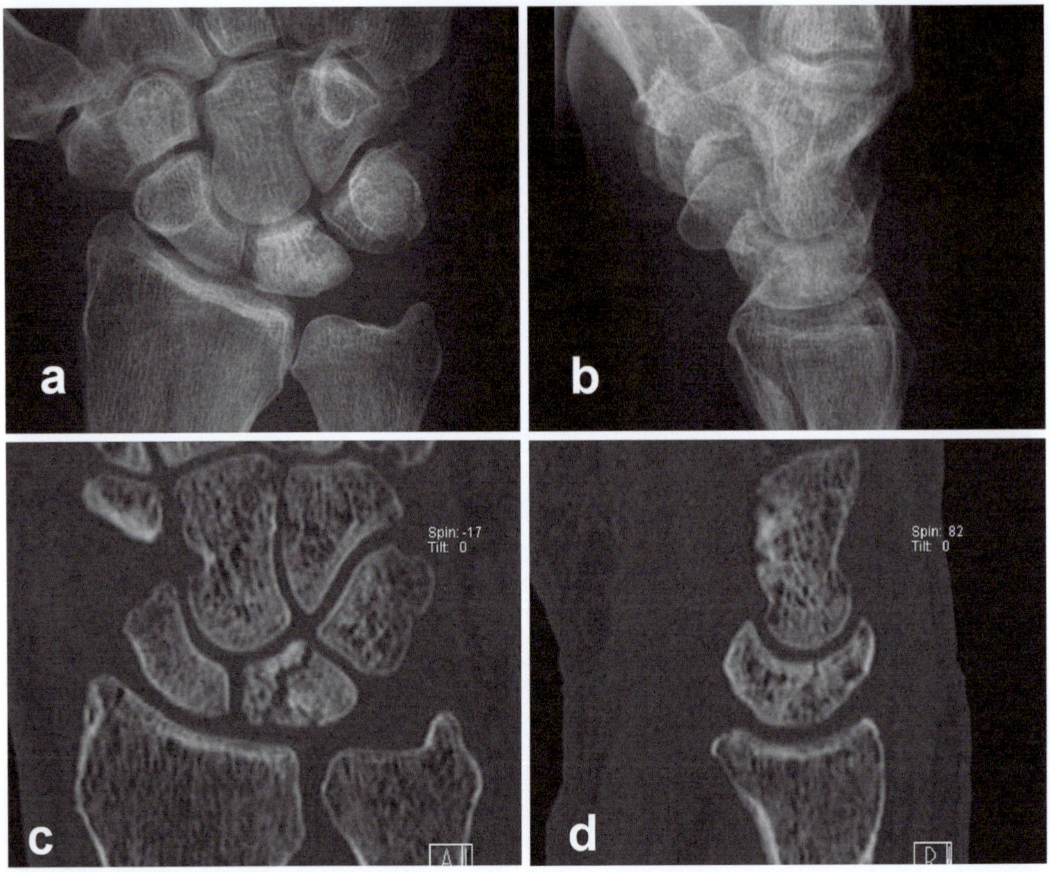


**Fig. 11.3** CT imaging for visualizing fracture lines in stage IIIa of Kienböck's disease. Patient is a 57-year-old male with painful wrist and reduced range of motion. (**a**, **b**) Dorsopalmar and lateral radiographs demonstrate a sclerotic lunate, but fracture lines are not clearly identified. (**c**, **d**) Coronal and sagittal MPR CT images (1-mm slices) reveal an oblique lunate fracture and dense osteosclerosis. An impacted fragment causes straightening of the proximal lunate

Kienböck's disease is discernible earlier and with more precision in CT imaging.

- *Evidence of stage IIIa*: CT imaging is useful to demonstrate fracture or fragmentation of the lunate. The early phase of stage IIIa is characterized by subtle linear fracture lines and small zones of impacted fragments at the proximal-radial circumference of the lunate. These findings can often be occult with plain radiography. Discrete fractures and impaction at the proximal circumference are reliably detected with high-resolution technique (Fig. 11.3). Osteosclerosis and lunate collapse may be the consequence of revascularization [18, 27]. However, it is not clear whether a fracture seen in advanced stages is the primary cause of Kienböck's disease or occurs later in the natural history as the result of revascularization, bone resorption, and structural weakness. Furthermore, CT imaging allows proper visualization of the coronal fracture, which can be overlooked with MRI, particularly when the signal height of the lunate is heavily compromised in the fracture area [23]. Coronal fractures are comprehensively depicted in sagittal MPR images. Evidence of proximal and/or sagittal fractures definitely confirms stage IIIa of Kienböck's disease. Carpal instability in Kienböck's disease (stage IIIb) does not constitute an indication for CT imaging, as instability criteria are sufficiently confirmed with the use of radiographs (Youm's index, radioscaphoid angle) for differentiating stages IIIa and IIIb [31–33].

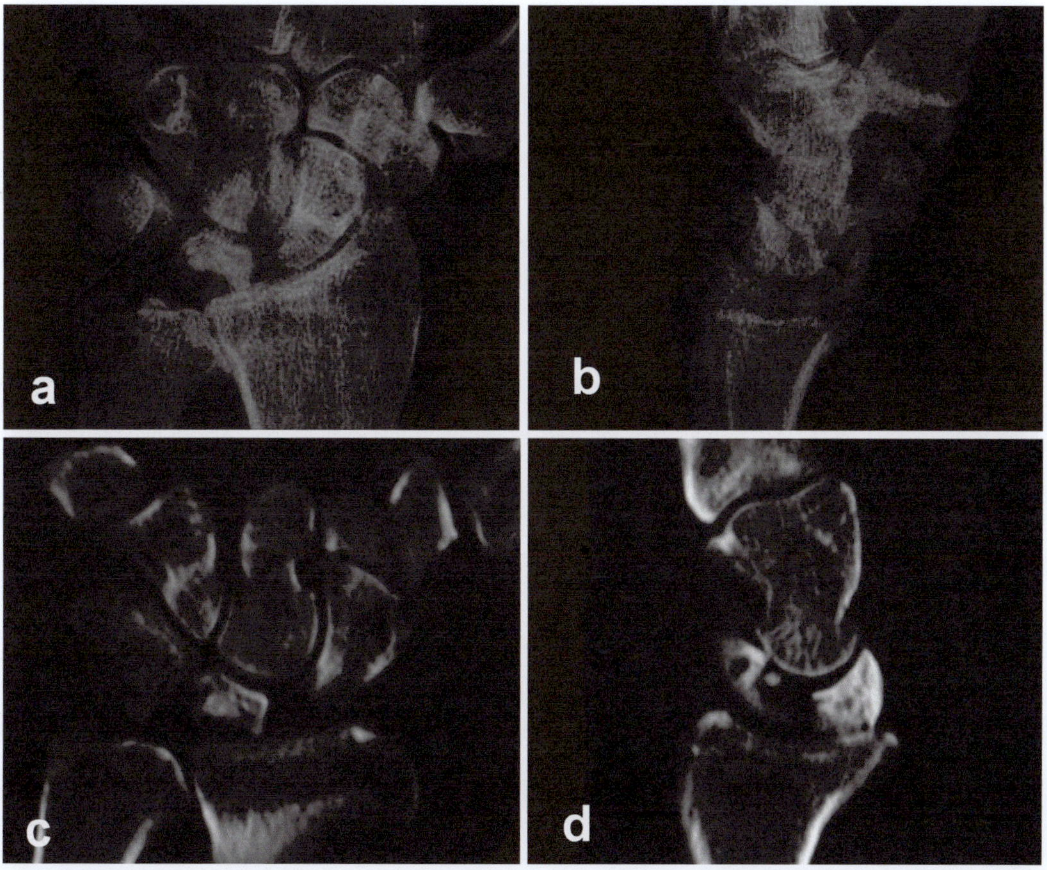

**Fig. 11.4** CT imaging for demonstrating osteoarthritis in stage IV of Kienböck's disease. Patient is a 57-year-old male with progressive wrist pain over the last 3 months, who now has a marked restriction in his range of motion. (**a**, **b**) Dorsopalmar and lateral radiographs demonstrate an osteosclerotic and fractured lunate, with loss of carpal height. Osteoarthritis of the distal radioulnar joint is a secondary finding. (**c**, **d**) Coronal and sagittal CT MPR images demonstrate advanced chondropathia of the palmar aspect of the radiolunate joint. The lunate is coronally fractured and osteosclerotic. *Note*: The visual impression of these MPR images is different from Figs. 11.1 and 11.2, because a slice thickness of 2 mm has been used in post-processing

- *Evidence of stage IV*: Initial stages of perilunar osteoarthritis are reliably detected with CT imaging demonstrating small osteophytes, subchondral osteosclerosis, cysts, and asymmetry of the radiocarpal and midcarpal joint spaces (Fig. 11.4). Thus, a CT exam should be ordered in suspected stage IIIb of Kienböck's disease when osteoarthritis (stage IV) must be ruled out in surgical treatment planning [23]. However, the CT exam is not required in advanced cases when osteoarthritis is clearly visible on plain radiographs.

In conclusion, CT identifies the advanced stages of Kienböck's disease more precisely than plain radiography and MRI. If osteonecrosis has already been diagnosed with another imaging procedure (i.e. X-ray, MRI), CT should also be performed to determine the exact disease stage according to the osseous morphologic criteria. Thus, CT imaging should be an inherent part of the diagnostic work-up in Kienböck's disease.

## Magnetic Resonance Imaging (MRI)

Magnetic resonance imaging (MRI) is used for imaging of the lunate bone marrow and for

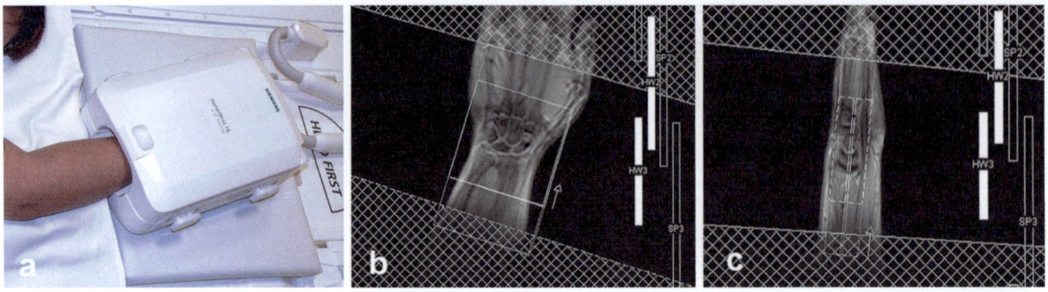


**Fig. 11.5** Acquisition technique of wrist MR imaging. (**a**) In-center positioning of the wrist. The patient is lying on the MRI table in the "superman position" (i.e., lying prone, with the arm overhead and the hand pronated). The hand is placed in a 16-channel, phased-array coil dedicated for high-resolution wrist and hand MRI. (**b**, **c**) Coronal and sagittal localizers (scouts) for planning a coronal acquisition volume ("slab") of 8 cm × 8 cm in-plane size. Active coil elements are displayed on the *right side*. Saturation pulses are placed proximal and distal to the acquisition volume to minimize vascular flow artifacts as well as fold-over artifacts. *Arrows* indicate the phase encoding direction

determining its viability in Kienböck's disease [16, 17, 22, 23, 34, 35].

## Acquisition Techniques in MRI

High-resolution MRI sequences must be applied to sufficiently visualize the bone marrow of the lunate. We recommend the following parameters [23]:

- The 1.5 or 3.0 T MRI scanner is required. The low- and midfield scanners (0.2–1.0 T) have a lower field strength, which do not provide adequate spatial and contrast resolution due to the poor signal-to-noise ratios (SNR) and contrast-to-noise ratios (CNR).
- The application of a multichannel, phased-array wrist coil has become standard in MRI of the extremities (Fig. 11.5). The phased-array coils have the advantage of "parallel imaging technology," which significantly expands the possibilities of MRI techniques by acquiring either high-resolution images in the same time or by producing the images with a reduced acquisition time. Of course, the high-resolution MRI of the wrist is favorable in Kienböck's disease.
- The optimal geometric scan parameters for wrist MRI are: Field of view 80 mm, slice thickness 2 mm without gap (interleaved acquisition order) when acquiring 2D sequences, and slice thickness 0.5 mm in acquisition of 3D sequences.
- The sequences should be acquired in all three orthogonal planes, with the coronal and sagittal being most important in Kienböck's disease.
- Acquisition of these sequence types is recommended:
  - PD-weighted FSE with fat-saturation (coronal plane)
  - PD-weighted FSE with fat-saturation (transaxial plane).
  - T1-weighted FSE nonenhanced (coronal plane)
  - T1-weighted FSE with fat-saturation after intravenous gadolinium (coronal plane)
  - T1-weighted FSE with fat-saturation after intravenous gadolinium (sagittal plane).

## MRI of the Normal Bone

With regard to the signal height in MRI, bone can be subdivided into two compartments [36]:

- The *calcified bone compartment* comprises the compact bone of the peripheral cortex and the central cancellous (trabecular) bone, which serves as architectural framework for bone marrow. The calcified bone substance which is mainly composed of the osteoid matrix and calcium phosphate complexes does not provide any signal with MRI, and has therefore a low ("dark") signal intensity on both T1 and T2-weighted sequence types.

- The *medullary bone compartment* is composed of the bone marrow and is embedded between the trabecular (cancellous) bone. The bone marrow consists of red (hematopoietic) and yellow (fatty, adipose) cells that are dispersed through the trabecular bone framework. The percentage of yellow marrow increases with age. MRI provides direct assessment of the hematopoietic and fatty marrow of cancellous bone. The yellow marrow has a similar MRI signal to subcutaneous fat—high on T1 and intermediate on T2-weighted images. Red marrow has lower signal intensity than yellow marrow on T1-weighted images. In the normal bone marrow, the high intensity MRI signal is due to the predominance of the medullary fat cells.
- The perfusion state of the bone marrow can be assessed with tissue-dependent relaxation times. In studies correlating MRI and pathohistologic findings of the bone, a close relationship has been found between the MRI signal heights of the calcified bone substance and the bone marrow [20]. Thus, any changes in the signal intensity of the bone marrow indirectly indicate an underlying pathology or disturbance of the bone metabolism. This phenomenon is one of the basic assumptions in reading MRI of Kienböck's disease.

## MRI in Kienböck's Disease

MRI is able to distinguish areas of viable and nonviable bone within the lunate. The capability of MRI in identifying osteonecrosis is based on the physical principle that magnetic relaxivity of the bone marrow is changed in ischemic, reparative as well as in necrotic tissue areas, allowing the differentiation of different states of bone viability [16, 17, 20, 23, 34, 36]:

- *Phase 1—Ischemia*: Ischemia leads to edema of the bone marrow. In the initial stage, signal intensity of the fatty bone marrow is increased in T2-weighted, fat-saturated sequences, and slightly decreased in T1-weighted sequences. Depending on the degree of the ischemic process, signal changes are either limited to the proximal circumference or extended throughout the entire lunate.
- *Phase 2—Necrosis*: The ischemic medullary fat cells survive for 2–5 days. After this time the medullary signal intensity decreases in T1- and T2-weighted images, to create hypointense signal height.
- *Phase 3—Repair*: The reparative process with mesenchymal neogenesis of fibrovascular repair tissue begins soon after onset of compromised vascular perfusion. This produces a further signal reduction in both T1- and T2-weighted sequences.
- *Phase 4—Remodeling*; Activated osteoblasts induce remodeling and osteosclerosis of the trabecular bone and thereby induce a further decrease of the signal intensity in T1- and T2-weighted sequences. Additionally, signal loss is generated by fragments at the proximal circumference of the lunate.

In the literature, two different MRI approaches have been reported for assessing the viability of the bone marrow: The traditional approach utilized standard MRI. The new approach utilizes intravenous gadolinium enhancement which creates a high intensity signal in the vascularized tissue.

### Unenhanced MRI

In traditional MRI [16, 17, 20, 34, 35], viability of the bone marrow is assumed in the presence of high-signal intensity in plain (unenhanced) T1- and T2-weighted sequences (Fig. 11.6). Viable bone marrow is also assumed in the presence of bone marrow edema, which presents with high signal intensity in fat-suppressed T2-weighted images. The underlying theory is that bone marrow edema can develop if the vascular supply is either unaffected or moderately compromised, only [17]. In contrast, nonviable bone marrow is assessed in unenhanced MRI by means of hypointense areas both in T1 and T2-weighted sequences indicating loss of the fatty marrow as well as the absence of any vascularity. Two degrees of signal defect can be differentiated on MRI [34, 35]: Focal signal loss on the radial half of the lunate

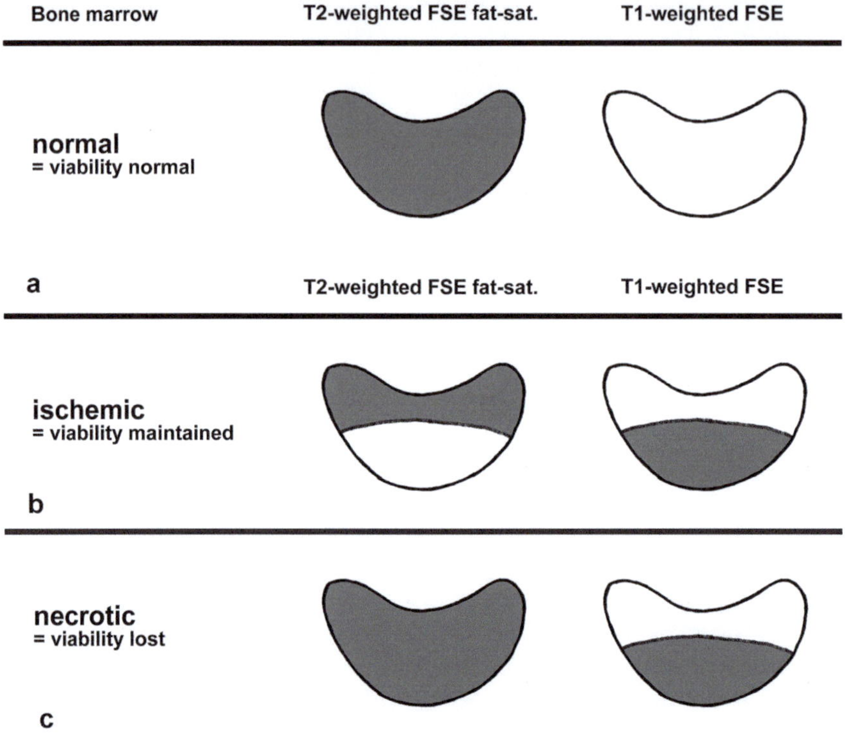


**Fig. 11.6** Schematic diagram of bone marrow viability in unenhanced (traditional) MRI. In the traditional MRI approach, normal, ischemic, and necrotic bone marrow is differentiated by means of plain T2- and T1-weighted FSE sequences. The lunate is shown in lateral views. (**a**) Normal bone marrow (viability unaffected). The signal height is homogeneously dark in fat-saturated T2-w FSE, and homogeneously bright in T1-w FSE. (**b**) Ischemic bone marrow (viability maintained). Mainly due to bone-marrow edema, the proximal pole of the lunate is hyperintense in fat-saturated T2-w FSE, and hypointense in T1-w FSE. Bone-marrow edema is regarded as an indirect sign of persistent perfusion in unenhanced MRI. (**c**) Necrotic bone marrow (viability lost). There is no bone-marrow present in fat-saturated T2-w FSE at the proximal circumference which is marked hypointense in T1-w FSE. In plain MRI, necrosis is characterized by the absence of both bone-marrow edema (T2-w) and fatty bone marrow (T1-w)

on T1-weighted images as well as normal or increased signal height on T2-weighted images suggests early ischemic involvement and a better prognosis, whereas generalized signal loss in T1 and T2-weighted images on the entire lunate is diagnostic for advanced osteonecrosis of the lunate.

Although proved only in scaphoid nonunion and not in Kienböck's disease, the concept of unenhanced MRI is limited in assessing osteonecrotic bone for several reasons [37, 38]. Firstly, unenhanced MRI uses the combination of T1- and T2-weighted sequences for determining bone-marrow viability, with the presumption that viability is maintained in the presence of bone-marrow edema. However, differentiation of intercellular (reversible) edema and intracellular (irreversible, cytotoxic) edema is not possible with T2-weighted sequences. Signal height on T2-weighted sequences does not allow the differentiation of necrotic, reparative, and normal bone marrow [37]. For this reason, high-signal areas in T2-weighted images are seen in viable as well as in nonviable bone marrow [38]. Secondly, the necrotic zone cannot be reliably discerned from the neighbored repair zone, because these zones can have the same signal intensity on both T1- and T2-weighted sequences. Low-signal-intensity areas on unenhanced T1-weighted images do not closely correlate with the extent of the necrotic areas and may oversize the necrotic area. Thus, with unenhanced T1-weighted images, the true osteonecrotic area will be overestimated, as the repair zone also appears to be necrotic [19]. Thirdly, the unenhanced MRI does not assess the repair zone which is considered essential in the pathoanatomy of osteonecrosis.

### Gadolinium-Enhanced MRI

In MRI, the perfusion state of the bone marrow can be assessed with tissue-dependent relaxation times and the effect of intravenous gadolinium [22, 37]. If there is significant contrast enhancement in the bone marrow, the T1 relaxation time is shortened by the influence of the paramagnetic gadolinium resulting in increased signal intensity in fat-saturated T1-weighted sequences.

By applying the intravenous contrast agent, a new concept was developed for assessing bone-marrow viability [22, 37]. The following section reviews the role of contrast-enhanced MRI (ceMRI) in the assessment of the pathoanatomic course of Kienböck's. This includes the three-layered zones, seen at the time of repair of the necrotic proximal lunate (Fig. 11.7).

#### Viable Bone Marrow

The bone marrow is viable in the following cases; normal bone marrow, ischemic bone marrow when it is initially compromised, (before necrosis) and reparative vascularized bone marrow. In ceMRI, areas of hyperenhancement are characteristic of reparative mechanisms in Kienböck's disease.

*Normal bone marrow*: In normal bone marrow, the yellow fat cells are exclusively responsible for the high signal in both T1- and T2-weighted images. An increased signal height is characteristic of the viable bone marrow displaying the bone marrow "white" in both unenhanced sequence types, and "dark" in fat-saturated sequences. With ceMRI, there is no contrast enhancement in the normal (unaffected) bone marrow.

*Repair tissue*: Viable bone tissue is also present in fibrovascular repair tissue which is located in the transition area between the necrotic zone and the zone of viable bone. The reparative area is characterized by the invasion of leucocytes, fibroblasts, and new vessels. The inflammation-like processes and the marked hyperemia, produce hyperenhancement in T1-weighted FSE sequences after 3–5 min following gadolinium injection [22, 37]. Its viability is measured by rating the degree of contrast-enhancement. Time-resolved, fast 2D- or 3D-GRE sequences can be applied for calculating a time-signal diagram over an interval of about 5 min (Fig. 11.8). These diagrams allow quantitative analysis of the local perfusion pattern and also the prognosis of the altered bone marrow in follow-up studies. However, the benefit of time-resolved enhanced MRI has recently been questioned, at least in assessing the bone-marrow viability in scaphoid nonunion [39].

#### Nonviable Bone Marrow

As stated above, the unenhanced T1-weighted images, may over-interpret the zone of bone marrow necrosis, as the zone of repair will also have a low signal intensity [19]. Following gadolinium, the repair zone will be enhanced and the nonperfused necrotic zone will still have a low signal intensity [23, 37].

Possible signal changes and patterns of contrast enhancement in Kienböck's disease are summarized in Table 11.1.

#### Three-Layered Anatomy

By determining bone marrow viability with the use of ceMRI, three geographic zones are discernable in the lunate [22, 23]:

- In the *proximal zone*, osteonecrosis is characterized by decreased signal height in T1-weighted sequences, and no hyperenhancement pattern after application of gadolinium.
- In the *middle zone*, fibrovascular repair tissue is visualized by means of an intensive hyperenhancement in T1-weighted fat-suppressed sequences after application of gadolinium—independent of the presence of a bone-marrow edema.
- The *distal zone* is displayed with normal signal heights of the unaffected bone marrow.

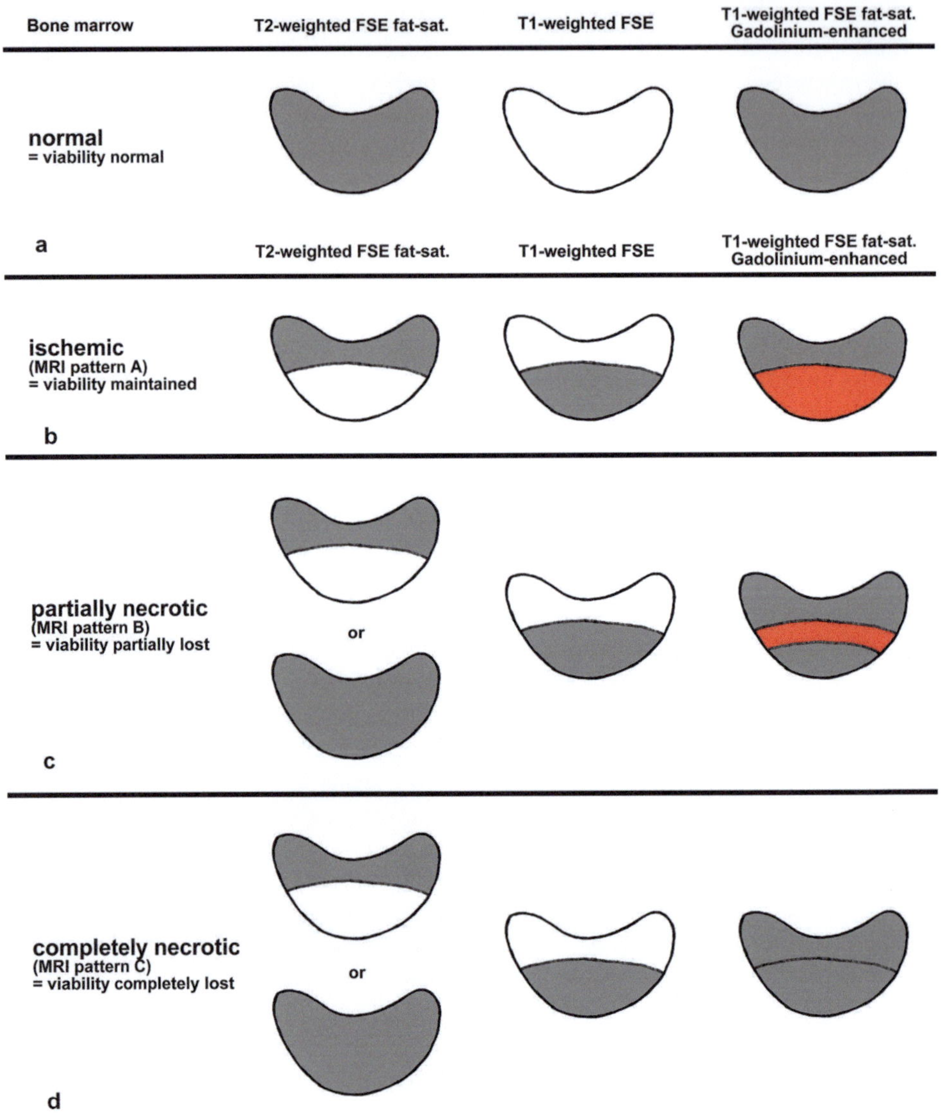


**Fig. 11.7** Schematic diagram of bone-marrow viability in gadolinium-enhanced MRI. In the contrast-enhanced MRI approach, normal, ischemic, partially necrotic, and completely necrotic bone marrow is differentiated by means of contrast enhancement in fat-saturated T1-weighted FSE sequences independent of the presence of bone-marrow edema in T2-weighted FSE sequences. The lunate is shown in lateral views. (**a**) Normal bone marrow (viability is unaffected). The signal height is homogeneously dark in fat-saturated T2-w FSE, and homogeneously bright in T1-w FSE. No contrast-enhancement within a homogeneously dark lunate is characteristic in fat-saturated T1-w FSE after intravenous gadolinium. (**b**) Ischemic bone marrow (viability is maintained, MRI pattern A). The proximal pole of the lunate is hyperintense in fat-saturated T2-w FSE, and hypointense in T1-w FSE due to bone-marrow edema. In fat-saturated T1-w FSE, there is a homogeneous gadolinium enhancement pattern of the entire proximal zone directly indicating maintained perfusion. (**c**) Partially necrotic bone marrow (viability is partially lost, MRI pattern B). The proximal pole of the lunate is hyperintense in fat-saturated T2-w FSE, and hypointense in T1-w FSE. Both necrotic and repairing zones are present. Differentiation is possible only on the basis of gadolinium enhancement: The repairing zone is marked by an intense enhancement, which characteristically is missing in the necrotic zone. (**d**) Completely necrotic bone marrow (viability is completely lost, MRI pattern C). Independent of present or missing bone-marrow edema in fat-saturated T2-w FSE, no enhancement is seen at all in fat-saturated T1-w FSE after gadolinium when compared to plain T1-w FSE

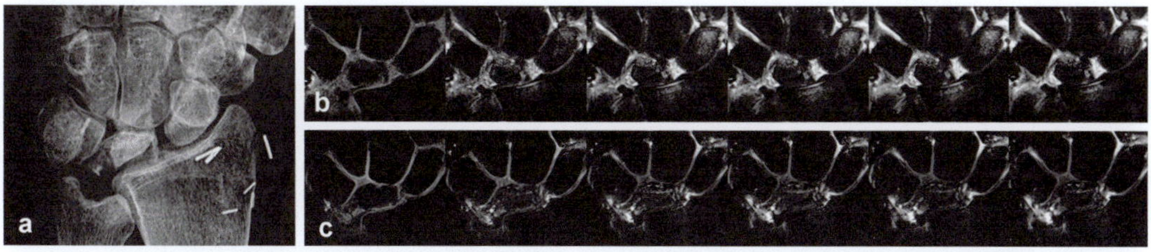


**Fig. 11.8** Dynamic perfusion MRI in stage IIIb of Kienböck's disease in the follow-up after free-vascularized osteochondral bone grafting. Patient is a 30-year-old female with advanced Kienböck's disease following vascularized bone grafting of the diseased lunate. (**a**, **b**) Dorsopalmar radiograph and MRI perfusion study (coronal 3D fast GRE sequence every 20 s after gadolinium injection) 4 months after grafting and hardware removal in the meantime. Contrast enhancement is inhomogeneous and increased at the ulnar side of the lunate where the vascular bundle inserts. (**c**) Perfusion study 9 months after grafting (same dynamic MRI sequence). Contrast enhancement has become more homogeneous. Later, a dorsal osteophyte was removed, and the lunate healed with moderate proximal deformity

**Table 11.1** Pathoanatomic processes in Kienböck's disease and their contribution to the signal height of the lunate

| Pathology | Signal intensity | | Contrast enhancement |
|---|---|---|---|
| | In T2 FSE | In Plain T1 FSE | T1 FSE gadolinium |
| Bone-marrow edema | Increased | Decreased | Homogeneous, territorial |
| Necrotic or emigrated fat cells | Decreased | Decreased | Dependent on viability state |
| Fibrovascular repair tissue | Decreased | Decreased | Homogeneous, zonal |
| Trabecular osteosclerosis | Decreased | Decreased | None |
| Pseudocysts | Increased | Decreased | Central none, peripheral rim |
| Fractures | Decreased | Decreased | None |

**Table 11.2** MRI patterns of Kienböck's disease in with contrast-enhancement

| MRI pattern | Signal intensity in | | Contrast enhancement in T1 FSE gadolinium | Pathology |
|---|---|---|---|---|
| | T2 FSE | T1 FSE | | |
| A | Increased | Decreased | Homogeneous, territorial | Bone-marrow edema |
| B | Increased or decreased | Decreased | Inhomogeneous, zonal | Partial osteonecrosis |
| C | Increased or decreased | Decreased | None | Complete osteonecrosis |

Accompanying joint effusions and a synovial thickening showing marked contrast enhancement are mostly seen in advanced MRI stages of Kienböck's disease. Characteristically, the radiolunate compartment is spared from osteoarthritis over a long period of time in the natural course.

### Viability Patterns in ceMRI

In Kienböck's disease, the degree of contrast enhancement in the endangered proximal segment constitutes the most relevant prognostic parameter [22, 23]. In close correlation to histopathological findings, three patterns of contrast enhancement of the lunate can be differentiated with plain (unenhanced) and enhanced T1-weighted MRI sequences (Table 11.2):

*MRI pattern A*: There is homogeneous, intense, and territorial enhancement after gadolinium at the proximal circumference or entire lunate (Fig. 11.9). The pathology is bone marrow edema with intact osteocyte function, maintained or reorganized perfusion of the bone marrow, and a normal bone structure.

*MRI pattern B*: An inhomogeneous contrast enhancement pattern is characteristic with three different zones of perfusion, (i.e. proximal necrosis, middle reparative, and distal

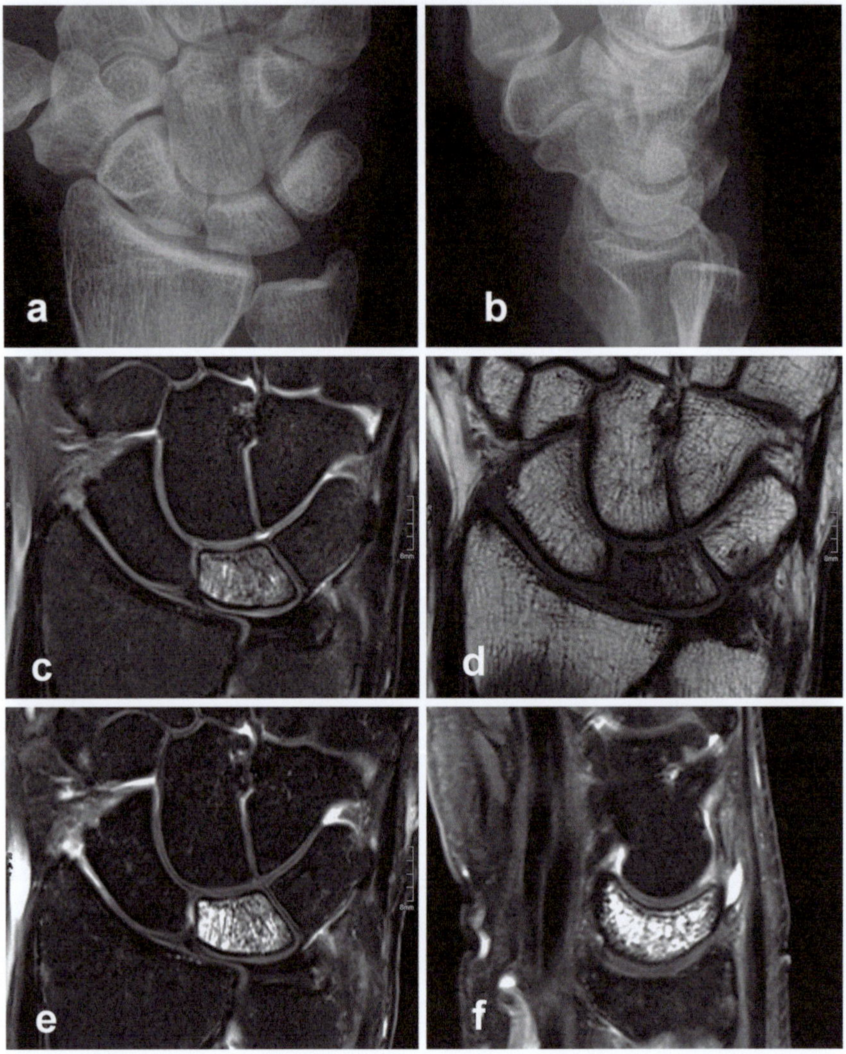


**Fig. 11.9** Ischemic lunate (MRI pattern A) in stage I of Kienböck's disease. Viability is maintained in edematous bone marrow of the lunate. 34-year-old male suffering from spontaneous onset of pain without previous wrist injury or overuse. (**a**, **b**) Dorsopalmar and lateral radiographs are normal and not suspicious of Kienböck's disease. Negative ulnar variance. (**c**) Territorial bone-marrow edema in the entire lunate (coronal PD-w FSE fat-saturated). (**d**) The radial and central parts of the lunate are of inhomogenously low signal (coronal T1-w FSE). (**e**, **f**) With intravenous gadolinium there is an intense enhancement within the lunate (coronal and sagittal T1-w FSE fat-saturated after gadolinium)

normal). The pathology is localized at the proximal lunate osteonecrosis with no vascular perfusion. Therefore there is no enhancement of the nonviable bone (Fig. 11.10). The middle reparative zone has dense cell proliferation and is hypervascular, therefore has marked contrast enhancement ("hyperenhanced" zone). The distal aspect of the lunate—particularly the dorsal and palmar poles—have normal signal height in unenhanced and enhanced MRI due to normal bone marrow, enhancement with contrast is not seen.

*MRI pattern C*: Generalized signal loss in T1-weighted sequences is seen in advanced necrosis cases with typically no contrast enhancement at all. Interestingly, bone-marrow edema can be found infrequently despite the

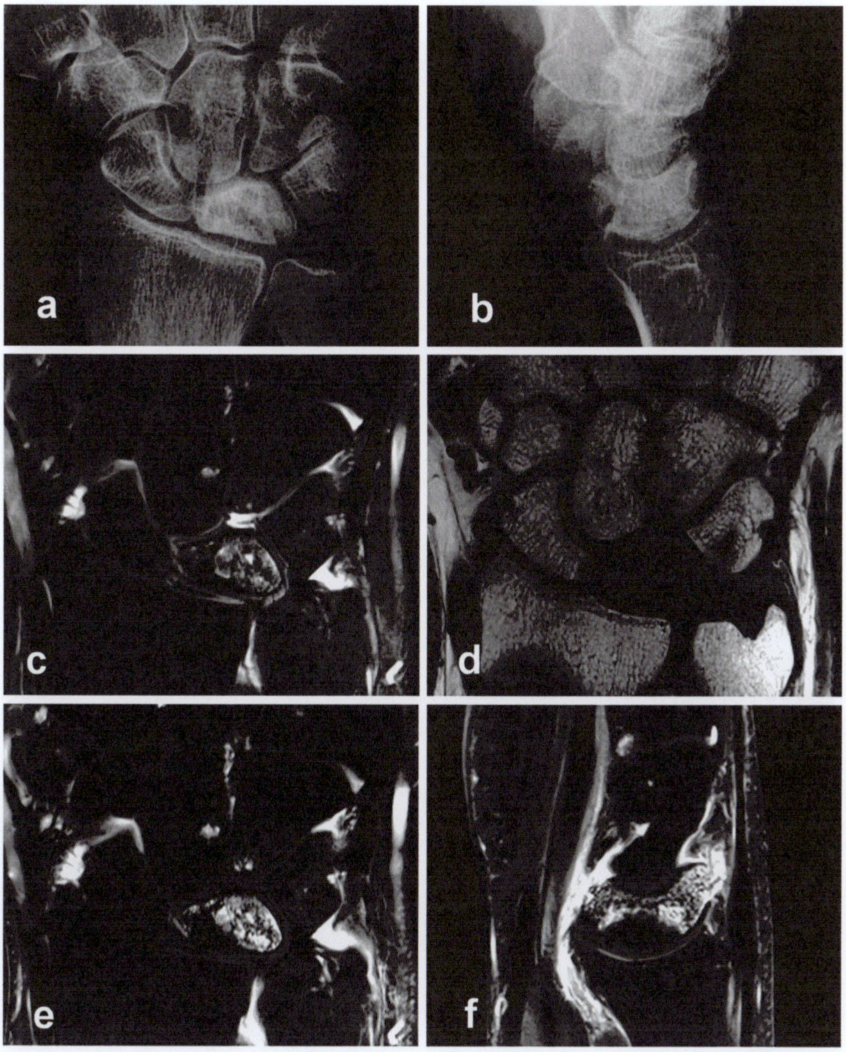


**Fig. 11.10** Partial lunate necrosis (MRI pattern B) in stage IIIb of Kienböck's disease. Patient is a 56-year-old male with a painful swollen wrist. Both necrotic and repair zones are located side by side. (**a, b**) In dorsopalmar and lateral radiographs, the lunate is diffuse osteosclerotic and flattened at its proximal circumference. (**c**) The hypointense proximal zone of the lunate is evident, while there is marked bone-marrow edema in the middle and distal parts (coronal PD-w FSE fat-saturated). Type II lunate with degeneration at the lunohamate joint. (**d**) In the T1-weighted sequence, the lunate is inhomogenously hypointense in its whole territory (coronal T1-w FSE). (**e, f**) With intravenous gadolinium, the proximal circumference of the lunate remains hypointense, whereas the middle part shows marked hyperenhancement, and the distal poles only have low hyperenhancement (coronal and sagittal T1-w FSE fat-saturated after intravenous gadolinium). Adjacent synovitis is remarkable

absence of perfusion and contrast enhancement (Fig. 11.11). In most cases of advanced Kienböck's disease however, there is also a signal loss in T2-weighted sequences (Fig. 11.12). Irreversible osteonecrosis of MRI pattern C is either focally limited to the proximal circumference or territorially extended to the entire lunate. Complete osteonecrosis ("dead bone") is present without any repairing areas. Histopathological slices are characterized by empty osteocyte vacuoles, territorial removal of debris, formation of bone cavities, and comminute fracture zones. The nonviable lunate has a poor prognosis, of course.

In advanced stages of Kienböck's disease, synovitis is present around the lunate in ceMRI.

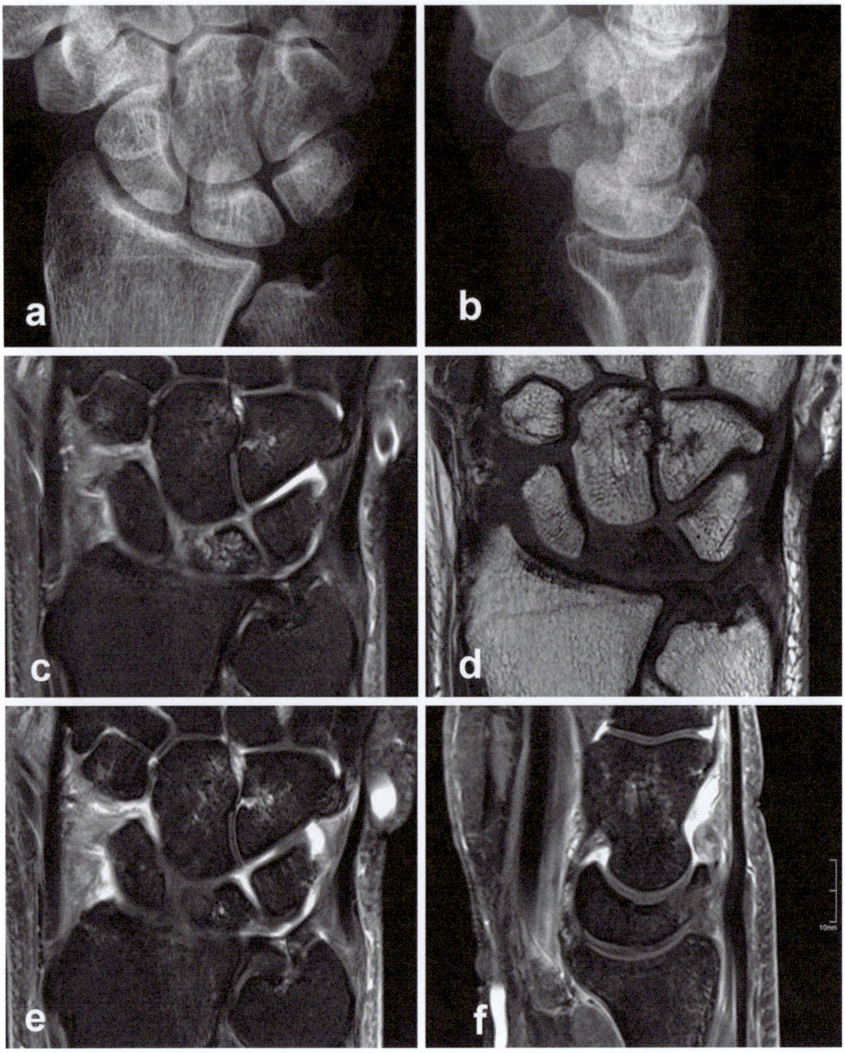


**Fig. 11.11** Complete lunate necrosis (MRI pattern C) in stage IIIc of Kienböck's disease. Patient is a 51-year-old male with a painful wrist and reduced range of motion as a result of a crushing injury of the hand 5 years before. Necrosis is manifest in the fractured lunate in the presence of bone-marrow edema. (**a**, **b**) Dorsopalmar and lateral radiographs show minor osteosclerosis and negative ulnar variance. (**c**) Patchy bone-marrow edema in the center of the lunate (coronal PD-w FSE fat-saturated). (**d**) The lunate, which is slightly changed in shape, is of inhomogeneous low signal (coronal T1-w FSE). (**e**, **f**) No hyperenhancement is present within the lunate, suggesting complete necrosis. The dorsal pole is fractured and displaced (coronal and sagittal T1-w FSE fat-saturated after intravenous gadolinium). Note diffuse carpal synovitis

## Classification Systems

The classic staging system of Kienböck's disease was introduced on the base of X-ray findings [7, 28]. Later, the X-ray-based classification has been modified several times with inserting imaging aspects of MRI and carpal biomechanics. Firstly, bone marrow edema identified on MRI [40]. Secondly, the subcategories of the stable and instable wrist were included, depending upon the radioscaphoid angle (RSA) [41]. The RSA is less than 60° in Lichtman stage IIIa, and greater than 60° in stage IIIb [32].

Thirdly, a new stage IIIc was introduced to assess the coronal fracture type of the lunate [33]. The inclusion of these different approaches led to

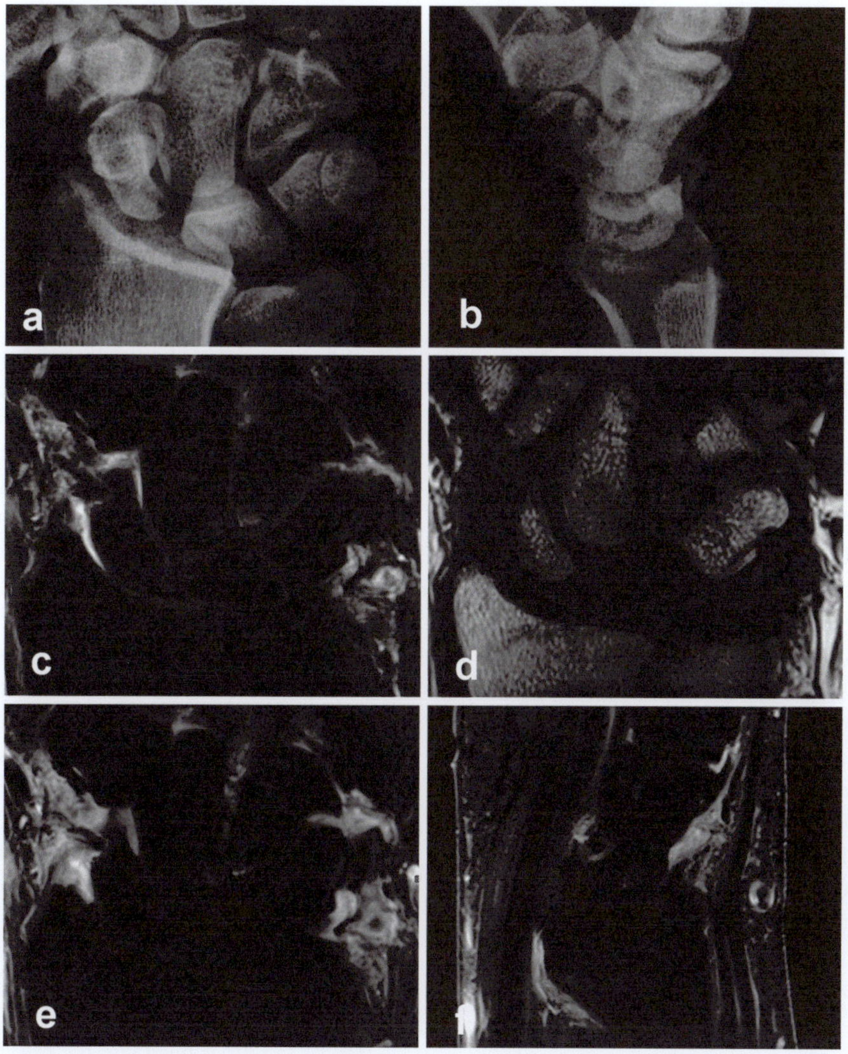

**Fig. 11.12** Complete lunate necrosis (MRI pattern C) in stage IIIc of Kienböck's disease. Patient is a 52-year-old male who has been suffering from severe wrist pain for 2 years. Necrosis is manifest in the absence of bone-marrow edema. (**a**, **b**) Dorsopalmar and lateral radiographs show slight lunate osteosclerosis. There is a negative ulnar variance and suspicion of a dorsal pole fracture. (**c**) The lunate is without any evidence of bone-marrow edema. The proximal pole is flattened, and horizontal fracture lines can be assumed. Hyperintense degenerative changes at the proximal poles of the hamate and capitate (coronal PD-w FSE fat-saturated). (**d**) On this T1-weighted image, the lunate has no signal, demonstrating there is no medullary fat (coronal T1-w FSE). (**e**, **f**) There is no hyperenhancement following gadolinium. The lunate is coronal fractured in the center and also at the proximal circumference. Marked synovitis is present (coronal and sagittal T1-w FSE fat-saturated after intravenous gadolinium)

the current osseous radiographic classification of Kienböck's disease. Indeed, this current classification is of value for clinical use and management decisions; however, it is incomplete with respect to assessing the vascularity of the lunate.

Other than the radiographic classification, the MRI patterns in signal intensity and contrast enhancement describe functional tissue parameters, i.e., the relaxivity of the bone marrow before and after application of gadolinium. Relaxivity is the ability of magnetic compounds to increase the relaxation rates of the surrounding water proton spins. Since different physical conditions are measured (X-ray absorption versus MRI relaxivity), there is no congruence between the radiographic and MRI classifications. While projection radiography and CT depict the osseous anatomy of the lunate and the perilunate joints, ceMRI exclusively covers the bone and bone-marrow viability. The assessment modalities do not compete in the evaluation of Kienböck's disease, but complement one another to achieve a comprehensive staging system of Kienböck's disease.

Therefore, it is recommended to apply both the X-ray classification [40] and the MRI classification system [22] side-by-side for exactly describing the stages of Kienböck's disease. For example, the pathoanatomic constellation of a proximal lunate fracture, with a stable wrist (RSA < 60°), and an active repair zone in the middle section of the lunate is classified in the proposed system as "Kienböck's stage IIIa, MRI pattern B".

There is actually the real necessity for a new and comprehensive classification system of Kienböck's disease [33]. Such a basically revised classification system should merge the traditional and all new imaging aspects (CT and contrast-enhanced MR imaging) as well as the arthroscopic evaluation of the articular cartilage for determining the exact degree of involvement in Kienböck's disease and for choosing appropriate treatment decisions [24].

## "Teenböck's": Pediatric and Juvenile

The prognoses of adult and younger Kienböck's disease are different. There is a high potential for spontaneous remodeling and revascularization in pediatric patients (up to 12 years) and juvenile patients (12 to skeleton maturity). In these patients, the condition is often self-limiting and the prognosis is considerably better, even in the advanced stages of the disease. In juvenile patients older than 16 years, this phenomenon is not as reliable as in the younger children. Unloading of the lunate is the treatment of choice [25, 26]. Usually there is bony healing of the lunate, but mostly with deformity. Temporary transfixation of the scaphotrapezoidal joint with titanium K-wires made from titanium is an ideal therapeutic option, as it allows MRI imaging and is reversible as soon as the lunate is healed [25]. Normalization of the MRI signal can be expected with the return of proximal blood flow, fat cells, and hematopoietic elements (Fig. 11.13).

## Differential Diagnoses

There is considerable variability of MRI presentation of Kienbock's disease (Fig. 11.14). However Kienböck's disease needs to be distinguished from other causes, particularly in the early stages, when radiographs may be negative. When interpreting MR images, one should keep in mind that only about 25 % of all signal-compromised lunates are caused by Kienböck's avascular necrosis [42]. There is a broad spectrum of differential diagnoses that account for the remaining 75 % [27, 42]. By evaluating the clinical, biomechanical, and imaging findings, the following pseudo-Kienböck's entities should be identified:

- *Ulnolunate impaction syndrome*: In contrast to Kienböck's disease, the maximum of the signal changes are located at the proximal-ulnar circumference of the lunate [43, 44]. Mostly, but not always, a positive ulnar variance is the cause of the biomechanical impaction of the ulnar head and the proximal-ulnar aspect of the lunate. For the same reason, degenerative TFC perforations are associated. Cystic and osteosclerotic lesions are accompanied by perifocal bone marrow edema in symptomatic patients. Figure 11.15a, b illustrates a case of ulnolunate impaction without positive ulnar variance and without perforated TFC.
- *Intraosseous ganglion cysts*: These cystoid lesions are located within the lunate, adjacent to the scapholunate (SL) and lunotriquetral (LT) ligaments inserts (Fig. 11.15c, d). Ganglion cysts develop from hypertrophy of the synovia enveloping the ligament, and form radiolucent cysts with a surrounding sclerotic rim. If there is a focal signal change on MRI,

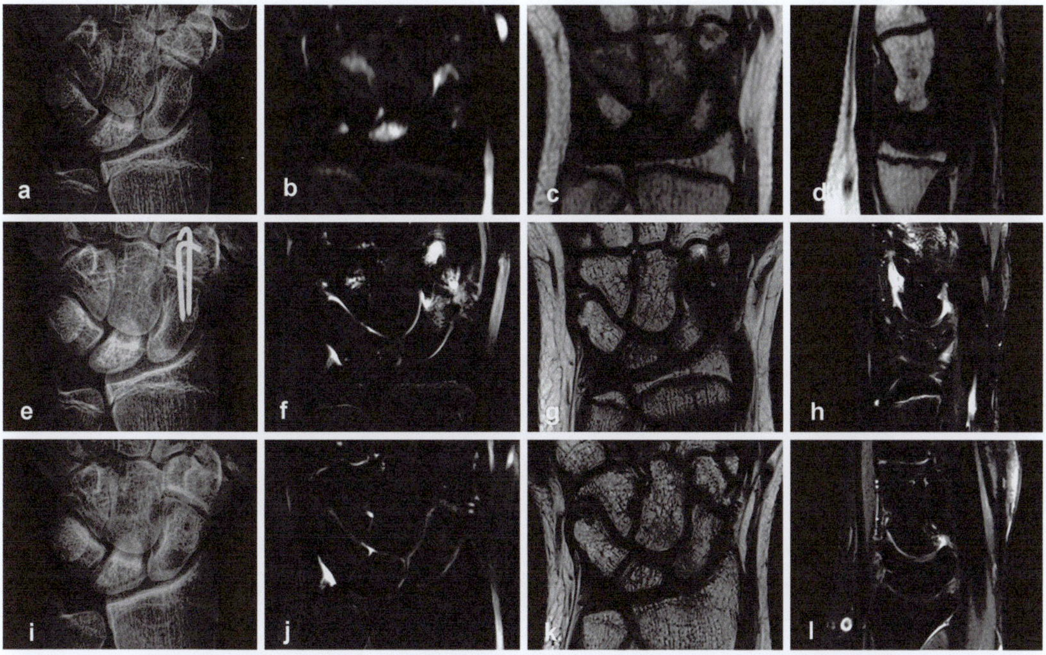


**Fig. 11.13** Healing of juvenile Kienböck's disease (stage I) in the follow-up after temporary STT fusion. Patient is a 14-year-old female adolescent with progressive wrist pain following a fall onto her outstretched hand 7 months before. (**a–d**) Pre-therapeutic baseline imaging (external MRI). Patchy osteosclerosis and bone-marrow edema of the lunate (hyperintense in T2-, hypointense in T1-weighted images) are eye-catching. (**e–h**) Imaging 4 months after temporary STT fusion. Osteosclerosis has advanced, but signal changes and gadolinium enhancement of the lunate are significantly improved. (**i–l**) Imaging 10 months after temporary STT fusion and hardware removal. Osteosclerosis has decreased, and signal changes and gadolinium enhancement of the lunate have completely normalized. Image order: Dorsopalmar radiographs in the left column, coronal PD-w FSE fat-saturated MRI in the second column, coronal T1-w FSE MRI in the third column, and sagittal plain T1-w FSE resp. T1-w FSE fat-saturated MRI after intravenous gadolinium in the fourth column

the differential diagnosis should include an intraosseous ganglion cyst. Then CT imaging should be performed for detailed visualization of the cystoid cavity surrounded by a sclerotic rim and connected to the interosseous ligament by a transcortical channel [45]. On MRI, a hyperintense, dumbbell-shaped lesion is obvious on T2-weighted images. In symptomatic cases, a perifocal edema is present.

- *Posttraumatic lesions*: Traumatic bone contusions ("bone bruises"), fractures, nonunions, and posttraumatic osteoarthritis (Fig. 11.15e, f) can mimic signal changes of Kienböck's disease [27]. Differentiation is usually possible by the history of a previous injury.
- *Lunotriquetral synchondrosis*: Characteristic of fibrocartilaginous coalition (Minaar type I) are irregularities of the subchondral bone substance, narrowed or absence of the LT joint space, and hyperintense signal changes of the subchondral bone marrow of the lunate and triquetrum (Fig. 11.15g, h) [46].
- *Inflammatory conditions*: With arthritis there are often subtle erosions surrounded by focal bone-marrow edema. Examples include rheumatoid arthritis, seronegative spondylarthropathies, and calcium pyrophosphate dehydrate (CPPD) arthropathy. Clinical presentation, typical involvement of several joints and pannus-like synovial thickening are indicative of the inflammatory arthritis.

Differentiation of the underlying pathology is possible in over 80 % of the signal-compromised lunates, when clinical, biomechanical, and imaging aspects are evaluated synoptically [42].

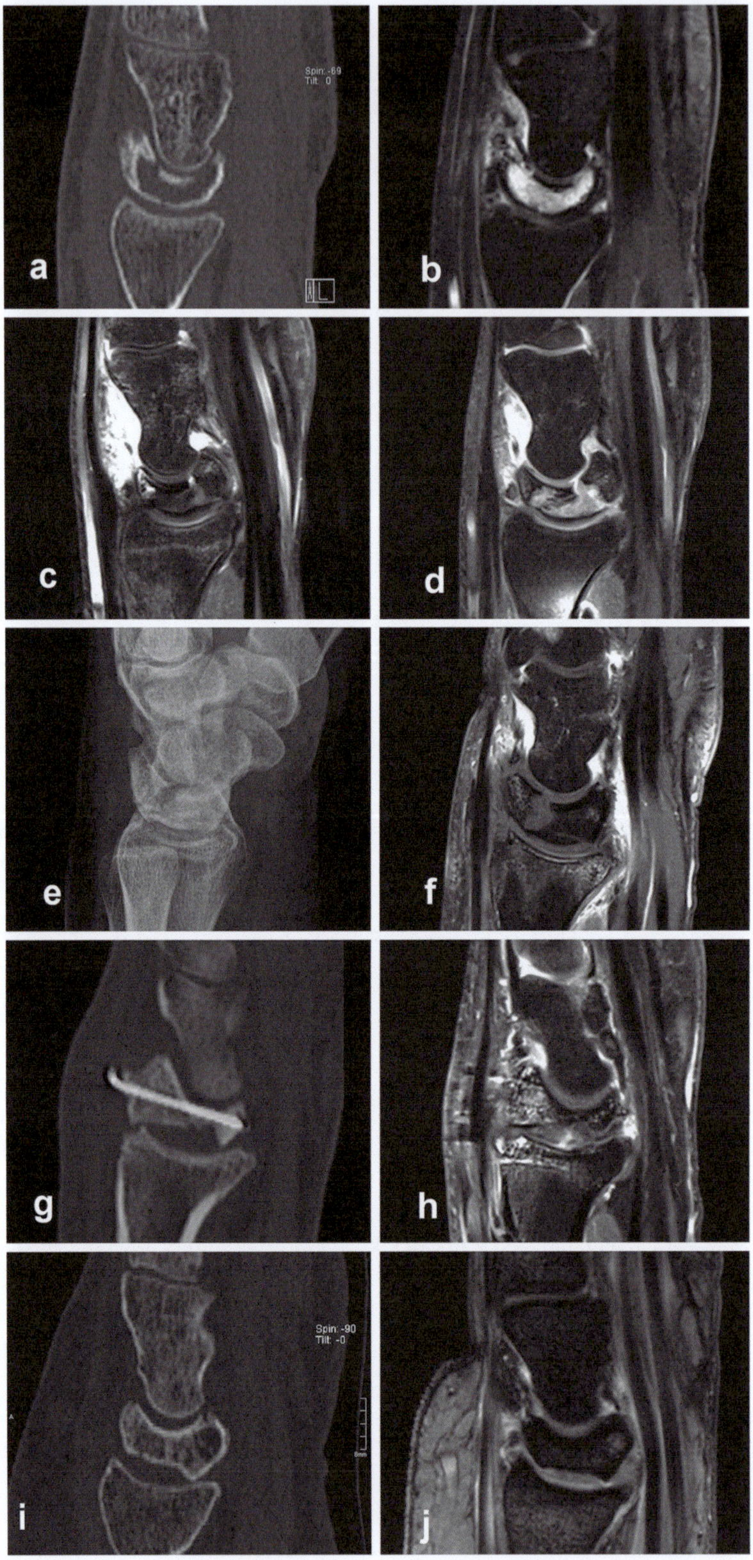


**Fig. 11.14** Collection of five different appearances of Kienböck's disease (all in stages IIIa or IIIb). (**a, b**) Hypervascularized repair zone (MRI pattern A). Sagittal CT and MRI (T1-w FSE fat-saturated after intravenous gadolinium) of a 24-year-old female suffering from wrist pain over 1 year. There is extensive central osteolysis and an impacted fragment at the distal circumference. The repair zone covering most of the lunate is extensively

## Limitations of Imaging

CT and MRI have significantly pushed the capabilities of advanced imaging in Kienböck's disease; however, some limitations are still present and evident:

Firstly, we strongly recommend high-resolution approaches for CT as well as for MR imaging with the use of thin slices (0.5 mm resp. 2 mm) and high image matrices (512×512 resp. 384×384) as introduced earlier in this chapter. The necessity of high-resolution imaging is anatomically based on the extension of the lunate of less than 2 cm. CT and MRI scans performed with lower resolution would potentially hide essential information required to accurately determine management.

Secondly, the necessity of including intravenous gadolinium in MRI for Kienböck's disease must be emphasized. As presented earlier in this chapter, there are compelling arguments for including contrast-enhanced MRI over plain MRI. However scientific evidence is yet to be provided with respect to gadolinium in the early stages and final outcome of Kienböck's disease. In the early stages of the disease, patients are often treated with immobilization, radial shortening, or STT fusion, so it has been difficult to obtain sufficient biopsies for histological correlation. However our unpublished data demonstrates an excellent correlation between the histology and three-zones seen with enhanced MRI.

Radiology-pathology correlation is much easier with the proximal fragment of a scaphoid nonunion. In a prospective study of 88 scaphoid nonunions, we compared the unenhanced MRI, contrast-enhanced MRI, and intraoperative bleeding from the proximal scaphoid [38]. Bone-marrow edema in unenhanced MRI was assessed as an inferior indicator of bone viability, and contrast-enhanced MRI provided significant higher sensitivity in detecting nonviable proximal fragments. A nearly equivalent approach has been reported for MRI and the tetracycline calcium complexes in the uptake of bone mineralization. Normal MRI signal of the bone marrow was shown to correlate with the presence of the osteoid and osteocytes, whereas absence of tetracycline label was noted in areas of focal osteonecrosis [16, 17].

And finally, we have suggested an expensive imaging protocol to diagnosis and stage Kienböck's disease. The costs are important, especially in the current health environment. However we believe cost-effectiveness is optimized when the best treatment is based on the best diagnostic information.

## Diagnostic Algorithm

Based on the different diagnostic capabilities of conventional radiography, CT, and MRI, the following algorithm is recommended for imaging and staging of Kienböck's disease:

**Fig. 11.14** (continued) vascularized. Bleeding bone marrow was found at surgery (cancellous bone grafting and temporary STT fusion). (**c**, **d**) Progressively vascularized repair zone (MRI pattern B). Preoperative and follow-up MRI (both exams with T1-w FSE fat-saturated after intravenous gadolinium) in an 18-year-old male with severe wrist pain. Extensive vascularized repair tissue and an ossified island have developed 7 months after temporary SST fusion and radial shortening (artifacts caused by the radial plate). Carpal synovitis is resolving. (**e**, **f**) Avascular repair zone (MRI pattern C). Lateral radiogram and sagittal MRI (T1-w FSE fat-saturated after intravenous gadolinium) in a 35-year-old male suffering from exertional wrist pain. Repair zones at coronal and proximal fractures are without any enhancement and thus avascular. Patchy enhancement is present in the dorsal pole of the lunate, only. (**g**, **h**) Free-vascularized osteochondral bone graft. Sagittal CT and MRI (T1-w FSE fat-saturated after intravenous gadolinium) in a 22-year-old male treated with osteochondral bone graft which is fixed with a dorsal k-wire to the remaining lunate (CT imaging 1 month after surgery). After hardware removal, MRI nicely depicts a central fissure in the articular cartilage of the lunate (20 months later). (**i**, **j**) Healed Kienböck's disease in an adult. Sagittal CT and MRI (T1-w FSE fat-saturated after intravenous gadolinium) in a 64-year-old female with carpal discomfort for decades. The concave defect of the proximal circumference of the lunate is partially covered by articular cartilage, but there is a deep chondral defect at the palmar pole. No signal changes were detectable on plain T1- and T2-weighted sequences (not shown)

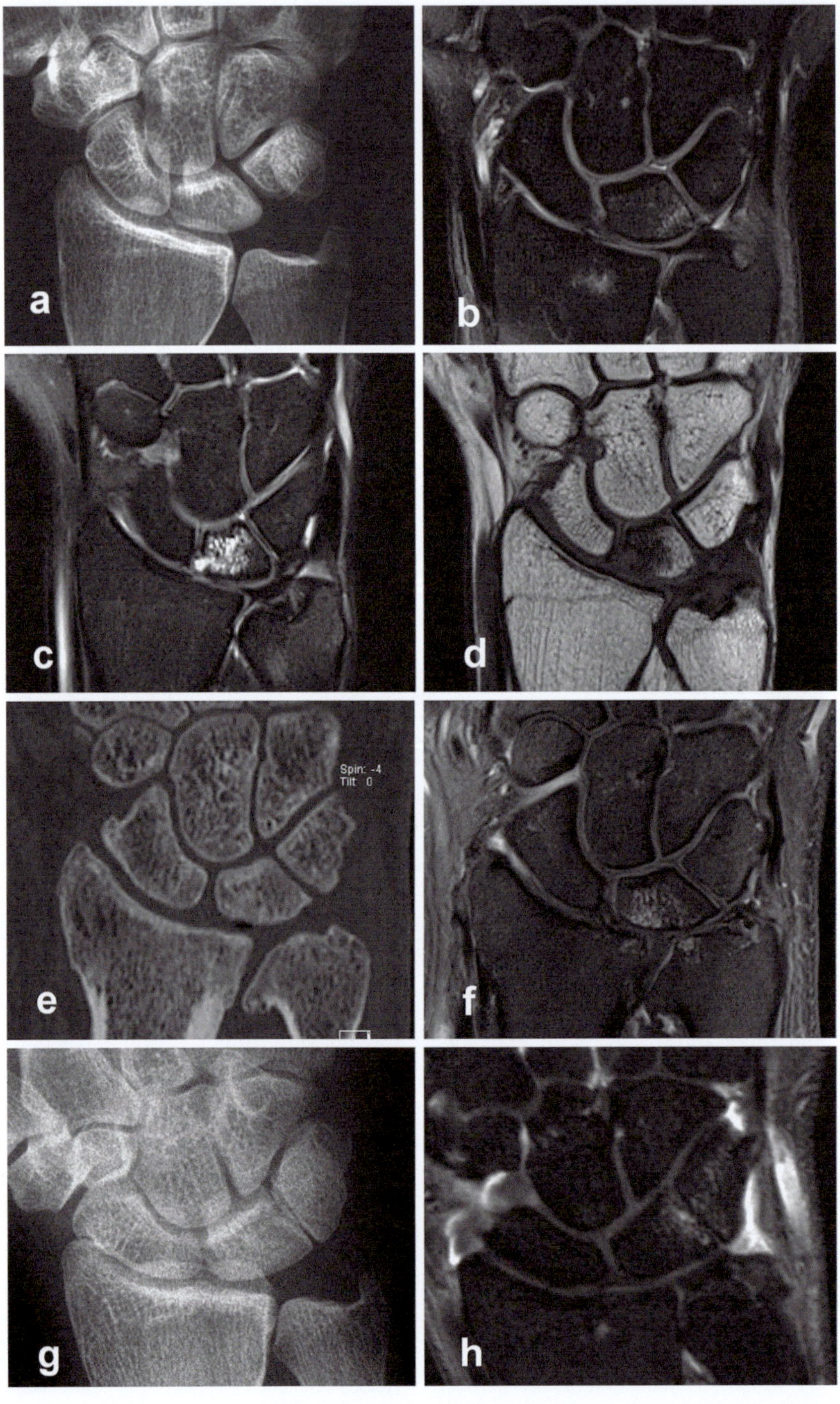


**Fig. 11.15** Differential diagnoses of Kienböck's disease. (**a**, **b**) Ulnar carpal impaction syndrome. Patient is a 44-year-old female with ulnar-sided wrist pain. Dorsopalmar radiograph is unremarkable. In fat-saturated PD-w FSE, subchondral bone-marrow edema is located at the proximal-ulnar circumference of the lunate. This ulnar-sided edema is different in localization from radial-sided signal changes in Kienböck's disease. Note, TFC is not perforated by degeneration. (**c**, **d**) Intraosseous ganglion cyst originating from the scapholunate ligament. Patient is a 16-year-old female with dorsal wrist pain. A 6-mm ganglion cyst, originating from the scapholunate ligament, is both extra- and intraosseous. Surrounding bone-marrow edema is seen in fat-saturated PD-w FSE (*left*),

- Historically, radiography is the first line of imaging. The radiographic views should be acquired in the neutral position to provide a standardized assessment of ulnar variance. The diagnosis of advanced Kienböck's disease is primarily established through radiographs. No further imaging is required in stage IV disease, because only salvage procedures would be indicated.
- Plain radiographs are also valuable in detecting or excluding a broad spectrum of the differential diagnoses.
- Plain radiography will not identify the early marrow changes of Kienböck's disease. An MRI is therefore recommended if Kienböck's disease is suspected, despite normal radiographs. In stage I Kienböck's disease, MRI is the only modality that will provide a diagnosis.
- Generally, ceMRI is useful in Kienböck's stages I to III to assess bone-marrow viability (MRI patterns A to C). It should be used in conjunction with X-rays and CT imaging which will provide a better appreciation of the macroscopic osseous changes. Additionally, ceMRI provides the unique capability to assess the perfusion and degree of repair, and can therefore is of some prognostic value in the healing process (see Fig. 11.8).
- Once the diagnosis of Kienböck's disease is established, determination of the degree of involvement should be made in order to guide the management options. In the intermediate stages, CT imaging is essential to determine the precise osseous changes of the lunate and the perilunar joints.
- This includes assessment of trabecular osteosclerosis (stage II), small fractures of the proximal lunate (stage IIIa), coronal fractures (stage IIIc) and identify perilunar osteoarthritis (stage IV).
- Bone scintigraphy is not currently recommended for assessing Kienböck's disease, because of its low specificity.

In summary, both contrast-enhanced MRI and high-resolution CT imaging are important in Kienböck's disease due to their different capabilities: CT imaging is needed for osseous morphology, MRI is essential for assessing bone and bone-marrow viability. Both procedures should be applied in equivocal diagnostic and therapeutic cases. Once armed with this advanced imaging information, the clinician is better placed to assess the differential diagnosis and stage the vascular, osseous, and articular cartilage of the lunate. This assists the clinician to interpret the clinical problem, assess the healing potential, and create an informed treatment algorithm. The individual treatment options are discussed in detail later in the book. Some examples are presented in Figs. 11.8, 11.13, and 11.15.

**Acknowledgement** We cordially thank Dr. Gregory Bain for enhancing the style of the original manuscript.

## References

1. Kienböck R. Über traumatische Malazie des Mondbeins und Kompressionsfracturen. Fortschr Röntgenstr. 1910;16:77–103.
2. Irisarri C. Aetiology of Kienböck's disease. J Hand Surg Br. 2004;29:281–7.
3. Lluch A, Garcia-Elias M. Etiology of Kienböck disease. Tech Hand Surg. 2011;15:33–7.
4. Gelberman RH, Bauman TH, Menon J, Akeson WH. The vascularity of the lunate bone and Kienböck's disease. J Hand Surg Am. 1980;5:272–8.
5. Panagis JS, Gelberman RH, Taleisnik J, Baumgaertner M. The arterial anatomy of the human carpus. Part

**Fig. 11.15** (continued) while a cortical defect at the communicating site is best visualized in plain T1-w FSE (*right*). (**e**, **f**) Osteoarthritis including the radiolunate and ulnolunate articulations. Patient is a 30-year-old male with malunited distal radius fracture. On the CT scan the subchondral changes of post-traumatic arthritis are seen at the radiolunate, ulnolunate and distal radioulnar joints. So-called "vacuum phenomenon" is seen in coronal CT. The MRI demonstrates the edema and the torn TFC (fat-saturated PD-w FSE). (**g**, **h**) Lunotriquetral coalition, fibrocartilaginous subtype (Minaar type I). Incidental finding in a 34-year-old male after crush injury of his midhand. Congenital synchondrosis is characterized by a narrowed and irregular lunotriquetral joint space as well as by hyperintense signal inclusions on the ulnar side of the lunate in fat-saturated PD-w FSE

II. The intraosseous vascularity. J Hand Surg Am. 1983;8:375–82.
6. Lee M. The intraosseous arterial pattern of the carpal lunate bone and its relation to avascular necrosis. Acta Orthop Scand. 1963;33:43–55.
7. Stahl F. On lunatomalacia (Kienböck's disease), a clinical and roentgenological study, especially on its pathogenesis and the late results of immobilization treatment. Acta Chir Scand. 1947;126(Suppl): 1–133.
8. Schiltenwolf M, Martini AK, Mau HC, Eversheim S, Brocai DR, Jensen CH. Further investigations of the intraosseous pressure characteristics in necrotic lunates (Kienböck's disease). J Hand Surg Am. 1996; 21:754–8.
9. Hultén O. Über anatomische Variationen der Handgelenkknochen. Acta Radiol. 1928;9:155–68.
10. Gelberman RH, Salamon RB, Jurist JM, Posch JL. Ulnar variance in Kienbock's disease. J Bone Joint Surg Am. 1975;57:674–6.
11. Antuna Zapico JM. Kienböck's disease. Rev Ortop Traumatol. 1993;37IB(Suppl I):100–13.
12. Nakamura R, Tanaka Y, Imaeda T, Miura T. The influence of age and sex on ulnar variance. J Hand Surg Br. 1991;16:84–8.
13. Chung KC, Spilson MS, Kim MH. Is negative ulnar variance a risk factor for Kienböck's disease? A meta-analysis. Ann Plast Surg. 2001;47:494–9.
14. Razemon JP. Kienböck's disease radiology. Ann Radiol. 1982;25:353–8.
15. Owers KL, Scougall P, Dabirrahmani G, Wernecke G, Jhamb A, Walsh WR. Lunate trabecular structure: a cadaveric radiograph study of risk factors for Kienböck's disease. J Hand Surg Eur Vol. 2010;35: 120–4.
16. Desser TS, McCarthy S, Trumble T. Scaphoid fractures and Kienböck's disease of the lunate: MR imaging with histopathologic correlation. Magn Reson Imaging. 1990;8:357–62.
17. Trumble TE, Irving J. Histologic and magnetic resonance imaging correlations in Kienböck's disease. J Hand Surg Am. 1990;15:879–84.
18. Aspenberg P, Wang JS, Jonsson K, Hagert CG. Experimental osteonecrosis of the lunate. Revascularization may cause collapse. J Hand Surg Br. 1994;19:565–9.
19. Hashizume H, Asahara H, Nishida K, Inoue H, Konishiike T. Histopathology of Kienboeck's disease. Correlation with magnetic resonance and other imaging techniques. J Hand Surg Br. 1996;21:89–93.
20. Ogawa T, Nishiura Y, Hara Y, Okamoto Y, Ochiai N. Correlation of histopathology with magnetic resonance imaging in Kienböck's disease. J Hand Surg Am. 2012;37:83–9.
21. Raffray M, Cohen GM. Apoptosis and necrosis in toxicology: a continuum or distinct modes of cell death? Pharmacol Ther. 1997;75:153–77.
22. Schmitt R, Heinze A, Fellner F, Obletter N, Strühn R, Bautz W. Imaging and staging of avascular osteonecroses at the wrist and hand. Eur J Radiol. 1997; 25:92–103.
23. Schmitt R, Kalb KH. Imaging in Kienböck's disease. Handchir Mikrochir Plast Chir. 2010;42:162–70.
24. Bain GI, Begg M. Arthroscopic assessment and classification of Kienböck's disease. Tech Hand Up Extrem Surg. 2006;10:8–13.
25. Kalb K, Pillukat T, Schmitt R, Prommersberger KJ. Die Lunatumnekrose im Kindes- und Jugendalter. Handchir Mikrochir Plast Chir. 2010;42:187–97.
26. Irisarri C, Kalb K, Ribak S. Infantile and juvenile lunatomalacia. J Hand Surg Eur Vol. 2010;35:544–8.
27. Arnaiz J, Piedra T, Cerezal L, Ward J, Thompson A, Vidal JA, et al. Imaging of Kienböck disease. Am J Roentgenol. 2014;203:131–9.
28. Decoulx P, Marchand M, Minet P, Razemon JP. La Maladie de Kienböck chez le mineur. Lille Chir. 1957;12:65–81.
29. Palmer AK, Glisson RR, Werner FW. Ulnar variance determination. J Hand Surg Am. 1982;7:376–9.
30. Friedman L, Yong-Hing K, Johnston GH. The use of coronal computed tomography in the evaluation of Kienböck's disease. Clin Radiol. 1991;44:56–9.
31. Youm Y, McMurtry RY, Flatt AE, Gillespie TE. Kinematics of the wrist. Part I – an experimental study of radial-ulnar deviation and flexion-extension. J Bone Joint Surg Am. 1978;60:423–31.
32. Goldfarb CA, Hsu J, Gelberman RH, Boyer MI. The Lichtman classification for Kienböck's disease: an assessment of reliability. J Hand Surg Am. 2003;28: 74–80.
33. Lichtman DM, Lesley NE, Simmons SP. The classification and treatment of Kienböck disease: the state of the art and a look at the future. J Hand Surg Eur Vol. 2010;35:549–54.
34. Reinus WR, Conway WF, Totty WG, Gilula LA, Murphy WA, Siegel BA, et al. Carpal avascular necrosis: MR imaging. Radiology. 1986;160:689–93.
35. Sowa DT, Holder LE, Patt PG, Weiland AJ. Application of magnetic resonance imaging to ischemic necrosis of the lunate. J Hand Surg Am. 1989;14:1008–16.
36. Vande Berg BC, Malghem J, Lecouvet FE, Maldague B. MRI of the normal bone marrow. Skeletal Radiol. 1998;27:471–83.
37. Cerezal L, Abascal A, Garcia-Valtuille R, García-Valtuille R, Bustamante M, del Piñal F. Usefulnes of gadolinium-enhanced MR imaging in the evaluation of the vascularity of scaphoid nonunions. Am J Roentgenol. 2000;174:141–9.
38. Schmitt R, Christopoulos G, Wagner M, Krimmer H, Fodor S, van Schoonhoven J, et al. Avascular necrosis (AVN) of the proximal fragment in scaphoid nonunion: is intravenous contrast agent necessary in MRI? Eur J Radiol. 2011;77:222–7.
39. Donati OF, Zanetti M, Nagy L, Bode B, Schweizer A, Pfirrmann CW. Is dynamic gadolinium enhancement needed in MR imaging for the preoperative assessment of scaphoidal viability in patients with scaphoid nonunion? Radiology. 2011;260:808–16.
40. Lichtman DM, Ross G. Revascularization of the lunate in Kienböck's disease. In: Gelberman RH, editor. The wrist. New York, NY: Raven; 1994. p. 363–72.

41. Lichtman DM, Alexander AH, Mack GR, Gunther SF. Kienböck's disease – update on silicone replacement arthroplasty. J Hand Surg Am. 1982;7:343–7.
42. Schmitt R, Christopoulos G, Kalb K, Coblenz G, Fröhner S, Brunner H, et al. Differential diagnosis of the signal-compromised lunate in MRI. Fortschr Röntgenstr. 2005;177:358–66.
43. Imaeda T, Nakamura R, Shionoya K, Makino N. Ulnar impaction syndrome: MR imaging findings. Radiology. 1996;201:495–500.
44. Cerezal L, del Piñal F, Abascal F, García-Valtuille R, Pereda T, Canga A. Imaging findings in ulnarsided wrist impaction syndromes. Radiographics. 2002; 22:105–21.
45. Magee T, Rowedder AM, Degnan GG. Intraosseous ganglia of the wrist. Radiology. 1995; 195:517–20.
46. Stäbler A, Glaser C, Reiser M, Resnick D. Symptomatic fibrous lunato-triquetral coalition. Eur Radiol. 1999;9:1643.

# Acute Lunate Fractures and Translunate Dislocations

# 12

Gregory Ian Bain, Vikas R. Singh, Joideep Phadnis, and Meenalochani Shunmugam

## Introduction

Lunate fractures and translunate fracture dislocations are rare (0.5 %) [1–4]. In a series of 157 perilunate dislocations there were no translunate fractures reported [4]. The only published data on acute lunate fractures are in the form of case reports and case series. In 1910, Robert Kienbock published a paper on perilunate dislocations (immediately following his landmark publication on lunate avascular necrosis). He states that isolated fractures of scaphoid are most frequent, followed by fractures of the scaphoid and radius. In addition, he described that when the scaphoid fractures, and the lunate dislocates, the proximal aspect of scaphoid stays with the forearm while the distal aspect remains with the hand [5] (Fig. 12.1).

G.I. Bain, MBBS, FRACS, FA(Ortho)A, PhD (✉)
Professor, Upper Limb and Research, Department of Orthopedic Surgery, Flinders University and Flinders Medical Centre, Bedford Park, Adelaide, SA, Australia

V.R. Singh, MBBS, MS, DNB
Department Orthopedic Surgery, Lyell Mcewin Hospital, Haydown Road, Elizabeth Vale, SA 5112, Australia

J. Phadnis, FRCS (Tr & Orth)
Department of Trauma and Orthopedics, Brighton and Sussex University Hospitals, NHS Trust, Eastern Road, Brighton, East Sussex BN1 6AG, UK

M. Shunmugam, MBBS, MSSc
Department of Orthopedic Surgery, Flinders University and Flinders Medical Centre, Adelaide, SA 5042, Australia
e-mail: greg@gregbain.com.au

## Lunate Fracture

Teisen and Hjarbaek reviewed 17 lunate fractures collected over 31 years. Based on plain radiological appearance and the vascularity of the lunate, they classified the lunate fractures into five types. However their classification does not incorporate the relationship between the lunate fracture, perilunate instability, or carpal instability [1]. Other investigators have discussed similar cases of translunate, perilunate fracture-dislocations (or subluxations) but have made no reference to the classification systems commonly used in the application of treatment principles [6–10].

## Perilunate Injuries

A perilunate dislocation involves dislocation of the carpus from the lunate, with associated osteoligamentous injuries [11–14]. In 1980, Johnson classified perilunate fracture dislocations according to the associated structures involved [12]. A lesser arc injury involves the ligaments that surround the lunate (scapholunate and lunotriquetral ligaments). A greater arc injury involves the

© Springer International Publishing Switzerland 2016

D.M. Lichtman, G.I. Bain (eds.), *Kienböck's Disease*, DOI 10.1007/978-3-319-34226-9_12

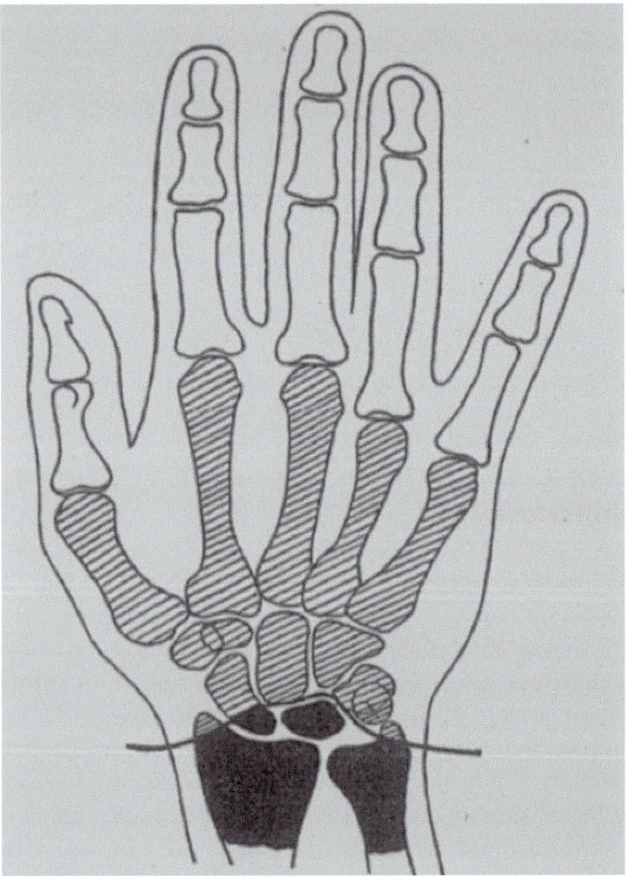

**Fig. 12.1** This is one of many fine images from Robert Kienbock's paper on perilunate injuries in 1910. He stated that, when the scaphoid fractures and the lunate dislocates, the proximal scaphoid remains attached to forearm while the distal part remains with the hand. From Kienböck R. Uber traumatische Malazie des Mondbeins und ihre Folgezustände: Entartungsformen und Kompressions-frakturen. Fortschr Roentgenstr 1910;16:78–103

carpal bones that surround the lunate (scaphoid, capitate, triquetrum, radial, and ulnar styloid). It is common for there to be a mix of greater and lesser arc injuries.

Mayfield described that perilunate dislocation could be reproduced with a progressive ligamentous injury that commenced on the volar radial side, and then around the lunate to the ulnar side of the wrist [12, 13]. This involves a combination of extension, intercarpal supination, and ulnar deviation [11–14], such as occurs with a fall onto the outstretched hand with a fixed pronated radius [11]. Mayfield classified perilunate dislocation into four stages, with a characteristic progression of the injury (Fig. 12.2) [12, 13]. The radiolunate ligament remains attached and allows the lunate to rotate 180°. Alternatively, the lunate remains in place and the remaining carpus translocates dorsally (dorsal perilunate dislocation).

## Translunate Instability

In 2008 Bain introduced the translunate arc concept in a series of three patients [15]. The arc is complementary to the greater and lesser arcs. It includes a zone of injury through the lunate producing a lunate fracture, with associated perilunate injuries. Graham introduced the concept of the inferior arc, in which the path of injury is through the radiocarpal plane [16] (Fig. 12.3). The traditional classification of greater and lesser arc injuries was expanded to a more inclusive classification of carpal fracture-dislocations, which included the translunate and radiocarpal arcs. This classification also assists in identifying the correct management plan.

The pathomechanics of the translunate perilunate dislocation is unclear. Mayfield did not

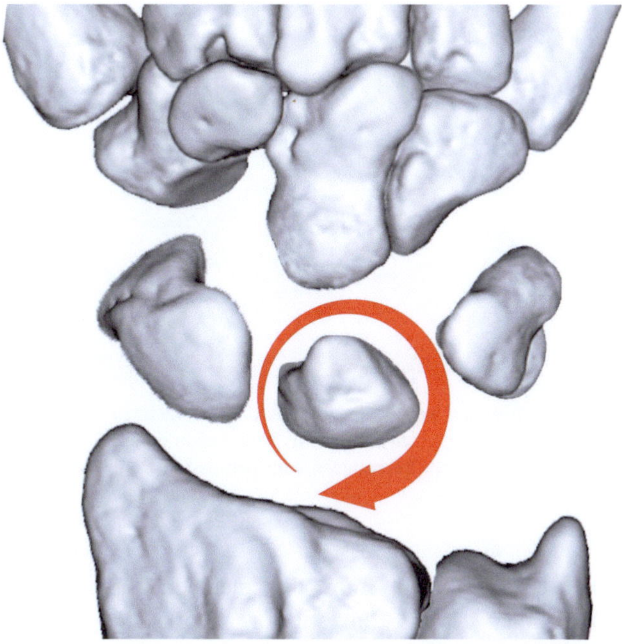

**Fig. 12.2** Mayfield's four stages of perilunate instability. Stage I—Scapholunate ligament disruption. Stage II—Capitolunate dislocation (usually dorsal). Stage III—Lunotriquetral ligament disruption. Stage IV—Dorsal radicarpal ligament disruption. Image created from information from Mayfield JK. Wrist ligamentous anatomy and pathogenesis of carpal instability. Orthop Clin North Am 1984:15:214

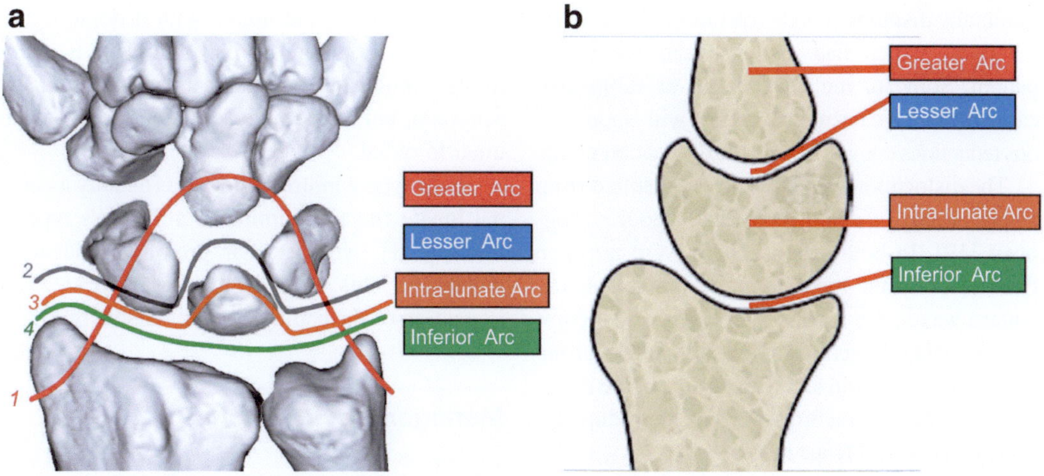


**Fig. 12.3** Spectrum of arc injuries of the wrist. (**a**) Coronal plane. (*1*) greater; (*2*) lesser; (*3*) translunate, and (*4*) inferior arcs. (**b**) Sagittal view of the central column, with the associated four arcs. Reproduced with permission from Bain GI, Pallapati S, Eng K. Translunate perilunate injuries—a spectrum of this uncommon injury. J Wrist Surg 2013; 02(01): 063–068. ©Georg Thieme Verlag KG

assess the effect of a lunate fracture; however, it is likely to be a variation of his description of perilunate instability. It is usually a high-velocity mechanism to create the lunate fracture and the associated carpal injuries [1, 11]. The degree of lunate displacement depends on the type of lunate fracture and the associated carpal fracture and ligament injuries.

Bain et al. divided carpal injuries with an associated lunate fracture into subluxation and dislocation. A total of 34 cases were identified from the literature over a period of 35 years from

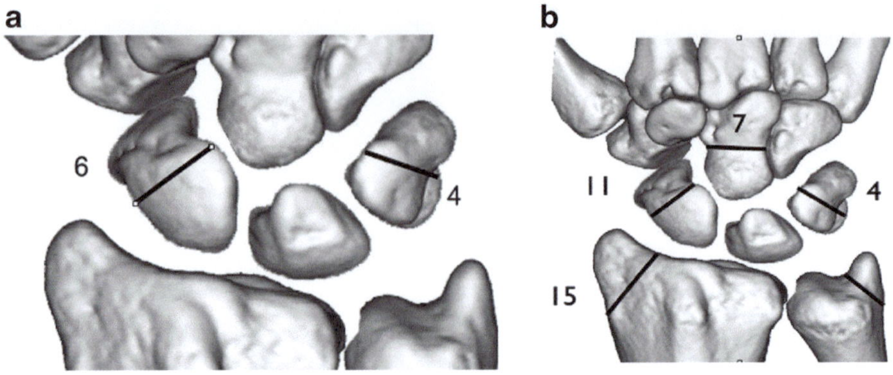


**Fig. 12.4** Location and incidence of associated fractures with translunate perilunate injuries. (**a**) Subluxation group. (**b**) Dislocation group. Reproduced with permission from Bain GI, Pallapati S, Eng K. Translunate perilunate injuries—a spectrum of this uncommon injury. J Wrist Surg 2013; 02(01): 063–068. ©Georg Thieme Verlag KG

1976 to 2011 and from the members of International Wrist Investigator Workshop (IWIW) [15, 17–19].

The subluxation group (ten cases) included minimally displaced lunate fractures to lunate subluxations, which had a translunate arc injury pattern. Some of the undisplaced or subluxated cases could have been dislocations with spontaneous reductions compared with the dislocation group.

The dislocation group (24 cases) resulted from a high-energy mechanism and had a poorer prognosis [19]. In both groups, there were no open fractures, and the most common lunate fracture pattern was in the coronal plane. The most common associated fractures in the subluxation group were of the scaphoid and triquetrum. In the dislocation group the fractures were of the radial styloid and scaphoid (Fig. 12.4).

In several cases, the lunate fracture was not identified initially and the presentation was delayed. This is particularly the case in the subluxation group, where the displacement was less obvious. To identify all the injuries preoperatively, we recommend a 2D and 3D CT scan, which provides great resolution. Traction radiographs provide an appreciation of the injuries, as it minimizes the overlap of the carpus and unmasks the zone of injury [18].

We have performed a further review of lunate fractures and found that the associated instabilities were either of the radiocarpal (type 1) or midcarpal joint (type 2) (Figs. 12.5 and 12.6). The injuries were further subdivided into carpal reduced, subluxated, and dislocated.

Type 1 injuries usually involved a transverse plane fracture of the lunate with a dorso-radial instability of the radiocarpal joint. This is likely to be similar to the mechanism reported by Mayfield, but in the reverse direction, i.e., from ulnar to radial.

In the type 2 injuries, there was usually a coronal lunate fracture, similar to a Teisen's type V fracture [1], with a volar proximal midcarpal instability. This is likely to be due to an axial impaction of the capitate on the lunate [1, 20].

## Management Principles

With a perilunate dislocation, the volar radiolunate ligament remains intact, stabilizing the lunate to the radius. Therefore, the key management principle of all perilunate dislocations is to stabilize the proximal carpal row to the "keystone" lunate (Fig. 12.7). The greater arc fractures are reduced and fixed and the lesser arc injuries are stabilized and the ligaments repaired. We also neutralize the midcarpal joint with a K wire from the distal scaphoid to the capitate.

When assessing a wrist injury that includes a lunate fracture, it is important to consider both the lunate fracture and the associated carpal

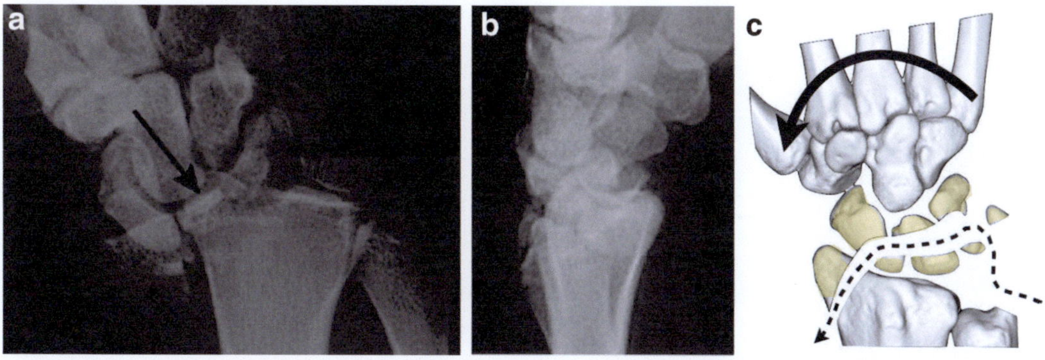


**Fig. 12.5** Translunate perilunate dislocation—type 1 (radiocarpal) dislocation. (**a**) Coronal plane; (**b**) sagittal plane; (**c**) diagram of type 1 translunate radiocarpal dislocation. (**a**) and (**b**) Reproduced with permission from Bain GI, McLean JM, Turner PC, Sood A, Pourgiezis N. Translunate fracture with associated perilunate injury: 3 case reports with introduction of the translunate arc concept. J Hand Surg Am 2008;33(10):1770–1776. Copyright 2008 American Society for the Surgery of the Hand. Published by Elsevier, Inc. All rights reserved. (**c**) Copyright Dr. Gregory Bain

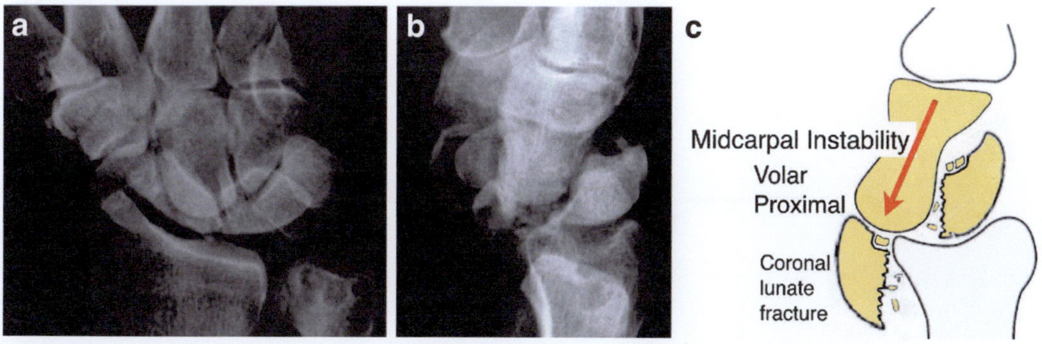


**Fig. 12.6** Translunate fracture with type 2 (midcarpal) instability. (**a**, **b**) Radiographs of trans-styloid, translunate, perilunate fracture–dislocation. (**c**) Diagram of type 2 translunate (midcarpal) dislocation. Copyright Dr. Gregory Bain

instability. If the lunate is also fractured, then the treatment algorithm must change, as the surgeon needs to stabilize the lunate "keystone" first, and then stabilize the proximal carpal row. The associated lunate fracture makes the stabilization process considerably more difficult.

Undisplaced lunate fractures can often be managed conservatively in a plaster cast. Translunate fracture dislocations are typically high-energy injuries. Consequently, these injuries are often more complex, more difficult to treat, and are more likely to have a poor prognosis. It may be difficult to achieve a satisfactory lunate reduction and fixation in the presence of co-existing lesser and/or greater arc injuries. We recommend fixing the lunate "keystone" first, and then the greater arc, and finally stabilizing the lesser arc ligament injuries.

This can be done via either a volar, dorsal, or combined approach. In complex cases, consideration should be given to add a neutralization device such as an external fixateur or bridging plate [21]. If there is a delayed presentation, or extensive comminution, or the above methods are unsuccessful, then a salvage procedure may be required. Salvage options include proximal row carpectomy (PRC), lunate excision, scaphocapitate fusion, wrist arthroplasty, and full wrist

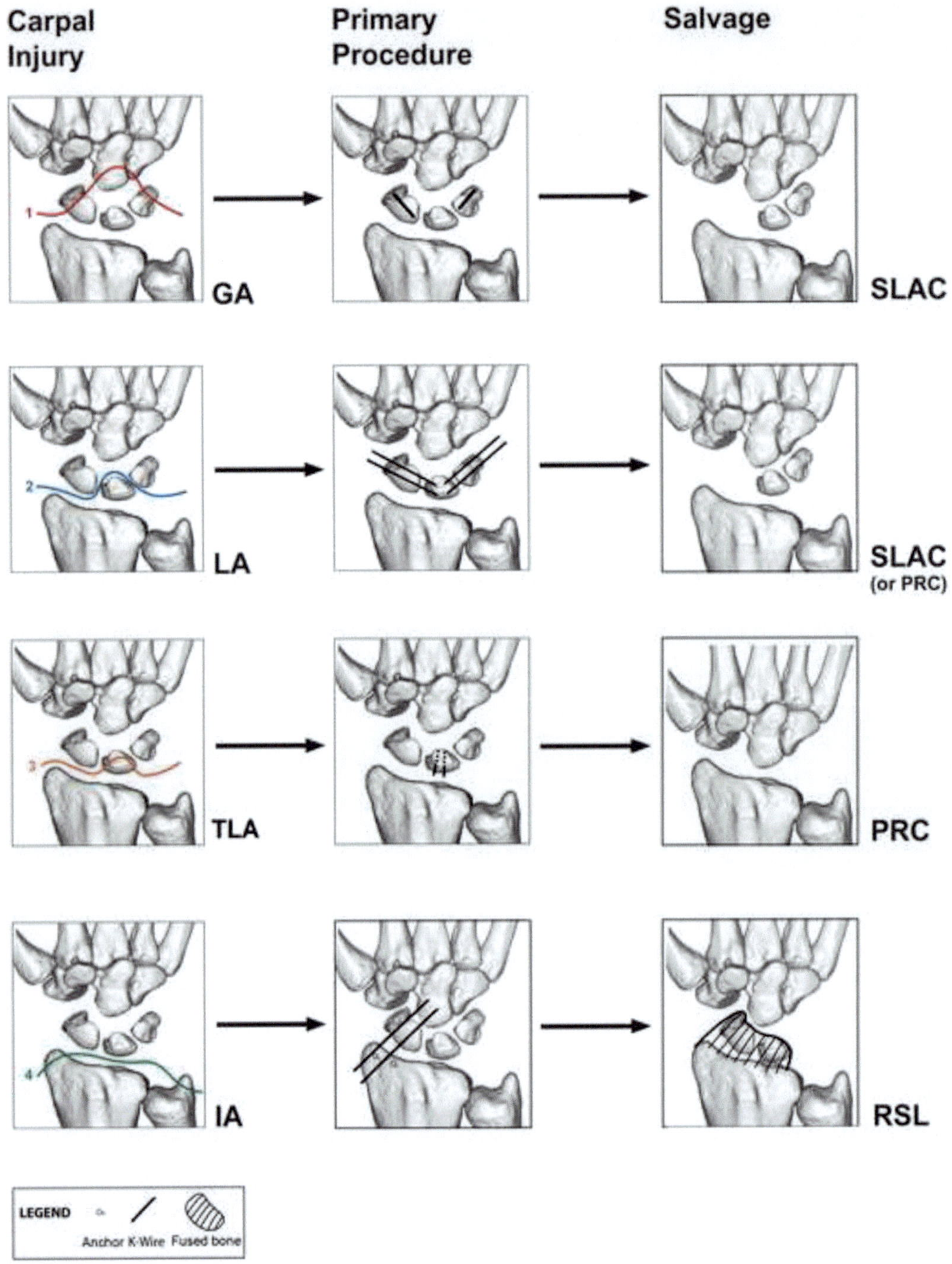


**Fig. 12.7** The "arcs" of complex carpal injuries are presented in diagrammatical form. The algorithm presents the path of instability through the wrist and the structures injured through each arc, followed by the preferred method(s) of fixation requiring repair, and the likely salvage procedure for each. *GA* greater arc, *LA* lesser arc, *TLA* translunate arc, *IA* inferior arc, *SLAC* scapholunate advanced collapse procedure, *PRC* proximal row carpectomy procedure, *RSL* radioscapholunate fusion procedure. Copyright Dr. Gregory Bain

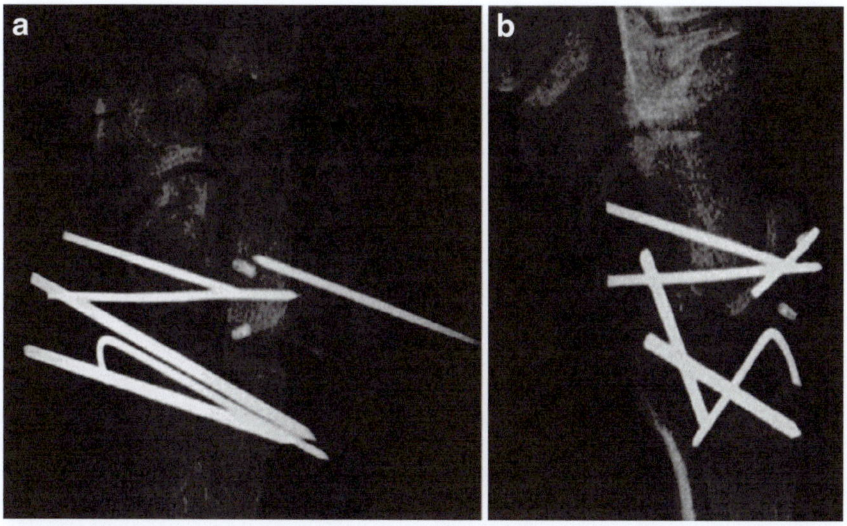


**Fig. 12.8** Failed K-wire internal fixation of the comminuted translunate fracture dislocation (see Fig. 12.3). Radiographs of (**a**) coronal plane and (**b**) sagittal plane. Reproduced with permission from Bain GI, McLean JM, Turner PC, Sood A, Pourgiezis N. Translunate fracture with associated perilunate injury: 3 case reports with introduction of the translunate arc concept. J Hand Surg Am 2008;33(10):1770–1776. Copyright 2008 American Society for the Surgery of the Hand. Published by Elsevier, Inc. All rights reserved. (c) Copyright Dr. Gregory Bain

fusion. A scaphocapitate fusion can be considered for an unsalvageable central column, in which case the load is transferred from the central column to the radial column. These salvage options may be required as a primary or secondary procedure (Fig. 12.8).

The principles of management of the translunate injuries are to stabilize the lunate keystone first, and then fix the greater arc injuries and finally the lesser arc injuries. If the injury is very severe or the diagnosis has been delayed, a salvage procedure may be a preferred option.

## Conclusion

Lunate fractures and translunate fracture dislocations are uncommon and are best assessed with CT scans, to allow a better understanding of the complexity of the injury.

Complex carpal dislocations can be classified by the arc of injury. The arcs include the greater, lesser, translunate, and inferior arcs. The intralunate arc injuries can be subclassified into midcarpal or radiocarpal instabilities, which can be in a dorsal or volar direction. The magnitude of instability is classified as a reduced, subluxation, and dislocation of the wrist.

## References

1. Teisen H, Hjarbaek J. Classification of fresh fractures of the lunate. J Hand Surg Br. 1988;13:458–62.
2. Kuderna H. Frakturen und luxationsfrakturen der hand-warzel. Orthopade. 1986;15:95–108.
3. Razemon JP. Fractures of the carpal bone with the exception of fractures of the carpal scaphoid. In: Razemon JP, editor. The wrist. Edinburgh: Churchill Livingstone; 1988. p. 126–9.
4. Sasaki T. Lunate body fractures. J Jpn Soc Surg Hand. 1991;8:635–9.
5. Kienböck R. Uber traumatische Malazie des Mondbeins und ihre Folgezustände: Entartungsformen und Kompressions- frakturen. Fortschr Roentgenstr. 1910;16:78–103.

6. Conway WF, Gilula LA, Manske PR, Kriegshauser LA, Rholl KS, Resnik C. Translunate, palmar perilunate fracture-subluxation of the wrist. J Hand Surg Am. 1989;14:635–9.
7. Mason GC, Bowman MW, Fu FH. Translunate, perilunate fracture-dislocation of the wrist. A case report. Orthopedics. 1986;9:1001–4.
8. Takase K, Yamamoto K. Unusual combined scaphoid and lunate fracture of the wrist: a case report. J Hand Surg Am. 2006;31:414–7.
9. Noble J, Lamb DW. Translunate scapho-radial fracture. A case report. Hand. 1979;11:47–9.
10. Vichard P, Tropet Y, Balmat P, Brientini JM, Pem R. Reflections on 4 cases of ante-lunar carpal luxations. Ann Chir Main Memb Super. 1991;10:331–6.
11. Johnson RP. The acutely injured wrist and its residuals. Clin Orthop Relat Res. 1980;149:33–44.
12. Mayfield JK. Patterns of injury to carpal ligaments. A spectrum Clin Orthop Relat Res. 1984;187:36–42.
13. Mayfield JK. Mechanism of carpal injuries. Clin Orthop Relat Res. 1980;149:45–54.
14. Garcia-Elias M, Geissler WB. Carpal instability. In: Green DP, Hotchkiss RN, Pederson MD, editors. Green's operative hand surgery. 5th ed. New York, NY: Churchill Livingstone; 2005. p. 591–602.
15. Bain GI, McLean JM, Turner PC, Sood A, Pourgiezis N. Translunate fracture with associated perilunate injury: 3 case reports with introduction of the translunate arc concept. J Hand Surg Am. 2008;33(10):1770–6.
16. Graham TJ. The inferior arc injury: an addition to the family of complex carpal fracture-dislocation patterns. Am J Orthop. 2003;32(9, Suppl):10–9.
17. Enoki NR, Sheppard JE, Taljanovic MS. Transstyloid, translunate fracture-dislocation of the wrist: case report. J Hand Surg Am. 2008;33(7):1131–4.
18. Blazar PE, Murray P. Treatment of perilunate dislocations by combined dorsal and palmar approaches. Tech Hand Up Extrem Surg. 2001;5(1):2–7.
19. Bain GI, Pallapati S, Eng K. Translunate perilunate injuries—a spectrum of this uncommon injury. J Wrist Surg. 2013;02(01):063–8.
20. Vasireddy A, Lowdon I. Lunate fracture in an amateur soccer player. J Orthop Sports Phys Ther. 2009;39(12):884.
21. Vichard P, Tropet Y, Balmat P, Brientini JM, Pem R. Reflections on 4 cases of ante-lunar carpal luxations. Ann Chir Main Memb Super. 1991;10:331–6.

# Arthroscopic Assessment and Treatment of Kienböck's Disease

# 13

Benjamin R. Graves, George S. Gluck, Gary G. Poehling, Terry L. Whipple, Francisco del Piñal, and Gregory Ian Bain

The purpose of this chapter is to discuss wrist arthroscopy and its value in the staging and treatment of Kienböck's disease. Tips and techniques for the use of arthroscopy in the diagnosis and treatment of Kienböck's disease are also presented.

Watanabe et al. first described the use of wrist arthroscopy in the evaluation of Kienböck's disease in 1995 [1]. They found the incidence of interosseous ligament tears correlated with radiographic stage; however, they noted that articular cartilage damage was underestimated based on preoperative radiographs. Since then, multiple authors [2–4] have reported that preoperative radiographic assessment does not necessarily correlate with articular anatomy seen during arthroscopy, with radiographs often underestimating the extent of chondral damage and degeneration. Wrist arthroscopy is also an important tool in the treatment of Kienböck's disease, with reported interventions that include synovectomy and debridement [5], lunate core decompression [6, 7], lunate bone grafting [8], and intercarpal arthrodesis [9]. In order to understand how wrist arthroscopy can be beneficial in Kienböck's disease, it is important to understand the etiology, natural history, and current management concepts. These topics have been reviewed in depth elsewhere in this book, so will not be reviewed here. Ultimately, the true etiology remains uncertain, but it is thought to be related to both vascularity and joint mechanics [10, 11]. Additionally, significant controversy remains in the treatment of this condition. The source of this uncertainty largely stems from the fact that the incidence is low, and that some patients may be asymptomatic [12].

B.R. Graves, MD (✉)
Hand and Upper Extremity, Department of Orthopedic Surgery, Wake Forest University Baptist Hospital, 1 Medical Center Blvd., Winston Salem, NC 27157, USA
e-mail: bgraves@wakehealth.edu

G.S. Gluck, MD
Hand and Upper Extremity, Department of Orthopedic Surgery, Wake Forest University Baptist Hospital, 1 Medical Center Blvd., Winston Salem, NC 27157, USA

8585 S. Eastern Avenue, Las Vegas, NV 89123, USA

G.G. Poehling, MD, PhD
Department of Orthopedic Surgery, Wake Forest University Baptist Hospital, 131 Miller St., Winston Salem, NC 27103, USA

T.L. Whipple, MD
Virginia Commonwealth University School of Medicine, PO Box 70386, Richmond, VA 23255, USA

F. del Piñal, MD, DrMed
Department of Hand and Plastic Surgery, Hospital Mutua Montañesa, Paseo de Pereda 20-1, Santander 39004, Spain

G.I. Bain, MBBS, FRACS, FA(Ortho)A, PhD
Professor, Upper Limb and Research, Department of Orthopedic Surgery, Flinders University and Flinders Medical Centrer, Bedford Park, Adelaide, SA, Australia

© Springer International Publishing Switzerland 2016
D.M. Lichtman, G.I. Bain (eds.), *Kienböck's Disease*, DOI 10.1007/978-3-319-34226-9_13

While the dominant or primary cause of Kienböck's disease has yet to be determined, the end result is necrosis and collapse. It is clear that the disease is associated with decreased grip strength and wrist motion, and there is a varying degree of lunate collapse [13].

Imaging is required, including plain radiographs for evaluating alignment and osseous structures. CT scans provide a better resolution of the osseous structures. Magnetic resonance imaging can assess vascularity and necrosis [14], but it is less reliable for evaluating articular cartilage [15]. Current staging and treatment algorithms would benefit from a greater understanding of the articular cartilage involvement in Kienböck's disease. For example, MRI can clearly delineate necrosis and fracture, but the integrity of the articular cartilage is better assessed through direct visualization and palpation, which can be provided by arthroscopy. Armed with this information, the surgeon can determine if there are functional articular surfaces, or if reconstructive or salvage procedures such as a proximal row carpectomy should be performed. Perhaps attempts at lunate preservation would be reasonable in a young patient if the lunate articular surfaces are intact despite fracture and underlying necrosis. This information can't reliably be obtained from MRI in the absence of complete joint collapse on plain radiographs or CT scan.

Arthroscopy of the wrist allows direct visualization and palpation of articular surfaces. This information can play a valuable role in staging and clinical decision making in Kienböck's disease. High-resolution MRI provides a great deal of information about the integrity of the radiocarpal and midcarpal articulations, but arthroscopy remains the gold standard against which all noninvasive diagnostic modalities are compared [15].

In an attempt to guide surgical decision making, and to potentially improve surgical outcomes, Bain and Begg have developed an arthroscopic staging system based on the number of nonfunctional articular surfaces (Fig. 13.1) [3]. The principle is to identify the articulations that are nonfunctional (compromised), and either excise or fuse them, to allow the wrist to be mobilized with the functional articulations. If all of the remaining articulations are functional, then the patient is more likely to have minimal pain and a functional range of motion [16].

*In grade 0*, all articular surfaces are functional. Therefore the surgical management is directed at the symptomatic synovium and attempting to alter the natural history. An arthroscopic synovectomy is performed [5]. An extra-articular unloading procedure may be indicated. If there is negative ulnar variance then a radial shortening osteotomy could be performed. For neutral or positive ulnar variance a capitate

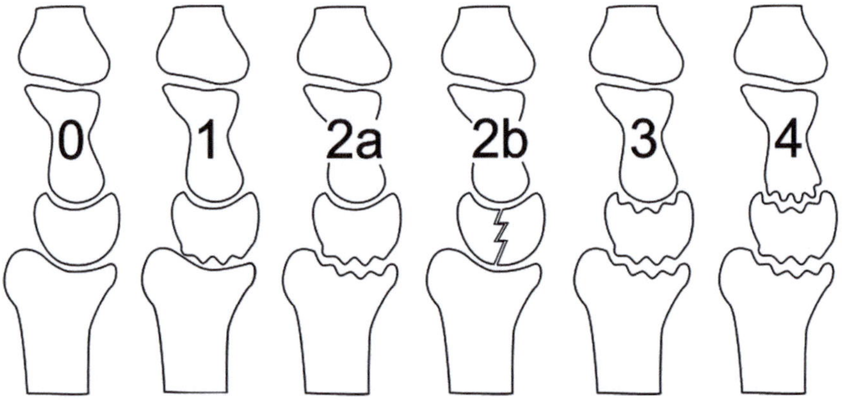


**Fig. 13.1** Bain and Begg arthroscopic classification of Kienböck's disease. The grade is determined by the number of nonfunctional articular surfaces. The grading system assists the surgeon to determine the best surgical option, based on the pathoanatomic findings. Reprinted with permission from Bain GI, Durrant A. An articular-based approach to Kienböck avascular necrosis of the lunate. Tech Hand Up Extrem Surg. 2011 Mar; 15(1):41–7

shortening procedure could be performed. A revascularization procedure could also be indicated in this group, especially if perfusion studies demonstrated marked necrosis. Other options are arthroscopic assisted drilling of the lunate [6, 7] and possibly arthroscopic bone grafting [8].

*In grade 1*, a nonfunctional proximal lunate articular surface is identified as the only articular abnormality. A healthy midcarpal joint and lunate facet of the distal radius are seen on arthroscopy. Proximal row carpectomy or radioscapholunate fusion may be indicated.

*In grade 2* there are two nonfunctional articular surfaces. This grade is subdivided based on the location of articular compromise. Grade 2a involves the proximal articular surface of the lunate and the lunate facet of the distal radius. A radioscapholunate fusion will eliminate both nonfunctional articular surfaces and enable the wrist to articulate through the normal midcarpal joint.

Grade 2b involves the proximal and distal articular surfaces of the lunate. This typically occurs when there is a coronal fracture in the lunate extending between the radiocarpal and midcarpal joints. The lunate fossa of the radius and the head of the capitate are normal. With the coronal fracture, of the avascular lunate, internal fixation is unlikely to be successful and a vascularized bone graft will be compromised as there are two fractured articular surfaces. In this case the lunate is not reconstructible; therefore a salvage procedure of the lunate is required, such as a lunate excision, lunate replacement, or proximal row carpectomy. If the lunate is left in situ, it will elute chemical factors from the necrotic lunate into the joint [17].

*In grade 3* there are three nonfunctional articular surfaces. The capitate articular surface will most likely remain functional. However the intact surface can be the lunate facet. This situation could be managed with a hemiarthroplasty. Alternatively, a salvage procedure such as a total wrist fusion or total wrist arthroplasty may be performed, depending on the patient's age and activity level.

*In grade 4*, all four articular surfaces are nonfunctional. In this case the wrist is not reconstructible; therefore a salvage procedure of the wrist is required, such as a total wrist fusion or arthroplasty. If the patient does not wish to proceed with a salvage procedure, then all other options can be considered (e.g., synovectomy +/− radial shortening); however that will leave compromised articulations and the patient is likely to have persistent pain.

Arthroscopy facilitates direct visual assessment of the articulations of the lunate and a probe is used to assess the degree of softening of the articular surfaces. Correlating the information gained through arthroscopy with preoperative imaging will assist the surgeon in making a better informed treatment decision. Bain and Begg reported that synovitis was present in all cases and that the degree of synovitis correlated with the degree of articular damage [3]. Plain radiographs often underestimated the severity of articular changes and arthroscopic findings commonly changed the recommended treatment. A fascinating statistic is that 82 % of cases had at least one nonfunctional articulation, and 61 % had at least two nonfunctional articulations. There were cases identified in which the chondral envelope was intact, although softening and collapse of the subchondral bone plate were noted. This was considered an important subgroup where attempts at revascularization and unloading of the lunate could potentially provide a good functional outcome.

From the spectrum of arthroscopic findings, an articular based classification of Kienböck's disease was created. Based on the articular based principles, a treatment algorithm was proposed (Table 13.1) [17]. The advantage of this method is that the distribution of functional articular surfaces determines treatment.

*A functional articular surface* will appear normal arthroscopically, which is to say it will have a smooth, glistening, "hard-boiled egg" appearance. The normal subchondral bone is firm to palpation without significant softening. Minor fibrillation is still considered a functional articular surface.

*Nonfunctional articular surface* would include those with extensive fibrillation, fissuring, localized or extensive loss, a floating articular surface, and fracture (Fig. 13.2). The aim of surgical treatment is to maintain functional wrist motion with the remaining functional articulations.

**Table 13.1** Articular based approach to avascular necrosis of the lunate[a]

| Grade | Description | Recommended treatment |
|---|---|---|
| Grade 0 | All articular surfaces are functional | Synovectomy[b] |
| | | Joint leveling |
| | | Vascularized BG |
| | | Forage |
| Grade 1 | One nonfunctional surface. Usually the proximal lunate | RSL fusion PRC |
| Grade 2a | Two nonfunctional surfaces. Proximal lunate and lunate facet of radius | RSL fusion |
| Grade 2b | Two nonfunctional surfaces. Proximal and distal surfaces of the lunate | PRC lunate replacement |
| Grade 3 | Three nonfunctional surfaces. Usually preserved capitate articular surface | Hemiarthroplasty |
| | | Total wrist fusion |
| | | Wrist replacement |
| Grade 4 | Four nonfunctional articular surfaces | Total wrist fusion |
| | | SC fusion |

*PRC* proximal row carpectomy, *RSL fusion* radioscapholunate fusion, *BG* bone graft

[a]Reprinted with permission from Bain GI, Durrant A. An articular-based approach to Kienböck avascular necrosis of the lunate. Tech Hand Up Extrem Surg. 2011 Mar;15(1):41–7

[b]Synovectomy is performed in all patients at the time of arthroscopy

The initial paper by Bain and Begg was titled "Arthroscopic Assessment and Classification of Kienböck's Disease" [3]. This paper was based on arthroscopic findings and defined the functional articulations, reported the clinical arthroscopic spectrum, and proposed a classification system, and an algorithm for each group. A subsequent paper titled "An Articular-based Approach to Kienbock Avascular Necrosis of the Lunate" highlighted that there will inevitably be new developments in assessment of the articular surfaces, and that critical factor in treating Kienböck's disease is to take into account the articular surfaces in determining management. It also detailed the patho-anatomical aspects of the development of Kienböck's avascular necrosis, and how it related to the subchondral bone plate, and the articular cartilage. Although many surgeons can perform arthroscopy, probably most hand surgeons are not comfortable or not trained in performing wrist arthroscopy. Therefore to have an articular based approach extends this concept to all surgeons, and does not lock them into an arthroscopic approach, rather engages them to respect the articular aspects of Kienböck's! To direct the hand surgeon who never does arthroscopy to scope the wrist can only lead to trouble. As MRI and other modalities evolve, this concept will become more important.

The articular based classification respects the articular aspects of the carpus, and uses it to guide treatment of the wrist based on patho-anatomical surgical principles. If all articular surfaces are intact, then a procedure that does not violate the integrity of the articular surface, such as synovectomy, drilling, vascularized bone grafting, or joint leveling, is indicated. If there is a mix of functional and non-functioning articular surfaces, a wrist-reconstructive procedure that maintains carpus mobility through the remaining functional articular surfaces is ideal. If the lunate is not reconstructible, then a lunate salvage/wrist-reconstructive procedure should be performed (e.g., proximal row carpectomy, radioscapholunate fusion, lunate replacement, or hemiarthroplasty).

If the entire wrist is not reconstructible, then a wrist salvage procedure should be performed (e.g., total wrist fusion or arthroplasty).

The above concepts are adopted in the management of degenerative disorders of the wrist [18]. It has puzzled one author (GIB) for some years that the commonly recommended principles of management of Kienböck's disease are different from other degenerative conditions of the wrist, such as scapholunate advanced collapse wrist [18]. As such, a more direct approach considering the integrity of the articular cartilage was developed. The functional status of articular cartilage is best appreciated when it is seen as part of the overall pathologic process. The classification and concepts presented in this study [17] are pathoanatomic, and not just anatomic. The approach that is presented takes into account the articular cartilage in patients with Kienböck's

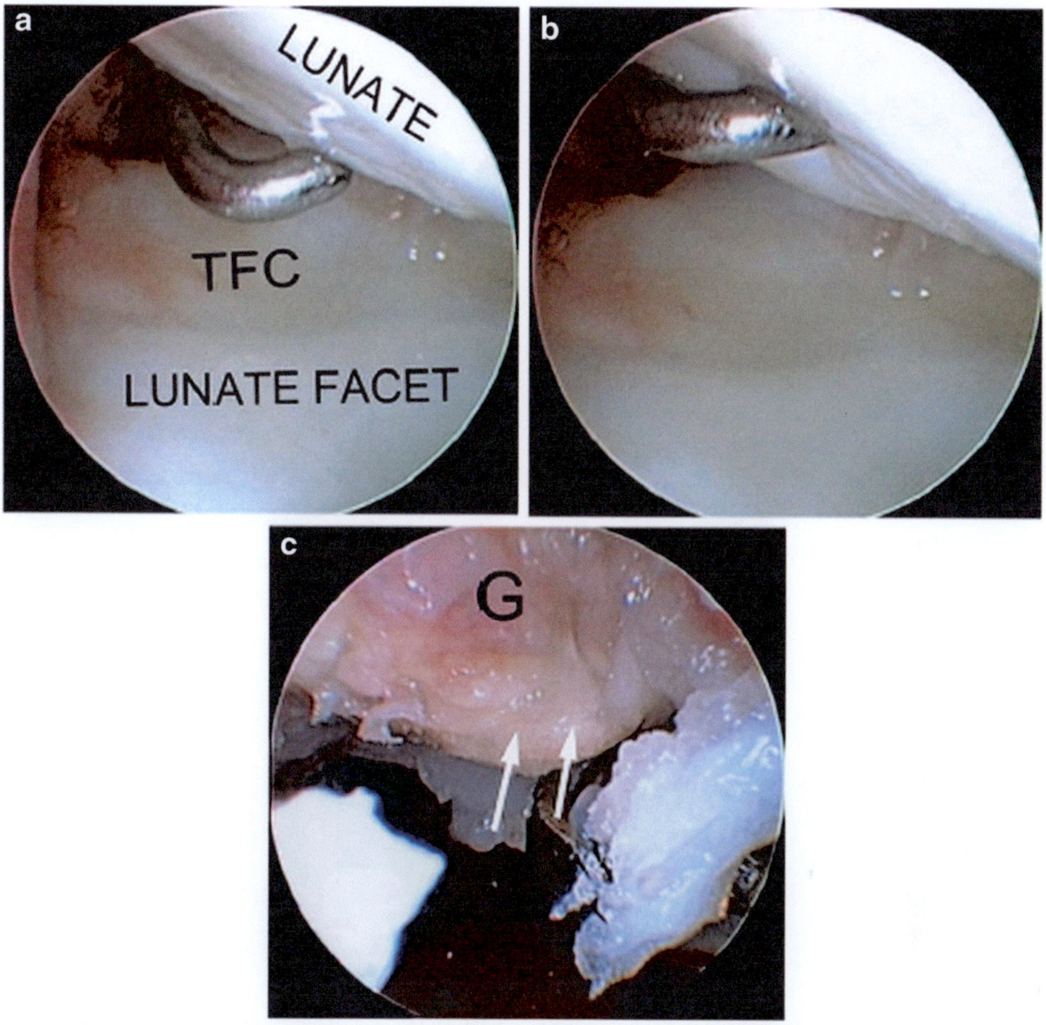


**Fig. 13.2** (**a**, **b**) "Bag of worms" sign, pathognomonic of Kienböck's. (**c**) After removing the cartilage shell of the lunate, necrotic bone (*arrows*) and granulating tissue (*G*) can be seen (scope in 3–4 and probe in 6R). Reprinted from Gluck GS et al. Wrist arthroscopy and its role in Keinböck's disease. In: del Piñal F et al. (eds.). Arthroscopic Management of Ulnar Pain. Berlin, Heidelberg: Springer-Verlag; 2012: 253–263, with kind permission from Springer Science and Business Media

disease and *emphasizes the importance of* the pathoanatomic aspects of articular cartilage in the decision-making process.

## Technique: Arthroscopic Assessment and Debridement

A standard wrist arthroscopy is performed with a tourniquet, traction tower, and a 2.7 mm 30° arthroscope. The lunate, adjacent articular surfaces, and interosseous ligaments are examined via the 6R portal with a probe in the 3–4 portal. The midcarpal joint is evaluated through the midcarpal radial and ulnar portals. The presence or absence of synovitis or loose bodies is noted. As seen in Fig. 13.3, the surfaces are palpated with a probe and the presence of softening, "floating" (unsupported) articular surface or gross degenerative changes are noted. The lunate is meticulously inspected for chondral integrity and fractures.

Debridement of the radiocarpal and midcarpal joints is performed with a full-radius oscillating shaver. First, synovectomy is performed to facili-

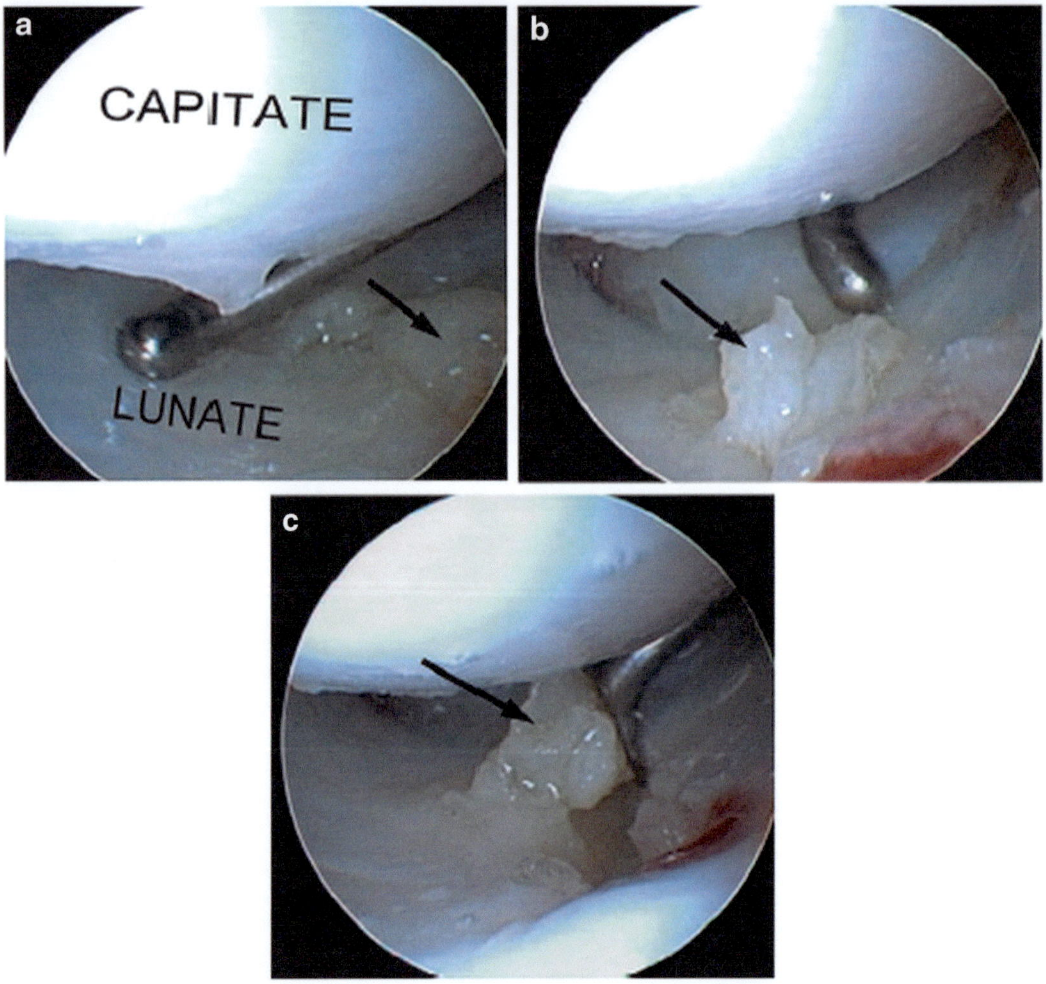


**Fig. 13.3** (**a**, **b**) In the midcarpal space, the lunate cartilage seems normal—only a loose body could be seen on first inspection (*arrow*). (**c**) When probing, a clear coronal fracture (*arrow*) can be seen at the junction of the dorsal and middle lunate thirds (scope in UMC and probe in RMC). In: del Piñal F et al. (eds.). Arthroscopic Management of Ulnar Pain. Berlin, Heidelberg: Springer-Verlag; 2012: 253–263, with kind permission from Springer Science and Business Media

tate visualization. Once a clear view is obtained, loose bodies, torn intercarpal ligaments, and unstable chondral surfaces are removed using arthroscopic shavers, suction baskets, and pituitary rongeurs. If no further surgical intervention is planned, arthroscopic debridement alone can help with symptoms and has been shown to be a valuable treatment option in those patients where the lunate has progressed to collapse or fracture. In 1999, Poehling's group reported on a small cohort of patients with Lichtman stage 3A and 3B Kienböck's disease [5]. Patients were managed with arthroscopic debridement of synovitis, loose bodies, unstable chondral surfaces, and torn intercarpal ligaments. All patients achieved significant improvements in pain, motion, and grip strength with minimal morbidity. Additionally, all patients reported resolution of mechanical symptoms. All patients returned to their prior level of activity or occupation within 4 weeks of surgery. After an average follow-up of 19 months, about half had progression of lunate sclerosis. Clinical results were maintained and none of the patients had further carpal collapse or

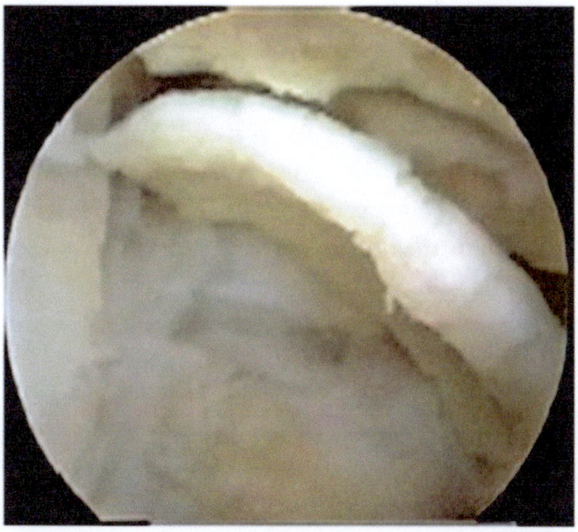

**Fig. 13.4** Loose lunate osteochondral fragment. Reprinted from Gluck GS et al. Wrist arthroscopy and its role in Keinböck's disease. In: del Piñal F et al. (eds.). Arthroscopic Management of Ulnar Pain. Berlin, Heidelberg: Springer-Verlag; 2012: 253–263, with kind permission from Springer Science and Business Media

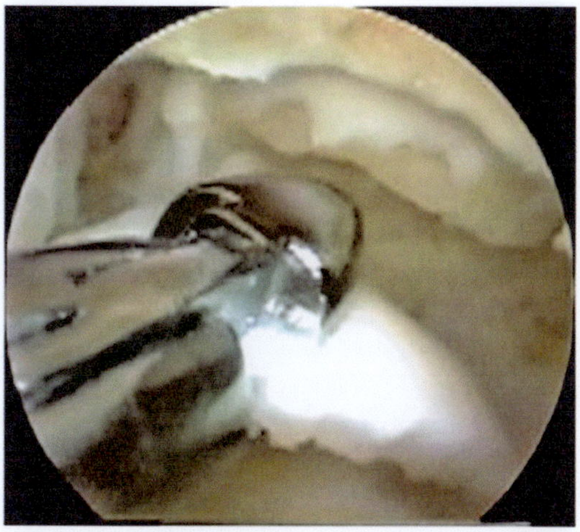

**Fig. 13.5** Removal of loose lunate osteochondral fragments. Reprinted from Gluck GS et al. Wrist arthroscopy and its role in Keinböck's disease. In: del Piñal F et al. (eds.). Arthroscopic Management of Ulnar Pain. Berlin, Heidelberg: Springer-Verlag; 2012: 253–263, with kind permission from Springer Science and Business Media

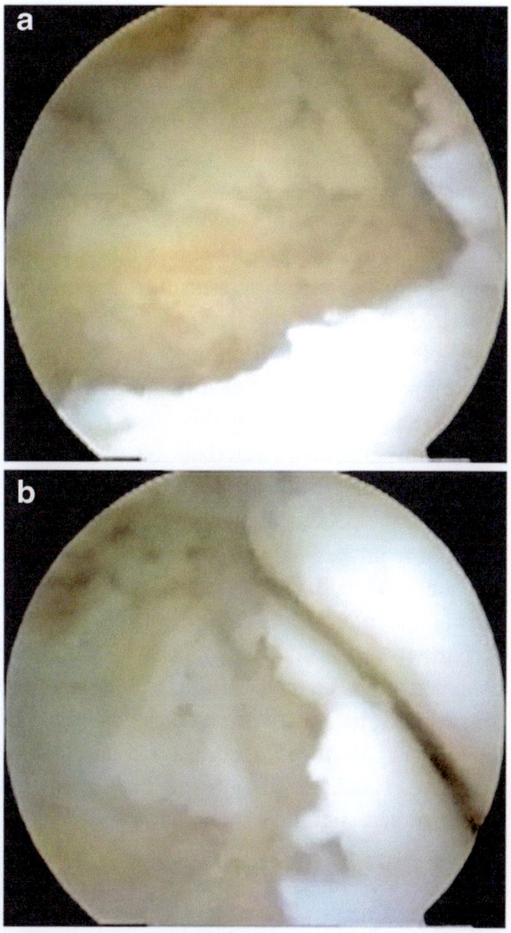

**Fig. 13.6** (**a**, **b**) Defect in the necrotic lunate after debridement of loose bodies. Reprinted from Gluck GS et al. Wrist arthroscopy and its role in Keinböck's disease. In: del Piñal F et al. (eds.). Arthroscopic Management of Ulnar Pain. Berlin, Heidelberg: Springer-Verlag; 2012: 253–263, with kind permission from Springer Science and Business Media

symptomatic instability during the study period (Figs. 13.4, 13.5, and 13.6).

In the early stages of Kienböck's disease, the goals of treatment should be to either halt progression or reverse osseous changes prior to compromise of subchondral support and subsequent articular degeneration. Arthroscopy, as a diagnostic tool, should ideally help the surgeon identify which patients fall into a truly reversible category. This would potentially allow for consistent alteration of the natural history, and also prevent unnecessary secondary or complex surgeries in a patient who would otherwise have similar long-term outcomes or symptom relief with either no intervention or a more simple intervention with more rapid recovery.

Arthroscopy can also be a valuable treatment tool in early, pre-collapse Kienböck's disease.

Forage has been used in the early stages of femoral head osteonecrosis as a minimally invasive osseous drilling to create revascularization [19]. Bain et al. published a small case series of arthroscopic/fluoroscopic guided drilling of the lunate for Kienböck's disease diagnosed prior to evidence of necrosis on MRI or sclerosis on plain radiographs [6]. These patients were managed with arthroscopic assisted drilling alone after failure of nonoperative treatment. This led to complete reversal of symptoms and imaging abnormalities after a 6-year follow-up period. Of note, a second patient in this case report had already progressed to sclerosis on plain radiographs but chose drilling as a less invasive option. Although the patient improved clinically during the follow-up period, radiographs showed progression and collapse in accordance with the natural history of the disease [17, 19].

Further supporting this approach, Mehrpour et al. performed an open drilling technique of the lunate in 20 patients with average follow-up of 5 years [7]. All of the stage 1 and 2 patients had objective, standardized outcome measures that demonstrated significant lasting improvement, and there was no radiographic progression. However, two of the four stage 3 patients later required a radial shortening osteotomy. The ideal patient for forage will have failed nonoperative treatment, have all articular surfaces intact (Bain and Begg grade 0), and have no fragmentation of the lunate (Lichtman grade 0 or 1). The minimally invasive arthroscopic technique is likely to have less morbidity and quicker rehabilitation. A joint-leveling procedure can be performed at the same time as the forage procedure, or as a secondary procedure if the patient has persistent pain despite the forage.

## Technique: Arthroscopic Assisted Drilling of the Lunate

Preoperative planning, based on the MRI to identify the correct trajectory into the area of necrosis, is important. The drill perforates the area of necrosis, creates a weep-hole for the venous hypertension, generates a regional reactive hyperemia, introduces an acute inflammatory response into the area of chronic inflammation, and opens a channel into which new granulation tissue and a cascade of vessels will proliferate.

A standard wrist arthroscopy is performed and once the integrity of the articular surfaces has been confirmed to be grade 0, attention is turned to drilling the lunate. A drill sleeve to protect the extensor tendons is introduced into the 3–4 portal, and positioned on the dorsal aspect of the lunate with arthroscopy and fluoroscopy guidance. Both the angle of the drill and the position of the wrist can be adjusted to strategically direct the drill to the areas of necrosis to encourage vascular ingrowth. Two or three passes of a 2.5 mm drill are made into the lunate (Fig. 13.7). Once the drill is removed, morselized bone graft can be tamped through the same drill sleeve, into the lunate under arthroscopic control [8]. Any debris should be lavaged from the joint. Postoperatively, patients are provided with a removable wrist splint and instructed to mobilize the wrist as

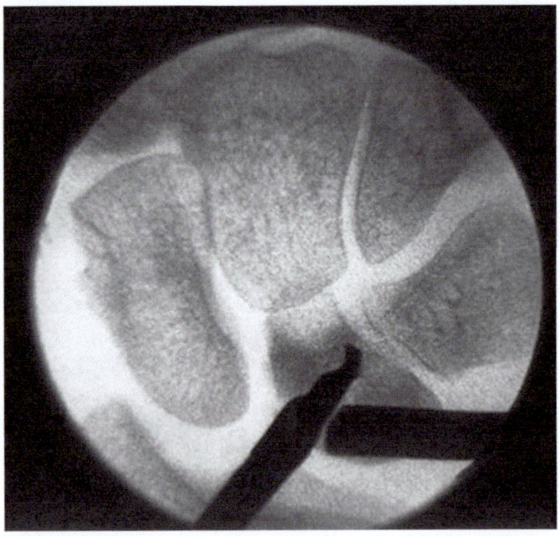

**Fig. 13.7** Forage of the lunate. Fluoroscopic image of the wrist, with the scope in the 6R portal and the drill within a sheath in the 3–4 portal. The drill is positioned under arthroscopic control, and confirmed to be satisfactory with fluoroscopy. Once positioned the drill is advanced. Arthroscopic-directed drilling of the lunate in a patient with arthroscopic grade 0 Kienböck's disease. Reprinted with permission from Bain GI, Durrant A. An articular-based approach to Kienböck avascular necrosis of the lunate. Tech Hand Up Extrem Surg. 2011 Mar;15(1):41–7

comfort allows. Hand therapy would only be required if postoperative progress is slow.

As arthroscopic techniques and technology have evolved, so do have the capabilities of the wrist arthroscopist to perform previously open procedures in a minimally invasive fashion. Proximal row carpectomy and intercarpal fusions are two examples of procedures that can be performed arthroscopically. Arthroscopic proximal row carpectomy is not only technically possible, but can provide a faster recovery and earlier range of motion than the open technique [20]. Limited intercarpal fusion, such as scaphocapitate fusion, can serve to prevent collapse of the distal carpal row and stabilize scaphoid rotation in the setting of Kienböck's disease. Resection of the proximal pole of the capitate can also serve to unload the lunate. A prospective, randomized study was performed to compare open versus arthroscopic scaphocapitate fusion in Kienböck's disease [9]. Patients in the open group also had a lunate revascularization procedure performed and the arthroscopic group included resection of the proximal pole of the capitate. The lunate was preserved in both groups. Sixteen patients with Lichtman stage III disease were reviewed at an average follow-up of 3 years. The arthroscopic group without revascularization had shorter surgical times and returned to regular daily activities quicker (6 weeks versus 15 weeks). The arthroscopic group had better Mayo wrist scores, but this did not reach statistical significance due to the small number of patients. Revascularization did not have a significant effect on clinical or radiographic outcome at 3 years. There were no nonunions.

## Technique for Arthroscopic Scaphocapitate Fusion

Following an arthroscopic assessment and debridement of the wrist, the capitate pole is excised using a shaver or burr until the midcarpal surface of the lunate does not abut the capitate (Fig. 13.8).

The arthroscope is directed toward the scaphocapitate joint through the ulnar midcarpal portal. The cartilage on the adjacent surfaces of the capitate and scaphoid is debrided through the radial midcarpal portal, until the subchondral bone is exposed. With the arthroscope in the scaphoid fossa, a guide wire is advanced through the anatomic snuffbox, onto the scaphoid, in preparation to be advanced into the capitate. It should be directed into the scaphoid in a ulnar, dorsal, and distal direction. The arthroscope is then re-positioned in the midcarpal joint, and the guide wire is advanced into the capitate under arthroscopic visualization. The wrist is placed in maximal extension and ulnar deviation to ensure scaphoid extension prior to crossing the arthrodesis site. With the arthroscope in the scaphocapitate joint

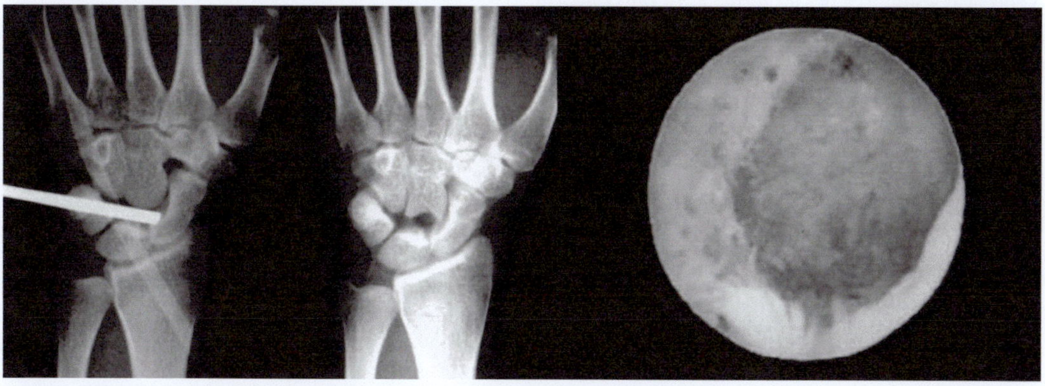

**Fig. 13.8** Radiograph of the arthroscope in the midcarpal joint and after arthroscopic resection of the head of the capitate. Republished with permission of Arthroscopy Association of North America and Elsevier, from Leblebicioğlu G, Doral MN, Atay öA, Tetik O, Whipple TL. Open treatment of stage III Kienböck's disease with lunate revascularization compared with arthroscopic treatment without revascularization. Arthroscopy. 2003 Feb;19(2):117–30

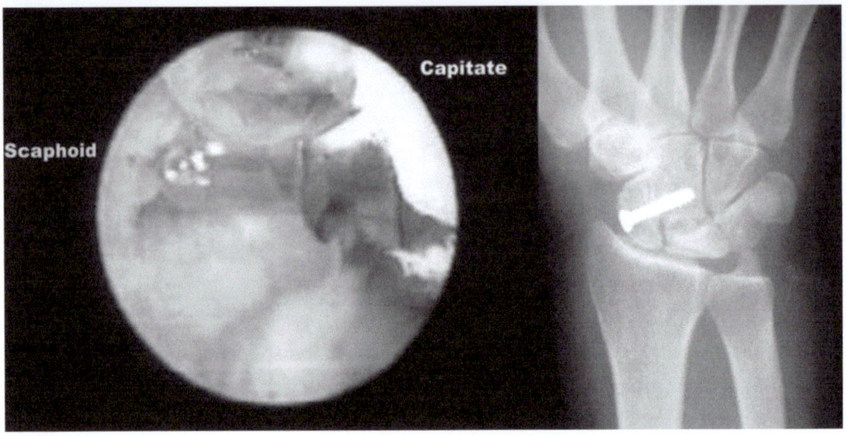


**Fig. 13.9** Screw across the scaphoid-capitate articulation as seen from the radial midcarpal portal and subsequent radiograph showing final fixation for the arthrodesis. *Arrow* denotes screw threads spanning the scaphocapitate joint. Republished with permission of Arthroscopy Association of North America and Elsevier, from Leblebicioğlu G, Doral MN, Atay öA, Tetik O, Whipple TL. Open treatment of stage III Kienböck's disease with lunate revascularization compared with arthroscopic treatment without revascularization. Arthroscopy. 2003 Feb;19(2):117–30

and the guide wire in place, the length of the screw is determined and the cannulated drill and screw are placed over the wire. The guide wire is deliberately made long to avoid it displacing. The precise positioning of the wire and screw can be confirmed with arthroscopy and intraoperative fluoroscopy. The arthroscope is then slightly withdrawn, and the screw is tightened to observe compression between the scaphoid and the capitate (Fig. 13.9). A second screw may be used for added fixation. The lunate is left in situ.

Postoperatively, the wrist is immobilized in a short arm splint in a position of 15° of dorsiflexion and 10° of ulnar deviation for 4 weeks. After removal of the splint, the patient is allowed to passively mobilize the wrist [9]. Follow-up radiographs are performed to confirm the position of carpal fixation and later to confirm union.

The majority of the literature regarding Kienböck's disease does not include wrist arthroscopy to determine the diagnosis or guide treatment. Hopefully, this chapter has helped demonstrate how wrist arthroscopy can serve as a valuable tool in the evaluation and management of this challenging disease. Arthroscopy provides direct evidence of articular surface involvement and allows the surgeon to design a logical solution to maintain a functional motion. Further studies are required before we have the appropriate information at the various stages of the disease that is consistently better than the natural history. The authors hope that arthroscopy will be incorporated into more future studies to provide valuable additional diagnostic information and facilitate less invasive treatment options for patients with Kienböck's disease.

## References


1. Watanabe K, Nakamura R, Imaeda T. Arthroscopic assessment of Kienböck's disease. Arthroscopy. 1995;11(3):257–62.
2. Salmon J, Stanley JK, Trail IA. Kienböck's disease: conservative management versus radial shortening. J Bone Joint Surg Br. 2000;82(6):820–3.
3. Bain GI, Begg M. Arthroscopic assessment and classification of Kienbock's disease. Tech Hand Up Extrem Surg. 2006;10(1):8–13.
4. Tatebe M, Hirata H, Shinohara T, Yamamoto M, Okui N, Kurimoto S, et al. Arthroscopic findings of Kienböck's disease. J Orthop Sci. 2011;16(6): 745–8.
5. Menth-Chiari WA, Poehling GG, Wiesler ER, Ruch DS. Arthroscopic debridement for the treatment of Kienbock's disease. Arthroscopy. 1999;15(1):12–9.
6. Bain GI, Smith ML, Watts AC. Arthroscopic core decompression of the lunate in early stage Kienbock disease of the lunate. Tech Hand Up Extrem Surg. 2011;15(1):66–9.

7. Mehrpour SR, Kamrani RS, Aghamirsalim MR, Sorbi R, Kaya A. Treatment of Kienböck disease by lunate core decompression. J Hand Surg Am. 2011;36(10):1675–7.
8. Pegoli L, Ghezzi A, Cavalli E, Luchetti R, Pajardi G. Arthroscopic assisted bone grafting for early stages of Kienböck's disease. Hand Surg. 2011;16(2):127–31.
9. Leblebicioğlu G, Doral MN, Atay öA, Tetik O, Whipple TL. Open treatment of stage III Kienböck's disease with lunate revascularization compared with arthroscopic treatment without revascularization. Arthroscopy. 2003;19(2):117–30.
10. Watson HK, Guidera PM. Aetiology of Kienböck's disease. J Hand Surg Br. 1997;22(1):5–7.
11. Lluch A, Garcia-Elias M. Etiology of Kienböck disease. Tech Hand Up Extrem Surg. 2011;15(1):33–7.
12. Mennen U, Sithebe H. The incidence of asymptomatic Kienböck's disease. J Hand Surg Eur Vol. 2009;34(3):348–50.
13. Keith PPA, Nuttall D, Trail I. Long-term outcome of nonsurgically managed Kienböck's disease. J Hand Surg Am. 2004;29(1):63–7.
14. Trumble TE. Avascular necrosis after scaphoid fracture: a correlation of magnetic resonance imaging and histology. J Hand Surg Am. 1990;15(4):557–64.
15. Haims AH, Moore AE, Schweitzer ME, Morrison WB, Deely D, Culp RW, et al. MRI in the diagnosis of cartilage injury in the wrist. AJR Am J Roentgenol. 2004;182(5):1267–70.
16. Palmer AK, Werner FW, Murphy D, Glisson R. Functional wrist motion: a biomechanical study. J Hand Surg Am. 1985;10(1):39–46.
17. Bain GI, Durrant A. An articular-based approach to Kienbock avascular necrosis of the lunate. Tech Hand Up Extrem Surg. 2011;15(1):41–7.
18. Bain GI, McGuire DT. Decision making for partial carpal fusions. J Wrist Surg. 2012;1(2):103–14.
19. Mont MA, Carbone JJ, Fairbank AC. Core decompression versus nonoperative management for osteonecrosis of the hip. Clin Orthop Relat Res. 1996;324:169–78.
20. Weiss ND, Molina RA, Gwin S. Arthroscopic proximal row carpectomy. J Hand Surg Am. 2011;36(4):577–82.

# Part III

# Management

# Minimally Invasive Techniques for the Treatment of Kienböck's Disease

# 14

William F. Pientka II, Timothy Niacaris, Marc A. Caragea, and David M. Lichtman

## Introduction

The treatment of osteonecrosis of the lunate has evolved considerably since first described by Kienböck in 1910 [1]. Surgical options include a variety of joint-leveling procedures, vascularized bone grafts, wrist arthrodeses with or without lunate excision, and excision of bones in the proximal carpal row. In 1993, the senior author recognized that treatment outcomes of Kienböck's disease vary based on disease severity and chronicity. He proposed a treatment algorithm based on the staging system he introduced in 1977 [2, 3]. Despite widespread use of this algorithm, surgical outcomes today still remain somewhat unpredictable and, as with all open procedures, have the potential for morbidity. To decrease complications associated with established surgical options, less invasive, surgical techniques are being investigated. These techniques include temporary scapho-trapezio-trapezoidal (STT) pinning, core decompression of the distal radius and ulna or lunate, balloon lunatoplasty, and immobilization using external fixation devices.

W.F. PientkaII , MD (✉)
Department of Orthopedic Surgery, John Peter Smith Hospital, 1500 S. Main St, Fort Worth, TX 76104, USA

6155 Highwoods Ct., Fort Worth, TX 76112, USA
e-mail: wpientka@jpshealth.org

T. Niacaris, MD, PhD
Department of Orthopedic Surgery, University of North Texas Health Science Center, 800, 5th Avenue, Suite 400, Fort Worth, TX 76104, USA

M.A. Caragea, BS
University of North Texas Health Science Center – Texas College of Osteopthic Medicine, 3500 Camp Bowie Blvd, Fort Worth, TX 76107, USA

D.M. Lichtman, MD
Rear Admiral (Retired), US Navy, Adjunct Professor, Department of Surgery, Uniformed Services University of the Health Sciences, Bethesda, MD, USA

Adjunct Professor, Department of Orthopedic Surgery, University of North Texas Health Sciences Center, Fort Worth, TX, USA

## Temporary Scapho-Trapezio-Trapezoidal Pinning

Yajima [4] originally described temporary STT pinning in adolescent patients with Kienböck's disease in 1998. This procedure decompresses the lunate by temporarily transferring forces from the radiolunate to the scaphocapitate and radioscaphoid joints. This allows temporary decompression of the lunate long enough to allow for revascularization without permanent alteration of anatomic joint relationships.

In addition to temporary STT fixation, Yajima advocated revascularization of the lunate using the second or third dorsal metacarpal artery and vein. He used a drill hole from dorsal to volar on the lunate to pass the vascular pedicle, then

© Springer International Publishing Switzerland 2016
D.M. Lichtman, G.I. Bain (eds.), *Kienböck's Disease*, DOI 10.1007/978-3-319-34226-9_14

secured the pedicle to the palmar joint capsule, and reinforced the tunnel with autograft bone. Following vascular bundle implantation, he inserted three 0.045-in. Kirschner wires. The first was placed from the dorsal scaphoid into the trapezium with the wrist in slight extension, the second from the dorsal trapezoid to the scaphoid, and the third from the trapezium to the trapezoid. Yajima later modified this technique with respect to K-wire placement. In the new configuration, he places two wires from the trapezoid to the scaphoid and one from the scaphoid to the trapezium. This eliminates the need for fixation between the trapezium and trapezoid. Yajima emphasizes the importance of ensuring that no K-wires cross the radiocarpal joint regardless of configuration (Fig. 14.1).

Following the procedure, the extremity is immobilized in a short arm cast for 4 weeks to allow soft-tissue healing and integration of the vascular pedicle. K-wires are removed upon radiographic evidence of lunate healing, usually between 4 and 6 months postoperatively. Wrist range of motion is not restricted after the initial 4-week period of cast immobilization. In the second month, isometric non-weight-bearing wrist exercises are started. Light lifting is allowed at 3 months postoperatively.

Yajima [4] reported complete pain resolution in 80 % of patients and increased grip strength following STT pinning with vascular augmentation. There was no difference in postsurgical wrist range of motion or mean carpal height in this study.

Several case reports also demonstrate the effectiveness of STT pinning. In 1998, Yasuda [5] et al. reported on a 12-year-old female with stage IIIB Kienböck's disease treated with temporary scaphotrapezoidal joint pinning. A postoperative MRI demonstrated revascularization of the lunate, along with healing of lunate fractures present preoperatively. Wrist extension and flexion both increased from 40° to 90° and grip strength increased from 9 to 21 kg following 4 months of splint immobilization and subsequent pin removal.

In 2004, Shigematsu [6] reported on an 11-year-old female with stage IIIA Kienböck's disease treated with temporary STT pinning. The patient underwent 4 weeks of cast immobilization and pin removal at 8 weeks. Wrist flexion improved from 60° to 90° and extension improved from 30° to 90°. Grip strength improved from 5 to 24 kg. Radiographs showed reconstitution of the lunate with a return to normal bone density. Furthermore, carpal height ratio improved from 0.45 to 0.51 postoperatively, compared to 0.54 in the unaffected wrist. A postoperative MRI showed evidence of revascularization at 10 months.

In 2005 Kazuki [7] performed temporary STT pinning on a 15-year-old girl followed by sequential MRI and plain radiographs monthly from 1 to 6 months, and at 9, 12, and 24 months postoperatively to evaluate lunate revascularization.

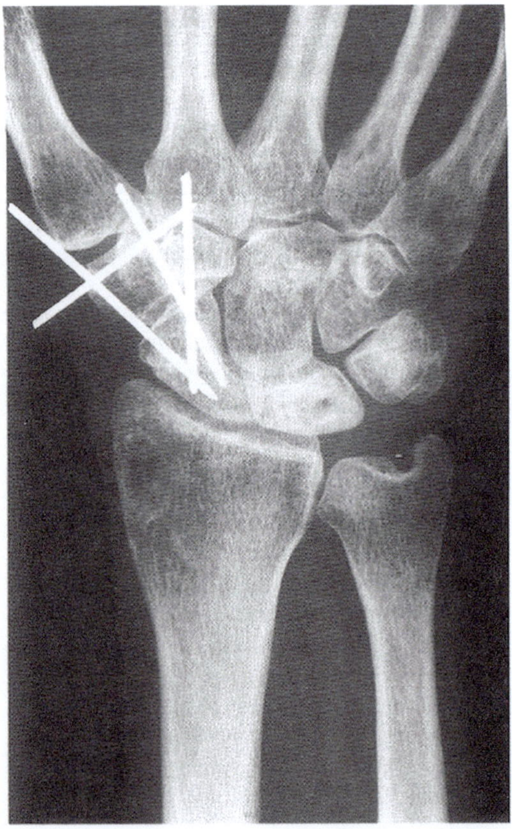

**Fig. 14.1** Postoperative PA radiograph of a 46-year-old woman who underwent temporary STT pinning for treatment of stage IIIa Kienböck's disease. Reprinted from Journal of Hand Surgery, 23(3), Yajima H, Ono H, Tamai S, Temporary internal fixation of the scaphotrapeziotrapezoidal joint for the treatment of Kienbock's disease: a preliminary study, 402–410, Copyright 1998

K-wires were removed at 6 months. The low-intensity area of the lunate on T1-weighted MRI demonstrated a notable increase in signal at 3 months and T1-weighted MRI of the lunate had normalized by 6 months. Radiographs showed decreased lunate sclerosis and cystic changes, with bony sclerosis eliminated by 9 months. The carpal height ratio did not change and lunate collapse did not progress.

Ando et al. [8], in 2009, presented a retrospective review of six adolescent patients with Kienböck's disease (three stage IIIA, three stage IIIB) treated with temporary ST joint fixation for between 3 and 6 months. They noted statistically significant increases in wrist flexion and extension postoperatively, as well as an increase in grip strength. A postoperative MRI noted improvement to a nearly normal lunate signal in all patients.

In summary, temporary ST joint immobilization effectively neutralizes forces across the lunate and heightens the regenerative potential of the skeletally immature lunate. We recommend this procedure in patients with good revascularization potential, such as adults with high signal intensity on preoperative gadolinium perfusion studies as well as for selected juveniles and adolescents. In children, temporary pinning results in restoration of carpal height in many cases and therefore represents a reasonable operative choice, even when X-rays demonstrate type IIIA or IIIB Kienböck's disease. Because the procedure is minimally invasive and non-destructive it is particularly well suited to younger patients.

## Balloon Lunatoplasty

In 2011 Chen [9] introduced the concept of using a balloon system to restore height (similar to what has been commonly used for vertebral compression fractures) in cases of Kienböck's disease with lunate collapse. He and his colleagues presented a cohort of five patients (two stage II, two stage IIIA, two stage IIIB) treated with balloon lunatoplasty. Immediate postoperative imaging showed lunate expansion to normal dimensions. At 24-month follow-up, significant improvements in pain, strength, and wrist range of motion were noted in all five patients. Follow-up imaging showed no progression or further lunate collapse, and all patients returned to their previous level of employment.

To perform balloon lunatoplasty, Chen uses an 11-gauge vertebroplasty needle positioned in the lunate from a dorsal approach and directed towards the center of the collapsed lunate in stage III or the center of the less dense cystic region of the lunate in stage II. Needle position is verified using c-arm fluoroscopy. A working cannula is placed using a guide wire and the entrance point is drilled for the balloon. Half of the balloon is inserted into the lunate and inflated to impact the necrotic bone. The balloon is subsequently removed and bone cement is injected under fluoroscopy using a kyphoplasty cement system. Extravasation of cement beyond the lunate is to be avoided and immediately removed through a minimal incision if identified fluoroscopically.

Chen's results indicate that balloon lunatoplasty is effective in the treatment of stage IIIA or early stage IIIB Kienböck's disease and allows restoration of lunate geometry, which may prevent carpal degeneration [9]. In addition, this procedure eliminates the need for joint fusion and prolonged immobilization and allows for earlier rehabilitation. The surgeon must recognize and remedy cement extravasation from the lunate, which was seen in up to 20 % of patients in Chen's study. Chen recommends using high-viscosity cement injected under low pressure to decrease the occurrence of cement extravasation.

In 2012 Ken [10] presented an in vitro study on percutaneous cement lunatoplasty. The procedure was performed in four cadavers, using the contralateral wrist as a paired control. Cement was injected at 200 psi and fluoroscopy was used to ensure no cement extravasation. The injected lunates and their contralateral-paired controls were then loaded to failure in axial compression. The results demonstrated an increase in the mean load to failure for treated lunates compared to their untreated counterparts (3.5 kN vs. 3.0 kN).

There is no information available regarding the long-term outcome of patients treated with balloon lunatoplasty. As in vertebroplasty, there is some concern that a cemented lunate may be exceedingly dense, potentially leading to wear and fragmentation of surrounding structures. Outside of investigational studies, we do not yet endorse this treatment use in Kienböck's disease.

## Core Decompression of the Radius

Illarramendi [11] in 2001 astutely noted spontaneous resolution of Kienböck's disease in patients experiencing non-displaced distal radius fractures. He theorized that the local biologic response to fracture healing alters the physiologic environment and stimulates revascularization of the lunate. As a surgical alternative to distal radius fracture, Illarramendi proposed distal radius and/or ulnar metaphyseal core decompression as a treatment for Kienböck's disease.

This procedure calls for a 3 to 4 cm longitudinal incision along the radial border of the distal radius metaphysis. Branches of the radial nerve are identified and protected. A bony window is created measuring 2 cm × 0.5 cm, located 2 cm proximal to the radial styloid. The distal radius metaphysis is curetted and subsequently impacted without removing any bone. The bone cortex removed is either broken into 5 mm fragments or impacted back into place as a single piece. The distal ulnar metaphysis is then approached with a longitudinal incision between the extensor and flexor carpi ulnaris tendons. A bone window is made 2 cm proximal to the ulnar styloid. The core decompression technique for the ulna matches the aforementioned technique used in the distal radius. The extremity is immobilized for 3 weeks in a short arm cast. Strenuous activities are avoided for 3 months, and monthly follow-ups are performed for the first 6 months, followed by annual visits.

Illarramendi [11] reported on 22 patients that underwent metaphyseal core decompression for stage I, II, or IIIA Kienböck's disease. At 10-year follow-up, no patient had required further surgical procedures; 72.7 % of patients were pain free and 18 % reported mild occasional pain. One patient reported worsening pain and had radiographic evidence of intercarpal arthritis and another had moderate pain that required modification of their occupation. Average grip strength was 75 % of the contralateral wrist and range of motion was 77 % of the contralateral wrist at final follow-up. Three of the 22 patients did not have core decompression of the ulna, and had equivalent outcomes at 10-year follow-up to those patients who had both the radius and ulna decompressed. Carpal height ratio was unchanged from preoperative measurements at final follow-up.

Biomechanical cadaver studies have been performed to evaluate the effect of distal radius metaphyseal core decompression on the wrist. Sherman [12] identified a significant decrease in the stiffness of the distal radius after distal radius metaphyseal core decompression, but no changes in the distribution of forces across the radiocarpal joint or in the ulnocarpal fossa were noted. Illarramendi attributed the immediate postoperative pain relief following core decompression to alteration of the local intraosseous pressure. In addition, he believed that revascularization of the lunate was enhanced by a regional vascular response secondary to surgical core decompression or injury from a fracture. Further studies on the vascular physiology of these structures are necessary to determine the cause-and-effect relationship behind these observations.

## Core Decompression of the Lunate

Increased intraosseous pressure secondary to venous congestion may also contribute to the development of avascular necrosis of the lunate [13]. This consideration led to experimentation with core decompression of the lunate, first described by Bain in 2011 [14]. Also in 2011, Mehrpour [15] published on lunate core decompression in a cohort of 20 patients with stage I–IIIb Kienböck's disease. The surgical procedure involved transverse dorsal and capsular incisions over the lunate. A high-speed burr was used to decompress the lunate. The cancellous bone from the lunate was not removed. Postoperatively, the extremities were splinted initially, and then immobilized in a short arm cast for a total of 6 weeks. Range-of-motion exercises were then initiated.

At 5-year follow-up, Mehrpour noted a significant decrease in pain, as well as improvement in DASH scores, flexion, extension, and radial and

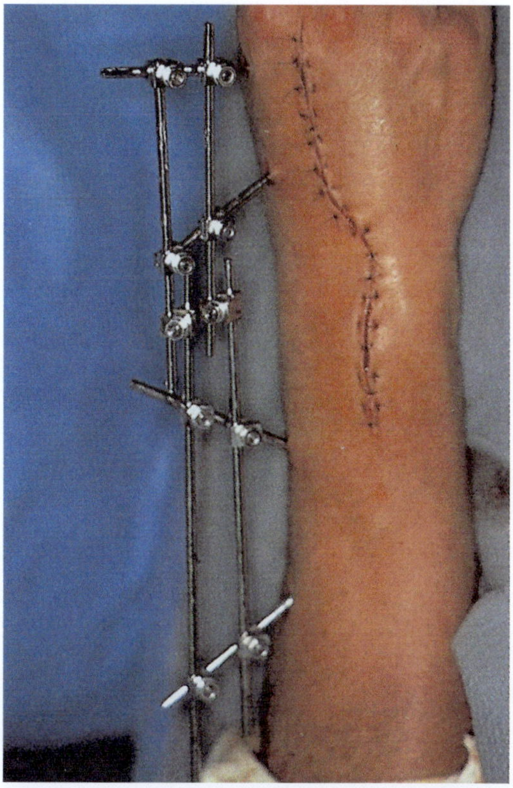

**Fig. 14.2** PA radiograph of a wrist that has been temporarily stabilized with an external fixator. Reprinted with permission from Gelberman RH, editor. Master Techniques in Orthopedic Surgery: The Wrist. 3rd ed. Philadelphia: Lippincott Williams & Wilkins; 2009

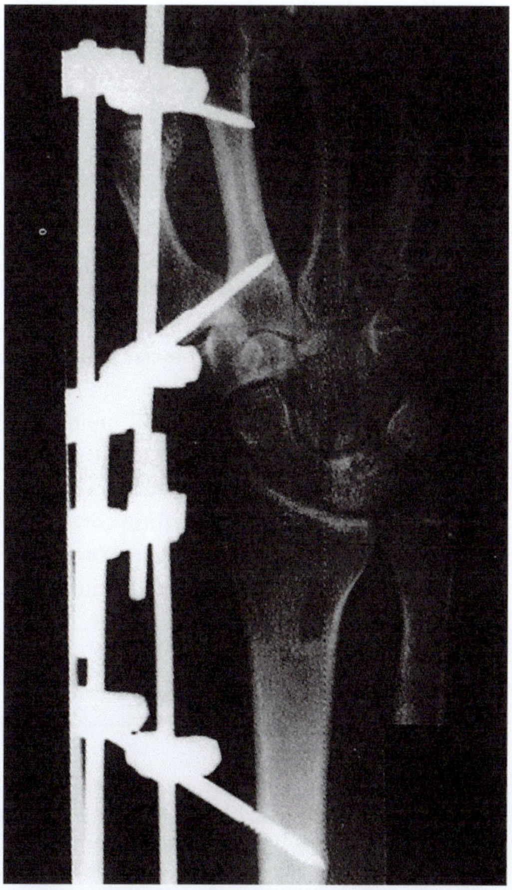

**Fig. 14.3** Clinical photograph of the same patient with a wrist external fixator in place for temporary immobilization after undergoing a lunate revascularization procedure. Reprinted with permission from Gelberman RH, editor. Master Techniques in Orthopedic Surgery: The Wrist. 3rd ed. Philadelphia: Lippincott Williams & Wilkins; 2009

ulnar deviation. There was no postoperative progression of disease stage, and no operative complications. Ten percent of patients (all with stage III disease) went on to radial shortening osteotomy due to continued pain. These results suggest that lunate core decompression may be a reasonable option for treatment of stages I and II Kienböck's, but may not lead to successful results in stage III where the lunate has already collapsed.

## External Fixation

External fixation has complemented many of the historical treatment options for Kienböck's disease. As an example, vascularized bone grafting is often supplemented by the addition of external fixation (or temporary STT pinning) to unload the lunate during the postoperative period [16, 17]. Both techniques may prevent compression of the lunate during the revascularization process when the lunate is highly susceptible to further collapse. The true effect of the fixator (or temporary pinning) is unknown, however, because the outcome of the combined procedures is largely dependent on the stage of the disease and the quality of the revascularization procedure itself (Figs. 14.2 and 14.3).

Although external fixation can provide similar change in force transmission across the lunate as STT pinning, it is more difficult for the patient to tolerate and is associated with an increased risk of local infection. Therefore, we do not recommended external fixation as an isolated procedure for the treatment of Kienböck's disease.

## Conclusion

In summary, minimally invasive procedures for Kienböck's disease can be effective under certain circumstances. As we learn more about the natural history of the disorder the precise indications for these procedures will become clearer. At present we recommend temporary STT pinning or external fixation as adjunctive procedures to provide stress transfer following direct revascularization of the lunate. We also perform core lunate decompression, followed by cancellous bone grafting, for questionable lesions of the lunate. In this instance, the procedure serves both a diagnostic and therapeutic function.

## References


1. Peltier LF. The classic. Concerning traumatic malacia of the lunate and its consequences: degeneration and compression fractures. Privatdozent Dr. Robert Kienbock. Clin Orthop Relat Res 1980;(149):4–8.
2. Lichtman DM, Mack GR, MacDonald RI, Gunther SF, Wilson JN. Kienbock's disease: the role of silicone replacement arthroplasty. J Bone Joint Surg Am. 1977;59(7):899–908.
3. Lichtman DM, Degnan GG. Staging and its use in the determination of treatment modalities for Kienbock's disease. Hand Clin. 1993;9(3):409–16.
4. Yajima H, Ono H, Tamai S. Temporary internal fixation of the scaphotrapezio-trapezoidal joint for the treatment of Kienbock's disease: a preliminary study. J Hand Surg Am. 1998;23(3):402–10.
5. Yasuda M, Okuda H, Egi T, Guidera PM. Temporary scapho-trapezoidal joint fixation for Kienbock's disease in a 12-year-old girl: a case report. J Hand Surg Am. 1998;23(3):411–4.
6. Shigematsu K, Yajima H, Kobata Y, Kawamura K, Nakanishi Y, Takakura Y. Treatment of Kienbock disease in an 11-year-old girl with temporary fixation of the scaphotrapeziotrapezoidal joint. Scand J Plast Reconstr Surg Hand Surg. 2005;39(1):60–3.
7. Kazuki K, Uemura T, Okada M, Egi T. Time course of magnetic resonance images in an adolescent patient with Kienbock's disease treated by temporary scapho-trapezoidal joint fixation: a case report. J Hand Surg Am. 2006;31(1):63–7.
8. Ando Y, Yasuda M, Kazuki K, Hidaka N, Yoshinaka Y. Temporary scaphotrapezoidal joint fixation for adolescent Kienbock's disease. J Hand Surg Am. 2009;34(1):14–9.
9. Chen W, Wang J, Pan J, Zhang Q, Shao X, Zhang Y. Primary results of Kienbock's disease treated using balloon kyphoplasty system. Arch Orthop Trauma Surg. 2012;132(5):677–83.
10. Ken CC, Singh VA, Luis GE. Kienbock's disease: percutaneous cement lunatoplasty--a cadaver study. J Hand Surg Eur Vol. 2012;37(1):81–2.
11. Illarramendi AA, Schulz C, De Carli P. The surgical treatment of Kienbock's disease by radius and ulna metaphyseal core decompression. J Hand Surg Am. 2001;26(2):252–60.
12. Sherman GM, Spath C, Harley BJ, Weiner MM, Werner FW, Palmer AK. Core decompression of the distal radius for the treatment of Kienbock's disease: a biomechanical study. J Hand Surg Am. 2008;33(9): 1478–81.
13. Jensen CH. Intraosseous pressure in Kienbock's disease. J Hand Surg Am. 1993;18(2):355–9.
14. Bain GI, Smith ML, Watts AC. Arthroscopic core decompression of the lunate in early stage Kienbock disease of the lunate. Tech Hand Up Extrem Surg. 2011;15(1):66–9.
15. Mehrpour SR, Kamrani RS, Aghamirsalim MR, Sorbi R, Kaya A. Treatment of Kienbock disease by lunate core decompression. J Hand Surg Am. 2011;36(10): 1675–7.
16. Botelheiro JC. Conservative versus operative treatment for Kienbock's disease. A retrospective study. J Hand Surg Br. 1999;24(1):139.
17. Luo J, Diao E. Kienbock's disease: an approach to treatment. Hand Clin. 2006;22(4):465–73. abstract vi.

# Capitate Shortening for Kienböck's Disease

# 15

Ahmadreza Afshar

## Introduction

In 1986, Almquist introduced capitate-shortening osteotomy to the armamentarium of treatments for Kienböck's disease [1–3]. He reported that revascularization and healing of the fragmented lunate occurred in 83 % of patients and that postoperative grip strength improved to 80 % of the opposite side [2, 3]. Subjective pain relief after surgical treatment in Kienböck's disease depends on multiple factors. Capitate-shortening osteotomy has mechanical and biological healing effects on the lunate. Innes et al. have postulated that a cortical disruption increases the local circulation to the lunate [4]. In accordance with this hypothesis Bekler et al. [5] performed capitate forage and Blanco and Blanco [6] performed radial osteotomy without shortening to treat Kienböck's disease. A study using magnetic resonance imaging (MRI) on nine patients demonstrated that the revascularization process of the lunate after capitate-shortening osteotomy began at an average of 4.7 months (3–7 months) postoperatively (Fig. 15.1) [7].

Of the carpal bones, the lunate bone bears the greatest load per unit surface [2]. Reducing load on the lunate probably prompts revascularization of the bone and prevents further changes in the shape of the lunate and collapse of the carpus. Capitate-shortening osteotomy efficiently decreases the load transfer across the lunate bone [8–11]. Horii et al. have demonstrated that the shortened capitate transferred less load (66 % reduction) across the radio-lunate joint than the shortened radius (45 % reduction) [8]. The load of the carpus pass through the three columns (radial, intermediate, and ulnar columns) across the wrist joint, to the forearm. Capitate-shortening osteotomy diverts the load from the intermediate column to the radial and ulnar columns and adjacent intercarpal joints [8, 11], therefore unloading and protecting the radiolunate articulation.

There is no consensus on the best surgical treatment for Kienböck's disease [12–22]; however, capitate-shortening osteotomy is a simple and straightforward procedure that has gained interest in recent years [1–3, 7, 23, 24, 27–31].

## Indications

Traditionally, surgical treatment for Kienböck's disease is based on the Lichtman stages [12, 13] of the disease and ulnar variance [14–17]. Capitate-shortening osteotomy usually has been offered to patients with ulnar neutral and positive variances in the early Lichtman stages (stage I, stage II, and stage IIIA) of Kienböck's disease [1–3]. However, capitate-shortening osteotomy

A. Afshar, MD (✉)
Department of Orthopedics, Urmia University of Medical Sciences, Imam Khomeini Hospital, Modaress Street, Ershad Boulevard, Urmia, West Azarbaijan 57157-81351, Iran
e-mail: afshar_ah@yahoo.com

© Springer International Publishing Switzerland 2016

D.M. Lichtman, G.I. Bain (eds.), *Kienböck's Disease*, DOI 10.1007/978-3-319-34226-9_15

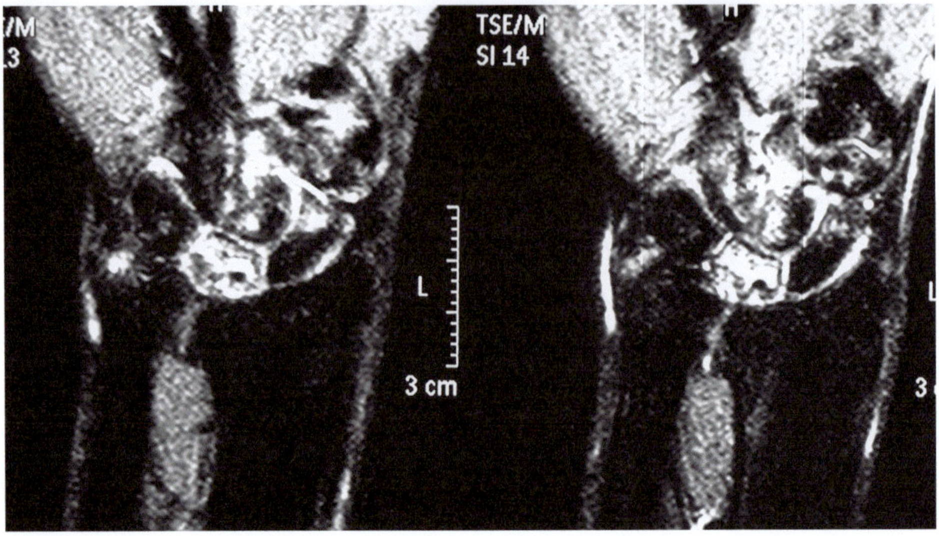


**Fig. 15.1** Three months postoperative fat suppression MRI image with high signal intensity and bone marrow edema in the capitate and lunate. The changes are highly suggestive of lunate revascularization and post-osteotomy of the capitate

is an independent procedure from ulnar variance, and it has also gained interest for ulnar-negative patients in recent years [23]. Capitate-shortening osteotomy does not affect the kinematics of the distal radioulnar joint and the risk of ulnar side pain does not increase [23, 24]. Significant fragmentations of the lunate and arthritic changes with cartilage loss around the lunate are contraindications for capitate-shortening osteotomy [3].

## Contraindications

There are a number of important contraindications for capitate shortening. Preoperative assessment with imaging modalities is essential. However, the final decision as to the correct surgical procedure should be made following inspection of the carpus at the time of surgery. These factors should be considered with the preoperative imaging and must be discussed with the patient before surgery. If at the time of surgery the capitate shortening is considered to be contraindicated, then the surgeon must have an alternative plan.

Contraindications include the following:

1. The lunate is too fragmented.
2. There are advanced arthritic changes of the lunate articular surfaces.
3. There are advanced arthritic changes of the articular surfaces adjacent to the lunate.

## Operative Techniques

Preoperative radiographs of the patient are performed (Figs. 15.2 and 15.3). A dorsal surgical approach which begins at the base of the third metacarpal and extends 4 cm proximally [2, 3]. The distal aspect of the fourth extensor compartment retinaculum may be incised to aid in retraction of the extensor tendons to the ulnar side. The dorsal interosseous nerve, located in the floor of the fourth extensor compartment, can be resected for de-innervation (Fig. 15.4). A longitudinal dorsal capsulotomy is performed, and the capsule is reflected to expose the capitate and lunate. A synovectomy may be required (Fig. 15.5). No imaging technique can be substituted for the direct observation of the lunate's condition. The distal concave articular surface of the lunate is inspected by traction along the middle finger. To observe the proximal surface of the lunate and radiolunate joint, the dorsal capsule over the lunate is dissected. This step provides a direct assessment and staging of the diseased lunate. The dorsal dissection should be limited so as not to further compromise the circulation to the avascular lunate.

At this point a decision is made as to whether the capitate shortening is appropriate, taking into the surgical observations, imaging, and the demands of the patient. Importantly the contraindications are considered.

To proceed with the osteotomy, use a fine-oscillating saw to make two parallel cuts in the capitate at the junction of its middle and distal thirds (Fig. 15.6). The osteotomy site is located in the capitate waist at the level of the distal dorsal articular surface of the scaphoid. The stepwise cuts are made 2 mm apart and the proximal cut is completed first. If the distal cut is completed first, it makes it diffiult to keep the proximal fragment stable during completion of the proximal cut. The attachment of the volar wrist capsule and ligaments to the proximal third of the waist of capitate is preserved. Then, a 2 mm wafer of bone is removed by prying it up (Fig. 15.7). The remnants of the proximal and distal volar cortexes may be removed by a small curet or rongeur to ensure that the two cut surfaces are aligned correctly. The two cut sur-

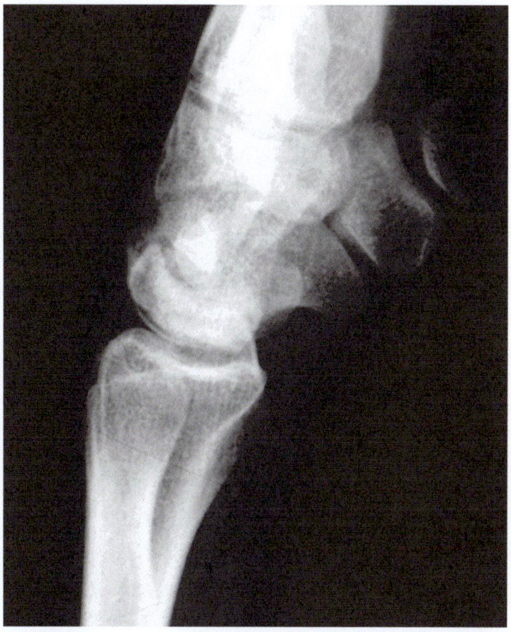

**Fig. 15.3** Preoperative lateral radiograph of the left wrist with Kienböck's disease

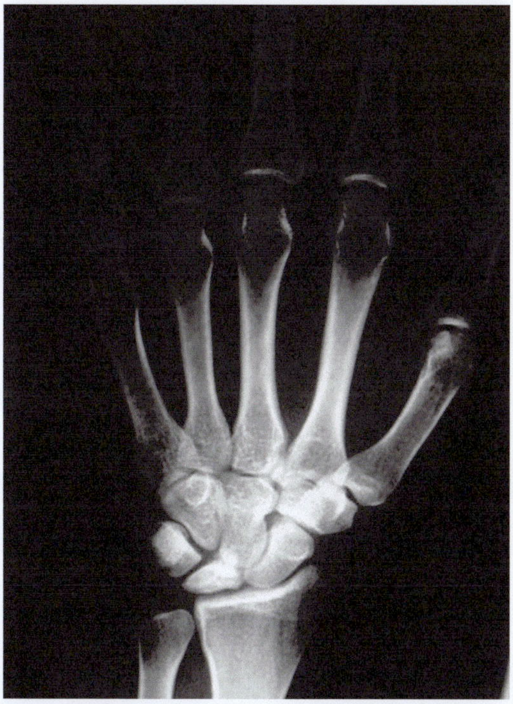

**Fig. 15.2** Preoperative anteroposterior radiograph of the left wrist with Kienböck's disease

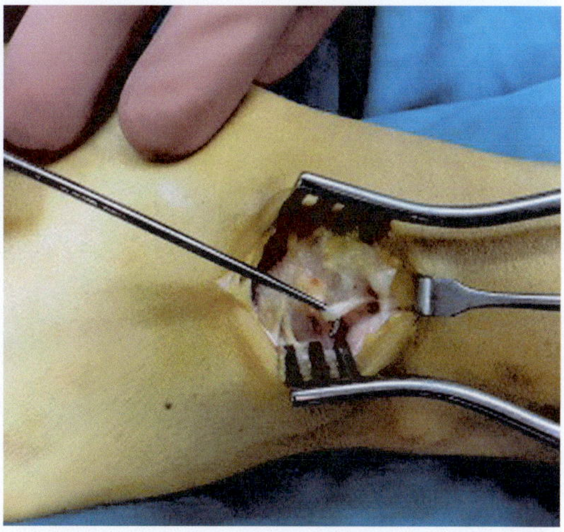

**Fig. 15.4** The fourth extensor compartment tendons are retracted to ulnar side. The hook at the distal level of the fourth extensor compartment shows the terminal branch of the dorsal interosseous nerve

faces are compressed manually by a curved blunt instrument inserted proximally (Fig. 15.8) and are fixed with two crossed 0.062 in K-wires. The wires are inserted percutaneously from distal to proximal (Fig. 15.9). The K-wires should not penetrate the proximal articular surface of the capitate. The K-wires may be placed on the ulnar and radial sides of the fingers' extensor tendons. The placement of the K-wires is confirmed with radiographs (Figs. 15.10 and 15.11). The wires may be left out of the skin, so they can be removed in the office easily. Alternatively, the osteotomy site may be fixed by a headless screw [23] or a staple [24]. The wounds are closed in layers and the wrist is protected with a short-arm splint.

Postoperatively, light activity of the fingers is advocated. After 1 week the short-arm splint is changed to a short-arm cast. The osteotomy site usually heals in about 6–8 weeks. When union is confirmed by radiographs, the pins and cast are removed and the patient increases his/her activity level and starts active and passive wrist range-of-motion exercises. The wrist should be protected by a wrist splint until the revascularization of the lunate is complete.

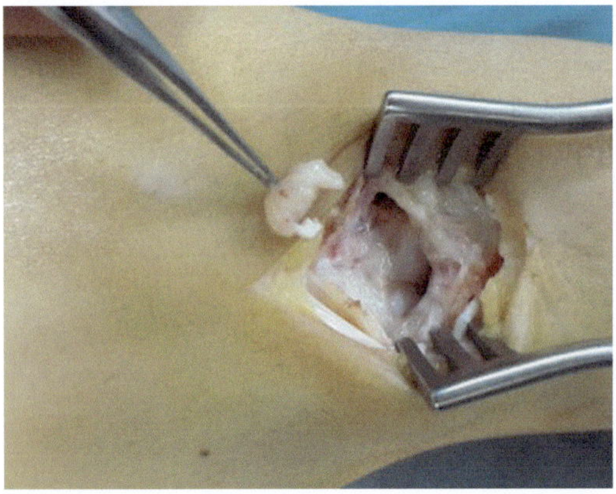

**Fig. 15.5** The wrist joint is opened and the proximal articular surface of the capitate is visualized. The hypertrophic synovium is removed

## Technical Alternatives

If there is a relatively long capitate waist, Almquist recommended removal of a thickness (e.g., 3–4 mm) bone wafer [2, 3]. Almquist did perform capitohamate arthrodesis along with capitate-shortening osteotomy [2, 3]. However, several studies failed to demonstrate an efficient load

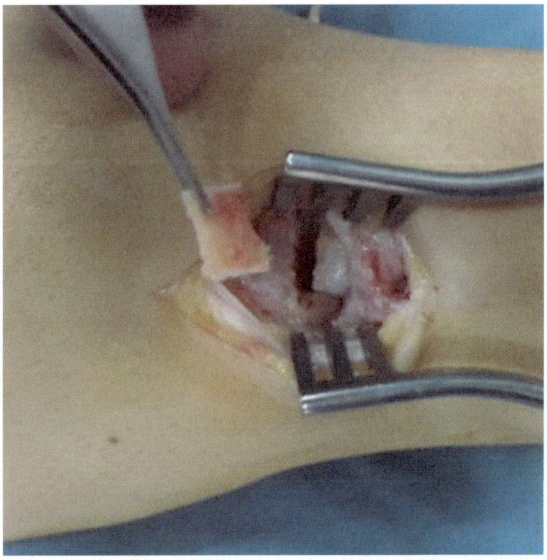

**Fig. 15.7** A 2 mm wafer of bone is removed

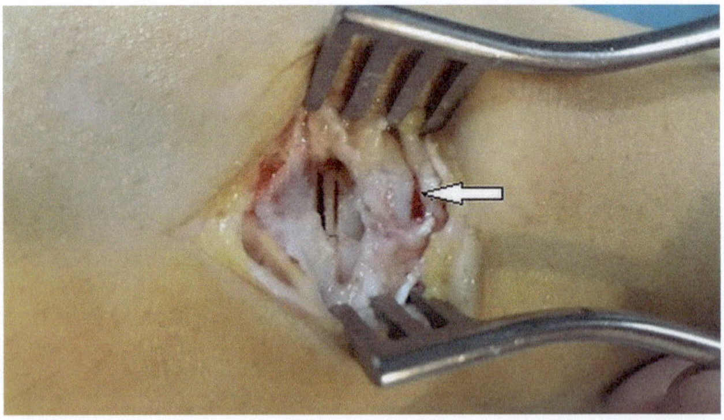

**Fig. 15.6** At the junction of middle and distal third of the waist of capitate bone two parallel cuts, with 2 mm intervals, are made using an oscillating saw. The arrow indicates the lunate bone

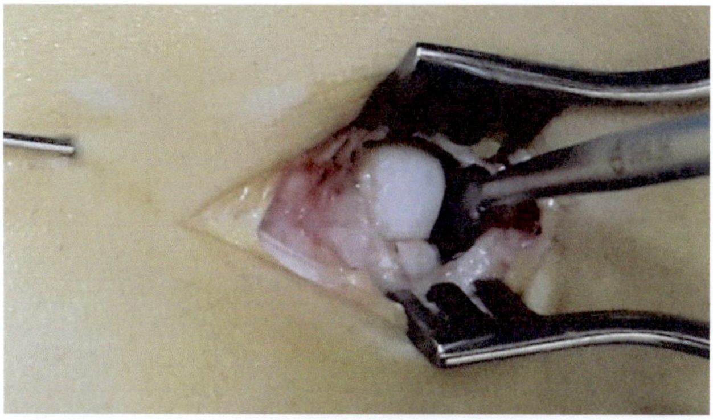

**Fig. 15.8** The osteotomy surfaces are compressed with a curved blunt instrument and then stabilized with two K-wires inserted percutaneously from distal to proximal. The arrow indicates the capitate's head

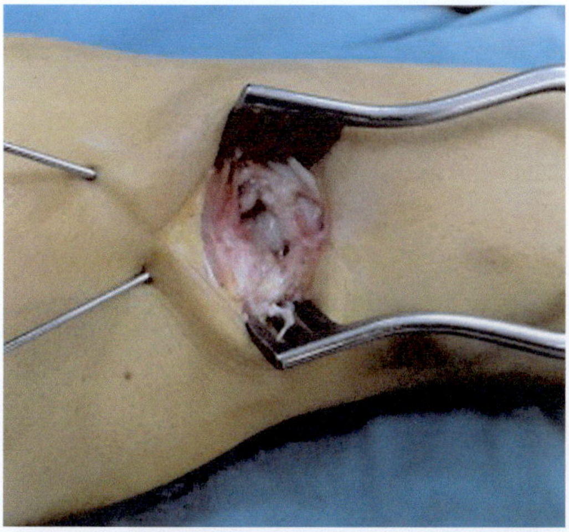

**Fig. 15.9** The osteotomy fixed with two crossed K-wires. The wires are inserted percutaneously from distal to proximal. The K-wires are placed ulnar and radial sides of the fingers' extensor tendons

reduction by adding a capitohamate arthrodesis to the capitate-shortening osteotomy [3, 24–26]. Therefore, subsequent authors have abandoned this part of the original procedure [7, 23, 24, 27].

Waitayawinyu et al. and Kakinoki et al. performed a vascularized bone graft for the lunate along with capitate-shortening osteotomy to expedite the revascularization process of the lunate [28, 29]. Waitayawinyu et al. also performed hamate shortening in some of their study subjects; however, the added benefit of this part to the procedure was not clear.

Okamoto et al. treated six Kienböck patients with capitate-shortening and capitate-hamate fusion. They noted a progressive scaphoid flexion in their patients. They believe that after capitate shortening the distal carpal row migrates proximally because of a shortened capitate and scaphoid adopts a palmar flexed position. The carpal collapse stops when the capitolunate contact is re-established [30]. Moritomo et al. [23] have suggested a reverse "L-shape" osteotomy to recess only the lunate facet of the capitate to circumvent the potential progression of carpal collapse that was noted by Okamoto et al. [30]. In this procedure, the length of the scaphoid facet of the capitate is not violated and this may help to preserve the normal position of the scaphoid bone in the wrist [23].

Fouly et al. performed a distal capitate shortening with capitometacarpal arthrodesis [31]. The third metacarpal is the most stable metacarpal at the wrist. Fouly et al. theorized that the arthrodesis of the base of the third metacarpal to the shortened distal capitate not only reduces the load to the intermediate column, but also prevents the proximal migration of the capitate and progression of carpal collapse [31].

## Outcomes

In cumulative data from 85 patients who underwent capitate osteotomy, the majority of patients demonstrated improvement in wrist pain, grip strength, and wrist range of motion [2, 3, 7, 24, 27–31]. There were no reported cases of nonunion or avascular necrosis of the proximal fragment [2, 7, 23, 24, 27–31]. In cumulative data from 67 patients who underwent capitate-

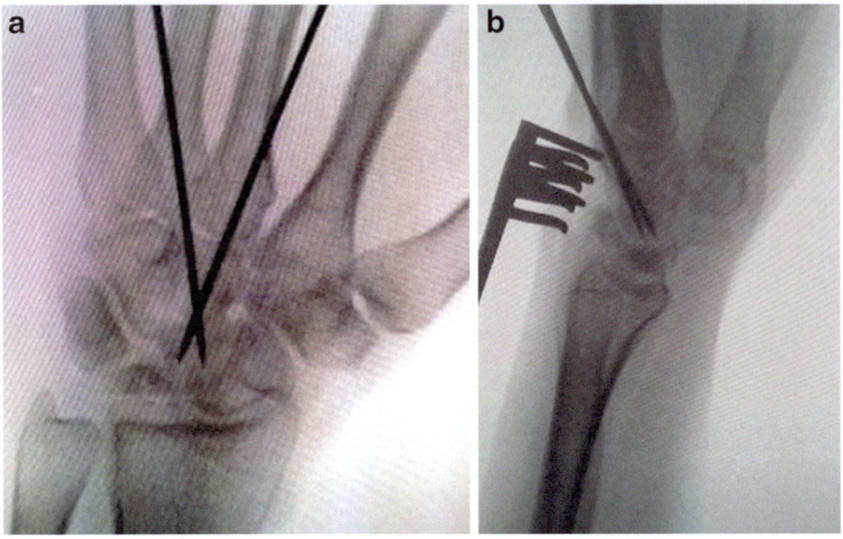


**Fig. 15.10** The placements of the K-wires are checked with intraoperative fluoroscopy. (**a**) Anteroposterior view. (**b**) Lateral view

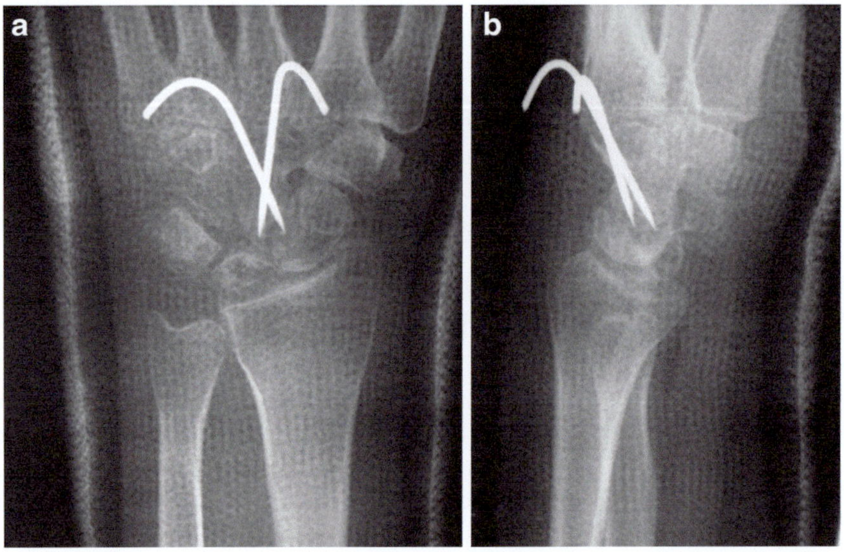


**Fig. 15.11** Anteroposterior radiographs of the left wrist 7 weeks postsurgery. (**a**) Anteroposterior view. (**b**) Lateral view

shortening osteotomy, no carpal malalignment was noted [2, 7, 24, 27–29].

Vander Grend et al. investigated the blood supply of the capitate bone [32]. They found three patterns of intraosseous circulation. The common denominator of the three vascular patterns was a retrograde flow from distal to proximal which may predispose to the non-union or avascular necrosis of the proximal fragment. These same concerns are also applicable to the scaphocapitate (Fenton) syndrome where there is a fractured scaphoid and capitate, with the proximal capitate fragment rotating up to 180°. In several series there were no reported cases of avascular necrosis or non-union of the capitate, as long as the proximal fragment was appropriately reduced and fixed [33–43].

## Conclusion

Capitate shortening is a technically simple method of unloading the lunate. It is indicated if the patient has an intact lunate and the articular surfaces are functional. It is contraindicated if the lunate is fragmented or if the articular surfaces of the lunate or adjacent articulations are not functional.

The decision to perform a capitate-shortening osteotomy is based on assessment of the lunate and articular surfaces of the carpus, with preoperative imaging and intraoperative examination.

Unlike the radial shortening, it can be used in either ulnar-positive or ulnar-negative variance, and it does not compromise the distal radioulnar joint. With the appropriate indications, the reported outcomes of this procedure are good.

## References


1. Almquist EE. Kienbock's disease. Clin Orthop Relat Res. 1986;202:68–78.
2. Almquist EE. Capitate shortening in the treatment of Kienböck's disease. Hand Clin. 1993;9(3):505–12.
3. Almqiust EE. Capitate shortening osteotomy. In: Blair WF, editor. Techniques in hand surgery. 1st ed. Baltimore, MD: Williams and Wilkins; 1996. p. 1067–74.
4. Innes L, Strauch RJ. Systematic review of the treatment of Kienböck's disease in its early and late stages. J Hand Surg Am. 2010;35(5):713–7. 717.e1–4.
5. Bekler HI, Erdag Y, Gumustas SA, Pehlivanoglu G. The proposal and early results of capitate forage as a new treatment method for Kienböck's disease. J Hand Microsurg. 2013;5(2):58–62.
6. Blanco RH, Blanco FR. Osteotomy of the radius without shortening for Kienböck disease: a 10-year follow-up. J Hand Surg Am. 2012;37:2221–5.
7. Afshar A. Lunate revascularization after capitate shortening osteotomy in Kienböck's disease. J Hand Surg Am. 2010;35(12):1943–6.
8. Horii E, Garcia-Elias M, Bishop AT, Cooney WP, Linscheid RL, Chao EY. Effect on force transmission across the carpus in procedures used to treat Kienböck's disease. J Hand Surg Am. 1990;15:393–400.
9. Kataoka T, Moritomo H, Omokawa S, Iida A, Wada T, Aoki M. Decompression effect of partial capitate shortening for Kienbock's disease: a biomechanical study. Hand Surg. 2012;17(3):299–305. doi:10.1142/S0218810412500219. PMID: 23061936.
10. Viola RW, Kiser PK, Bach AW, Hanel DP, Tencer AF. Biomechanical analysis of capitate shortening with capitate hamate fusion in the treatment of Kienböck's disease. J Hand Surg Am. 1998;23:395–401.
11. Werber KD, Schmelz R, Peimer CA, Wagenpfeil S, Machens HG, Lohmeyer JA. Biomechanical effect of isolated capitate shortening in Kienbock's disease: an anatomical study. J Hand Surg Eur Vol. 2013;38(5):500–7. doi:10.1177/1753193412458996. PMID: 22918882.
12. Lichtman DE, Mack GR, MacDonald RI, Gunther SF, Wilson JN. Kienböck's disease: the role of silicone replacement arthroplasty. J Bone Joint Surg Am. 1977;59:899–908.
13. Lichtman DE, Degnan GG. Staging and its use in the determination of treatment modalities for Kienböck's disease. Hand Clin. 1993;9:409–16.
14. Beredjiklian P. Kienböck's disease. J Hand Surg Am. 2009;34:167–75.
15. Schuind F, Eslami S, Ledoux P. Kienbock's disease. J Bone Joint Surg Am. 2008;90:133–9.
16. Allan CH, Josbi A, Lichtman DE. Kienbock's disease: diagnosis and treatment. J Am Acad Orthop Surg. 2001;9:128–36.
17. Afshar A, Aminzadeh-Gohari A, Yekta Z. The association of Kienbock's disease and ulnar variance in the Iranian population. J Hand Surg Eur Vol. 2013;38(5): 496–9.
18. Afshar A, Eivaziatashbeik K. Long-term clinical and radiological outcomes of radial shortening osteotomy and vascularized bone graft in Kienböck disease. J Hand Surg Am. 2013;38(2):289–96.
19. Paksima N, Canedo A. Kienböck's disease. J Hand Surg Am. 2009;34:1886–9.
20. De Smet L, Degreef I. Treatment options in Kienbock's disease. Acta Orthop Belg. 2009;75(6):715–26.
21. Afshar A. Lunate resection and vascularized os pisiform transfer in Kienböck's disease. J Hand Surg Am. 2006;31(3):50.
22. Afshar A. Long-term subjective and radiological outcome after reconstruction of Kienböck's disease stage 3 treated by a free vascularized iliac bone graft. J Hand Surg Am. 2008;33(7):1247.
23. Moritomo H, Murase T, Yoshikawa H. Operative technique of a decompression procedure for Kienböck's disease: partial capitates shortening. Tech Hand Up Extrem Surg. 2004;8(2):110–5.
24. Gay A, Parratte S, Glard Y, Mutaftschiev N, Legre R. Isolated capitate shortening osteotomy for early stage of Kienböck's disease with neutral ulnar variance. Plast Reconstr Surg. 2009;124:560–6.
25. Werner FW, Palmer AK. Biomechanical evaluation of operative procedures to treat Kienböck's disease. Hand Clin. 1993;9:431–43.
26. An K. The effect of force transmission in the carpus after procedures used to treat Kienböck's disease. Hand Clin. 1993;9:445–54.
27. Rabarin F, Saint Cast Y, Cesari B, Raimbeau G, Fouque PA. Capitate osteotomy in Kienböck's disease in twelve cases. Clinical and radiological results at five years follow-up. Chir Main. 2010;29(2):67–71. doi:10.1016/j.main.2010.02.001. PMID: 20299261.
28. Waitayawinyu T, Chin SH, Luria S, Trumble TE. Capitate shortening osteotomy with vascularized bone grafting for the treatment of Kienböck's disease

in ulnar positive wrist. J Hand Surg Am. 2008;33: 1267–73.
29. Kakinoki R, Matsumoto T, Suzuki T, Funakoshi N, Okamoto T, Nakamura T. Lunate plasty for Kienböck's disease: use of a pedicled vascularised radial bone graft combined with shortening of the capitate and radius. Hand Surg. 2001;6(2):145–56.
30. Okamoto M, Abe M, Shirai H, Ueda N, Kagawa Y. Capitate shortening for Kienböck's disease. J Jpn Soc Surg Hand. 1999;15:674–6.
31. Fouly EH, Sadek AF, Amin MF. Distal capitate shortening with capitometacarpal fusion for management of the early stages of Kienböck's disease with neutral ulnar variance: case series. J Orthop Surg Res. 2014;9(1):86.
32. Vander Grend R, Dell PC, Glowczewskie F, Leslie B, Ruby LK. Intraosseous blood supply of the capitate and its correlation with aseptic necrosis. J Hand Surg Am. 1984;9(5):677–83.
33. Sabat D, Dabas V, Suri T, Wangchuk T, Sural S, Dhal A. Trans-scaphoid transcapitate transhamate fracture of the wrist: case report. J Hand Surg Am. 2010;35(7):1093–6.
34. Sabat D, Arora S, Dhal A. Isolated capitate fracture with dorsal dislocation of proximal pole: a case report. Hand. 2011;6(3):333–6.
35. Leung YF, Ip SP, Wong A, Ip WY. Transscaphoid transcapitate transtriquetral perilunate fracture-dislocation: a case report. J Hand Surg Am. 2006;31(4):608–10.
36. Schliemann B, Langer M, Kösters C, Raschke MJ, Ochman S. Successful delayed surgical treatment of a scaphocapitate fracture. Arch Orthop Trauma Surg. 2011;131(11):1555–9.
37. Apergis E, Darmanis S, Kastanis G, Papanikolaou A. Does the term scaphocapitate syndrome need to be revised? A report of 6 cases. J Hand Surg Br. 2001;26(5):441–5.
38. Kim YS, Lee HM, Kim JP. The scaphocapitate fracture syndrome: a case report and literature analysis. Eur J Orthop Surg Traumatol. 2013;23 Suppl 2:S207–12.
39. Hamdi MF. The scaphocapitate fracture syndrome: report of a case and a review of the literature. Musculoskelet Surg. 2012;96(3):223–6.
40. Sawant M, Miller J. Scaphocapitate syndrome in an adolescent. J Hand Surg Am. 2000;25(6):1096–9.
41. Thomsen NO. A dorsally displaced capitate neck fracture combined with a transverse shear fracture of the triquetrum. J Hand Surg Eur Vol. 2013;38(2):210–1.
42. Yoshihara M, Sakai A, Toba N, Okimoto N, Shimokobe T, Nakamura T. Nonunion of the isolated capitate waist fracture. J Orthop Sci. 2002;7(5):578–80.
43. Osti M, Zinnecker R, Benedetto KP. Scaphoid and capitate fracture with concurrent scapholunate dissociation. J Hand Surg Br. 2006;31(1):76–8.

# Radial-Shortening and Ulnar-Lengthening Operations for Kienböck's Disease

16

Anuj P. Netto and Robert M. Szabo

## Introduction

The most common procedures to treat Kienböck's disease involve osteotomies of the radius or ulna and are frequently referred to as joint-leveling procedures. The rationale for these osteotomies comes from the belief that abnormal association between the lunate and radius leads to altered mechanics at the radiocarpal joint which predispose those individuals to developing Kienböck's disease. This theory was first proposed by Hultén in 1928 who observed a greater preponderance of ulnar minus variance in his patients with Kienböck's disease (78 %) compared to the normal population (23 %) [1]. Despite these and other observations supporting Hultén's theory, there have been further studies casting doubt on his concept, suggesting racial differences between ulnar variance and the development of Kienböck's disease [2, 3]. As such, these studies have still demonstrated improved functional outcomes in these patient populations with joint-leveling procedures suggesting that outcomes are likely related to the alteration of force transmission across the lunate rather than the resolution of a specific anatomic causal factor.

A number of biomechanical studies have since been performed which further support the observations of Hultén. Horii et al. demonstrated in their rigid body spring model that joint-leveling procedures resulted in a 45 % reduction in force through the radiolunate joint [4]. Cadaveric studies by Werner and Palmar have also demonstrated similar reduction of force across the radiolunate joint with radial-shortening and ulnar-lengthening osteotomies [5]. The exact amount of resection or lengthening has been of some debate. In vitro analysis by Trumble et al. through sequential radial shortening or ulnar lengthening led them to conclude that change of approximately 2 mm in length led to maximal decompression of the lunate while minimizing complications of ulnocarpal impingement or incongruity of the distal radioulnar joint [6].

## Osteotomy Options

Several joint-leveling procedures have been described with the goal of achieving ulnar-neutral variance. Hultén in 1935 described a radial-shortening osteotomy [7] and Persson soon followed with a ulnar-lengthening procedure [8]. Both techniques have demonstrated improvement of symptoms and share the advantage of

A.P. Netto, MD, MPH • R.M. Szabo, MD, MPH (✉)
Department of Orthopedics, Davis Health Care System, University of California, 4860 Y Street, Suite 3800, Sacramento, CA 95817, USA
e-mail: rmszabo@ucdavis.edu

© Springer International Publishing Switzerland 2016
D.M. Lichtman, G.I. Bain (eds.), *Kienböck's Disease*, DOI 10.1007/978-3-319-34226-9_16

being extra-articular should disease progression warrant further intra-articular intervention. Some have postulated that a radial-shortening osteotomy effectively lengthens the extrinsic musculotendinous units crossing the carpus, subsequently decreasing the force across the lunate [9]. Radial-shortening osteotomy is generally favored as ulnar lengthening has the disadvantage of associated morbidity with autograft harvesting, typically from the iliac crest. Additionally, ulnar lengthening has an increase in nonunion rates as union is required at two bone-graft interfaces and the ulnar diaphysis is more difficult to obtain union even without bone grafting with nonunion rates as high as 9 % [10]. This complication was even observed in early iterations of the radial-shortening osteotomy, which employed a 3.5 mm plate to stabilize a diaphyseal-based osteotomy. Subsequently, a distally based osteotomy at the metaphyseal/diaphyseal junction was employed utilizing a T-plate, which also had nonunion problems, and now the preferred fixation for stabilization and compression is a volar locking distal radius plate.

While radial-shortening and ulnar-lengthening osteotomies have offered treatment options for patients with ulnar-negative variance, they are of little utility for patients with ulnar-neutral or -positive variance. Kojima et al. in 1984 described a radial closing wedge osteotomy for patients with ulnar-positive variance [11], which decreased radial inclination while minimally affecting ulnar variance. They effectively demonstrated reduced axial load across the lunate through distribution of contact stress over a great surface area of the lunate. Their work was followed by Tsumura et al. who demonstrated in a rigid body spring model that the optimal lateral closing wedge angle in which the force transmitted through the lunate was evenly distributed across the radius and ulna at 15° [12].

The biomechanical data supporting radial wedge osteotomies has not been consistent. Studies published by Watanabe et al., employing a rigid body spring model, demonstrated a decrease in the force through the radiolunate and ulnolunate joints by 10 % and 36 %, respectively [13]. Their osteotomy model was theoretically similar to a lateral closing wedge osteotomy, effectively reducing the radial inclination. Cadaveric studies performed by Werner and colleagues analyzed the effect of medial closing, lateral opening, and lateral closing wedge osteotomies of the radius on the force transmitted across the radiolunate and ulnolunate joints [5]. With respect to the lateral opening wedge osteotomy, they demonstrated a decrease in pressure across the radiolunate joint at 4° of angulation, which was completely eliminated at 8° of angulation. A corresponding increasing in ulnolunate pressure was observed at increasing angles. This same relationship was seen with the medial closing wedge osteotomy. Ulnolunate pressure dramatically reduced with lateral closing wedge osteotomies; however there was a corresponding increase in radiolunate pressure. Kam et al. demonstrated a 26 % decrease in lunate cortical strain with a radial opening wedge osteotomy and a 24 % increase with a radial closing wedge osteotomy [14].

## Indications

Traditionally, indications for radial or ulnar osteotomies have been limited to patients with early symptomatic disease with the absence of degenerative changes and the maintenance of normal lunate architecture, stages I, II, and IIIA. However, these indications have slowly expanded to include those patients with stage IIIB disease as long-term follow-up studies have demonstrated equivalent outcomes. Previous concern over degenerative changes of the lunate resulting in further arthrosis of the carpus led many to believe that further intra-carpal procedures were required to alleviate symptoms and improve outcomes. However, most patients with stage IIIB disease treated with a radial or ulnar osteotomy experience improved symptoms and objective outcome measures, despite radiographic progression of disease [15–21]. While there is still some debate as to the inclusion of patients with stage IIIB disease, it is still widely felt that radial and ulnar osteotomies are a relative contraindication in patients with stage IV disease where wrist fusion, proximal row carpectomy, and denervation procedures are more predictable.

Radial-shortening and ulnar-lengthening osteotomies are only considered in patients with ulnar-negative variance. The concern for ulnar impingement and decreased forearm rotation precludes patients with ulnar-neutral or -positive variance. In those patients, a wedge osteotomy of the radius can be utilized instead to offset the force on the lunate while maintaining preoperative ulnar variance.

## Technique

### Radial-Shortening Osteotomy

The patient is placed supine on the operative table and after induction of anesthesia, the operative extremity is draped over a hand table with a pneumatic tourniquet placed high up on the extremity. After Esmarch exsanguination, the tourniquet is typically inflated to 250 mmHg.

A longitudinal incision is carried out in the interval between the flexor carpi radialis tendon and the radial artery. The incision typically starts at the wrist flexion crease and extends proximally approximately 7–10 cm. An incision is made through the anterior flexor carpi radialis tendon sheath, in line with the superficial skin incision. A fascial incision is made between the radial artery and the flexor carpi radialis (FCR) tendon sheath instead of directly through the floor of the FCR sheath in order to protect the palmar cutaneous branch of the median nerve, which is sometimes located more radially. The flexor pollicis longus tendon and the finger flexor tendons and median nerve are retracted ulnarly while the brachioradialis muscle and radial artery are retracted radially. The pronator quadratus is incised sharply and subperiosteally elevated along its radial and distal borders.

A Synthes™ (DePuy Synthes Trauma, West Chester, PA, USA) 2.4 mm volar locking distal radius T-plate with dynamic compression holes proximally is placed along the volar cortex of the radius. We like this particular plate for this indication because of the ability to obtain compression of the osteotomy site with the compression holes in this plate. After configuring the position radiographically such that the osteotomy will not violate the distal radial ulnar joint, two screws are placed in the distal most holes. The osteotomy location is planned such that three dynamic compression slots are available through the plate in the proximal fragment. The plate and distal screws are removed and a transverse osteotomy is templated on the cortical bone. The distance between the two osteotomy sites should theoretically correlate to the degree of ulna-negative variance such that post-osteotomy variance is neutral. Typically, this is between 2 and 3 mm. Nakamura et al. demonstrated that radial shortening greater than 4 mm led to significantly less satisfactory patient outcomes [22]. The osteotomy is performed using stacked blades in an oscillating saw [23] with careful attention paid towards avoiding over-resection (Fig. 16.1).

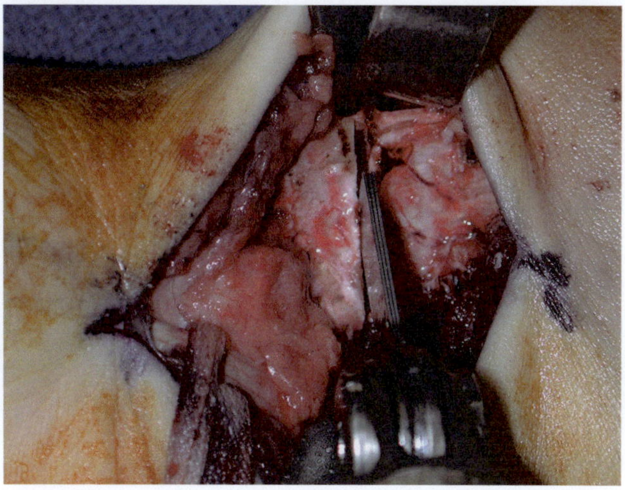

**Fig. 16.1** Radial osteotomy performed using stacked blade technique

After completion of the osteotomy, the plate is fixed to the distal fragment through the previously drilled holes. The proximal and distal fragments are apposed and compressed through the dynamic compression holes in the proximal portion of the plate. Using image intensifier, apposition and compression are confirmed on both the volar and dorsal cortices in addition to adequate correction of ulnar variance (Fig. 16.2).

Range of motion consisting of wrist flexion/extension and forearm pronation/supination is checked intraoperatively to ensure no loss in motion as a result of the plate/screw construct or osteotomy. The pronator quadratus is repaired over the plate and screws to help prevent attritional rupture of flexor tendons. The tourniquet is released, adequate hemostasis is achieved, and the wound is irrigated. The skin and subcutaneous tissues are closed with absorbable suture.

## Radial Wedge Osteotomy

Two types of wedge osteotomies of the radius have been described, employing a similar approach and procedure, when compared to a radial-shortening osteotomy. The first involves a z-type osteotomy in two planes [24] while the other involves a more simple lateral closing wedge osteotomy [25]. Both are presented in brief.

The step-cut or z-osteotomy is typically performed in the distal one-quarter of the radius and is done by first making a longitudinal osteotomy along the long axis of the radius. Trapezoidal segments of bone are subsequently resected on the distal/volar and proximal/dorsal segments of bone allowing the radius to translate in two planes resulting in radial deviation of the distal carpus and reduction of the radial inclination angle. Internal fixation is typically accomplished with 2 × 3.5 mm cortical screws in the anterior-posterior plane (Fig. 16.3).

We prefer the simpler, lateral closing wedge osteotomy, which is performed approximately 5 cm proximal to the radial styloid. A 15°, laterally based, closing wedge osteotomy is templated on the exposed bone. Kirschner wires can be used along the axis of each cut to increase precision of the osteotomy. The osteotomy is performed and the resulting segments of radius are internally fixed with a 4-hole LC/DC plate in compression (Fig. 16.4).

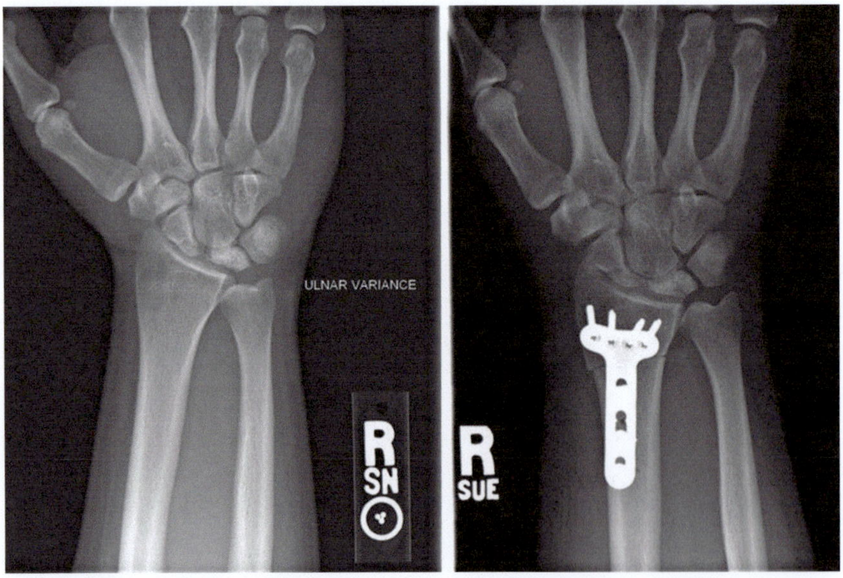


**Fig. 16.2** Preoperative (*left*) and postoperative (*right*) radiographs confirming correction of ulnar variance

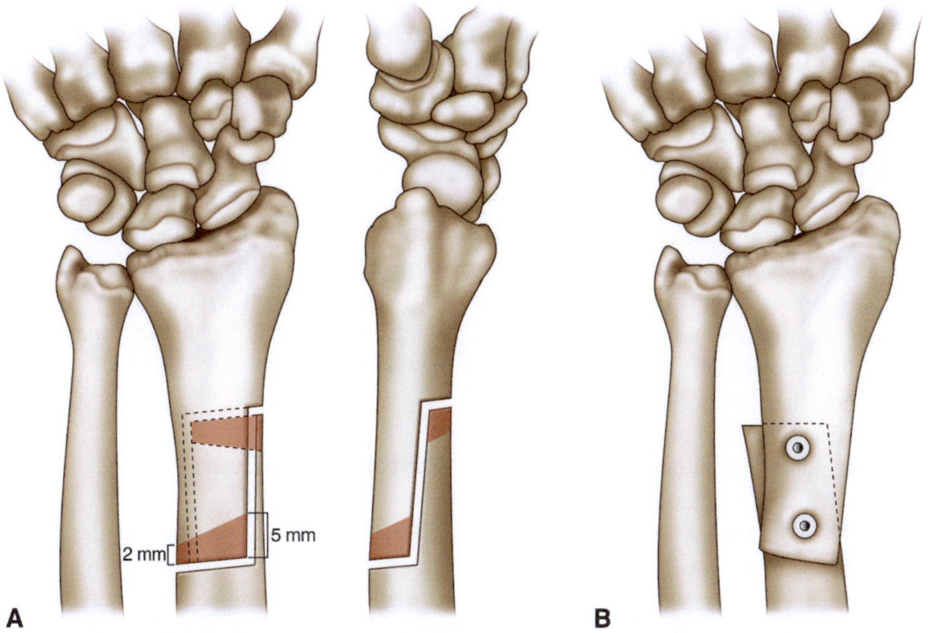


**Fig. 16.3** (**a**, **b**) Schematic of z-type radial wedge osteotomy

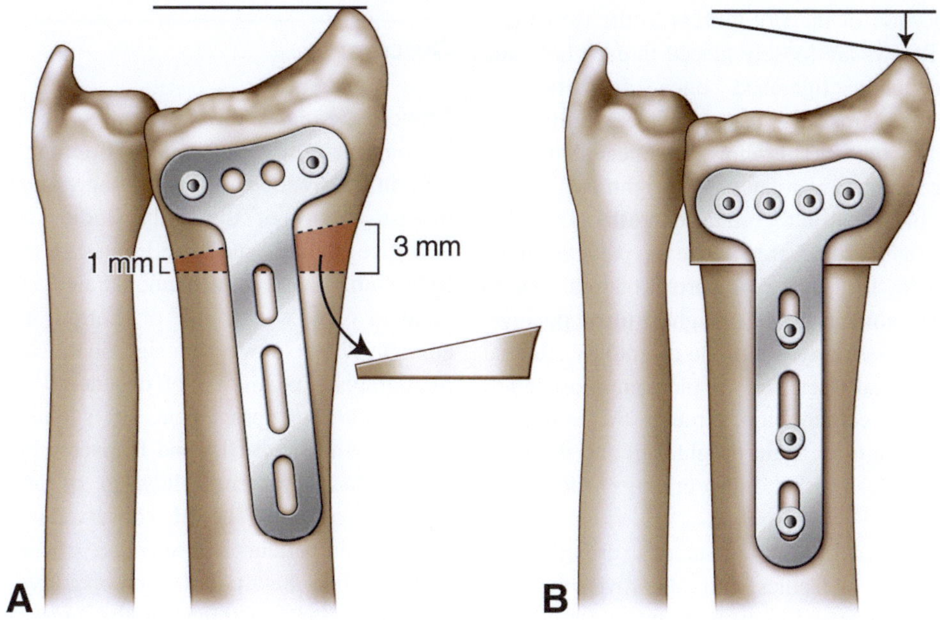


**Fig. 16.4** (**a**, **b**) Schematic of lateral closing wedge radial osteotomy

## Ulnar-Lengthening Osteotomy

The ulnar-lengthening osteotomy has been modified from the initial description by Persson, in which he used cerclage wire to secure an oblique osteotomy [8], to a simpler technique illustrated below, initially described by Armistead et al. [26]. This classic description can be modified with newer plating options and more modern techniques.

Ulnar lengthening is performed with similar preoperative patient positioning and preparation with the addition of sterilely preparing the ipsilateral anterior iliac crest. After induction of anesthesia, exsanguination, and tourniquet inflation, a longitudinal incision approximately 7–10 cm is made over the subcutaneous border of the distal ulna. The soft tissues are subperiosteally elevated over the distal third of the ulna. The flexor carpi ulnaris and extensor carpi ulnaris are reflected in their respective directions.

A transverse osteotomy is performed through the medial three-fourths of the distal ulna in a location sufficient to allow distal fixation of a four-hole plate with slotted holes. The plate is placed on the ulna and all four holes are drilled in the portion of the slot closest to the osteotomy site. Screws are loosely placed in each hole and subsequently tightened once distraction is achieved across the osteotomy site utilizing a lamina spreader. This allows for linear distraction while minimizing rotatory malalignment.

A bicortical autograft is harvested from the anterolateral iliac crest. Size is predetermined based on the degree of correction required to achieve ulnar neutral or slightly ulnar positive. The graft is inserted into the osteotomy site and the proximal screws on the plate are loosened to allow for compression through the autograft. Screws are once again retightened and the graft trimmed flush with the surrounding cortical bone (Fig. 16.5).

Correction of ulnar variance is verified utilizing image intensifier. Intraoperative range of motion is assessed to evaluate full wrist flexion/extension and forearm pronation/supination. Ulnar deviation might be reduced as a result of ulnar lengthening. Additionally, loss in pronation/supination can occur in patients who undergo ulnar-lengthening or radial-shortening osteotomy and who have a reverse obliquity of the sigmoid notch of the radius where the angle between the radiocarpal and distal radioulnar joints is increased. In these instances, a lateral closing wedge osteotomy of the radius can be combined with the associated joint-leveling procedure to correct for this impingement [27]. As an alternative, some surgeons trim the protruding bone of the proximal sigmoid notch with a narrow osteotome or rongeur to accommodate the ulnar head in its new location.

## Postoperative Course

The postoperative care for all the osteotomies described here are essentially the same. The extremity is immobilized for a period of 6 weeks while the patient is instructed on exercises for the thumb and digits. After 6 weeks, the patient is started on range-of-motion and strengthening exercises for the wrist and forearm with return to normal activities expected by 3–6 months.

## Outcomes

Numerous studies have been published highlighting the efficacy of radial-shortening osteotomy in the treatment of early-stage Kienböck's disease. Many of the early studies assessed objective findings and were limited in length of follow-up. Weiss et al. demonstrated improvement in pain, wrist range of motion, and grip strength while showing no significant change in radiographic parameters of degeneration. They demonstrated improvement of symptoms in patients with stage IIIA and B disease but were limited to short-term follow-up of less than 4 years on average. They also observed improved outcomes in patients whose degree of correction was less than the amount of preoperative ulnar-negative variance highlighting the importance of unloading the lunate in the treatment of Kienböck's disease [15]. Rock and colleagues had similar short-term objective findings but interestingly showed no difference between

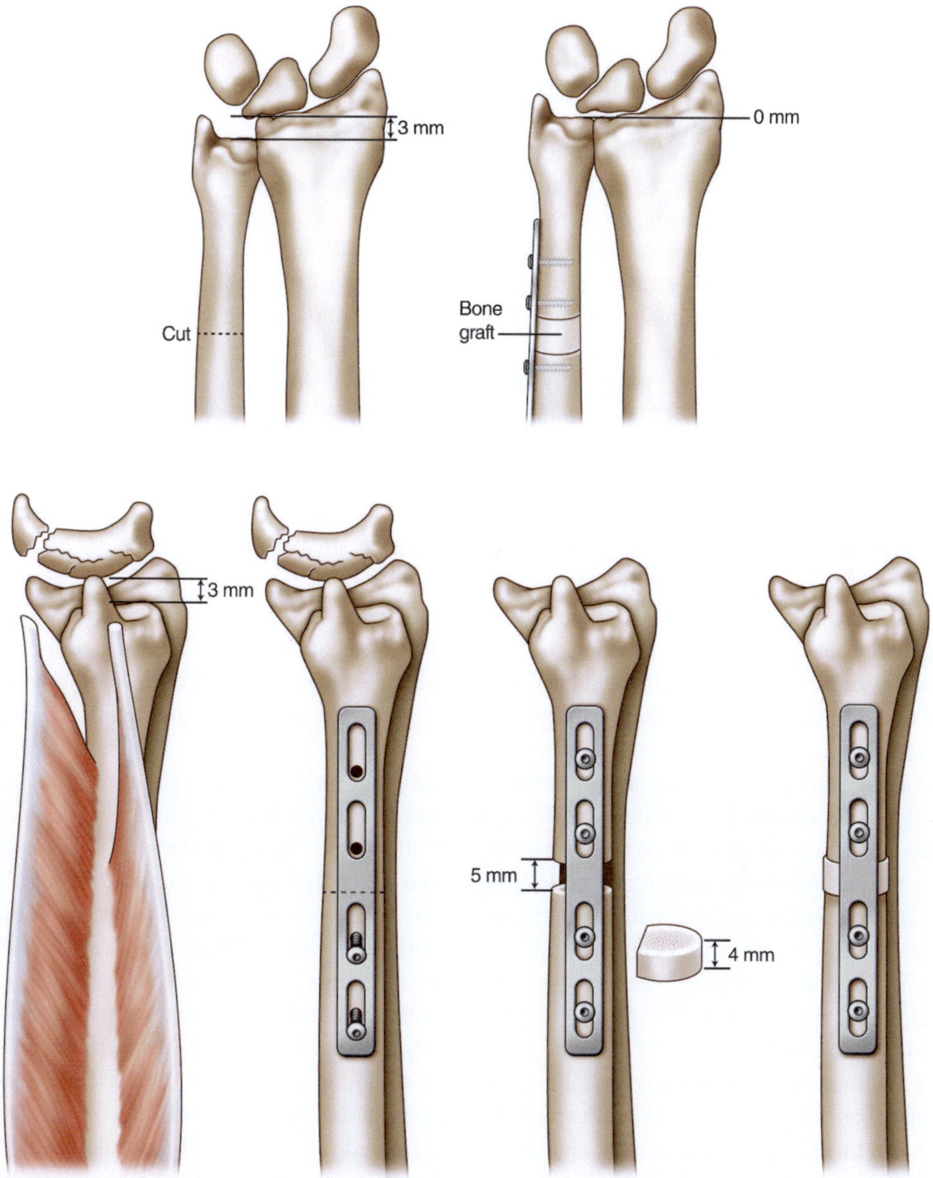


**Fig. 16.5** Schematic of ulnar lengthening osteotomy (the lateral view images)

patients with stage II or stage IV disease treated with radial-shortening osteotomy [16]. They acknowledged their average follow-up time of 4.5 years as likely not capturing disease progression but illustrated that radial-shortening osteotomies may be of some benefit in the short term. Calfee et al. demonstrated similar improvements in patients with stage II/IIIA compared to stage IIIB with slightly longer average follow-up at 7 years [17]. In addition to objective findings, they analyzed validated patient-based outcome measures (VAS for pain and function, QuickDASH, modified Mayo wrist scores) to demonstrate no clinically relevant differences between stage II/IIIA and IIIB Kienböck's disease.

As previously mentioned, Nakamura and colleagues evaluated factors affecting operative results of radial-shortening osteotomy [22]. In addition to highlighting the amount of radial shortening predictive of satisfactory results, they also demonstrated no difference in clinical or radiographic findings at an average follow-up of 5.5 years with respect to ulnar variance or stage of disease. Age less than 30 years was the only other variable predictive of satisfactory results.

More recently, several long-term studies have emphasized the resiliency of previously published short-term results of radial osteotomies in the treatment of Kienböck's disease. Koh et al. showed improvement of pain, wrist range of motion, and grip strength at 5-year follow-up, which was subsequently maintained at a minimum of 10 years [18]. Although radiographic changes worsened at final follow-up, these changes did not affect clinical outcome in their patients. Watanabe et al. utilized a validated outcome measure (DASH) in addition to objective clinical measures to demonstrate reliable outcomes at an average of 21 years in patients with stage II and III disease [19]. Patients with stage IIIB disease tended to have worse functional outcomes at final follow-up. Matsui and colleagues went one step further and obtained magnetic resonance imaging in their small cohort of patients with stage III and IV disease, preoperatively and at final follow-up of at least 10 years [20]. They successfully showed increased T1 signal intensity of the lunate in 7 out of 10 wrists likely correlating to long-term preservation of the lunate.

Good clinical and radiographic outcomes have been demonstrated in short- and long-term studies involving radial wedge osteotomies. Nakamura et al. reported improved pain, wrist flexion-extension, and radiographic parameters at an average of 2.5 years [28]. Given the design of the step-cut osteotomy, they did notice a trend towards decreased pronation but was not significant. They also analyzed factors influencing their results and found that patients who had 10–15° of radial deviation of the distal part of the radius after osteotomy had better outcomes than those with 5–9°. Younger patients less than 30 years old trended towards better outcomes but were not significant. Ulnar variance, presence or absence of radial shortening, stage of disease, or duration of follow-up did not correlate with outcome.

Similar objective clinical results were observed at long-term follow-up of 14 years on average, despite radiographic progression of disease [29]. When comparing wedge to shortening osteotomy of the radius, Iwasaki and colleagues showed similar improvement in pain, range of motion, and grip strength in patients with stage IIIB and IV disease [21]. Both treatment groups were similar with respect to age, stage of disease, and duration of follow-up with closing wedge osteotomy reserved for ulnar neutral or positive variance while radial shortening utilized for ulnar-negative patients.

There are few outcome studies concerning ulnar-lengthening procedures. Persson first described the ulnar-lengthening procedure in 1945 and subsequently reported his additional experiences with 5-year follow-up [8, 30]. He was able to demonstrate superior results in 23 patients including improved pain, grip strength, and preservation of radiographic parameters of the lunate. Tillberg, in 1968, reported his experiences on nine patients and further validated Persson's findings with 13.5-year follow-up on average [31]. Armistead and colleagues at the Mayo Clinic reported their successful findings in 20 patients treated with an ulnar osteotomy. They found improved symptoms of pain, preservation of wrist motion between 70 and 86 % of the contralateral wrist, and a 17 % increase in grip strength compared to preoperative values [26]. Ulnar deviation was the only wrist motion significantly affected with only 53 % of the contralateral value. Quenzer and Linscheid reported on the largest sample of patients treated with ulnar-lengthening osteotomy [32]. With an average follow-up of 94 months, they found 90 % satisfaction rate with surgery, 86 % pain relief, and 70 % of their patients had returned to their original job. Despite comparable outcomes, ulnar-lengthening procedures have largely fallen out of favor when compared to radial-sided procedures secondary to increased complication rates, particularly nonunions and need for additional bone graft [9].

Weiss et al. described two main complications attributed to radial shortening osteotomy [15]. By far, the most prevalent complication was nonunion of the osteotomy, which they noted around 3–4 % in their patient population. Additionally, they cautioned against over shortening the radius leading to incongruity of the distal radioulnar joint and ulnar impaction syndrome. For this, they recommended resection of less than 4 mm to avoid pain associated with pronation/supination and ulnar deviation, respectively.

In their large cohort of patients treated with ulnar lengthening, Quenzer and Linscheid found an overall complication rate of 22 % with most attributed to hardware removal secondary to painful implants (44 %) [32]. Their delayed union and nonunion rate was 14 % and they observed ulnocarpal impingement in 8 % of patients. Although their patients had technically satisfactory ulnar-lengthening osteotomies, they noted that 11 % of patients at final follow-up had further procedures for relief of wrist pain. Due to the relatively large number of complications, many advocate for radial shortening procedures, as highlighted in a comparative study from the Mayo Clinic [33].

## Conclusion

While the exact role of ulnar variance in the pathogenesis of Kienböck's disease remains unclear, the acceptance that ulnar variance does play a role in its natural history has led to the popularization of various joint-leveling procedures. Since Hultén's observations in 1928, numerous biomechanical and outcome studies have illustrated the benefits of unloading the force witnessed by the lunate in the overall progression of disease. As was mentioned before, both radial-shortening and ulnar-lengthening osteotomies provide equivalent results with respect to pain, wrist range of motion, and grip strength and as such are increasingly being used in patients with severe disease as a temporizing procedure. Despite the complications associated with ulnar-lengthening osteotomies, it along with radial-shortening osteotomies offers the added benefit of staying extra-articular should further intra-articular salvage procedures be required in the future.

## References


1. Hultén O. Uber anatomische Variationen der Handgelenkknochen. Acta Radiol. 1928;9:155–68.
2. D'Hoore K, De Smet L, Verellen K, Vral J, Fabry G. Negative ulnar variance is not a risk factor for Kienböck's disease. J Hand Surg Am. 1994;19(2):229–31.
3. Muramatsu K, Ihara K, Kawai S, Doi K. Ulnar variance and the role of joint levelling procedure for Kienböck's disease. Int Orthop. 2003;27(4):240–3.
4. Horii E, Garcia-Elias M, Bishop AT, Cooney WP, Linscheid RL, Chao EY. Effect on force transmission across the carpus in procedures used to treat Kienböck's disease. J Hand Surg Am. 1990;15(3):393–400.
5. Werner FW, Palmer AK. Biomechanical evaluation of operative procedures to treat Kienböck's disease. Hand Clin. 1993;9(3):431–43.
6. Trumble T, Glisson RR, Seaber AV, Urbaniak JR. A biomechanical comparison of the methods for treating Kienböck's disease. J Hand Surg Am. 1986; 11(1):88–93.
7. Hultén O. Uber die entstechung and behandlung der lunatummalazie (morbus Kienbock). Acta Chir Scand. 1935;76:121–35.
8. Persson M. Pathogenese und behandlung der Kienbockschen lunatummalazie: die frakturtheorie im lichte der erfolge operativer radiusverkurzung (Hultén) und einer neuen operationsmethodeulnaverlangerung. Acta Chir Scand. 1945;92 Suppl 98:1–58.
9. Weiss AP. Radial shortening. Hand Clin. 1993;9(3): 475–82.
10. Constantine KJ, Tomaino MM, Herndon JH, Sotereanos DG. Comparison of ulnar shortening osteotomy and the wafer resection procedure as treatment for ulnar impaction syndrome. J Hand Surg Am. 2000;25(1):55–60.
11. Kojima TKM, Tsumura H, Himeno S, Shinohara N. Wedge osteotomy of radius for Kienböck's disease. J Jpn Soc Surg Hand. 1984;1:431–4.
12. Tsumura H, Himeno S, Morita H, Sasaki Y, Ueda Y, Morishita K, et al. The optimum correcting angle of wedge ostetomy at the distal end of the radius for Kienböck's disease. J Jpn Soc Surg Hand. 1984;1:435–9.
13. Watanabe K, Nakamura R, Horii E, Miura T. Biomechanical analysis of radial wedge osteotomy for the treatment of Kienböck's disease. J Hand Surg Am. 1993;18(4):686–90.
14. Kam B, Topper SM, McLoughlin S, Liu Q. Wedge osteotomies of the radius for Kienböck's disease: a

biomechanical analysis. J Hand Surg Am. 2002;27(1): 37–42.
15. Weiss AP, Weiland AJ, Moore JR, Wilgis EF. Radial shortening for Kienbock disease. J Bone Joint Surg Am. 1991;73(3):384–91.
16. Rock MG, Roth JH, Martin L. Radial shortening osteotomy for treatment of Kienböck's disease. J Hand Surg Am. 1991;16(3):454–60.
17. Calfee RP, Van Steyn MO, Gyuricza C, Adams A, Weiland AJ, Gelberman RH. Joint leveling for advanced Kienböck's disease. J Hand Surg Am. 2010;35(12):1947–54.
18. Koh S, Nakamura R, Horii E, Nakao E, Inagaki H, Yajima H. Surgical outcome of radial osteotomy for Kienböck's disease-minimum 10 years of follow-up. J Hand Surg Am. 2003;28(6):910–6.
19. Watanabe T, Takahara M, Tsuchida H, Yamahara S, Kikuchi N, Ogino T. Long-term follow-up of radial shortening osteotomy for Kienbock disease. J Bone Joint Surg Am. 2008;90(8):1705–11.
20. Matsui Y, Funakoshi T, Motomiya M, Urita A, Minami M, Iwasaki N. Radial shortening osteotomy for kienbock disease: minimum 10-year follow-up. J Hand Surg Am. 2014;39(4):679–85.
21. Iwasaki N, Minami A, Oizumi N, Suenaga N, Kato H, Minami M. Radial osteotomy for late-stage Kienböck's disease. Wedge osteotomy versus radial shortening. J Bone Joint Surg Br. 2002;84(5):673–7.
22. Nakamura R, Imaeda T, Miura T. Radial shortening for Kienböck's disease: factors affecting the operative result. J Hand Surg Br. 1990;15(1):40–5.
23. Labosky DA, Waggy CA. Oblique ulnar shortening osteotomy by a single saw cut. J Hand Surg Am. 1996;21(1):48–59.
24. Calandriello B, Palandri C. The treatment of lunatomalacia by radius shortening. Z Orthop Grenzgeb. 1966;101(4):531–4.
25. Miura H, Sugioka Y. Radial closing wedge osteotomy for Kienböck's disease. J Hand Surg Am. 1996;21(6): 1029–34.
26. Armistead RB, Linscheid RL, Dobyns JH, Beckenbaugh RD. Ulnar lengthening in the treatment of Kienböck's disease. J Bone Joint Surg Am. 1982;64(2):170–8.
27. Quenzer DE, Dobyns JH, Linscheid RL, Trail IA, Vidal MA. Radial recession osteotomy for Kienböck's disease. J Hand Surg Am. 1997;22(3):386–95.
28. Nakamura R, Tsuge S, Watanabe K, Tsunoda K. Radial wedge osteotomy for Kienbock disease. J Bone Joint Surg Am. 1991;73(9):1391–6.
29. Wada A, Miura H, Kubota H, Iwamoto Y, Uchida Y, Kojima T. Radial closing wedge osteotomy for Kienböck's disease: an over 10 year clinical and radiographic follow-up. J Hand Surg Br. 2002;27(2): 175–9.
30. Persson M. Causal treatment of lunatomalacia; further experiences of operative ulna lengthening. Acta Chir Scand. 1950;100(6):531–44.
31. Tillberg B. Kienboeck's disease treated with osteotomy to lengthen ulna. Acta Orthop Scand. 1968;39(3): 359–69.
32. Quenzer DE, Linscheid RL. Ulnar lengthening procedures. Hand Clin. 1993;9(3):467–74.
33. Trail IA, Linscheid RL, Quenzer DE, Scherer PA. Ulnar lengthening and radial recession procedures for Kienböck's disease. Long-term clinical and radiographic follow-up. J Hand Surg Br. 1996;21(2): 169–76.

# Radial Closing Wedge Osteotomy for Kienböck's Disease

# 17

Masahiro Tatebe, Ryogo Nakamura, and Hitoshi Hirata

## Historical Perspectives

The lunate is the central bone of the proximal carpal row and the keystone of the wrist. Kienböck's disease is a progressive disorder characterized by aseptic necrosis of the lunate bone. The precise etiology remains unknown; however, Kienböck's disease is multifactorial and (1) overload, (2) vascularity, and (3) mechanical predisposition cause lunatomalacia. Currently, there is no consensus on treatment for Kienböck's disease. Although the lunate overloading theory is insufficient to explain the etiology of Kienböck's disease [1], mechanical factors also have been theorized to contribute to the development of osteonecrosis [2]. Therefore several procedures have been reported to unload the lunate and to prevent a progressive condition [2].

M. Tatebe, MD, PhD (✉)
Hand and Microsurgery Center, Anjo Kosei Hospital, 28 Higashihirokute, Anjocho, Anjo 446-8602, Japan
e-mail: tatebe@med.nagoya-u.ac.jp; masahirottb@gmail.com

R. Nakamura, MD, PhD
Department of Orthopedic Surgery, Nagoya Hand Center, Chunichi Hospital, 3-12-3 Marunouchi, Nakaku, Nagoya 460-0002, Japan

H. Hirata, MD, PhD
Department of Hand Surgery, Nagoya University Graduate School of Medicine, 65 Tsurumaicho, Showaku, Nagoya 466-8550, Japan

Radial osteotomy is an extra-articular and lunate-preserving procedure. A lateral closing wedge osteotomy of the distal radius that decreases radial inclination has been recommended for Kienböck's disease based on clinical investigations [3].

## Biological Effect

Several investigators have reported on the biomechanical effects of radial wedge osteotomy [4–7]. Nakamura advocated a radial closing osteotomy to increase the radiolunate contact surface, producing a more uniform distribution of forces and thus reducing load on the lunate [8]. The radial closing osteotomy in this situation decreases the radial inclination of the distal radius and increases the contact area between the radius and the lunate [9–11]. By doing so, contact stress and force transmission across both the radiolunate and the capitolunate articulations are decreased [12]. A radial closing wedge osteotomy could shift the loading vector and ulnar deviation of the carpus, extending the scaphoid (Fig. 17.1). Recent reports mentioned that the radial open wedge osteotomy had better biological effects than the radial closing wedge osteotomy [7]. However, most biomechanical analyses simulate a certain position that does not apply to all daily activities or sports activities, and do not assess actual motion. Therefore the precise biomechanical consequences of radial wedge

© Springer International Publishing Switzerland 2016
D.M. Lichtman, G.I. Bain (eds.), *Kienböck's Disease*, DOI 10.1007/978-3-319-34226-9_17

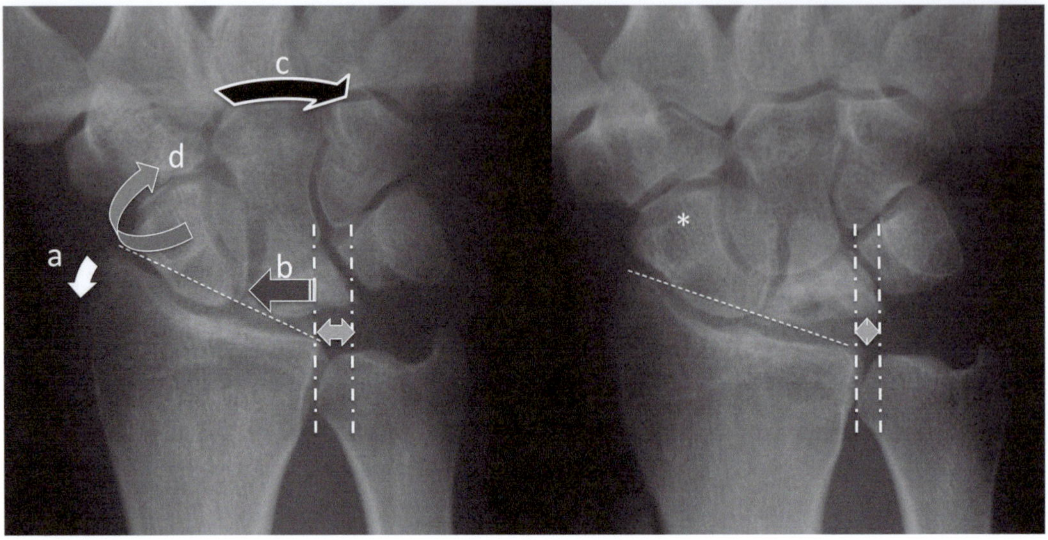


**Fig. 17.1** The symbols depict the anatomic changes following radial closing wedge osteotomy: *solid white arrow* (**a**), carpus shifts radially; *outlined dark short arrow* (**b**), carpus deviates ulnarly; *outlined dark long arrow* (**c**), scaphoid extends (**d**); asterisk (*), ring sign improves

osteotomy remain unclear. Indeed, the radial closing wedge osteotomy had good results in clinical settings. Soejima et al. reported that the satisfactory clinical outcome of the lateral closing wedge osteotomy of the distal radius for advanced-stage Kienböck's disease can be attributed to the effects of the increased lunate-covering ratio (LCR: Fig. 17.2) and the improved radioscaphoid angle on carpal alignment [13].

## Osteotomy Effect: Revascularization

Given the vascularity of the wrist as a network of vascular anastomoses encircling the radius and extending across the carpus, osteotomy of the radius may incite sufficient hyperemia to accelerate revascularization of the lunate [14, 15]. Theoretically, any surgical procedure near the lunate may induce changes in arterial inflow or venous drainage, resulting in pain relief and occasionally in changes in the architecture of the lunate [1]. The aim of surgical intervention in the early stages of Kienböck's disease is to improve lunate circulation by unloading the bone [16], and the radial closing wedge osteotomy achieves this.

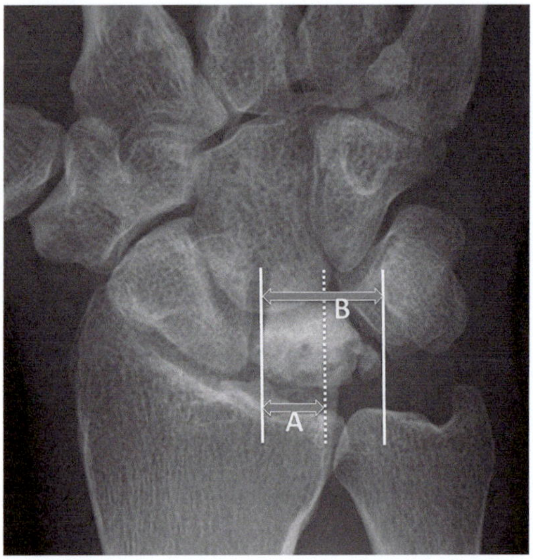


**Fig. 17.2** Measurement of lunate covering ratio (LCR). LCR = A/B

## Surgical Anatomy and Indications

The proximal lunate contacts the lunate fossa of the radius and triangular fibrocartilage complex (TFCC), and distally is in contact with the capitate and hamate [17]. There are two types of lunate described by Viegas: the distal lunate contacts the capitate (type I lunate) or the hamate (type II lunate) [18]. Arthroscopic examination showed a higher incidence of type 1 lunates in patients with Kienböck's disease than in patients without Kienböck's disease [19]. Historically, anatomical factors associated with Kienböck's disease are negative ulnar variance, and a small and radially inclined lunate. More recent studies have called this into question, noting no difference in ulnar variance between normal wrists and those with Kienböck's disease, and that negative ulnar variance occurs with equal frequency in patients both with and without Kienböck's disease [2, 20]. A radial closing wedge osteotomy does not change ulnar variance and can be used for ulnar plus variance. For minus variance, a radial closing wedge and shortening (combined) osteotomy, or only radial shortening osteotomy, are recommended.

## Examination and Imaging

Patients have wrist pain, tenderness, and occasional swelling over the lunate, decreasing grip strength and decreasing wrist motion. Plain X-rays show sclerosis, fragmentation, and loss of height of the lunate. Carpal malalignment occurs in the advanced stage. MRI is the most sensitive and specific test and may detect very early disease. Lichtman's classification is frequently used in the assessment and management of Kienböck's disease. Good indications for the radial closing osteotomy are Lichtman stage 1,2,3a, and 3b with ulnar-positive and neutral wrist. Imaging of Kienböck's disease has some problems. First, the difference between Lichtman stage 3a and 3b is not reliable [17]. Second, radiographic severity does not always correlate with the degree of symptoms, which contributes further to the difficulty in assessing the natural history of this condition [17].

Wrist arthroscopy provides a valuable preoperative evaluation [21, 22]. Wrist arthroscopy revealed that younger patients had fewer cartilage lesions, which may explain the better clinical results in younger patients [22]. Once cartilage is destroyed, full recovery will not occur, which may be why the severity of cartilage lesions affects the clinical outcome [11, 22].

## Surgical Procedure

The procedure is usually performed under an axial block or general anesthesia and tourniquet control. Originally, the surgical approach from the dorsolateral aspect of the radius was used, but now we prefer a palmar FCR approach, between the flexor carpi radialis and brachioradialis. The flexor carpi radialis is retracted radially, and the other flexor tendons ulnarly, to expose the pronator quadratus muscle. The pronator quadratus is incised at its radial insertion, and the distal third of the radius is exposed subperiosteally. The optimal correction angle is 15° according to the study done by Tsumura et al. [23] using a rigid-body spring model [3]. Historically, a step-cut osteotomy and screw fixation 5 cm proximal to the tip of the radial styloid process is used. Now, when using volar locking plate or locking compression plate, a simple wedge osteotomy is performed 3 cm proximal to the tip of the radial styloid process, so as not to obstruct the distal radioulnar joint (DRUJ) (Fig. 17.3). Preoperatively, we designed the osteotomy line to decrease the radial inclination from 5 to 10° (the final radial inclination was 10–15° postoperatively). Nakamura et al. reported that the results were better for younger patients than older ones and that 10–15° of radial deviation was better than 5–9° [8]. The proximal setting volar locking plate system is used for easy handling and stable fixation (Fig. 17.4). An additional procedure, such as a vascularized bone graft, could be combined with this procedure. Cast or splint fixation is applied for several weeks postoperatively. Complications after a radial closing osteotomy include nonunion, delayed union, ulnar impaction syndrome, and DRUJ arthrosis.

## Expected Outcomes

The literature contains several reports of good long-term results with these procedures in Kienböck's disease, and the factor that most affects clinical results after radial shortening is patient age. Our results include 47 cases (34 males and 13 females, average age 34.8, range 14–64). The average grip strength increased from 64 to

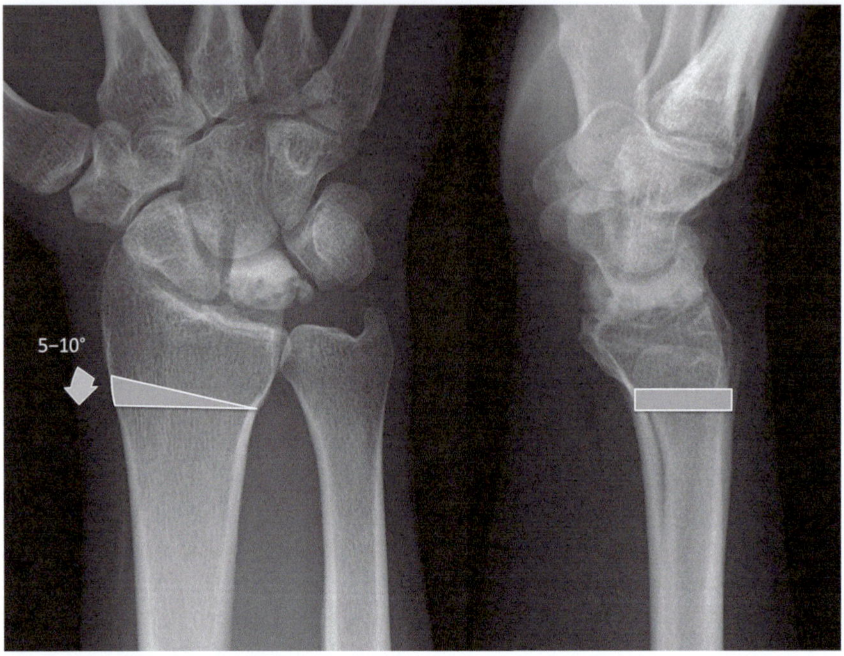


**Fig. 17.3** Preoperative surgical design. Simple closing wedge osteotomy located 3 cm proximal to the radial styloid

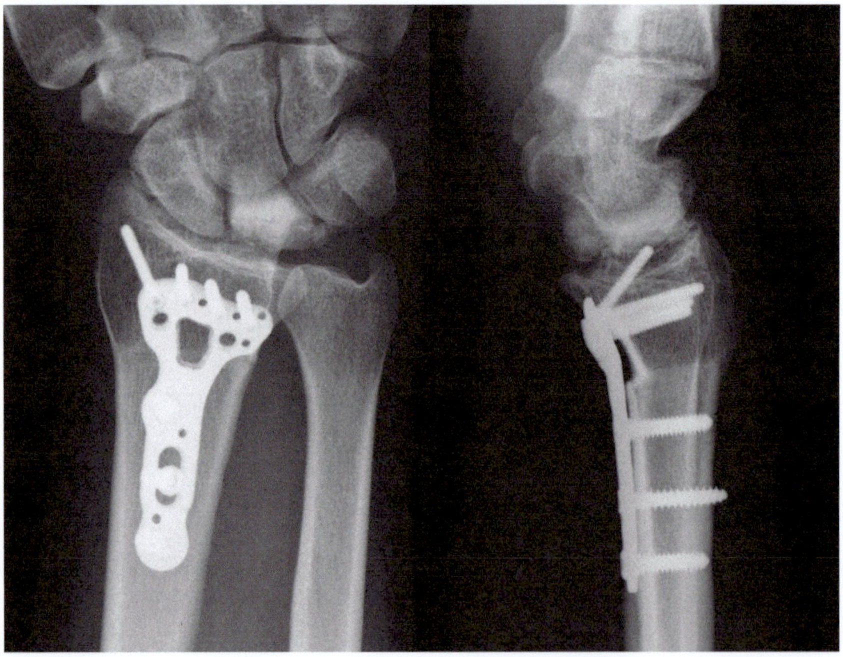

**Fig. 17.4** Postoperative plain X-ray. Osteotomy stabilized with a volar locking plate

87 % and the range of flexion–extension increased from 88 to 100°. Although many patients had mild wrist pain after surgery, most patients had decreased pain and regained powerful grip strength. Using the Lichtman's radiological classification, there were 8 stage 2; 26 stage 3a; and 13 stage 3b. Postoperative carpal geometry did not significantly improve, nor did they progress toward carpal collapse (pre-op ulnar variance [UV] −0.1, radial inclination [RI] 28.1, carpal height ratio [CHR] 0.51, radioscaphoid angle [RSA] 64°, Ståhl index [SI] 0.35, LCR 0.52, post-op UV 1.9, RI 17.3, CHR 0.486, RSA 66.1, SI 0.296, LCR 0.58). Preoperatively, 21 cases had lunate fragmentation, and 9 of 21 cases had bony union postoperatively. Most patients were clinically improved, but radiological improvement was not marked. A long-term follow-up study showed that degenerative change around the scaphoid might occur after a closing wedge osteotomy [10]. Regarding radial osteotomy procedures, Schuind et al. stated that these offer "durable pain relief and may improve grip strength," but do not offer a cure. At best, they can "slow down" the development of the disease [24].

## References


1. Blanco RH, Blanco FR. Osteotomy of the radius without shortening for Kienböck disease: a 10-year follow-up. J Hand Surg Am. 2012;37:2221–5.
2. Luo J, Diao E. Kienböck's disease: an approach to treatment. Hand Clin. 2006;22:465–73.
3. Miura H, Sugioka Y. Radial closing wedge osteotomy for Kienböck's disease. J Hand Surg Am. 1996;21:1029–34.
4. Horii E, Garcia-Elias M, Bishop AT, Cooney WP, Linscheid RL, Chao EY. Effect on force transmission across the carpus in procedures used to treat Kienböck's disease. J Hand Surg Am. 1990;15:393–400.
5. Viola RW, Kiser PK, Bach AW, Hanel DP, Tencer AF. Biomechanical analysis of capitate shortening with capitate hamate fusion in the treatment of Kienböck's disease. J Hand Surg Am. 1998;23:395–401.
6. Watanabe K, Nakamura R, Horii E, Miura T. Biomechanical analysis of radial wedge osteotomy for the treatment of Kienböck's disease. J Hand Surg Am. 1993;18:686–90.
7. Kam B, Topper SM, McLoughlin S, Liu Q. Wedge osteotomies of the radius for Kienböck's disease: a biomechanical analysis. J Hand Surg Am. 2002;27:37–42.
8. Nakamura R, Tsuge S, Watanabe K, Tsunoda K. Radial wedge osteotomy for Kienböck disease. J Bone Joint Surg Am. 1991;73:1391–6.
9. Hayashi O, Sawaizumi T, Ito H. Closing radial wedge osteotomy for Preiser's combined with Kienböck's disease: two case reports. Hand Surg. 2009;14:57–62.
10. Koh S, Nakamura R, Horii E, Nakao E, Inagaki H, Yajima H. Surgical outcome of radial osteotomy for Kienböck's disease-minimum 10 years of follow-up. J Hand Surg Am. 2003;28:910–6.
11. Tatebe M, Horii E, Majima M, Koh S, Nakamura R, Hirata H. Radial osteotomy for Kienböck's disease with displaced fracture of the lunate. J Hand Surg Am. 2007;32:1343–7.
12. Lamas C, Mir X, Llusà M, Navarro A. Dorsolateral biplane closing radial osteotomy in zero variant cases of Kienböck's disease. J Hand Surg Am. 2000;25:700–9.
13. Soejima O, Iida H, Komine S, Kikuta T, Naito M. Lateral closing wedge osteotomy of the distal radius for advanced stages of Kienböck's disease. J Hand Surg Am. 2002;27:31–6.
14. Illarramendi AA, Schulz C, De Carli P. The surgical treatment of Kienböck's disease by radius and ulna metaphyseal core decompression. J Hand Surg Am. 2001;26:252–60.
15. Nakamura R, Watanabe K, Tsunoda K, Miura T. Radial osteotomy for Kienböck's disease evaluated by magnetic resonance imaging. 24 cases followed for 1-3 years. Acta Orthop Scand. 1993;64:207–11.
16. Gay A, Parratte S, Glard Y, Mutaftschiev N, Legre R. Isolated capitate shortening osteotomy for early stage of Kienböck's disease with neutral ulnar variance. Plast Reconstr Surg. 2009;124:560–6.
17. Lutsky K, Beredjiklian PK. Kienböck disease. J Hand Surg Am. 2012;37:1942–52.
18. Viegas SF, Wagner K, Patterson R, Peterson P. Medial (hamate) facet of the lunate. J Hand Surg Am. 1990;15:564–71.
19. Tatebe M, Imaeda T, Hirata H. The impact of lunate morphology on Kienbock's disease. J Hand Surg Eur Vol. 2015;40:534.
20. Allan CH, Joshi A, Lichtman DM. Kienböck's disease: diagnosis and treatment. J Am Acad Orthop Surg. 2001;9:128–36.
21. Bain GI, Begg M. Arthroscopic assessment and classification of Kienbock's disease. Tech Hand Up Extrem Surg. 2006;10:8–13.
22. Tatebe M, Hirata H, Shinohara T, Yamamoto M, Okui N, Kurimoto S, Imaeda T. Arthroscopic findings of Kienböck's disease. J Orthop Sci. 2011;16:745–8.
23. Tsumura H, Himeno S, Morita H, Sasaki Y, Ueda Y, Morihisa K, et al. The optimum correcting angle of wedge osteotomy at the distal end of the radius for Kienböck's disease. J Jpn Soc Surg Hand. 1984;1:435–9.
24. Schuind F, Eslami S, Ledoux P. Kienböck's disease. J Bone Joint Surg Br. 2008;90:133–9.

# 18 Vascularized Pedicle Flaps for Kienböck's Disease

William R. Aibinder and Alexander Y. Shin

## Introduction

Conventional nonvascularized cancellous or corticocancellous bone grafts, whether allograft or autograft, heal by creeping substitution whereby remodeling with trabecular resorption precedes revascularization and new bone formation [1]. This process relies on vascular ingrowth from the periphery, which allows for osteogenic cells to invade the graft site. Resorption significantly weakens the bone during this slow process leading to an increased rate of fatigue fractures over time [2].

Vascularized bone grafting provides several distinct advantages over conventional bone grafting. Firstly, osteocytes are preserved with an intact blood supply, decreasing the risk of graft resorption as viable osteoclasts and osteoblasts are delivered to regions of dead bone [3, 4]. Thus, bone heals without creeping substitution. This leads to a decreased risk of fatigue fracture with consistent graft incorporation and union [5, 6]. With less remodeling, bone mass and strength are preserved with less osteopenia seen [7]. Davis et al. demonstrated increased strength, toughness, and modulus of elasticity compared to conventional bone grafts when stressed in torsion [8]. Furthermore, blood flow to the vascularized bone graft (VBG) is maintained and increases over time as demonstrated in an experimental canine model [9, 10]. The blood flow in the pedicled graft immediately after elevation was 8.42 mL/min/100 g compared to 16.53 mL/min/100 g on the contralateral side. Two weeks later a hyperemic response was noted with a flow rate of 33.72 mL/min/100 g, while the contralateral limb's flow rate remained unchanged. This was significantly higher than the flow rate observed with a conventional graft, which was 0.62 mL/min/100 g.

Based on these findings, pedicled VBGs have been used for over a century in the treatment of avascular necrosis and bone defects throughout the body [11–13]. Pedicled VBGs are used increasingly for various carpal pathologies, including Kienböck's disease [14–18].

Three principles confer the effectiveness of a pedicled VBG. The pedicle must be long enough to reach the recipient site without tension, the nutrient vessels must supply cortical and cancellous bone, and the vessels must have sufficient blood flow to maintain bone viability [14].

In 1971, Beck described the first use of a VBG in the treatment of Kienböck's disease with the transfer of a vascularized decorticated pisiform, which was later modified by Saffar [19, 20]. In 1979, Hori et al. published on the transplantation a dorsal metacarpal arteriovenous pedicle into the necrotic lunate bone [21]. Palmar-based distal radius grafts offer additional options [22]. In

W.R. Aibinder, MD • A.Y. Shin, MD (✉)
Department of Orthopedic Surgery, Mayo Clinic, 200 First Street SW, Rochester, MN 55905, USA
e-mail: shin.alexander@mayo.edu

© Springer International Publishing Switzerland 2016

D.M. Lichtman, G.I. Bain (eds.), *Kienböck's Disease*, DOI 10.1007/978-3-319-34226-9_18

1995, Sheetz et al. described the blood supply of the dorsal distal radius, which gave rise to the use of reverse-flow VBGs for the treatment of multiple carpal pathologies [14, 23–25]. Specifically, the 4 + 5 ECA was described for the treatment of Kienböck's disease. A modification with the ECA vessels included within a capsular flap has been reported [26]. In 2001, Bengoechea-Beeby et al. reported on the use of an index finger metacarpal VBG [27].

The purpose of this chapter is to review the anatomy, surgical technique, and outcomes of pedicled VBGs for Kienböck's disease, in particular the 4 + 5 ECA.

## Anatomy

The dorsal distal radius is a common source of VBGs for the treatment of Kienböck's disease. Sheetz et al. described the extraosseous and intraosseous blood supply of the distal radius which serves as the basis for several donor grafts [23]. By evaluating 35 fresh cadaveric limbs the authors showed that the dorsal vessels have a constant pattern with a consistent relationship to anatomic landmarks. The four arteries that supply the distal radius and ulna are the radial, ulnar, anterior interossesous, and posterior interosseous arteries. Four vessels reliably branch from these arteries and are important in the design of pedicled VBGs. Two vessels are superficial to the extensor retinaculum and reside between the extensor compartments. They are thus aptly named the 1,2 and 2,3 intercompartmental supraretinacular arteries (1,2 and 2,3 ICSRA). Two vessels are deep and reside on the floor of the fourth and fifth compartments, and are thus appropriately named the fourth and fifth extensor compartmental arteries (ECA) (Fig. 18.1).

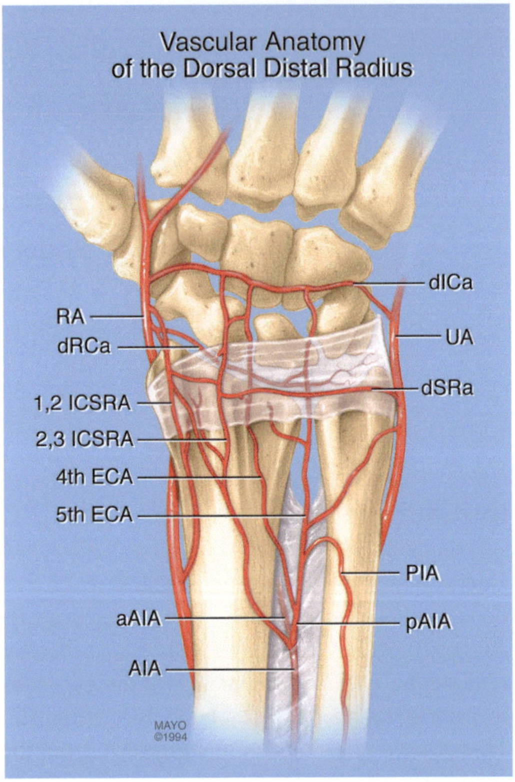


**Fig. 18.1** Vascular anatomy of the dorsal distal radius. 1,2 ICSRA (1,2 intercompartmental supraretinacular artery), 2,3 ICSRA (2,3 intercompartmental supraretinacular artery, fourth ECA (fourth extracompartmental artery), fifth ECA (fourth extracompartmental artery), aAIA (anterior branch of anterior interosseous artery), AIA (anterior interosseous artery), pAIA (posterior branch of the anterior interosseous artery), PIA (posterior interosseous artery), dSRa (dorsal supraretinacular arch), UA (ulnar artery), dICa (dorsal intercarpal arch), RA (radial artery), dRCa (dorsal radiocarpal arch). Used with permission from the Mayo Foundation for Medical Education and Research. All rights reserved

Sheetz et al. noted the characteristics of the nutrient vessels related to each graft [23] (Table 18.1).

The 1,2 ICSRA originates from the radial artery an average of 48 mm proximal to the radiocarpal joint. In 2001, Zaidemberg et al. described the anatomic basis for a pedicled VBG based on this vessel for the treatment of scaphoid nonunions [24]. The authors termed it a "periosteal vessel," but it actually lays over the retinaculum. After branching, the vessel travels deep to the brachioradialis muscle and then courses superficial to the 1,2 intercompartmental septum of the extensor retinaculum before entering the anatomic snuffbox to anastomose with either the radial artery, the radiocarpal arch, and/or the intercarpal arch [23]. Some authors have reported using the 1,2 ICSRA to treat Kienböck's disease, however, because of the superficial location, short arc of rotation of the pedicle, and a small

**Table 18.1** Nutrient artery characteristics[a]

| Artery supplying nutrient arteries | Number of nutrient arteries (mean [range]) | Nutrient artery internal diameter (mm) (mean [range]) | Distance from nutrient artery penetration to RC joint (mm) (mean [range]) | Percentage of nutrient arteries that penetrate cancellous bone (%) |
|---|---|---|---|---|
| 1,2 ICSRA | 3.2 [0–9] | <0.10 [<0.05–0.15] | 15 [4–26] | 6 |
| Second EC br of 1,2 ICSRA | 1 [1] | 0.16 [0.14–0.19] | 21 [17–28] | 57 |
| 2,3 ISCRA | 1.8 [0–5] | 0.11 [0.07–0.19] | 13 [3–24] | 22 |
| Second EC br of 2,3 ICSRA | 1.4 [1–4] | 0.19 [0.09–0.28] | 18 [14–32] | 48 |
| Fourth ECA | 3.2 [1–6] | 0.16 [0.07–0.29] | 11 [3–19] | 45 |
| Fourth EC br of fifth ECA | 1.2 [1–2] | 0.15 [0.15] | 10 [6–12] | 43 |

*ICSRA* intercompartmental supraretinacular artery, *EC* extensor compartment, *ECA* extensor compartmental artery, *br* branch

[a]Reprinted with permission from The Journal of Hand Surgery, 20A, Sheetz KK, Bishop AT, Berger RA, The arterial blood supply of the distal radius and its potential use in vascularized pedicle bone grafts, 902–914, Copyright 1995, with permission from Elsevier

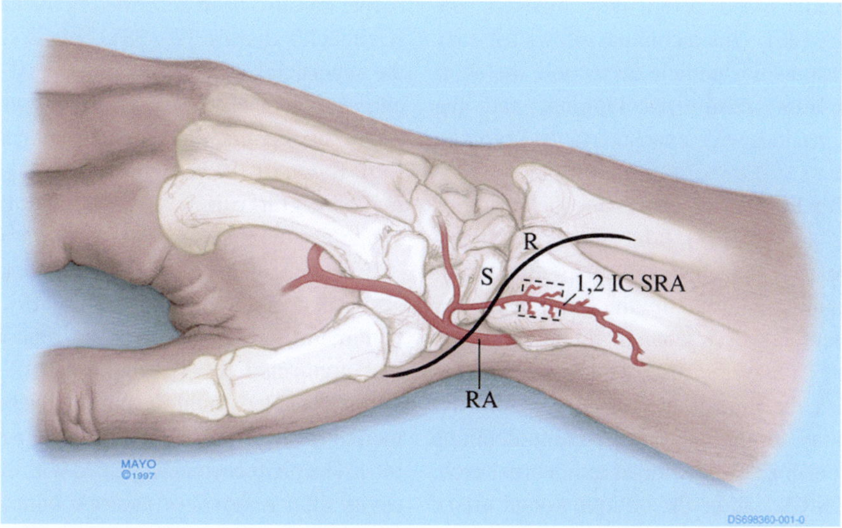


**Fig. 18.2** Anatomic representation of the 1,2 ICSRA (1,2 intercompartmental supraretinacular artery) VBG. S (scaphoid), R (radius), RA (radial artery). Used with permission from the Mayo Foundation for Medical Education and Research. All rights reserved

mean internal diameter of 0.3 mm, it is not favorable [28] (Fig. 18.2).

The 2,3 ICSRA originates from the anterior interosseous artery (AIA) proper 48 % of the time, the posterior division of the AIA 48 % of the time, or from the anterior division of the AIA the remaining 4 % of the time [23]. As its name indicates, the vessel courses superficial to the extensor retinaculum over Lister's tubercle to anastomose with the dorsal intercarpal arch, the dorsal radiocarpal arch, and/or the fourth ECA. It may also have transverse anastomoses with the 1,2 ICSRA. Compared to the 1,2 ICSRA, a greater percentage of the 2,3 ICSRA nutrient vessels penetrate into cancellous bone (see Table 18.1). Additionally, it has a larger mean internal diameter at 0.35 mm, and a larger arc of rotation making a pedicled VBG based on the 2,3

ICSRA more suitable for the treatment of Kienböck's disease [29]. Imai et al. presented a case report on the successful use of the 2,3 ICSRA-based VBG for the treatment of avascular necrosis of the capitate [30].

The fourth ECA originates most commonly from the posterior division of the AIA, but can also be supplied by the fifth ECA 45 % of the time [23]. It lies adjacent to the posterior interosseous nerve on the radial aspect of the fourth extensor compartment. This relationship was observed 70 % of the time, with the artery found in the 3,4 septum in the remainder of specimens. It anastomoses with the dorsal intercarpal arch, the dorsal radiocarpal arch, the 2,3 ICSRA, and/or the fifth ECA. This branch gives rise to an average of 3.2 nutrient vessels that penetrate into cancellous bone. Sotereanos et al. described a large capsular-based VBG that includes the fourth ECA [26]. This technique allows for easy graft harvest, avoids pedicle dissection, the short arc of rotation minimizes kinking, and the approach provides wide exposure to the scaphoid and lunate.

The fifth ECA originates from the posterior division of the AIA [23]. It has the largest diameter of the four dorsal vessels. It is most commonly found radially in the fifth extensor compartment, however, it can be found within the 4,5 septum 33 % of the time. This vessel anastomoses with the dorsal intercarpal arch consistently. It may additionally have communications with the fourth ECA, the dorsal radiocarpal arch, the 2,3 ICSRA, and/or the oblique dorsal artery of the distal ulna. Unlike the other dorsal vessels, the fifth ECA does not commonly provide any nutrient vessels to the distal radius.

As mentioned, multiple arterial arches in the dorsum of the hand connect intercompartmental and compartmental vessels allowing for retrograde flow VBGs, such as the 4+5 ECA, to be harvested.

Sheetz et al. also described the blood supply to the palmar distal radius [23]. The radial and ulna arteries are connected by the palmar metaphyseal and the palmar carpal arches. The palmar metaphyseal arch has a very short arc of rotation and is located within the pronator quadratus muscle belly with a variable location, diameter, and nutrient vasculature [23]. The radial portion of the palmar carpal arch has been utilized as part of a muscle-pedicle-bone graft using the distal radial bone and pronator quadratus musculature [22, 31]. Its use is limited by the variable vascular anatomy, short arc of rotation, and risk of disrupting the palmar radiocarpal ligaments during dissection with resultant instability [32]. Multiple modifications have been proposed, however, this graft is infrequently supported at present for the treatment of Kienböck's disease [33–36]. Haerle et al. performed an anatomic study of the palmar distal radius vascularity and endorsed a longer pedicle utilizing a retrograde graft based on the anterior branch of the AIA and the palmar carpal arch [37].

A pedicled VBG based on the second metacarpal has also been described in the treatment of Kienböck's disease [27, 38]. This is supplied by the superficial artery of the first dorsal intermetacarpal artery, which anastomoses with the deep artery of the first dorsal intermetacarpal space [39]. Based on the vascularity, a distal and proximal bone graft can be harvested with the superficial artery feeding the graft by retrograde flow.

First described in 1971, the pisiform bone has also been utilized as a VBG [19]. In 1982 Kuhlmann et al. performed an anatomic study that confirmed the dorsal branch of the ulnar artery provided multiple nutrient vessels to the medial pisiform from a large diameter vessel [40]. The pisiform can be placed within the lunate cavity after removal of necrotic bone to address the pathology in Kienböck's disease [41]. Heymans and Koebke also determined that a 90° palmar rotation of the pisiform within the lunate cavity places the longitudinal diameter in the dorsopalmar direction to maintain the carpal height [42]. The ulnar nerve is at risk during harvesting of the graft [43].

## Decision-Making

The treatment algorithm for Kienböck's disease is based on stage, ulnar variance, and status of the cartilage of the lunate, as well as, at the radiocarpal and midcarpal joints. Lunate revascularization is an appropriate option in patients with stage II and IIIA disease with intact lunate cartilage shells. Limited data has been promising for this treatment in stage IIIB disease [28, 29, 44, 45]. An intact cartilaginous shell is more predictive of successful revascularization as opposed to the presence of carpal collapse [46]. Bain and Begg described a classification based on the arthroscopic appearance and functionality of four articular surfaces: the lunate facet of the distal radius, the proximal and distal lunate articular surfaces, and the capitate [47]. A normal surface is defined as one that has a glistening appearance or only minor fibrillations. In cases of ulna neutral and positive variance where joint-leveling procedures are contraindicated because of the risk of ulnar impaction syndrome, vascularized bone grafting is a particularly attractive option. Similarly, in patients with ulna negative variance, revascularization is indicated in conjunction with additional procedures such as a radial shortening osteotomy. Lunate expansion with resultant restoration of the carpal height ratio is usually useful in instances of lunate volume loss. VBGs are favored after failure of alternative procedures. Revascularization in addition to mechanical unloading with intercarpal arthrodesis can also be considered.

Absolute contraindications to revascularization in Kienböck's disease include a displaced coronal fracture through the lunate, fragmentation of the cartilaginous shell, and adjacent intercarpal degenerative changes (stage IV disease). Previous surgery requiring exposure of the extensor retinaculum is a relative contraindication for dorsally based distal radius VBGs due to potential compromise of the vascularity. When the cartilage shell is disrupted or advanced degenerative disease is evident, salvage procedures such as limited wrist fusion (scaphocapitate fusion) or proximal row carpectomy should be considered.

High-risk patients, such as those with a current or recent smoking history, chronic steroid use, and those with peripheral vascular disease should be counseled appropriately.

There is no clear evidence in favor of one pedicled VBG to another. Consequently, the decision to use one graft over another is largely based on surgeon experience and preference. Our preferred graft is the 4+5 ECA because of the pedicle's long length, large diameter, and relative ulnar location. The latter allows for access to the lunate with minimal risk to the pedicle itself.

## Outcomes

There is limited data comparing vascularized bone grafting to unloading or salvage procedures [15]. Similarly, no studies have directly compared one type of vascularized graft to another. The paucity of such data makes evidence-based decision-making difficult, if not impossible.

Hori et al. reported on their use of a dorsal metacarpal arteriovenous pedicle in the treatment of Kienböck's disease [21]. They noted symptomatic improvement and revascularization in eight of nine patients with resolution of sclerosis. Tamai et al. found a loss of carpal height in 31 % of patients treated with an arteriovenous pedicle; however, 50 of 51 patients showed improvement in pain and grip strength [48]. Moneim and Duncan reported on 11 patients with stage II and IIIA disease treated with a second dorsal metacarpal arteriovenous pedicle and cancellous bone grafting [49]. Nine patients had successful results with significant pain relief, improved function, and no additional surgery. Two patients went on to require a proximal row carpectomy, while only one patient showed any signs of radiographic progression. Jones et al. reported on a patient with stage IIIA disease who underwent first dorsal metacarpal arteriovenous pedicle grafting with the use of a bone morphogenetic protein adjunct [50]. At final follow-up the patient was pain free with signs of revascularization on magnetic resonance imaging (MRI) and no signs of radiographic progression.

Several authors have described the use of a second metacarpal VBG for the treatment of carpal pathology [27, 38, 45, 51]. Bengoechea-Beeby et al. presented a case report of stage IIIA disease treated with an index metacarpal VBG based on the superficial artery of the first dorsal intermetacarpal space and retrograde flow from the deep artery of the first intermetacarpal space

[27]. At 3 years postoperatively, the patient was pain free with radiographic and MRI evidence of revascularization.

Several authors have reported on a metacarpal VBG in conjunction with additional procedures [45, 52]. Zafra et al. reported on five patients with stage IIIA (two patients) and IIIB (three patients) disease who underwent a second metacarpal VBG and a radius closing wedge osteotomy [45]. Four of five patients had no pain at final follow-up, and one patient showed radiographic evidence of further lunate collapse. Waitayawinyu et al. reported on 14 patients with stage II (six patients) and IIIA (eight patients) disease and ulna neutral or ulna positive variance who were treated with a capitate shortening osteotomy and third metacarpal VBG [52]. With a mean follow-up of 41 months, the authors demonstrated a significant improvement in grip strength, satisfaction, and arc of motion. Carpal height was maintained and there was no radiographic progression of disease. Patients with stage II disease had significantly better grip strength and satisfaction scores compared to those with stage IIIA disease. Fujiwara et al. reported on 18 patients with stage IIIA and IIIB disease who underwent VBG alone or VBG with a joint-leveling procedure [28]. Revascularization alone was reserved for patients with isolated stage IIIA disease. Eleven patients underwent a metacarpal VBG—nine based on the third, and two on the second; seven patients either underwent a 1,2 ICSRA or 2,3 ICSRA graft. The authors reported an improvement in the Mayo Modified Wrist Score in all patients. Two patients with stage IIIA disease progressed to stage IIIB disease, but none advanced to stage IV disease. Grip strength improved significantly. There was no significant change in carpal height or Stahl index in those with stage IIIA disease, however, those with stage IIIB disease who also underwent a joint-leveling procedure showed a significant improvement in those parameters.

Braun described the use of a palmar radius VBG on a pronator quadratus pedicle for the treatment of carpal pathology [22]. Such a graft has been used for the treatment of scaphoid nonunions and Kienböck's disease by several authors [33, 35, 36]. The pronator pedicle has a constant branch of the AIA which confers its utility [53]. Gong et al. reported on 41 patients with stage IIIB (13 patients) or stage IV (28 patients) disease at a mean follow-up of 3 years who underwent lunate excision with placement of a radial bone flap with a vascularized wrapping of the pronator quadratus [54]. All patients showed improvement in symptoms with 20 patients being pain-free. There was no significant change in carpal height. In 2009, Mathoulin and Wahegaonkar reported on 22 patients with stage II, IIIA, and IIIB disease at an average follow-up of 74 months who were treated with the modified volar distal radius VBG previously described by Haerle et al. and a joint leveling procedure, if indicated [55]. At final follow-up, 18 patients were pain free with improvement in range of motion and grip strength. MRI evidence of revascularization was noted in 17 patients (77 %). Two patients underwent reoperation.

Beck was the first to describe the vascularized pisiform graft [19]. Kuhlmann et al. described a modification to the technique whereby the graft was based on the dorsal branch of the ulnar artery [41]. Daecke et al. reported on the long-term outcomes of patients who underwent a vascularized pisiform graft for early stage and late stage disease [43, 56]. Early stage disease was treated by a pedicled pisiform VBG, while late disease was treated with excision of the lunate and interposition of the pisiform [20]. Twenty-three patients with early stage disease (II and IIIA) were followed for an average of 12 years. Fourteen had arrest of disease progression. Twenty patients were noted to have improvement in pain. Range of motion and grip strength also improved. In those with late stage disease, pain improved in 16 of 21 patients. There was no improvement in range of motion or grip strength. Eight patients showed progression of their disease stage and nearly half had signs of arthritic changes. Kuhlmann et al. showed similar results for early stage disease [41]. Von Maydell and Bruser reported on seven patients with stage IIIB disease who were treated with the Saffar procedure [57]. All had significant pain improvement with four patients reporting no pain. Grip strength and active range of motion were 77 % and 72 % of the contralateral limb, respectively. Five patients had progression of disease with advanced intercarpal arthritis. Despite radiographic progression, the use of a pisiform VBG results in a high rate of patient satisfaction and pain relief.

Moran et al. reported on 26 patients treated with the 4+5 ECA for stage II (12 patients), stage IIIA (ten patients), and stage IIIB (four patients) disease [44]. The lunate was unloaded temporarily in 20 patients with midcarpal pinning in 12 and external fixation in 8. Twenty-four patients (92 %) had significant improvement at 3 months postoperatively. There was no disease progression in 20 patients (77 %). Grip strength improved from 50 to 89 % of the contralateral limb. There was MRI evidence of revascularization at a mean follow-up of 20 months in 12 out of 17 patients (71 %). Two patients had complications related to pin tract infections. Two others had failures of their reconstruction and went on to total wrist arthrodesis.

Kirkeby et al. described a small series of five patients with stage II (four patients) and IIIA disease who underwent a 4+5 ECA VBG with a mean follow-up of 7.4 years [58]. None had any radiographic evidence of disease progression and four patients were fully employed.

Afshar and Eivaziatashbeik compared nine patients who underwent a radial shortening osteotomy to seven patients who underwent a 4+5 ECA for stage II and IIIA disease with a minimum follow-up of 5 years [59]. The authors noted no significant difference in pain relief, motion, grip strength, or radiographic assessment. However, the Cooney wrist function scores were significantly better in the VBG group.

As outlined previously, there are no prospective studies comparing different types of VBGs (Table 18.2).

## Preferred Technique

Our preferred technique in the treatment of stage II, IIIA, and IIIB Kienböck's disease is a VBG based on the fourth and fifth extracompartmental arteries in lunates that have an intact cartilage shell.

## Preoperative Planning

Preoperative planning begins with a radiographic assessment. Computed tomography (CT) allows the surgeon to assess the extent of necrosis and understand the lunate geometry. It is an imperative study for this reason. It aids in disease staging, as well as conceptualizing a plan to inset the graft. In our opinion, MRI provides little additional benefit other than the initial use to diagnose marrow signal changes in the lunate.

As described above, an intact cartilaginous shell is essential for the effectiveness of any vascularized graft. Arthroscopy is an effective tool to determine the status of the cartilage. When performing arthroscopy, the 4–5 or midcarpal ulnar portal is avoided to prevent potential injury to the fourth or fifth ECA pedicle. The radiocarpal joint is assessed by either the 3–4, 6U, or 6R portal, while the midcarpal joint is assessed by the midcarpal radial portal. The Bain classification can be used to assess the integrity of the cartilage [47]. If there is no fracture of the lunate cartilage, and minimal to no chondral injury of the adjacent surfaces, a revascularization procedure is performed. If there is evidence of cartilage wear or arthrosis, salvage procedures such as proximal row carpectomy or intercarpal arthrodesis are indicated. A discussion should be undertaken preoperatively with the patient regarding the possibility of a salvage procedure based on the observed findings.

Lastly, consideration should be given to the need for concomitant unloading of the lunate either with a temporary scaphocapitate pinning or scaphocapitate arthrodesis. For severely collapsed lunates, our preference has recently been for scaphocapitate arthrodesis secondary to the long time necessary for revascularization. Temporary scaphocapitate pinning is ideal in stage II Kienböck's disease or in lunates that do not need significant expansion in the distal-proximal direction.

**Table 18.2** Study designs of included studies

| Study | Year | Stage (Patients [*n*]) | Procedure | Mean follow-up (Months [Range]) | Outcomes |
|---|---|---|---|---|---|
| Hori et al. [21] | 1979 | Unknown (9) | Dorsal metacarpal AV pedicle graft | Unknown (4–36) | ROM, radiographic analysis |
| Tamai et al. [48] | 1993 | I (1); II (5); III (39); IV (6) | Dorsal metacarpal AV pedicle graft +/− ICBG +/− temporary unloading or STT fusion | 71 (12–181) | Pain, ROM, grip strength, radiographic analysis |
| Moneim and Duncan [49] | 1998 | II (6); IIIA (5) | Dorsal metacarpal AV pedicle graft | 72 (15–180) | Pain, ROM, grip strength, radiographic analysis |
| Jones et al. [50] | 2008 | I (1) | Dorsal metacarpal AV pedicle graft + BMP | 8 (8) | Pain, ROM, grip strength, radiographic and MRI analysis |
| Bengoechea-Beeby et al. [27] | 2001 | IIIA (1) | Second metacarpal VBG | 36 (36) | Pain, ROM, radiographic and MRI analysis |
| Zafra et al. [45] | 2005 | IIIA (2); IIIB (3) | Second metacarpal VBG + radial shortening osteotomy | 21.2 (16–25) | Pain, ROM, grip strength, radiographic analysis |
| Waitayawinyu et al. [52] | 2008 | II (6); IIIA (8) | Third metacarpal VBG + capitate shortening osteotomy | 41 (26–65) | Pain, ROM, satisfaction scores, radiographic analysis |
| Fujiwara et al. [28] | 2013 | IIIA (10); IIIB (8) | Second metacarpal, third metacarpal, 1,2 ICSRA, or 2,3 ICSRA +/− radial or capitate shortening osteotomy | 147 (122–186) | Pain, Mayo Modified Wrist Score, ROM, grip strength, radiographic and MRI analysis |
| Gong et al. [54] | 2006 | IIIB (13); IV (28) | Arthroplasty (radial VBG with pronator quadratus muscle) | 6.1 (3–22) | Pain, ROM, radiographic analysis |
| Mathoulin and Wahegaonkar [55] | 2009 | II (8); IIIA (10); IIIB (4) | Pedicled pronator VBG +/− joint leveling procedure | 74 (60–124) | Pain, ROM, grip strength, radiographic and MRI analysis |
| Kuhlmann et al. [41] | 2003 | III (7) | Pisiform VBG | Unclear | ROM, grip strength, radiographic analysis |
| Daecke et al. [56] | 2005 | II (13); IIIA (6); IIIB (1) | Pisiform VBG +/− joint leveling procedure | 150 (61.2–266.4) | Pain, ROM, grip strength, DASH, Cooney wrist score, radiographic analysis |
| Daecke et al. [43] | 2005 | II (1); IIIA (4); IIIB (10); IV (2) | Lunate resection + Vascularized pisiform os interposition +/− joint leveling procedure | 118.8 (66–178.8) | Pain, ROM, grip strength, DASH, Cooney wrist score, radiographic analysis |

(continued)

**Table 18.2** (continued)

| Study | Year | Stage (Patients [*n*]) | Procedure | Mean follow-up (Months [Range]) | Outcomes |
|---|---|---|---|---|---|
| von Maydell and Bruser [57] | 2008 | IIIB (7) | Lunate resection + Vascularized pisiform os interposition | 229.2 (144–276) | Pain, ROM, grip strength, DASH, radiographic analysis |
| Moran et al. [44] | 2005 | II (12); IIIA (10); IIIB (4) | 4+5 ECA VBG +/– temporary unloading | 31 (12–74) | Pain, Mayo Modified Wrist Score, ROM, grip strength, radiographic and MRI analysis |
| Kirkeby et al. [58] | 2014 | II (4); IIIA (1) | 4+5 ECA VBG | 88.8 (60–108) | DASH, ROM, grip strength, radiographic and MRI analysis |
| Afshar and Eivaziatashbeik [59] | 2013 | II (5); IIIA (11) | 4+5 ECA VBG versus radial shortening osteotomy | 78 (60–121) | Pain, ROM, grip strength, Cooney wrist score, Nakamura score, radiographic analysis |

*AV* arteriovenous, *VBG* vascularized bone graft, *BMP* bone morphogenetic protein, *ROM* range of motion, *MRI* magnetic resonance imaging, *ECA* extracompartmental artery

## Procedure

Once a determination is made to proceed with surgery, the patient is positioned supine with a hand table. The arm is exsanguinated and a standard dorsal midline incision is performed in line with the third metacarpal. Harvesting of the graft begins by identifying the fifth ECA in the fifth dorsal extensor compartment. The artery and venae commitantes are generally located in the floor of the compartment radially, often adjacent to or within the septum between the fourth and fifth extensor compartments. Occasionally, the vessels can course in and out of the compartment, making dissection challenging. A radially based extensor retinaculum flap is elevated from the fifth to the third compartment (Fig. 18.3a). The fifth ECA is traced proximally to its origin from the AIA and elevated. The fourth ECA is then identified, traced distally, and elevated (see Fig. 18.5a). A ligament sparing capsulotomy is performed along the radioscaphoid joint, the dorsal intercarpal ligament, and the dorsal radiocarpal ligament [60]. If the lunate was not initially inspected via arthroscopy, it should be inspected at this point (see Fig. 18.3c). If an intact cartilaginous shell is noted, with no fragmentation or adjacent degenerative changes, then the surgeon can proceed with vascularized bone grafting. Necrotic bone in the lunate is then removed under direct visualization and fluoroscopic imaging. This is done by the use of a high-speed burr and curettes through a dorsal burr hole (Fig. 18.4a, b). Care must be taken to preserve an intact cartilage shell and subchondral bone. If some collapse is noted, a small blunt-ended spreader should be used to expand the lunate to its normal dimensions (see Fig. 18.4a).

A bone graft centered 1.1 cm proximal to the radiocarpal joint and overlying the fourth ECA is marked to include the maximum number of nutrient vessels (see Fig. 18.3b). The excavated defect in the lunate is measured to determine the size of the graft necessary. The proximal-distal length corresponds to the depth of the defect and the radioulnar width corresponds to the anteroposterior

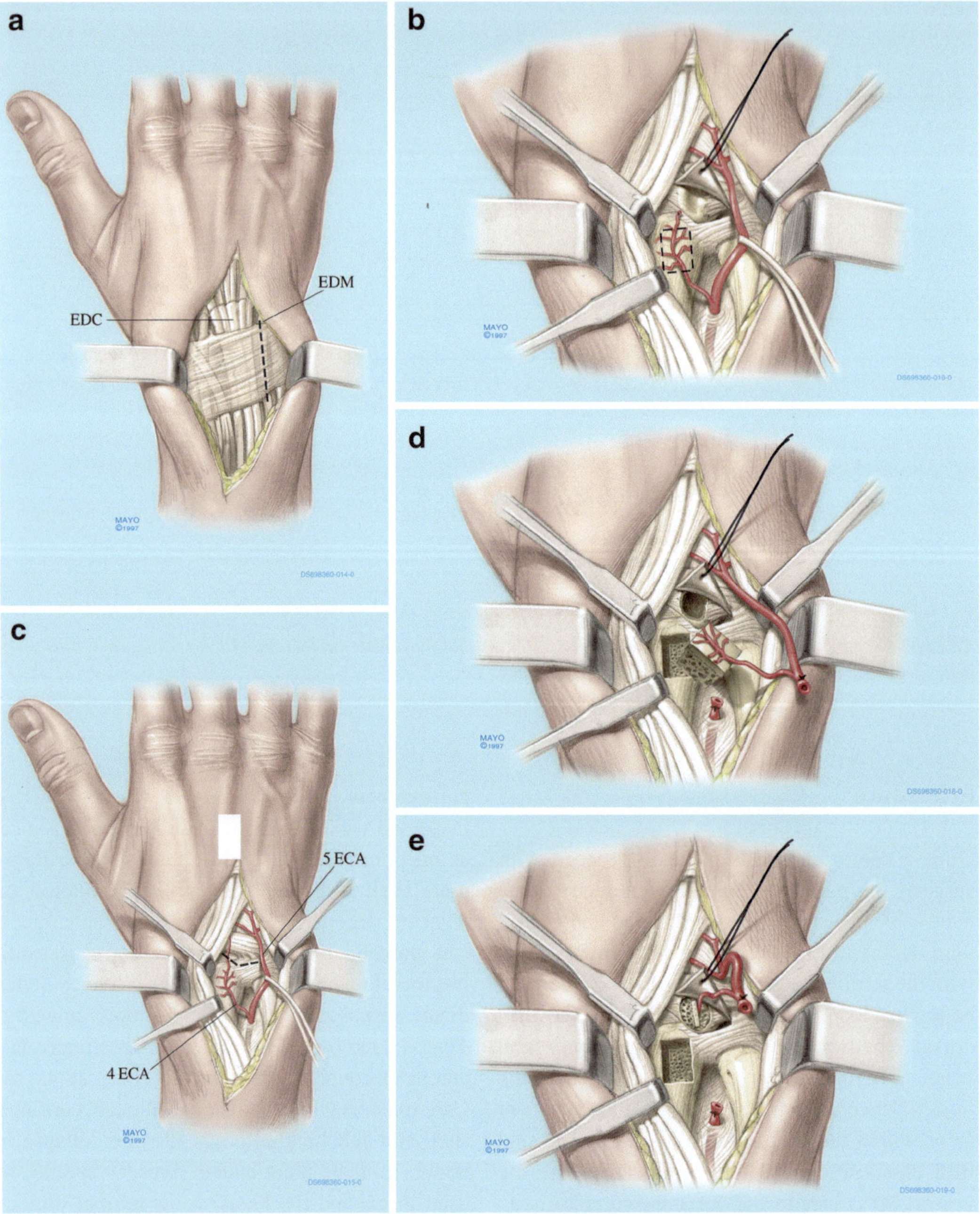


**Fig. 18.3** (**a**) Elevation of a dorsal retinacular flap over the fifth compartment. EDC (extensor digitorum communis), EDM (extensor digiti minimi). (**b**) Representation of the 4+5 ECA VBG. (**c**) Arthrotomy performed to expose lunate. ECA (extracompartmental artery). (**d**) Harvested 4+5 ECA VBG with ligation of vessel proximally to create a long pedicle with retrograde flow through the fifth ECA. (**e**) Insetting of the 4+5 VBG into the lunate cavity. Used with permission from the Mayo Foundation for Medical Education and Research. All rights reserved

dimension of the defect (see Fig. 18.3b). The graft is elevated with sharp osteotomes. The posterior division of the AIA is ligated proximal to the fourth and fifth ECA origins to ensure an adequate length of the pedicle to permit tension-free insetting (see Figs. 18.3d and 18.5b, c) The tourniquet may be deflated to assess graft vascularity, however, we often skip this step.

Cancellous bone graft is harvested from the dorsal distal radius and packed into the lunate

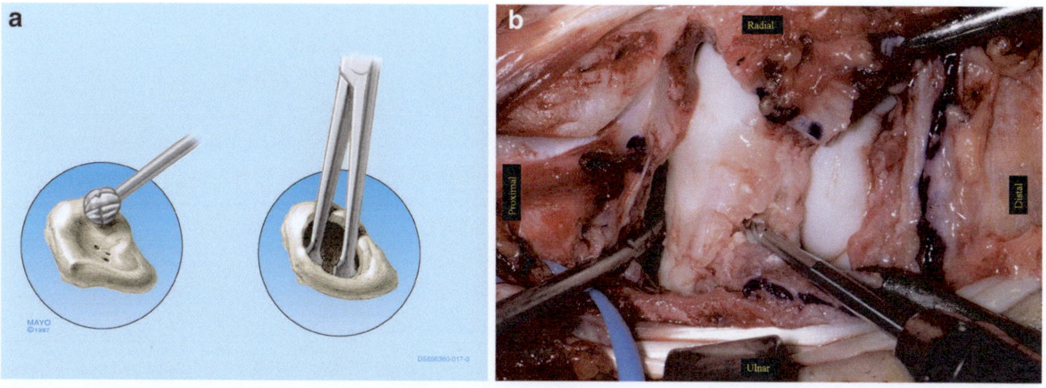


**Fig. 18.4** (**a**) High-speed burr and curette used to remove necrotic bone from the lunate. A blunt-ended spreader used to expand the lunate to its normal dimensions. Used with permission from the Mayo Foundation for Medical Education and Research. All rights reserved. (**b**) High-speed burr and curette used to remove necrotic bone from the lunate. A blunt-ended spreader used to expand the lunate to its normal dimensions

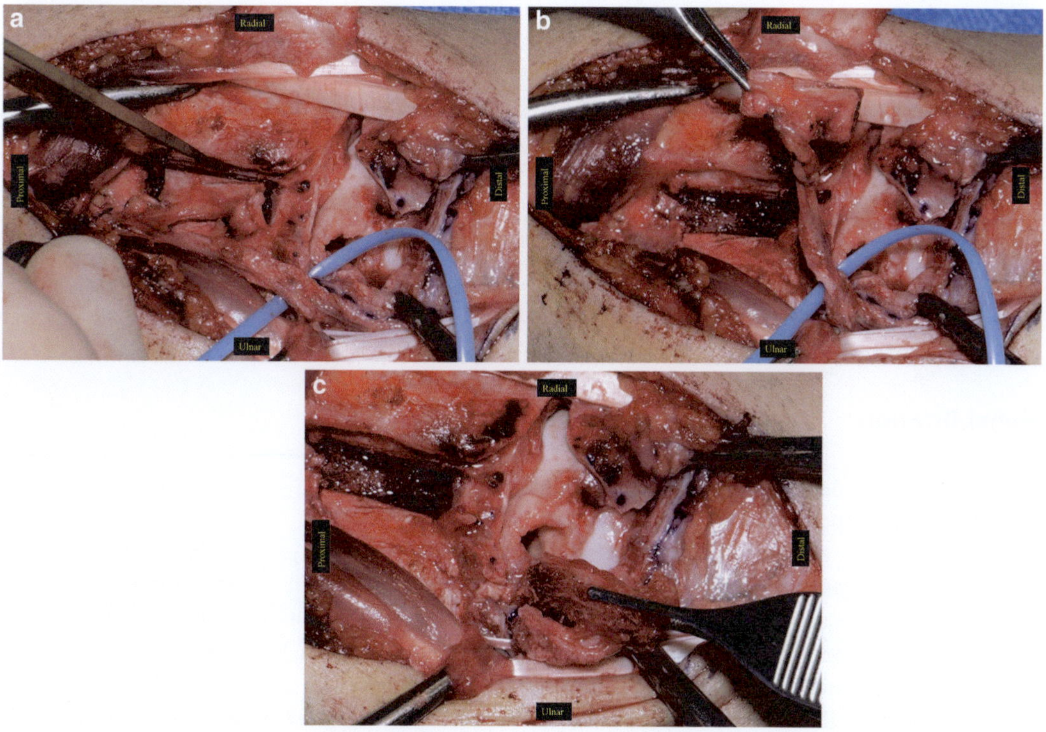


**Fig. 18.5** (**a**) Elevation of 4+5 ECA graft. Note long pedicle length. (**b**) Elevation of 4+5 ECA graft. Note long pedicle length. (**c**) Insetting of 4+5 ECA graft into lunate

defect leaving a path for the VBG. The VBG is then inset with the cortical surface oriented proximal to distal so that lunate height is maintained (see Fig. 18.3e). The graft should originally be made slightly larger than necessary to allow for trimming and an adequate fit. Internal fixation is has not been necessary in our series.

Unloading of the lunate is performed to help with revascularization and graft incorporation [14, 44, 61, 62]. This can be done with external fixation or midcarpal pinning. It is our preference to perform a scaphocapitate pinning with two 0.0625-in. Kirschner wires placed percutaneously while applying ten pounds of longitudinal

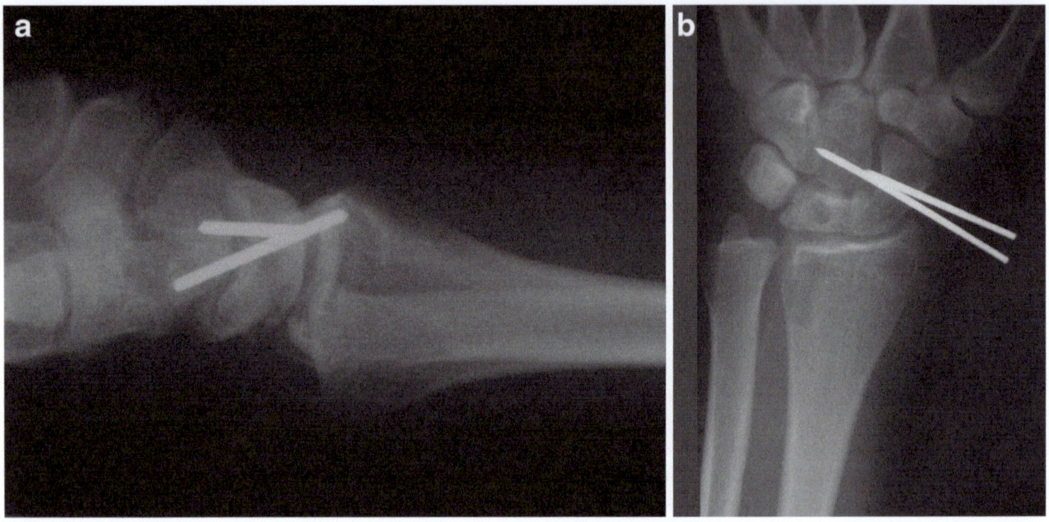

**Fig. 18.6** (**a**) Antero-posterior radiograph depicting temporary unloading of lunate via a scaphocapitate pinning with Kirschner wires. (**b**) Lateral radiographic depicting temporary unloading of lunate via a scaphocapitate pinning with Kirschner wires

traction for stage II Kienböck's disease (Fig. 18.6a, b). Permanent unloading with a scaphocapitate arthrodesis is performed for cases with higher degrees of collapse.

The wrist capsule and retinaculum are repaired and a long-arm postoperative splint is applied.

## Rehabilitation

The long-arm postoperative splint is removed at 10–14 days postoperatively and changed to a long-arm cast for an additional 4 weeks. At 6 weeks postoperatively, the cast is removed and gentle supervised wrist flexion and extension exercises are prescribed. The wrist is protected with a custom Orthoplast splint (Johnson and Johnson, New Brunswick, NY) for an additional 8 weeks. If utilized, the scaphocapitate Kirschner wires are removed at 12 weeks. At that point, strengthening exercises are initiated. The patient is weaned out of the splint symptomatically and followed for several years. Repeat radiographs are obtained at scheduled intervals to assess progression of disease, as well as revascularization.

## Complications

Complications related to this particular procedure include pin tract infections and injury to the fourth and/or fifth ECA if the 4–5 portal is used for arthroscopic assessment. Some patients may experience persistent pain, loss of motion, or loss of grip strength.

## Conclusion

Vascularized bone grafting has been proven to provide symptomatic relief, revascularization of the lunate, and arrest of radiographic progression in stage II and IIIA Kienböck's disease. Several authors support its use in stage IIIB disease, as well. An intact cartilaginous shell is the most important determinant of the effectiveness of this technique. Pedicled VBGs may be used as the sole treatment in ulna neutral and ulna positive variance, or as an adjunct to joint leveling procedures in those with an ulna negative variance. Stage IV disease is best treated with a salvage procedure. Although future studies are needed to elucidate the ideal VBG, we prefer the 4+5 ECA because of its long pedicle length, large pedicle diameter, and relative ulnar location. We also favor temporary or permanent unloading given the theoretical risk that early loads may hinder bone graft incorporation and revascularization. Regardless, these are technically demanding procedures and though attractive, technical error and pedicle injury are thought to contribute to failed revascularization attempts.

## References


1. Burchardt H. The biology of bone graft repair. Clin Orthop Relat Res. 1983;174:28–42.
2. Burchardt H. Biology of bone transplantation. Orthop Clin North Am. 1987;18(2):187–96.
3. Chacha PB. Vascularised pedicular bone grafts. Int Orthop. 1984;8(2):117–38. doi:10.1007/BF00265834.
4. Berggren A, Weiland AJ, Dorfman H. Free vascularized bone grafts: factors affecting their survival and ability to heal to recipient bone defects. Plast Reconstr Surg. 1982;69(1):19–29.
5. Weiland AJ, Moore JR, Daniel RK. Vascularized bone autografts. Experience with 41 cases. Clin Orthop Relat Res. 1983; (174):87–95.
6. Han CS, Wood MB, Bishop AT, Cooney WP. Vascularized bone transfer. J Bone Joint Surg Am. 1992;74(10):1441–9.
7. Cutting CB, McCarthy JG. Comparison of residual osseous mass between vascularized and nonvascularized onlay bone transfers. Plast Reconstr Surg. 1983;72(5):672–5.
8. Davis PK, Mazur JM, Coleman GN. A torsional strength comparison of vascularized and nonvascularized bone grafts. J Biomechanics. 1982;15(11):875–80.
9. Tu YK, Bishop AT, Kato T, Adams ML, Wood MB. Experimental carpal reverse-flow pedicle vascularized bone grafts. Part I: the anatomical basis of vascularized pedicle bone grafts based on the canine distal radius and ulna. J Hand Surg Am. 2000;25(1):34–45. doi:10.1053/jhsu.2000.jhsu025a0034.
10. Tu YK, Bishop AT, Kato T, Adams ML, Wood MB. Experimental carpal reverse-flow pedicle vascularized bone grafts. Part II: bone blood flow measurement by radioactive-labeled microspheres in a canine model. J Hand Surg Am. 2000;25(1):46–54. doi:10.1053/jhsu.2000.jhsu025a0046.
11. Davis JB. The muscle-pedicle bone graft in hip fusion. J Bone Joint Surg Am. 1954;36(4):790–9.
12. Farmer AW. The use of a composite pedicle graft for pseudoarthrosis of the tibia. J Bone Joint Surg Am. 1952;24(3):591–600.
13. Meyers MH, Harvey JP, Moore TM. Treatment of displaced subcapital and transcervical fractures of the femoral neck by muscle-pedicle-bone graft and internal fixation. A preliminary report on one hundred and fifty cases. J Bone Joint Surg Am. 1973;55(2):257–74.
14. Shin AY, Bishop AT. Pedicled vascularized bone grafts for disorders of the carpus: scaphoid nonunion and Kienböck's disease. J Am Acad Orthop Surg. 2002;10(3):210–6.
15. Payatakes A, Sotereanos DG. Pedicled vascularized bone grafts for scaphoid and lunate reconstruction. J Am Acad Orthop Surg. 2009;17(12):744–55.
16. Moran SL, Shin AY. Vascularized bone grafting for the treatment of carpal pathology. Orthop Clin North Am. 2007;38(1):73–85. doi:10.1016/j.ocl.2006.10.010.
17. Rizzo M, Moran SL. Vascularized bone grafts and their applications in the treatment of carpal pathology. Semin Plast Surg. 2008;22(3):213–27. doi:10.1055/s-2008-1081404.
18. Derby BM, Murray PM, Shin AY, Bueno RA, Mathoulin CL, Ade T, et al. Vascularized bone grafts for the treatment of carpal bone pathology. Hand. 2013;8(1):27–40. doi:10.1007/s11552-012-9479-0.
19. Beck E. Transfer of pisiform bone on vascular pedicle in the treatment of lunatomalacia. Handchirurgie. 1971;3(2):64–7.
20. Saffar P. Replacement of the semilunar bone by the pisiform. Description of a new technique for the treatment of Kienboeck's disease. Ann Chir Main. 1982;1(3):276–9.
21. Hori Y, Tamai S, Okuda H, Sakamoto H, Takita T. Blood vessel transplantation to bone. J Hand Surg Am. 1979;4(1):23–33. doi:10.1016/S0363-5023(79)80101-X.
22. Braun RM. Pronator pedicle bone grafting in the forearm and proximal carpal row. Orthop Trans. 1983;7(1):35.
23. Sheetz KK, Bishop AT, Berger RA. The arterial blood supply of the distal radius and ulna and its potential use in vascularized pedicled bone grafts. J Hand Surg Am. 1995;20(6):902–14. doi:10.1016/S0363-5023(05)80136-4.
24. Zaidemberg C, Siebert JW, Angrigiani C. A new vascularized bone graft for scaphoid nonunion. J Hand Surg Am. 1991;16(3):474–8.
25. Shin AY, Bishop AT. Vascularized bone grafts for scaphoid nonunion and Kienböck's disease. Orthop Clin North Am. 2001;32(2):263–77.
26. Sotereanos DG, Darlis NA, Dailiana ZH, Sarris IK, Malizos KN. A capsular-based vascularized distal radius graft for proximal pole scaphoid pseudarthrosis. J Hand Surg Am. 2006;31(4):580–7. doi:10.1016/j.jhsa.2006.01.005.
27. Bengoechea-Beeby MP, Cepeda-Uña J, Abascal-Zuloaga A. Vascularized bone graft from the index metacarpal for Kienböck's disease: a case report. J Hand Surg Am. 2001;26(3):437–43. doi:10.1053/jhsu.2001.24137.
28. Fujiwara H, Oda R, Morisaki S, Ikoma K, Kubo T. Long-term results of vascularized bone graft for stage III Kienböck disease. J Hand Surg Am. 2013;38(5):904–8. doi:10.1016/j.jhsa.2013.02.010.
29. Özalp T, Yercan HS, Okçu G. The treatment of Kienböck disease with vascularized bone graft from dorsal radius. Arch Orthop Trauma Surg. 2009;129(2):171–5. doi:10.1007/s00402-008-0586-x.

30. Imai S, Uenaka K, Matsusue Y. Idiopathic necrosis of the capitate treated by vascularized bone graft based on the 2, 3 intercompartmental supraretinacular artery. J Hand Surg Br. 2014;39(3):322–3. doi:10.1177/1753193412468396.
31. Fontaine C, Millot F, Blancke D, Mestdagh H. Anatomic basis of pronator quadratus flap. Surg Radiol Anat. 1992;14(4):295–9.
32. Shin AY, Bishop AT. Vascular anatomy of the distal radius: implications for vascularized bone grafts. Clin Orthop Relat Res. 2001;383(383):60–73.
33. Kawai H, Yamamoto K. Pronator quadratus pedicled bone graft for old scaphoid fractures. J Bone Joint Surg Br. 1988;70(5):829–31.
34. Kuhlmann JN, Mimoun M, Boabighi A, Baux S. Vascularized bone graft pedicled on the volar carpal artery for non-union of the scaphoid. J Hand Surg Br. 1987;12(2):203–10.
35. Leung PC, Hung LK. Use of pronator quadratus bone flap in bony reconstruction around the wrist. J Hand Surg Am. 1990;15(4):637–40.
36. Rath S, Hung LK, Leung PC. Vascular anatomy of the pronator quadratus muscle-bone flap: a justification for its use with a distally based blood supply. J Hand Surg Am. 1990;15(4):630–6.
37. Haerle M, Schaller HE, Mathoulin C. Vascular anatomy of the palmar surfaces of the distal radius and ulna: its relevance to pedicled bone grafts at the distal palmar forearm. J Hand Surg Br. 2003;28:131. doi:10.1016/S0266-7681(02)00279-6.
38. Makino M. Vascularized metacarpal bone graft for scaphoid non-union and Kienböck's disease. J Reconstr Microsurg. 2000;16(4):261–6. doi:10.1055/s-2000-7331. discussion 6-8.
39. Brunelli F, Brunelli G, Nanfito F. An anatomical study of the vascularisation of the first dorsal interosseous space in the hand, and a description of a bony pedicle graft arising from the second metacarpal bone. Surg Radiol Anat. 1991;13(1):73–5.
40. Kuhlmann JN, Guerin-Surville H, Chretien Y. Vascularization of the pyramidal and pisiform bones. Bull Assoc Anat. 1982;66(192):79–88.
41. Kuhlmann JN, Kron C, Boabighi A, Baux S, Mimou M. Vascularised pisiform bone graft. Indications, technique and long-term results. Acta Orthop Belg. 2003;69(4):311–6.
42. Heymans R, Adelmann E, Koebke J. Anatomical bases of the pediculated pisiform transplant and the intercarpal fusion by Graner in Kienböck's disease. Surg Radiol Anat. 1992;14:195. doi:10.1111/joa.12235.
43. Daecke W, Lorenz S, Wieloch P, Jung M, Martini A-K. Lunate resection and vascularized os pisiform transfer in Kienböck's disease: an average of 10 years of follow-up study after Saffar's procedure. J Hand Surg Am. 2005;30(4):677–84. doi:10.1016/j.jhsa.2005.02.015.
44. Moran SL, Cooney WP, Berger RA, Bishop AT, Shin AY. The use of the 4+5 extensor compartmental vascularized bone graft for the treatment of Kienböck's disease. J Hand Surg Am. 2005;30(1):50–8. doi:10.1016/j.jhsa.2004.10.002.
45. Zafra M, Carrasco-Becerra C, Carpintero P. Vascularised bone graft and osteotomy of the radius in Kienböck's disease. Acta Orthop Belg. 2005;71(2):163–8.
46. Elhassan BT, Shin AY. Vascularized bone grafting for treatment of Kienböck's disease. J Hand Surg Am. 2009;34(1):146–54. doi:10.1016/j.jhsa.2008.10.014.
47. Bain GI, Begg M. Arthroscopic assessment and classification of Kienbock's disease. Tech Hand Up Extrem Surg. 2006;10(1):8–13.
48. Tamai S, Yajima H, Ono H. Revascularization procedures in the treatment of Kienböck's disease. Hand Clin. 1993;9(3):455–66.
49. Moneim MS, Duncan GJ. Kienbock's disease: treatment by implantation of vascular pedicle and bone grafting. Iowa Orthop J. 1998;18:67–73.
50. Jones NF, Brown EE, Vogelin E, Urist MR. Bone morphogenetic protein as an adjuvant in the treatment of Kienbock's disease by vascular pedicle implantation. J Hand Surg Br. 2008;33(3):317–21. doi:10.1177/1753193408090394.
51. Mathoulin C, Brunelli F. Further experience with the index metacarpal vascularized bone graft. J Hand Surg Br. 1998;23(3):311–7.
52. Waitayawinyu T, Chin SH, Luria S, Trumble TE. Capitate shortening osteotomy with vascularized bone grafting for the treatment of Kienböck's disease in the ulnar positive wrist. J Hand Surg Am. 2008;33(8):1267–73. doi:10.1016/j.jhsa.2008.04.006.
53. Lee JC, Lim J, Chacha PB. The anatomical basis of the vascularized pronator quadratus pedicled bone graft. J Hand Surg Br. 1997;22(5):644–6.
54. Gong HS, Chung MS, Lee YH, Lee S. Arthroplasty for advanced Kienböck's disease using a radial bone flap with a vascularised wrapping of pronator quadratus. J Bone Joint Surg Br. 2006;88:623. doi:10.1302/0301-620X.88B5.
55. Mathoulin C, Wahegaonkar AL. Revascularization of the lunate by a volar vascularized bone graft and an osteotomy of the radius in treatment of the Kienböck's disease. Microsurgery. 2009;29(5):373–8. doi:10.1002/micr.20657.
56. Daecke W, Lorenz S, Wieloch P, Jung M, Martini A-K. Vascularized os pisiform for reinforcement of the lunate in Kienböck's disease: an average of 12 years of follow-up study. J Hand Surg Am. 2005;30(5):915–22. doi:10.1016/j.jhsa.2005.03.019.
57. von Maydell B, Brüser P. Long-term results after lunate replacement by the vascularised os pisiform for treatment of Kienböck's disease III b. Handchir Mikrochir Plast Chir. 2008;40(3):182–8. doi:10.1055/s-2007-965733.
58. Kirkeby L, von Varfalva Palffy L, Hansen TB. Long-term results after vascularised bone graft as treatment of Kienböck disease. J Plast Surg Hand Surg. 2014;48(1):21–3. doi:10.3109/2000656X.2013.793601.
59. Afshar A, Eivaziatashbeik K. Long-term clinical and radiological outcomes of radial shortening osteotomy and vascularized bone graft in Kienböck disease.

J Hand Surg Am. 2013;38(2):289–96. doi:10.1016/j.jhsa.2012.11.016.
60. Berger RA, Bishop AT, Bettinger PC. New dorsal capsulotomy for the surgical exposure of the wrist. Ann Plast Surg. 1995;35(1):54–9.
61. Gabl M, Lutz M, Reinhart C, Zimmermann R, Pechlaner S, Hussl H, et al. Stage 3 Kienböck's disease: reconstruction of the fractured lunate using a free vascularized iliac bone graft and external fixation. J Hand Surg Br. 2002;27(4):369–73. doi:10.1054/jhsb.2002.0766.
62. Yajima H, Ono H, Tamai S. Temporary internal fixation of the scaphotrapezio-trapezoidal joint for the treatment of Kienböck's disease: a preliminary study. J Hand Surg Am. 1998;23(3):402–10. doi:10.1016/S0363-5023(05)80457-5.

# 19 Osteochondral Free Flap Reconstruction of Advanced Kienböck's Disease

James P. Higgins and Heinz K. Bürger

## Introduction

The descending geniculate artery has been used increasingly as a versatile tool in reconstructive microsurgery. It has been most widely employed as the vascular pedicle for the medial femoral condyle (MFC) corticoperiosteal or corticocancellous flap used to address challenging cases of nonunion of long bones, tubular bones of the hand, carpal and tarsal bones, and the craniofacial skeleton. In addition to providing bone from the apex of the condyle, the vessel branches have demonstrated the capability of providing a cutaneous [1], osteocutaneous [2–4], or osteotendinous combinations [5], and have even served as a useful recipient vessel in extremity reconstruction [6].

The vascular pattern of this system also includes periosteal vessels supplying the cartilage-bearing trochlea of the medial patellofemoral joint. The utility of harvesting this convex cartilaginous surface as a vascularized flap was described in a case report of scaphoid reconstruction of a recalcitrant proximal pole nonunion in 2008 [7]. A subsequent clinical series described the promising early outcomes of use of the osteochondral medial femoral trochlea flap for proximal pole scaphoid nonunions [8]. Cadaveric studies have described the pertinent vascular arcade supplying this bone and cartilage [9, 10] and an anatomic study elucidated the similarities between the greater curvatures of the proximal lunate with the medial femoral trochlea [9].

J.P. Higgins, MD (✉)
Curtis National Hand Center, Union Memorial Hospital, 3333 N. Calvert St., Baltimore, MD 21218, USA
e-mail: jameshiggins10@hotmail.com

H.K. Bürger, MD
Department of Hand and Microsurgery, Private Clinic Maria Hilf, Klagenfurt, Carinthia 9020, Austria

## Anatomy

The DGA vascular system provides a dense filigree of blood vessels invested in the periosteum of the medial column of the distal femur. The DGA divides into two major periosteal branches: the longitudinal branch and the transverse branch. The longitudinal branch, which courses to the condyle, is used as the source vessel for the corticoperiosteal flap commonly used for osseous nonunions not requiring cartilage. The transverse branch, which courses anteriorly, is invested in the periosteum surrounding the medial femoral trochlea (MFT) [9, 10] (Fig. 19.1). Hugon et al. have observed that this site is a source of a convex osteochondral flap with a curvature similar to that of the proximal lunate on the sagittal and coronal plane [9]. This observation, as well as numerous cadaveric trials, led the authors to apply this segment of osteochondral bone to replace the collapsed lunate in cases of advanced Kienböck's disease with carpal collapse.

© Springer International Publishing Switzerland 2016
D.M. Lichtman, G.I. Bain (eds.), *Kienböck's Disease*, DOI 10.1007/978-3-319-34226-9_19

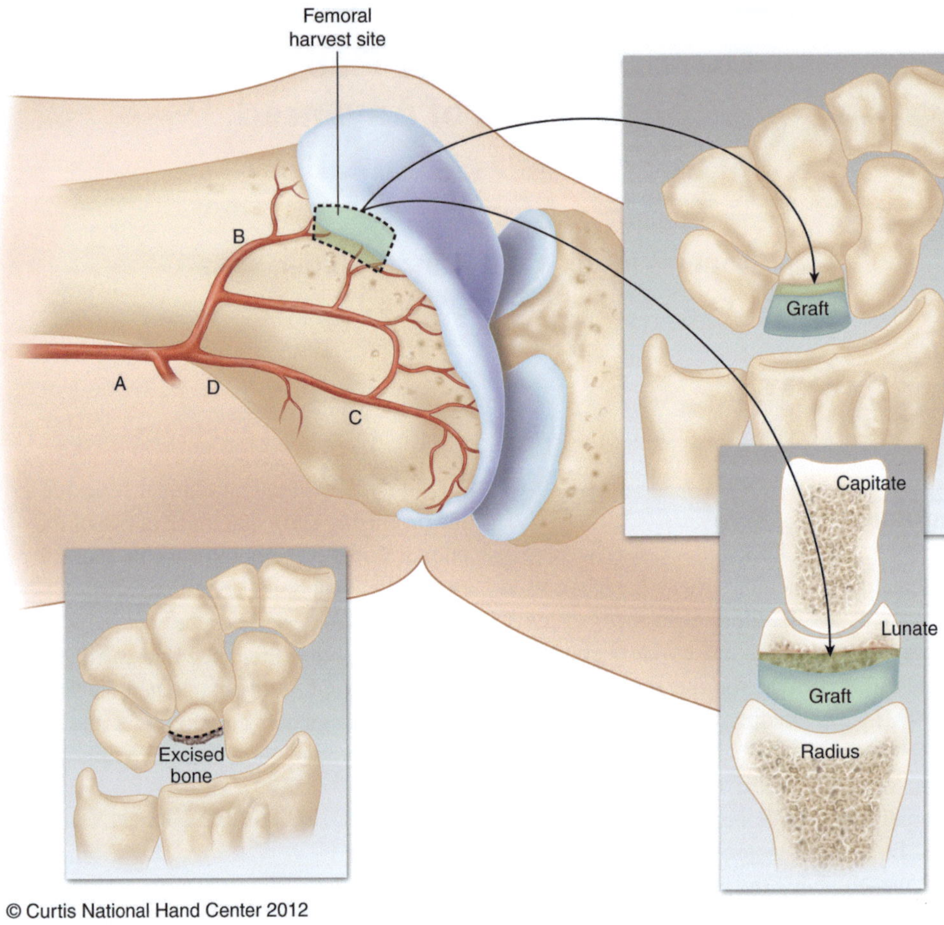


**Fig. 19.1** Representation of MFT and the planned portion of reconstructed proximal lunate. Portion of MFT harvested to provide vascularized osteocartilaginous reconstruction of the proximal lunate. Note the preservation of the native cartilage effacing the midcarpal joint. Vascular anatomy demonstrates branching pattern and supply of trochlea periosteum. (*A*) Descending geniculate artery. (*B*) Transverse branch to MFT. (*C*) Longitudinal branch. (*D*) Superomedial geniculate artery. © Copyright The Curtis National Hand Center

The authors have performed collectively a series of greater than 40 osteochondral lunate reconstructions. Their early experience in the use of this flap in the initial 16 patients was reported resulting in good intermediate-term results at a minimum of 12-month follow-up [11]. A summary of the technique and results of the study follows.

## Surgical Technique

### Wrist Exposure

The procedure begins with an exploration of the wrist to insure that the quality of the lunate fossa is adequate to pursue lunate reconstruction, and

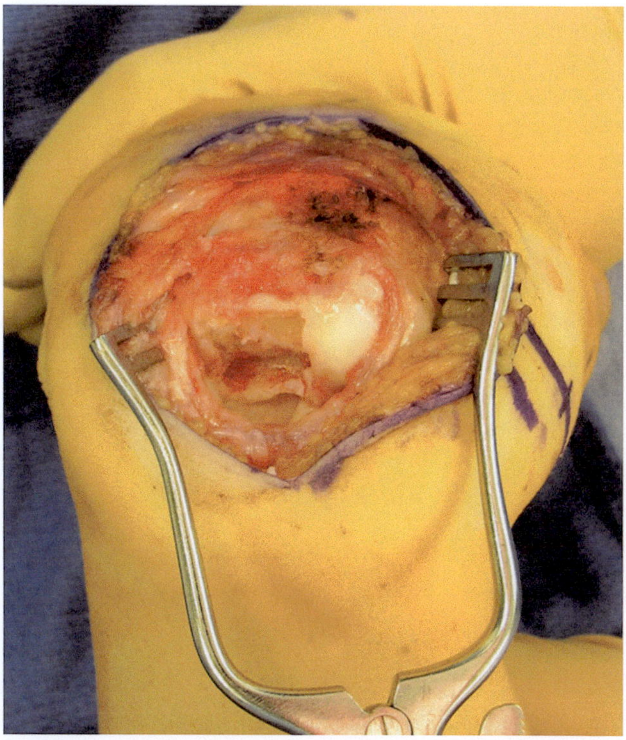

**Fig. 19.2** Intraoperative photo of dorsal left wrist dissection after the necrotic proximal lunate is resected while preserving cartilage effacing midcarpal joint. Wrist is in flexion demonstrating the extent of the lunate resection. Fingers are toward the top of the photo. Reprinted from The Journal of Hand Surgery, 39(7), Bürger HK, Windhofer C, Gaggl AJ, Higgins JP, Vascularized medial femoral trochlea osteochondral flap reconstruction of advanced Kienböck disease, 1313–22, Copyright 2014, with permission from Elsevier

to determine the dimensions of the osteochondral segment needed after lunate reconstruction. The wrist may be approached via either a volar or dorsal approach according to the surgeon's preference. The dorsal approach provides better visualization and ease of reconstruction. We have utilized a volar approach only in cases demonstrating a coronal split of the distal articular cartilage where there is a large segment of intact volar horn of the lunate that can accommodate screw fixation. If there is no obvious size superiority of the intact volar or dorsal lunate segments, we have preferred the dorsal approach.

## Lunate Preparation

The lunate fossa is inspected to confirm that it has remained adequately preserved to warrant lunate reconstruction. The lunate is then subtotally resected (Fig. 19.2). Its diseased and collapsed proximal portion can be excavated with a scalpel and rongeur while carefully preserving the (usually more preserved) distal-most portions of the scapholunate and lunotriquetral ligaments and the distal cartilage surface of the native lunate (Figs. 19.1 and 19.3). This maintains both the valuable linkage of the proximal row and the concave cartilage surface effacing the midcarpal joint. If a significant coronal split with displacement exists, interosseous wire or fiber-wire coaptation of these segments may be performed to provide complete cartilage coverage of the midcarpal surface. If there is no coronal split or the split is non-displaced a variety of fixation techniques may be planned (Fig. 19.4). The authors have used buried K-wire fixation across the lunotriquetral joint and scapholunate joints, respectively (affixing the osteochondral flap), mini-screw fixation between larger segments of the native distal lunate into the flap, or complete absence of fixation with dependence on a tightly fashioned flap and the defect. After careful measurement and sizing of the graft the surgeon will indeed find a satisfying and tight congruency between the flap and the evacuated lunate fossa.

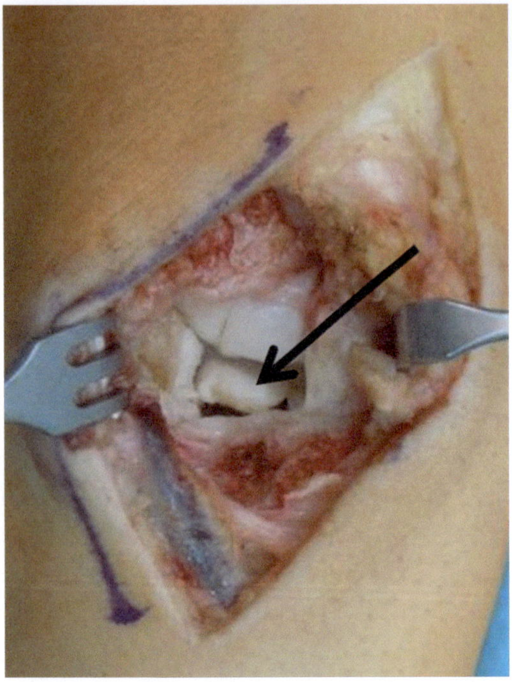

**Fig. 19.3** Intraoperative photo of the dorsal left wrist dissection after the necrotic proximal lunate is resected while preserving thin distal cartilage of the lunate which articulates with the midcarpal joint. Fingers are toward the top of the photo. Reprinted from The Journal of Hand Surgery, 39(7), Bürger HK, Windhofer C, Gaggl AJ, Higgins JP, Vascularized medial femoral trochlea osteochondral flap reconstruction of advanced Kienböck disease, 1313–22, Copyright 2014, with permission from Elsevier

## Preparation of Wrist Vessels

Prior to proceeding to the leg, the vessels are prepared for anastomosis in the wrist. When using a dorsal approach this is commonly the radial artery in the snuffbox (end-to-side) and its venae comitans (end to end). If a volar approach is used, the palmar branch of the radial artery and its venae are prepared for end-to-end anastomoses. The tourniquet is then released and attention is turned to the leg.

## Flap Exposure

The surgical markings are started at a location midpoint between the medial aspect of the patella and the palpable apex of the medial condyle of the femur. From this location a line is drawn coursing proximally in an oblique path toward the adductor canal (Fig. 19.5). This incision is taken through subcutaneous fat and directly through the fascia of the vastus medialis muscle. The vastus medialis is retracted anteriorly and the fascia posteriorly (Fig. 19.6). The medial column of the femur is rapidly made visible. At the depth of the dissection, immediately adjacent to the adductor tendon courses the DGA (Fig. 19.7).

The DGA can be traced distally along the medial column of the femur to feed a broad filigree of blood vessels intimately adherent into the periosteum of the medial distal femur (Fig. 19.8). The longitudinal branch supplies the region commonly used for harvest of the medial femoral condyle osteoperiosteal flap. The perpendicular transverse branch typically traverses the metaphyseal region and densely supplies the periosteum surrounding the medial femoral trochlea both on its medial aspect and proximal aspect (Figs. 19.1 and 19.9). This is the vessel that is utilized for MFT osteochondral reconstruction.

## Flap Harvesting

The DGA may be followed proximally to the adductor canal to its origin off the superficial femoral artery (SFA). As dissection progresses proximally the surgeon will obtain both increasing pedicle length and caliber. The surgeon may elect to limit this proximal dissection if less length or caliber is required.

After ligating the pedicle from the SFA, the DGA is reflected distally. The longitudinal branch to the condyle may be ligated. Harvest continues using the transverse branch that can be traced towards the medial trochlea. The periosteal vessels are left adherent to the territory of bone and cartilage desired for harvest. A sagittal saw and osteotomies may be used to harvest the proximal-most portion of the cartilage-bearing segment of the medial femoral trochlea. The dimensions correspond as follows:

1. The proximal-to-distal harvest is measured to recreate the radial-to-ulnar dimensions of the lunate in the wrist.

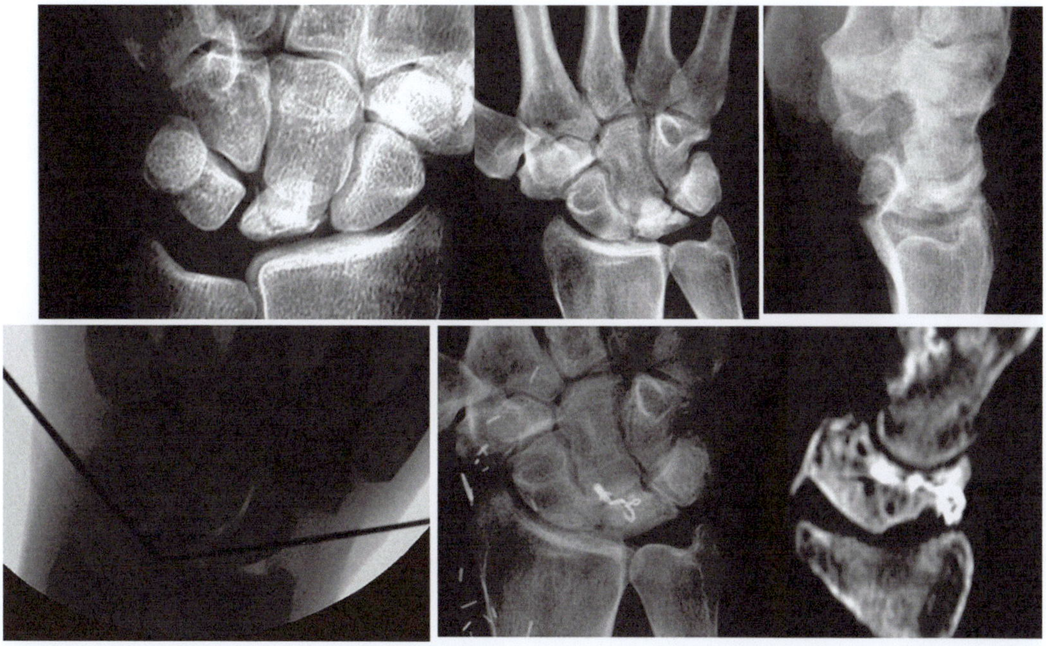

**Fig. 19.4** X-rays demonstrating two of the techniques commonly used for fixation of the reconstructed lunate. *Left*: Preoperative and postoperative AP radiographs of a case where K-wires were driven across lunotriquetral and scapholunate joints. No fixation is used to capture the remaining distal wafer of native lunate. Center: Preoperative and postoperative AP radiographs of a fragmented lunate with a displaced coronal split. Interosseous wire fixation is used to correct a displaced coronal split in the distal native lunate cartilage. The MFT segment is then tightly inserted without additional fixation. Carpal height was restored. *Right*: Preoperative lateral radiograph and postoperative coronal sagittal CT scan demonstrating the correction of the displaced coronal split in the distal native lunate. The CT image demonstrates the congruity of the midcarpal joint and the healing of the MFT to the distal native cartilage remnant. Also note the characteristic appearance of the reconstructed proximal flap on the coronal CT scan. The only visible contour is the V-shaped interface of the subchondral bone and cartilage. The more proximal cartilage layer is congruent with the lunate fossa. *Left bottom figure*: Reprinted from The Journal of Hand Surgery, 39(7), Bürger HK, Windhofer C, Gaggl AJ, Higgins JP, Vascularized medial femoral trochlea osteochondral flap reconstruction of advanced Kienböck disease, 1313–22, Copyright 2014, with permission from Elsevier

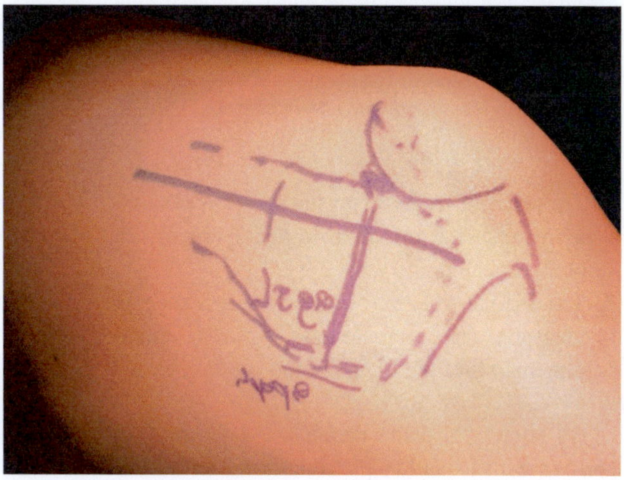

**Fig. 19.5** Intraoperative markings for harvest of the MFT flap. A straight incision is created from the interval between the medial patella and the palpable prominence of the medial femoral condyle. The length of the proximal extension toward the adductor canal can be varied according to the length of pedicle harvest desired. Patella is shown superiorly and distal leg is toward the right of the image

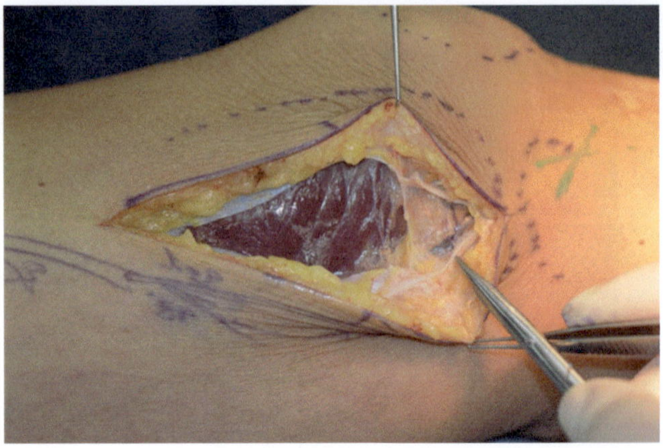

**Fig. 19.6** Immediately after skin dissection an incision is made through the fascia of the vastus medialis. The subsequent deeper dissection will proceed in this subfascial plane. The tip of the scissors is pointing to the reflected edge of the vastus medialis fascia. The distal leg is to the right

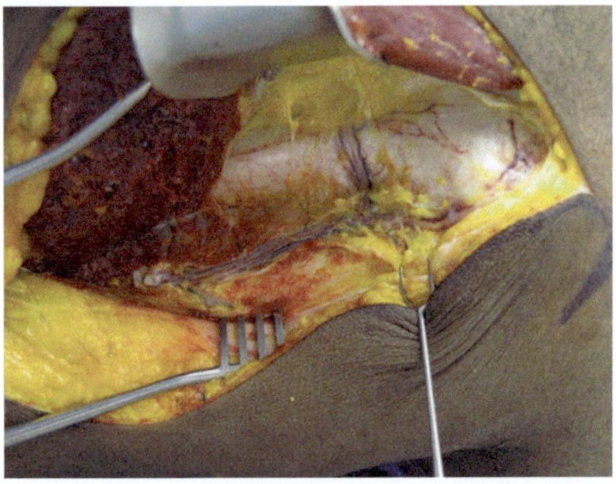

**Fig. 19.7** Exposure of the DGA is afforded by anterior reflection of the vastus medialis and dissection down to level of adductor tendon deep to the fascia of the vastus medialis. Proximally (*left*) the DGA courses parallel to the adductor tendon. Distally (*right*) it separates into two major branches: transverse and longitudinal. The transverse branch travels anteriorly below the vastus medialis toward the medial trochlea of the femur. Reprinted from The Journal of Hand Surgery, 37(5), Iorio ML, Masden DL, Higgins JP, Cutaneous angiosome territory of the medial femoral condyle osteocutaneous flap, 1033–41, Copyright 2012, with permission from Elsevier

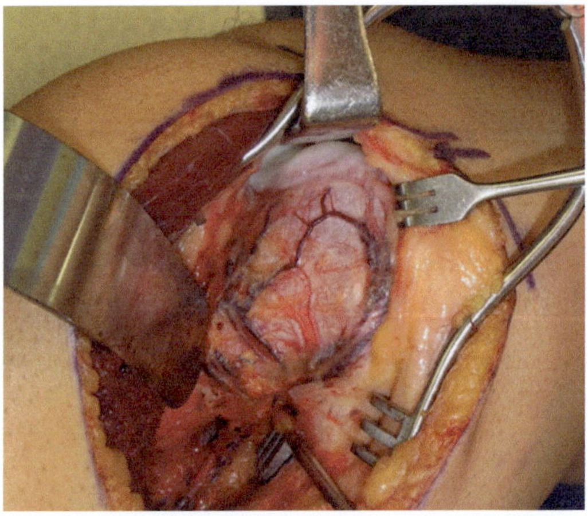

**Fig. 19.8** Intraoperative image of a typical branching pattern of the transverse branch of the DGA. As it courses anteriorly it approaches the cartilage-bearing trochlea proximally, often demonstrating an arcade of vessels along the osteochondral rim of the trochlea. Convex proximal trochlea to serve as proximal lunate is shown in situ. The distal leg is to the right

2. The anterior-to-posterior harvest is measured to recreate the proximal-to-distal dimension of the lunate in the wrist.
3. The medial-to-lateral harvest in the knee is measured to recreate the volar-to-dorsal dimensions of the lunate in the wrist.

An attempt is made to make the arthrotomy and harvest as small as possible to minimize the disturbance to the knee joint. The resultant defect is coated with bone wax to limit postoperative hemarthrosis. The capsule is closed. A minimal incision in the proximal-most aspect of the medial patellofemoral ligament is often needed to gain access for creation of the bone cuts. This ligament is repaired anatomically, taking great care not to make it excessively tight. A closed suction drain is placed in the subcutaneous tissue and the skin closed. No brace is required postoperatively and patients may ambulate as comfort permits.

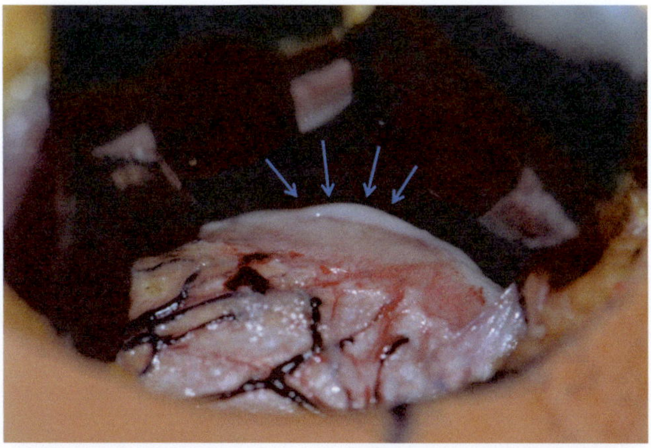

**Fig. 19.9** Intraoperative image showing typical filigree of periosteal vessels originating from transverse branch of descending geniculate artery and supplying the medial trochlea. Convex surface of the cartilage (indicated by *arrows*) can be seen under the retracted vastus medialis muscle. Reprinted from The Journal of Hand Surgery, 39(7), Bürger HK, Windhofer C, Gaggl AJ, Higgins JP, Vascularized medial femoral trochlea osteochondral flap reconstruction of advanced Kienböck disease, 1313–22, Copyright 2014, with permission from Elsevier

## Fixation of Flap to Lunate

The osteocartilaginous segment is then fashioned so as to fit into the defect created from resection of the lunate. The convex cartilage-bearing surface of the flap faces the concave lunate fossa of the radius. The remaining cancellous surfaces face the adjacent scaphoid and triquetrum as well as the preserved distal concave cartilaginous midcarpal articulation of the distal native lunate. Fixation may be achieved with any of the methods described above.

## Anastomosis of Flap Vessels

With the segment oriented as described the periosteal vascular pedicle will drape distally (Fig. 19.10). In the more common dorsal approach this will require draping the pedicle in a gentle curving fashion subcutaneously into the anatomic snuffbox. With the tourniquet released the microvascular anastomoses are performed. With release of the clamps generous bleeding may be observed along the periosteum and vascular leash as it dives deeply toward the reconstructed lunate. The skin is mobilized generously in all directions and closed loosely to avoid constriction of the pedicle.

## Postoperative Care

The patient typically remains in the hospital overnight for comfort and application of a warming blanket for vasodilation. After discharge they are maintained on 325 mg of aspirin daily for 3 weeks. The postoperative splint is exchanged for casting at week 2. Casting is maintained for 12 weeks, followed by a variable course of hand therapy as required. If buried hardware requires removal this is usually performed at 12 weeks postop. A CT scan is performed 12 weeks after surgery to confirm osseous union of the osteochondral segment to the distal native lunate segment. Therapy is not usually required for the knee donor site, but may be requested if the patient requires assistance with rehabilitation.

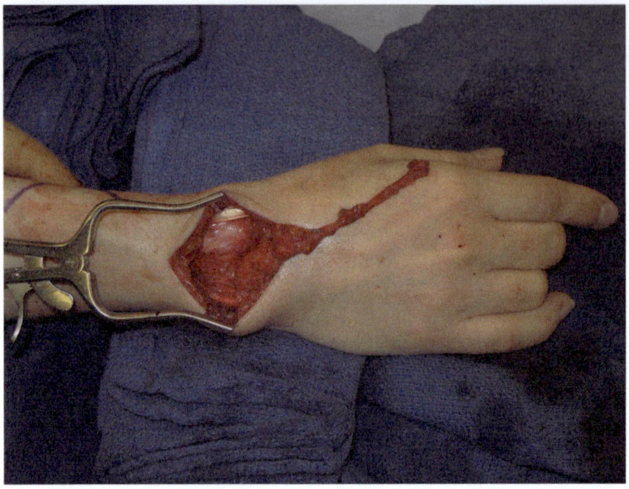

**Fig. 19.10** After inset of the MFT into the lunate fossa with the cartilage seated in the lunate fossa, the periosteum and vascular pedicle will drape distally. In the more common dorsal approach this is then gently routed in the subcutaneous plane radially into the anatomic snuffbox. Here the anastomoses will be performed to the radial artery (end to side) and vena comitans (end to end)

## Reported Results

The authors' initial series of 16 osteochondral lunate reconstructions has previously been reported [11, 12]. Union of the reconstructed lunates was confirmed in 15/16 with computed tomography (Figs. 19.11 and 19.12). There was little change in the mean carpal height (Stahl's indices) from preoperative (0.46) to postoperative (0.48). Lichtman staging remained unchanged in ten patients, improved in four patients (3a or 3b to 2), and worsened in two patients (3a to 3b). Radiographic progression of radiocarpal collapse was seen in these two patients. Asymptomatic midcarpal radiographic joint space narrowing was witnessed in one patient despite improvement in Lichtman grade (see Fig. 19.11).

The mean wrist motion at follow-up was 50° extension (range 30–80°) and 38° flexion (30–60°). This was not statistically different from the mean preoperative range of motion (45° extension and 38° flexion). Pronosupination and digital ROM were unaffected. Grip strength achieved at follow-up was 85 % of the contralateral side.

All but one patient experienced improvement in wrist pain (12/16 complete relief, 3/16 incomplete relief). The remaining patient had persistent pain and failed to achieve osseous healing. This patient ultimately underwent a salvage total wrist arthrodesis. All patients experienced donor-site discomfort ranging from 4 weeks to 3 months after surgery. All patients had resolution of knee pain and returned to preoperative activities including athletics.

## Discussion

As the authors have gained increasing experience with this technique we have learned several lessons. This is a challenging surgical technique that may demand more from the patient and surgeon than other reported surgical treatments of Kienböck's disease. This procedure provides reliable pain relief for patients with Kienböck's disease, as have many other reported surgical modalities for this disease. Like many other procedures, the indications are difficult to define when the techniques reported are multiple and the disease process is poorly understood.

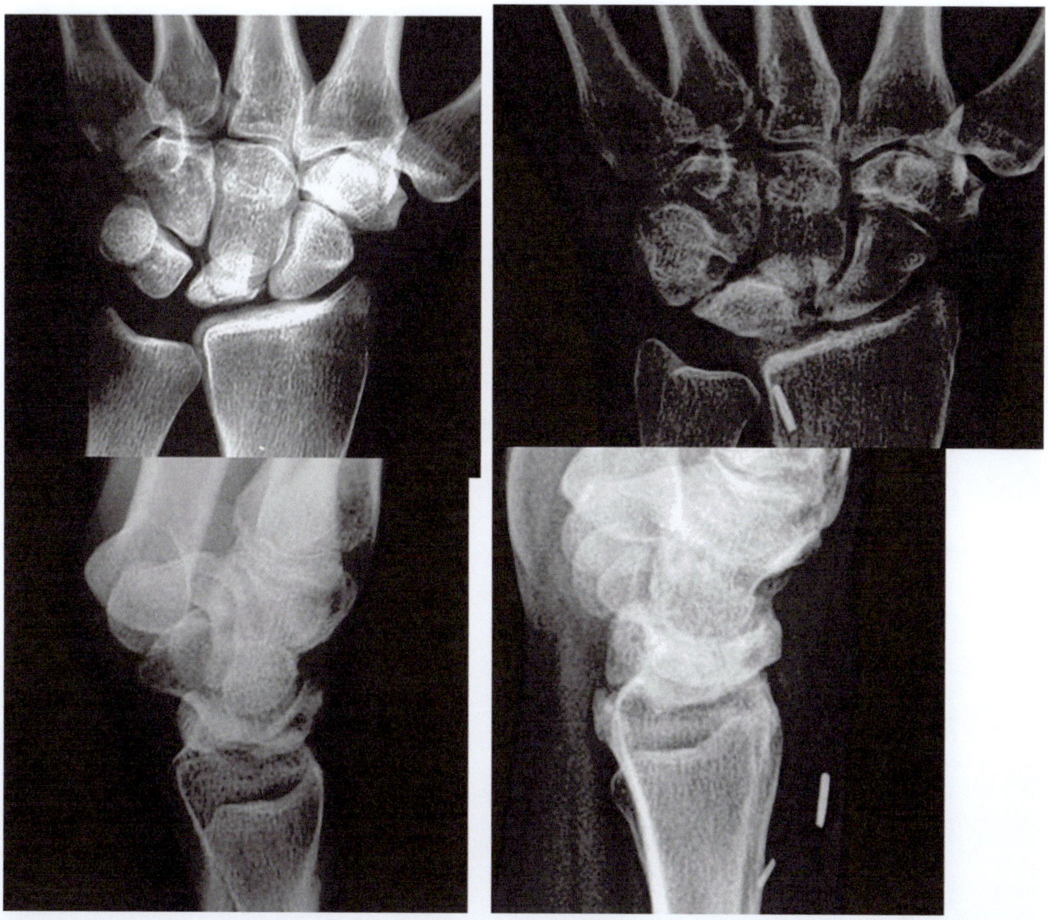

**Fig. 19.11** Preoperative radiograph (*left*) of a 30-year-old patient with stage 3A Kienböck's disease without scaphoid flexion or radiocarpal arthritis. At 39 months after MFT reconstruction (*right*), radiographs demonstrate improved carpal height, Stahl's Index, and lunate substance, converting to stage 2 disease. Reprinted from The Journal of Hand Surgery, 39(7), Bürger HK, Windhofer C, Gaggl AJ, Higgins JP, Vascularized medial femoral trochlea osteochondral flap reconstruction of advanced Kienböck disease, 1313–22, Copyright 2014, with permission from Elsevier

We have concluded that this technique can reliably provide the most profound impact in the treatment of advanced Kienböck's disease (stage 3a or 3B) where carpal collapse is demonstrated, a highly fragmented lunate is observed, and conventional treatment options were limited to ablative salvage operations (i.e., proximal row carpectomy). In these circumstances, the MFT may provide the sole means of autologous restoration of the lunate, restoration of carpal height, and reversal of Lichtman staging. In such a case, particularly in younger patients, the MFT provides an important alternative that can change conventional treatment algorithms.

MFT osteochondral reconstruction provides a resurfacing of the proximal cartilage surface of the lunate, and can re-establish lunate morphology in the presence of a coronal split of the distal lunate surface (see Fig. 19.4). It does not address chondral deficiencies of the proximal capitate or the lunate fossa. The indications for this reconstruction can thus be defined according to the articular approach advocated by Bain and Begg [13] as being a treatment (and means of reversal) of grade 1 and grade 2b Kienböck's disease, where conventional management would offer salvage procedures alone.

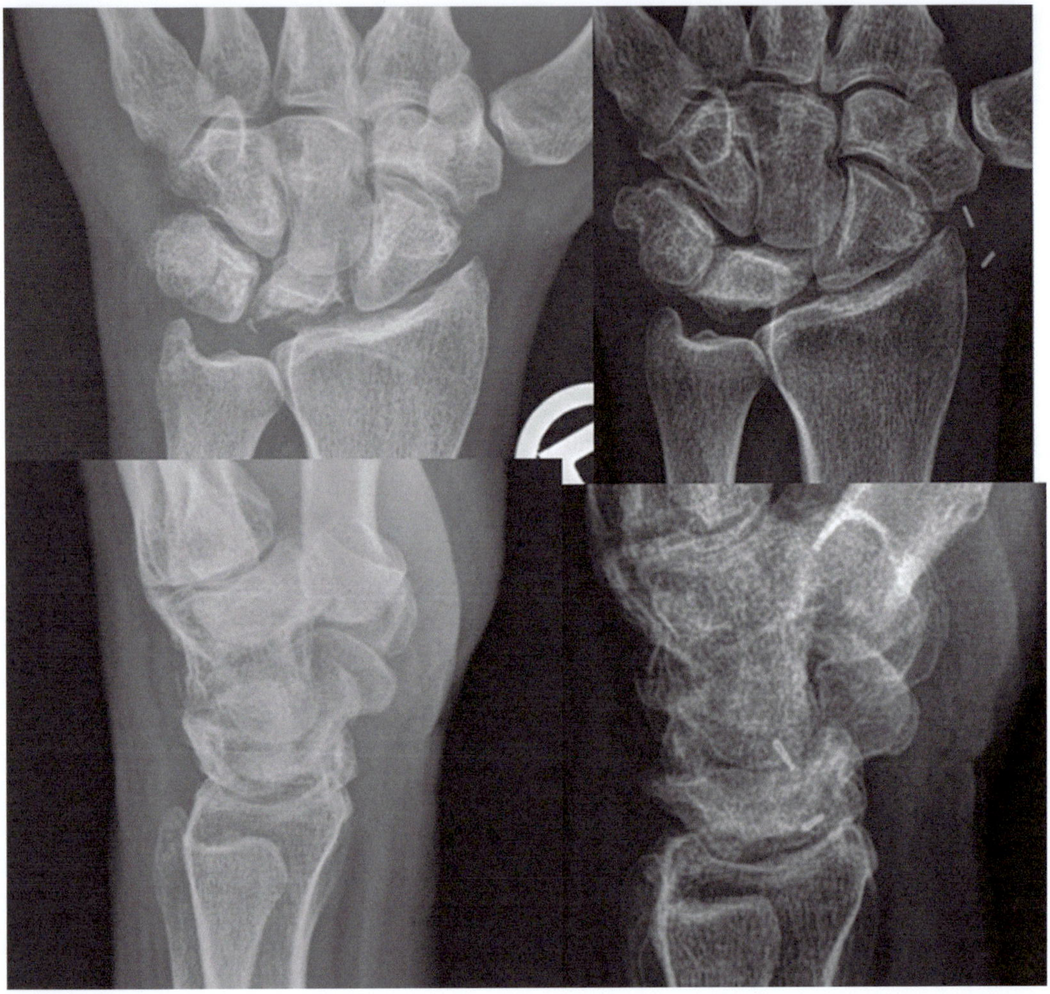

**Fig. 19.12** A 29-year-old patient with stage 3A Kienböck's disease. MFT reconstruction via dorsal approach using K-wire fixation. At 28 months after surgery, he has achieved improved carpal height and lunate substance, converting to stage 2 disease. *Top left*: Preoperative AP X-ray. *Bottom left*: Preoperative lateral X-ray. *Top right*: Postoperative AP X-ray. *Bottom right*: Postoperative lateral X-ray

Much investigation is still required to elucidate the natural history of cartilage survival in an intrasynovial environment with periosteal and subchondral blood supply. Rare opportunities for subsequent cartilage assessment in our patient series have arisen. One such case enabled arthroscopic MFT cartilage biopsy of a reconstructed lunate more than 3 years after surgery. This demonstrated uniformly viable chondrocytes in a normal-appearing cartilaginous stroma (this case report was in publication submission process at the time of this installment) (Fig. 19.13). The relative importance of the vascular pedicle (and its provided subchondral perfusion of the cartilage) and the synovial diffusion is of interest. The authors are completing an investigation on the histologic performance of these flaps with or without vascular pedicle nutrition in an analogous animal survival model with promising results (yet to be published). Finally, long-term follow-up on the donor-site morbidity both radiographically and subjectively is under way.

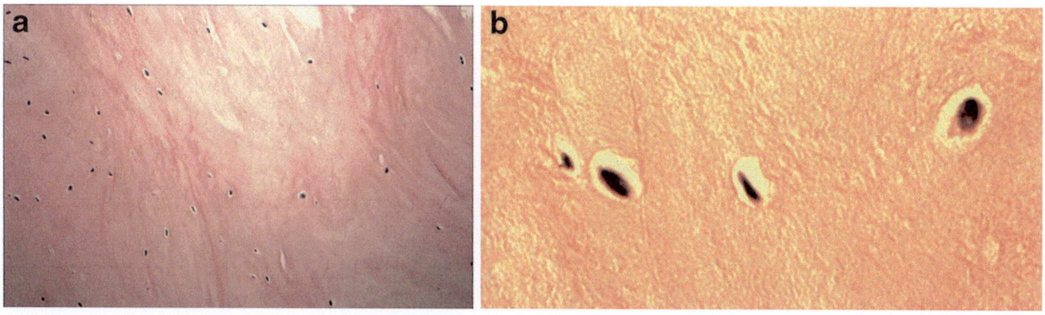


**Fig. 19.13** Hematoxylin and eosin-stained histology specimen arthroscopically obtained from the transferred cartilage of an MFT reconstruction of a lunate 39 months after surgery. Slides demonstrate viable chondrocytes in a normal-appearing cartilage matrix under 10× (**a**) and 40× (**b**) magnification

## References

1. Acland RD, Schusterman M, Godina M, Eder E, Taylor GI, Carlisle I. The saphenous neurovascular free flap. Plast Reconstr Surg. 1981;67(6):763–74.
2. Iorio ML, Masden DL, Higgins JP. Cutaneous angiosome territory of the medial femoral condyle osteocutaneous flap. J Hand Surg Am. 2012;37(5):1033–41.
3. Pelzer M, Reichenberger M, Germann G. Osteo-periosteal-cutaneous flaps of the medial femoral condyle: a valuable modification for selected clinical situations. J Reconstr Microsurg. 2010;26(5):291–4.
4. Martin D, Bitonti-Grillo C, De BJ, Schott H, Mondie JM, Baudet J, Peri G. Mandibular reconstruction using a free vascularised osteocutaneous flap from the internal condyle of the femur. Br J Plast Surg. 1991;44(6):397–402.
5. Huang D, Wang HW, Xu DC, Wang HG, Wu WZ, Zhang HR. An anatomic and clinical study of the adductor magnus tendon-descending genicular artery bone flap. Clin Anat. 2011;24(1):77–83.
6. Higgins JP. Descending geniculate artery: the ideal recipient vessel for free tissue transfer coverage of below the knee amputation wounds. J Reconstr Microsurg. 2011;27(9):525–30.
7. Kalicke T, Burger H, Muller EJ. A new vascularized cartilague-bone-graft for scaphoid nonunion with avascular necrosis of the proximal pole. Description of a new type of surgical procedure. Unfallchirurg. 2008;111(3):201–5.
8. Burger HK, Windhofer C, Gaggl AJ, Higgins JP. Vascularized medial femoral trochlea osteocartilaginous flap reconstruction of proximal pole scaphoid nonunions. J Hand Surg Am. 2013;38(4):690–700.
9. Hugon S, Koninckx A, Barbier O. Vascularized osteochondral graft from the medial femoral trochlea: anatomical study and clinical perspectives. Surg Radiol Anat. 2010;32(9):817–25.
10. Iorio ML, Masden DL, Higgins JP. The limits of medial femoral condyle corticoperiosteal flaps. J Hand Surg Am. 2011;36:1592–6.
11. Bürger HK, Windhofer C, Gaggl AJ, Higgins JP. Vascularized medial femoral trochlea osteochondral flap reconstruction of advanced Kienböck disease. J Hand Surg Am. 2014;39(7):1313–22.
12. Higgins JP, Bürger HK. Osteochondral flaps from the distal femur: expanding applications, harvest sites, and indications. J Reconstr Microsurg. 2014;30(7):483–90.
13. Bain GI, Begg M. Arthroscopic assessment and classification of Kienböck's disease. Tech Hand Upper Extrem Surg. 2006;10(1):8–13.

# Proximal Row Carpectomy for the Treatment of Kienböck's Disease

# 20

Harvey Chim and Steven L. Moran

## Introduction

Proximal row carpectomy (PRC) is an established and widely used procedure for treatment of degenerative conditions of the wrist. The procedure involves excision of the scaphoid, lunate, and triquetrum, with formation of a new articulation between the lunate fossa of the distal radius and the proximal aspect of the capitate. The procedure is particularly attractive for patients with Kienböck's disease as it avoids complicated surgery and allows one to remove the fragmented and avascular lunate. In addition, the rehabilitation can be initiated rapidly as there is no need to wait for bone healing or bone fusion as in other methods of wrist salvage for Kienböck's disease. This chapter reviews the literature specific to PRC when used in Kienböck's disease and tries to examine factors predictive for a successful outcome.

PRC has been a described procedure for wrist arthritis since the 1940s and as such the procedure has been extensively studied. Relief of pain and preservation of wrist range of motion have been demonstrated in multiple studies [1–3]. A functional arc of wrist motion can be maintained for over two decades following surgery [4–6]. Downsides to the surgery include a significant decrease in grip strength, which have led some researchers to suggest that PRC may be better for patients who are not engaged in heavy manual labor [6–8]. Depending upon the distribution of the joint degeneration, other salvage options may be preferred (e.g., RSL, 4-corner fusion, and scaphotrapezioumtrapeoidal [STT] fusion). Despite these newer options, no study has yet to show a significant improvement in upper extremity function over that achieved with PRC [6]. Concern still exists when performing PRC, as a substantial number of patients will go on to develop radiographic arthritic changes at the capitate radius interface. This is a particular concern in Kienböck's disease, as the fragmented lunate may produce some cartilage damage to the radius or capitate prior to diagnosis.

Indications for PRC include

1. Patients with persistent pain despite nonoperative management
2. Intact lunate fossa and capitate articular surfaces.
3. Advanced-stage disease in less active or older patients

Contraindications for PRC include

H. Chim, MD
Division of Plastic Surgery, University of Miami Miller School of Medicine, Clinical Research Building, 1120 N.W. 14th St, 4th Floor, Miami, FL 33136, USA

S.L. Moran, MD (✉)
Division of Plastic Surgery, Mayo Clinic, 200 First St. SW, Rochester, MN 55905, USA
e-mail: moran.steven@mayo.edu

© Springer International Publishing Switzerland 2016
D.M. Lichtman, G.I. Bain (eds.), *Kienböck's Disease*, DOI 10.1007/978-3-319-34226-9_20

1. Arthritis of the lunate fossa and/or capitate
2. Pathology involving the base of the capitate
3. Severe pancarpal arthritis (advanced stage IV disease)

If a PRC is contraindicated due to compromise of the capitate or lunate fossa cartilage, we prefer a scaphocapitate fusion. Other researchers recommend a PRC with a dorsal capsular interposition.

## Long-Term Outcomes of Proximal Row Carpectomy

An inevitable consequence of proximal row carpectomy is the development of arthritis at the radiocapitate joint. In a review of 82 patients in five studies where radiographic data was available [6], 65 had evidence of radiocapitate degenerative joint disease (79.3 %). However, radiographic changes did not correlate significantly with clinical findings or objective and subjective outcome measures. The significance of radiologic changes is a matter of debate, and a link between radiographic changes and pain or decreased function has not been established.

In the normal wrist, the load of the capitate is distributed to the scaphoid, lunate, and then to the radius. With a PRC the load is transferred directly from the capitate to only the lunate fossa. The capitate has a radius of curvature of only 64 % of the lunate fossa on anteroposterior radiographs and 60 % on true lateral radiographs [9]. This results in reduced contact area (21–26 %) and a 3.8 times increased contact pressure [10]. Also, the capitate both translates and rotates on the radius leading inevitably to radiologic evidence of arthritis.

In a systematic review of PRCs with more than 10 years of follow-up [6], it was found that the mean postoperative flexion/extension arc was 73.5° (preoperative 73.4°) and postoperative grip strength was 68.4 % of the contralateral side. A total wrist fusion was required in 14 % (21 of 147) at a mean of 53.4 months [6]. Interestingly, failures tend to occur prior to radiographic evidence of radiocapitate arthritis. Adjunctive procedures such as posterior interosseous nerve (PIN) neurectomy, radial styloidectomy, proximal capitate excision, or dorsal capsule interposition have been suggested to improve outcomes after PRC, but only PIN neurectomy has been shown to improve pain in long-term outcome studies [11, 12].

In a review of PRCs with a minimum of 20-year follow-up, 35 % of the (6/17) required a radiocarpal arthrodesis, at a mean of 11 years (8 months to 20 years) [13]. There was a higher incidence of conversion to total wrist fusion in the more active patients who were younger than 40 years of age.

## Proximal Row Carpectomy for Kienböck's Disease

It has been suggested that PRC failures may occur more often in patients with Kienböck's disease due to the presence of capitate or lunate fossa injury [14]. However a systematic review of PRCs with at least 10-year follow-up has demonstrated that Kienböck's disease did not have a worse prognosis [6, 15].

PRC is indicated as a salvage procedure for advanced Kienböck's disease, such as Lichtman's stages 3B and 4 [16]. Most studies have reported good short-term outcomes, with two series [14, 15] reporting results with at least 10-year follow-up.

Croog and Stern reported minimum 10-year results, with a mean flexion-extension arc of 105° and grip strength of 87 % of the contralateral side. There was a conversion rate of 14.3 % (3/21) to full wrist fusion at a mean of 23 months (5–53) [14]. Two of these patients had stage 4 disease, and the other with stage 3A disease had abutment between the radial styloid and trapezium and trapezoid. There was no association between Lichtman stage at the time of PRC and any objective or subjective outcome parameters. Like other long-term studies following PRC, degeneration of the radiocapitate articulation on radiographs was found in the majority of patients (87 %); however, there was no correlation between the radiographic changes and outcome measurements. Lumsden et al. [17] reported similar results with an average 15-year follow-up.

## Surgical Technique for Proximal Row Carpectomy

Our technique is similar to that used by most hand surgeons [11]. A dorsal longitudinal incision is made in line with the third metacarpal. The extensor retinaculum is then opened over the third dorsal extensor compartment and the extensor pollicis longus (EPL) tendon is released and transposed radially. Then, retinacular flaps are raised over the second and fourth dorsal compartments. A posterior interosseous nerve neurectomy is performed. A ligament-sparing capsulotomy along the fibers of the dorsal intercarpal ligament (DIC) and dorsal radiocarpal ligament (DRC) is then made, exposing the carpus (Fig. 20.1). The scaphoid, lunate, and triquetrum are then excised either en bloc or in piecemeal fashion (Figs. 20.2 and 20.3). Care is taken to avoid damage to the radioscaphocapitate ligament. Then, the wrist capsule and extensor retinaculum are repaired, followed by the skin. A volar splint is applied with the wrist in slight dorsiflexion and the metacarpophalangeal joints

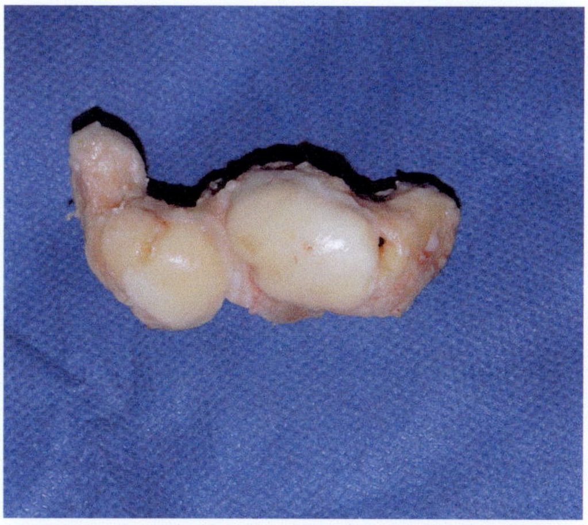

**Fig. 20.2** Intraoperative image of the proximal carpal row following en bloc resection. The specimen shows the lunate centrally with scaphoid to the left and triquetrum to the right

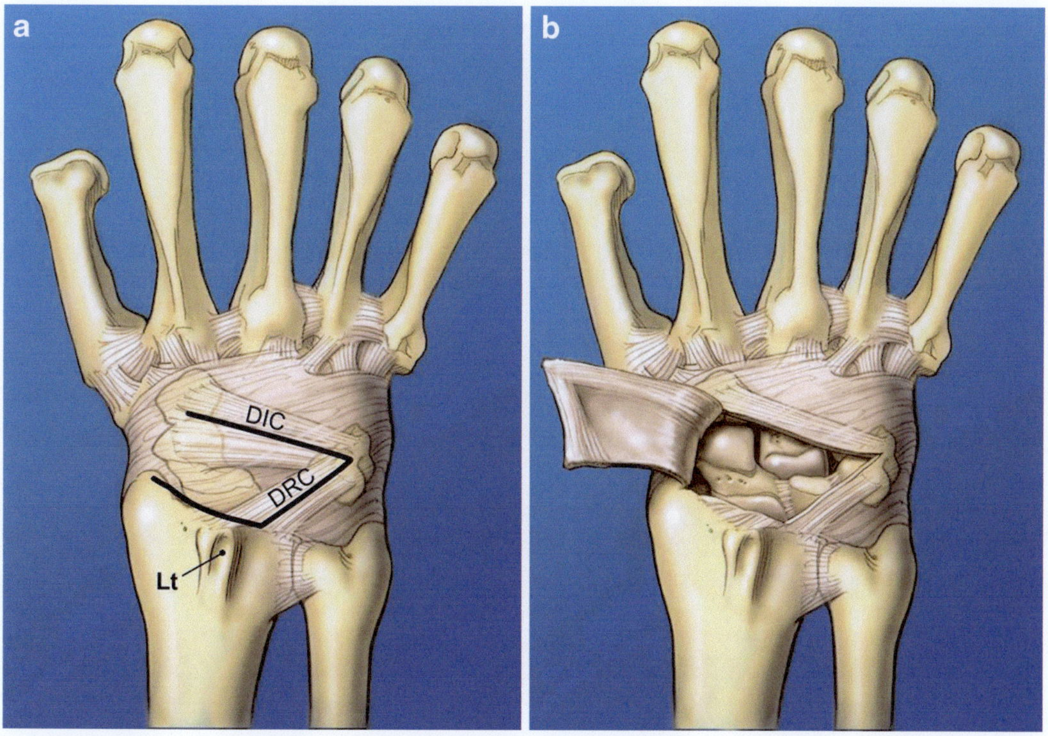


**Fig. 20.1** (**a**, **b**) Our approach for a standard PRC begins with a ligament-sparing dorsal capsulotomy, splitting the dorsal intercarpal and dorsal radiocarpal ligament. This allows excellent exposure of the midcarpal and radiocarpal joint. If a capsular interposition is planned, a large rectangular proximal based flap is interposed into the lunate fossa of the radius. Used with permission of Mayo Foundation for Medical Education and Research

free. Postoperative protocols vary in our institutions, with wrist immobilization time varying from 3 to 10 weeks depending on the presence of instability and the condition of the soft tissue. A temporary k-wire across the remaining wrist joint can be considered if the joint is unstable, such as if the radioscaphocapiate ligament is incompetent (Fig. 20.4).

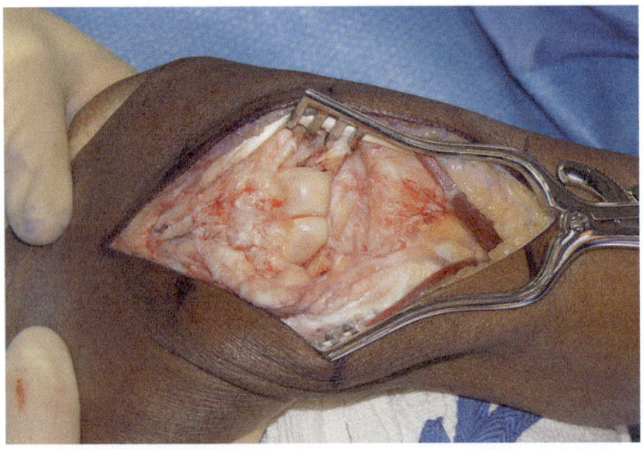

**Fig. 20.3** Intraoperative photo of capitate and hamate head following removal of proximal carpal row

## Proximal Row Carpectomy with Interposition

Nanavati et al. [18] found that the use of a meniscal interposition allograft after a PRC can normalize pressures at the radiocapitate articulation. This concept can be applied through the interposition of soft tissue to normalize peak pressures and increase the longevity of PRC [18, 19]. This theoretically extends the indications of PRC, with the capacity of using PRC as a treatment modality even in the presence of midcarpal arthritis or degeneration of the base of the capitate [20].

With interposition of the joint capsule [20], the surgical technique for exposure is similar to that for conventional proximal row carpectomy. However, a large proximally based U-shaped flap of the joint capsule is raised. The width is from the radial styloid to the distal radio-ulnar joint, and it extends to the second and fourth carpometacarpal joints. The proximal carpal row is then excised, and the dorsal capsular flap is then

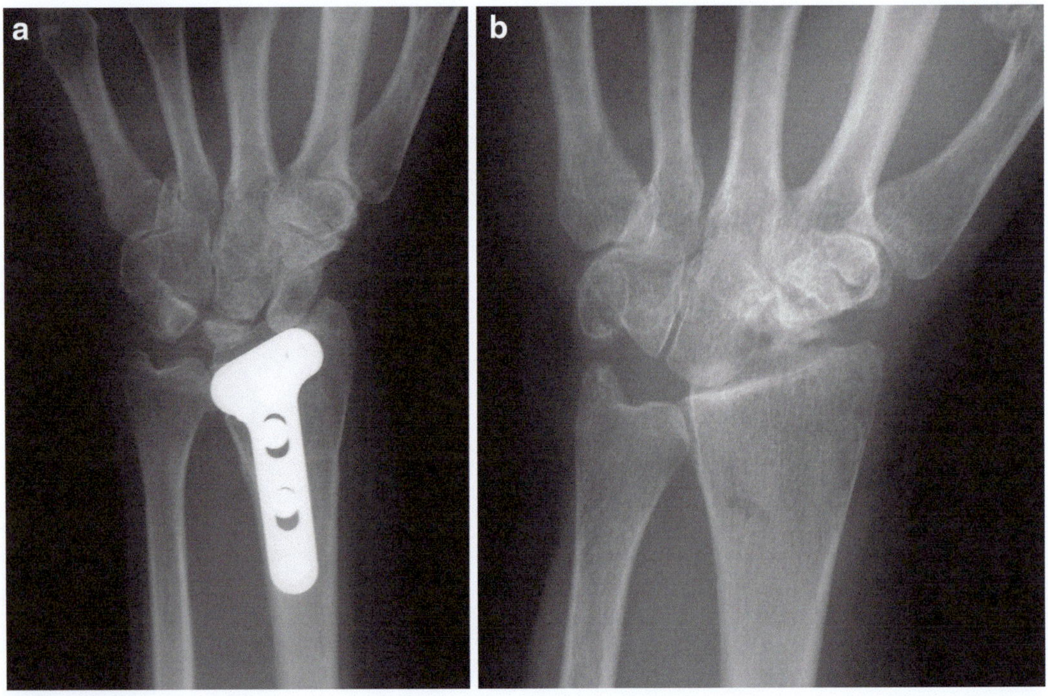


**Fig. 20.4** (**a**) Clinical example of a 45-year-old male who underwent radial-shortening osteotomy for Kienböck's disease. Patient continued to have pain with progression of lunate collapse. Patient elected to undergo hardware removal, radial styloidectomy, and proximal row carpectomy. (**b**) AP radiograph 3 years following PRC and hardware removal with stable radius-capitate interface

sutured to the volar wrist capsule to act as an interposition. Care is required to ensure that the flap is well secured and properly centered so that the capitate will articulate with the capsule over the lunate fossa. Closure of the joint capsule (if possible), extensor retinaculum, and skin is then performed in the usual fashion.

A review of eight patients with PRC and capsular interposition for degeneration of the capitate or lunate fossa identified progression of radiographic arthritis in 3/8 patients at 41-month follow-up [21]. However the radiological signs were not related to the pain, motion, grip, and functional scores. All patients had relief of pain with maintenance of preoperative motion (mean flexion-extension arc 71.9°) and grip strength (66.8 % of contralateral).

Use of the dorsal wrist capsule as an interposition material has the advantage of being well vascularized, obviating the need for distraction to protect the interposed tissue until revascularization. Diao et al. [12] found a well-preserved interposed capsule during arthroscopy in a patient who had previously undergone PRC with capsular interposition 9 months previous.

## Improving Preoperative Selection

Most recently, Wagner and colleagues evaluated 144 patients who had undergone PRC for a variety of wrist pathologies [22]. Patients were evaluated with the DASH as well as the PRWE. Improved pain, function, and survival outcomes were seen in those who underwent PRC after the age of 40, had a preoperative diagnosis of Kienböck's disease, underwent a concomitant neurectomy procedure, were non-laborers, and underwent surgery after 1990. At present we reserve PRC for patients with advanced (stage 3 and greater) Kienböck's disease who are greater than 40 years of age and have low demands for their wrist.

## Conclusion

Proximal row carpectomy is an effective salvage procedure for advanced Kienböck's disease (Lichtman stages 3 and 4). Indications for PRC include patients with persistent pain despite nonoperative management, with an intact capitate and lunate fossa. Careful patient selection is critical, and optimal results are obtained in patients older than 40 years of age who do not engage in heavy manual labor. A PRC is contraindicated if there is arthritis of the lunate fossa and/or capitate, in which case other options including scaphocapitate fusion or a dorsal capsular interposition can be performed.

Long-term studies have shown maintenance of good outcomes and relief of symptoms, despite the presence of degenerative changes at the new articulation. Long-term studies are required to determine the durability of capsular interposition in the presence of cartilage wear and arthritis.

## References


1. Crabbe WA. Excision of the proximal row of the carpus. J Bone Joint Surg Br. 1964;46:708–11.
2. Green DP. Proximal row carpectomy. Hand Clin. 1987;3:163–8.
3. Culp RW, McGuigan FX, Turner MA, Lichtman DM, Osterman AL, McCarroll HR. Proximal row carpectomy: a multicenter study. J Hand Surg Am. 1993;18:19–25.
4. Ryu JY, Cooney 3rd WP, Askew LJ, An KN, Chao EY. Functional ranges of motion of the wrist joint. J Hand Surg Am. 1991;16:409–19.
5. Palmer AK, Werner FW, Murphy D, Glisson R. Functional wrist motion: a biomechanical study. J Hand Surg Am. 1985;10:39–46.
6. Chim H, Moran SL. Long-term outcomes of proximal row carpectomy: a systematic review of the literature. J Wrist Surg. 2012;1:141–8.
7. Baumeister S, Germann G, Dragu A, Tränkle M, Sauerbier M. Functional results after proximal row carpectomy (PRC) in patients with SNAC-/SLAC-wrist stage II. Handchir Mikrochir Plast Chir. 2005;37:106–12.
8. Dacho AK, Baumeister S, Germann G, Sauerbier M. Comparison of proximal row carpectomy and midcarpal arthrodesis for the treatment of scaphoid nonunion advanced collapse (SNAC-wrist) and scapholunate advanced collapse (SLAC-wrist) in stage II. J Plast Reconstr Aesthet Surg. 2008;61:1210–8.
9. Imbriglia JE, Broudy AS, Hagberg WC, McKernan D. Proximal row carpectomy: clinical evaluation. J Hand Surg Am. 1990;15:426–30.
10. Hawkins-Rivers S, Budoff JE, Ismaily SK, Noble PC, Haddad J. MRI study of the capitate, lunate, and lunate fossa with relevance to proximal row carpectomy. J Hand Surg Am. 2008;33:841–9.
11. Ali MH, Rizzo M, Shin AY, Moran SL. Long-term outcomes of proximal row carpectomy: a minimum of 15-year follow-up. Hand. 2012;7:72–8.

12. Diao E, Andrews A, Beall M. Proximal row carpectomy. Hand Clin. 2005;21:553–9.
13. Wall LB, Didonna ML, Kiefhaber TR, Stern PJ. Proximal row carpectomy: minimum 20-year follow-up. J Hand Surg Am. 2013;38:1498–504.
14. Croog AS, Stern PJ. Proximal row carpectomy for advanced Kienböck's disease: average 10-year follow-up. J Hand Surg Am. 2008;33:1122–30.
15. DiDonna ML, Kiefhaber TR, Stern PJ. Proximal row carpectomy: study with a minimum of ten years of follow-up. J Bone Joint Surg Am. 2004;86:2359–65.
16. Lichtman DM, Lesley NE, Simmons SP. The classification and treatment of Kienböck's disease: the state of the art and a look at the future. J Hand Surg Eur Vol. 2010;35:549–54.
17. Lumsden BC, Stone A, Engber WD. Treatment of advanced-stage Kienböck's disease with proximal row carpectomy: an average 15-year follow-up. J Hand Surg Am. 2008;33:493–502.
18. Nanavati VN, Werner FW, Sutton LG, Klena J. Proximal row carpectomy: role of a radiocarpal interposition lateral meniscal allograft. J Hand Surg Am. 2009;34:251–7.
19. Eaton RG. Proximal row carpectomy and soft tissue interposition arthroplasty. Tech Hand Up Extrem Surg. 1997;1:248–54.
20. Ilyas AM. Proximal row carpectomy with a dorsal capsule interposition flap. Tech Hand Up Extrem Surg. 2010;14:136–40.
21. Kwon BC, Choi SJ, Shin H, Baek GH. Proximal row carpectomy with capsular interposition arthroplasty for advanced arthritis of the wrist. J Bone Joint Surg Br. 2009;91:1601–6.
22. Wagner ER, Bravo D, Elhassan B, Moran SL. Factors associated with improved outcomes following Proximal Row Carpectomy; a long-term outcome study of 144 patients. J Hand Surg Eur Vol. 2016; 41:484.

# 21 Scaphotrapeziotrapezoid and Scaphocapitate Fusion in Kienböck's Disease

Daniel J. Mastella and H. Kirk Watson

## Rationale

The lunate represents the central load-bearing column of the wrist and is critical to wrist function [1]. The osteonecrosis of Kienböck's disease compromises the load bearing capabilities of the lunate [2–6]. The patient's ability to use the wrist in Kienböck's disease is first limited by synovitis that produces pain and stiffness [7–9]. As the disease progresses, the collapse and fragmentation of the lunate produce additional mechanical limitations, with the end result being destruction of the radiolunate joint and collapse of the surrounding carpus due to loss of the keystone function of the lunate.

Preservation of the function of the wrist in the face of Kienböck's disease is the goal of treatment. The integrity of the lunate and the architecture of the carpus cannot be restored once lost; once progression of the disease threatens the integrity of the carpus, indication for surgical treatment exists [7, 9, 10]. Without treatment, irreversible fracture and fragmentation of the lunate and the collapse of the remainder of the carpus around the fragmented lunate destroys the function of the wrist. The principle of treatment for Kienböck's disease, therefore, is to preserve the lunate and the architecture of the surrounding carpus by redirecting the loads traversing the wrist around the lunate rather than through it [11–15]. The wrist loads can only be redirected around the lunate by forcing those loads through bone rather than relying on the natural ligament-bone system that directs the loads to the lunate. If we simplify the representation of the load bearing forces of the wrist, we find that the aggregate hand load can be represented as a vector oriented along the middle finger metacarpal [1, 4, 11]. This load is transmitted to the capitate, then to the lunate and on to the radius. Without the load bearing ability of the lunate, those forces seek another route [16, 17]. The ligamentous anatomy of the carpus is set to send those forces to the lunate and cannot, in the absence of the lunate, effectively transmit those forces to the radius via another route. Without the lunate, the loads across the carpus will cause it to collapse.

The scaphoid and scaphoid fossa have a bony contact surface area sufficient to accept the loads transmitted from the hand to the radius. Anatomically, however, the position of the scaphoid is out of line with the loads transmitted along the central ray of the middle finger metacarpal. However, using limited wrist arthrodesis techniques, the pathway of those loads can be redirected from the middle finger meacarpal, to the scaphoid and then to the radius. Two patterns of limited wrist arthrodesis can accomplish this

**Electronic supplementary material:** The online version of this chapter (doi:10.1007/978-3-319-34226-9_21) contains supplementary material, which is available to authorized users. Videos can also be accessed at http://link.springer.com/chapter/[10.1007/978-3-319-34226-9_21].

D.J. Mastella, MD (✉) • H.K. Watson, MD
The Hand Center, University of Connecticut, 195 Eastern Boulevard, Suite 200, Glastonbury, CT 06033, USA
e-mail: djmastella@gmail.com

© Springer International Publishing Switzerland 2016

D.M. Lichtman, G.I. Bain (eds.), *Kienböck's Disease*, DOI 10.1007/978-3-319-34226-9_21

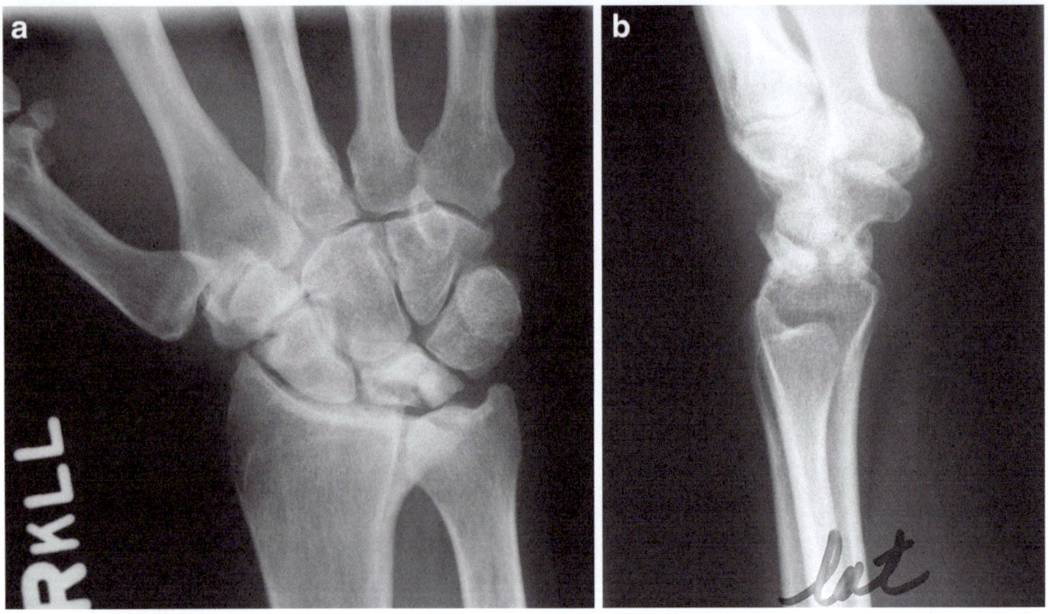


**Fig. 21.1** (**a**, **b**) Right wrist of 54-year-old male with stage 3b Kienböck's disease. STT fusion will unload the lunate to allow for potential healing and prevent secondary collapse of the wrist. Note the typical coronal split of the lunate in Kienböck's disease, seen on the lateral image

redirection: scaphotrapeziotrapezoid (STT) arthrodesis and scaphocapitate (SC) arthrodesis (Figs. 21.1 and 21.2) [12, 16–21].

The biomechanics of limited wrist arthrodesis are well established [2, 11, 19, 20, 22, 23]. It is critical to follow the principles to redirection of the loads through the wrist that will unload the diseased lunate in Kienböck's disease. Our goal in Kienböck's disease is to redirect the wrist loads into the scaphoid fossa of the radius. The ulnar wrist anatomy is unable to take up the loads across the wrist and any residual load will pass into the lunate, worsening the destruction of the wrist. STT or SC arthrodesis can unload the lunate by redirecting the forces into the scaphoid fossa.

## Indications

In Kienböck's disease, the lunate will often heal and ultimately remain a load-bearing member of the carpus. The long-term outcome of the wrist depends in part on the condition of the lunate. As a result, the optimal time to operate to redistribute loads through the wrist is before collapse of the external dimensions of the lunate. Therefore, we immobilize the wrist at the time of diagnosis of Kienböck's, but will proceed to STT fusion upon radiographic or clinical progression of disease.

In more advanced Kienböck's disease (3B or 4), after collapse of the external dimensions of the lunate, STT fusion can redirect essentially all the wrist loads through the scaphoid and unload the collapsed lunate [11, 19, 20, 23]. Even with a fragmented lunate, redirection the wrist loads through the scaphoid will reduce patient symptoms and improve function of the wrist.

We uniformly retain the fragmented lunate, as wrist ligament function is better with the lunate in place; excision of the lunate may contribute to ulnar translation of the carpus. If the patient has late synovitis related to a fragmented lunate, it may be excised even years after healing of the fusion.

## Principles

The principles of intercarpal fusion are [16, 20, 24, 25]:

1. *Maintain the external dimensions of the carpus*. This principle is especially important in

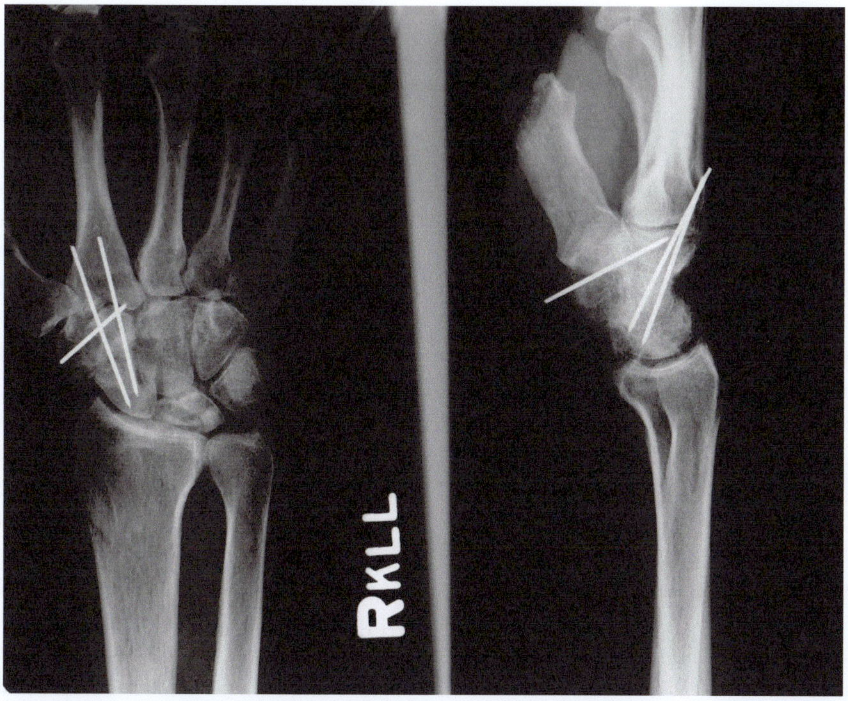


**Fig. 21.2** Patient from Fig. 21.1, s/p STT fusion. Pins are ready for removal. The volar to dorsal pin from the trapezium to the trapezoid is not necessary and is no longer used. Two 0.045 in. c-wires from the trapezoid to the scaphoid are sufficient with thumb spica cast immobilization

STT and SC fusions, as the remaining carpus requires normal alignment to provide functional motion. In STT fusion we use a 5 mm spacer, in addition to precise positioning of the wrist during pinning, to maintain the normal external dimensions of the STT joint after fusion. This principle also makes obvious the findings that STT fusion requires more bone graft than SLAC wrist reconstruction (where collapse of the capitate and hamate into the lunate and triquetrum is acceptable due to the lack of a scaphoid), and that compression screws are not desirable in STT fusion as they will reduce the external dimensions of the STT joint resulting in compromised wrist motion.

2. *Fuse only the joints necessary*; *do not fuse joints that are not involved.* Uninvolved, adjacent joints should not be pinned during STT or SC arthrodesis. The micro motion that occurs at the unfused joints will dissipate forces that would otherwise travel through the arthrodesis. Pinning of uninvolved joints results in added stress to the fusion site and potentiates a nonunion. By maintaining the articular surface of normal joints, wrist motion after limited wrist arthrodesis is maximized. Even joints with little motion under normal circumstances (e.g., the trapezoid-capitate joint) will allow some additional motion.
3. *Maximize surface area for arthrodesis.* All bones to be fused must be cut back to good cancellous bone, with all subchondral bony plate being removed. The entire fusion surface must be exposed and, in the case of STT fusion, the dorsal, non-articular cortex of the trapezium and trapezoid is included to augment the surface area. The larger the surface area, the better force transmission through the fusion site. Too small a fusion area, though healed, may result in pain with loading due to insufficient bone to carry the loads.
4. *Use dense cancellous autograft.* We use cancellous autograft from the distal radius almost

exclusively. Donor site morbidity is extremely low and the volume of bone available is adequate for use in the wrist and hand. The bone graft is densely packed into the fusion site to help with stability and provide a substrate for healing. Use of a dental amalgam tamp is essential to achieve the high density of bone graft for optimal fusion.

5. *Immobilize until fused, and then mobilize fully*. The fusion mass must be protected with immobilization until it has united. Early motion before it has united, compromises the stability, and threatens development of a nonunion. Once it has united, it can then be actively mobilized to optimize function.

## Surgical Technique for STT Fusion

The procedure can be seen in the accompanying video (Video 21.1).

STT fusion is approached using a transverse incision at the level of the STT joint [13, 14, 16, 18]. Transverse incisions at the dorsal wrist are far superior to longitudinal incisions as they allow for fewer adhesions to the extensor tendons and dorsal radial sensory nerve. The transverse incision crosses these structures at one point, rather than along their course as a longitudinal incision does. The transverse incision is, however, not extensile, so the incision must be correctly placed to provide proper exposure for a dorsal wrist procedure. Landmarks for the transverse incision for STT or SC fusion are found by palpating the distal radius.

The surgeon's thumb is placed on the tip of the radial styloid and the index finger on Lister's tubercle as our points of reference on the radius. A transverse incision is made at the level of the styloid. Dissection is carried down first to the level of the radiocarpal joint and the radioscaphoid articulation is inspected. If there is significant arthrosis at the proximal portion of the radioscaphoid articulation, not just at the dorsal ridge, but throughout the central portion of the proximal pole's articulation at the scaphoid facet, then a proximal row carpectomy, wrist fusion or total wrist arthroplasty may be a more appropriate procedure [16]. There may be eburnation or loss of cartilage at the dorsal edge of the scaphoid facet in cases of scaphoid instability. This finding does not contraindicate going forward with an STT fusion, as the STT fusion will control the dorsal skidding of the scaphoid, which causes the cartilage erosion. With improved stability, the scaphoid will no longer articulate at the marginal arthrosis. Similarly, arthritis that is limited to the distal scaphoid facet can be successfully treated with STT fusion as the styloid is excised as a portion of the procedure [26]. After inspection of the joint, the radial styloid is excised up to a maximum of 5 mm, preserving the origins of the radioscaphocapitate and long radiolunate upslope ligaments [27].

Attention is then turned to the STT joint. Approach is performed through the second dorsal compartment, between the extensor carpi radialis longus (ECRL) and extensor carpi radialis brevis (ECRB) tendons. These tendons are retracted and dorsal capsulectomy is performed. Curettes and rongeurs are used to take down the distal articular surface of the scaphoid, and the proximal articular surfaces at the trapezium and trapezoid. The amount of bone resection at the joint is critical. The entire cartilage surface is removed, as well as the subchondral plate of all three bones. Bony excision proceeds on the articular and nearby non-articular portions of the scaphoid, trapezium and trapezoid. The excision of all the subchondral bone exposes good cancellous bone, which is appropriate for fusion. Using a rongeur to lever distally along the trapezoid and trapezium enables the tip of the rongeur to curve around to the volar articular surface of the distal scaphoid to effectively resect this portion of the joint as well. The proximal half of the articulation between the trapezium and trapezoid is resected and the distal half is maintained.

At this juncture, the bone graft is taken from the ipsilateral distal radius [28]. A second transverse incision is made over the distal radius just proximal to Lister's tubercle, and subcutaneous tissues are dissected down to the interval between the first and second dorsal compartments. The first and second dorsal compartments are elevated subperiosteally, exposing sufficient distal radius just proximal to the styloid for bone graft harvesting. A 4 mm osteotome is then used to create a teardrop-shaped window with the apex of the tear aimed proximally. The window is removed and bone graft is curetted out. The window is then replaced and the first and second dorsal compartments fall back into their normal position.

This bone is then taken distally to the STT fusion site and a portion of the bone graft is placed in the volar aspect of the arthrodesis. Once volar graft is in place, the joints are pinned. Two 0.045 in. K-wires are drilled through the trapezoid. These are placed parallel to one another through the trapezoid in line with the scaphoid. Care is taken to angle them so that they are parallel to the scaphocapitate distal articulation.

Next, the more ulnar pin is advanced to the proximal bony surface of the trapezoid. A 5-mm spacer (we use the handle of a small double skin hook) is placed between the dorsal surface of the scaphoid and trapezoid and the wrist is placed in full radial deviation, 45° extension, with the surgeon's thumb pressing up on the volar tubercle of the scaphoid to stabilize it. This position gives the appropriate level of reduction of the scaphoid to approximately a 60° scapholunate angle [16, 29]. The more radial wire in the trapezoid is advanced into the scaphoid, the spacer removed, and the ulnar pin advanced into the scaphoid. This completes the fusion as the trapezium is rigidly attached to the trapezoid. A third pin can be placed through the trapezium into the scaphoid, if needed. A third pin is needed in cases where the finished construct seems less than stable or there are other negative factors such as heavy smoking, less than reliable patient cast care, etc. The rest of the bone graft is then packed densely with a dental amalgam tamp into the space between the scaphoid, trapezium, and trapezoid. A relatively large amount of bone graft is required for STT fusion as the external dimensions of the joint need to be maintained rather than collapsing the joint down in order to get fusion. By maintaining the height of the joint, the STT fusion becomes a loading column in the radial aspect of the wrist rather than collapsing down and allowing the load to move through the lunate. The lunate itself is never excised at the index procedure to prevent ulnar translation of the carpus. If symptoms occur due to a retained fragment of lunate, it can be removed later. This maintenance of height is in contradistinction to the SLAC wrist reconstruction where, due to the entire mid-carpal joint being involved, the bones can be collapsed into the space provided by the resection thus requiring less bone graft [20].

After bone graft is complete, ECRL and ECRB tendons are returned to their normal positions and the wound is closed with monofilament absorbable suture. The hand is dressed from fingertip to mid forearm with bulky, fluff gauze dressing to achieve soft tissue stabilization. It is critical that enough soft goods are used to make the anteroposterior dimension of the hand in the dressing as large as the width of the hand to avoid compression of the metacarpus when wrapping the hand. Bias cut hand wrap is used to give firm static compression and elastic bandages are to be avoided. This dressing is standard in reconstructive hand surgery, and critical to preserving the soft tissues of the hand. A long-arm thumb spica splint is applied in the operating room and, at 2 days postoperative, this dressing is converted to a long arm thumb spica cast. Long arm casting is continued for 3 weeks postoperatively. At the 3-week postoperative visit, the patient is converted from the long arm cast to a short arm thumb spica cast with the interphalangeal joint included. The patient is allowed finger motion from early on postoperatively as tolerated. Once adequate healing is seen on X-ray, which is typically at the 6-week mark, the pins are removed. The patient is started on range of motion for the wrist and continues range of motion for the digits (Figs. 21.3 and 21.4).

The technique for scaphocapitate fusion is similar to that of STT fusion [12, 17, 30–32]. The level of incision is the same as for STT fusion, but is placed more ulnarly and the wrist is approached between the second and fourth dorsal compartments. All of the principles of limited wrist arthrodesis must be followed, in particular

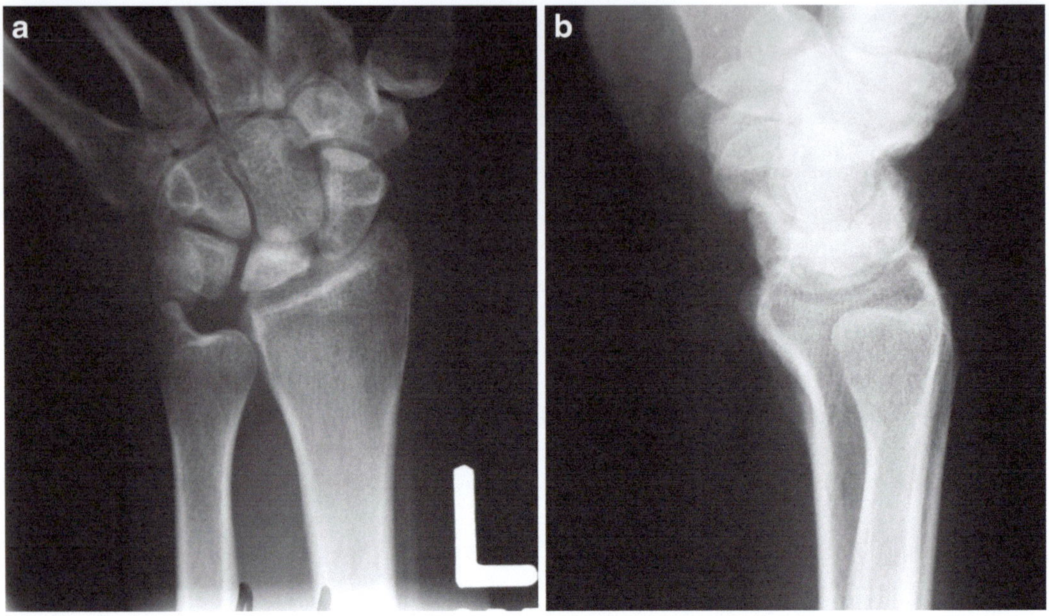


**Fig. 21.3** (**a**, **b**) Preoperative: 40-year-old female with Kienböck's disease, stage 3b

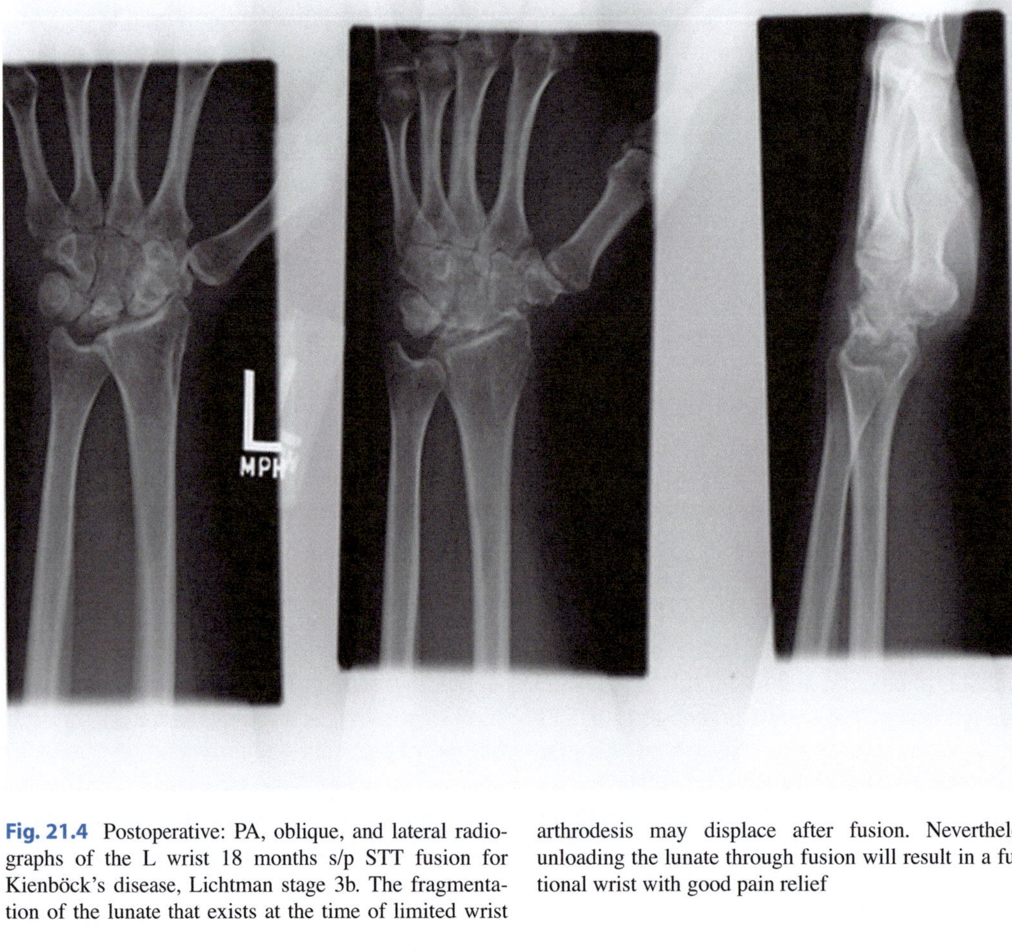


**Fig. 21.4** Postoperative: PA, oblique, and lateral radiographs of the L wrist 18 months s/p STT fusion for Kienböck's disease, Lichtman stage 3b. The fragmentation of the lunate that exists at the time of limited wrist arthrodesis may displace after fusion. Nevertheless, unloading the lunate through fusion will result in a functional wrist with good pain relief

maintaining the height of the carpus. The slope of the scaphocapitate joint tends to encourage proximal collapse of the joint after decortication. Care must me taken to preserve the external dimensions of the scaphocapitate joint to successfully transmit loads through the scaphoid facet. The correct position of the S-C fusion is best maintained by pins perpendicular to the plane of the fusion. We prefer the STT fusion to the S-C fusion; the fusion site is perpendicular to the loads and additional motion may be attained post op, as the joint between the trapezoid and the capitate will allow.

## Results

The results of both STT and SC fusion have shown them to effectively unload the lunate and transmit loads through the scaphoid [6, 12, 21, 30, 33–35]. There is a similar decrease in wrist motion after both procedures along with a decrease in pain and improvement in function [36].

## Conclusion

The ability to adjust the scaphoid and then stabilize it with STT and SC fusion allows the scaphoid to take a load through the radial column of the wrist and effectively unload the lunate in Kienböck's disease, improving force transmission across the wrist and, therefore, grip strength [14, 18, 37, 38]. Limited wrist arthrodesis is indicated in stage I when there is clinical or imaging progression of disease despite immobilization. When there is significant deterioration of the lunate, certainly by stage 2, limited wrist arthrodesis is strongly indicated. Grades 3a and 3b are good indications for a STT or SC fusion. In grade 4, the disease is advanced disease, so therefore a full wrist fusion is indicated.

## References


1. Viegas SF, Tencer AF, Cantrell J, Chang M, Clegg P, Hicks C, et al. Load transfer characteristics of the wrist. Part I. The normal joint. J Hand Surg Am. 1987;12(6):971–8.
2. Viegas SF, Tencer AF, Cantrell J, Chang M, Clegg P, Hicks C, et al. Load transfer characteristics of the wrist. Part II. Perilunate instability. J Hand Surg Am. 1987;12(6):978–85.
3. Tencer AF, Viegas SF, Cantrell J, Chang M, Clegg P, Hicks C, et al. Pressure distribution in the wrist joint. J Orthop Res. 1988;6(4):509–17.
4. Viegas SF, Patterson R, Peterson P, Roefs J, Tencer A, Choi S. The effects of various load paths and different loads on the load transfer characteristics of the wrist. J Hand Surg Am. 1989;14(3):458–65.
5. Patterson RM, Viegas SF, Elder K, Buford WL. Quantification of anatomic, geometric, and load transfer characteristics of the wrist joint. Semin Arthroplasty. 1995;6(1):13–9.
6. Iwasaki N, Genda E, Minami A, Kaneda K, Chao EY. Force transmission through the wrist joint in Kienböck's disease: a two-dimensional theoretical study. J Hand Surg Am. 1998;23(3):415–24.
7. Allan CH, Joshi A, Lichtman DM. Kienböck's disease: diagnosis and treatment. J Am Acad Orthop Surg. 2001;9(2):128–36.
8. Taniguchi Y, Yoshida M, Iwasaki H, Otakara H, Iwata S. Kienböck's disease in elderly patients. J Hand Surg Am. 2003;28(5):779–83.
9. Cross D, Matullo KS. Kienböck disease. Orthop Clin North Am. 2014;45(1):141–52.
10. Akelman E. Arthrodesis of the hand and wrist. In: Chapman MW, editor. Chapman's orthopaedic surgery. 3rd ed. Philadelphia, PA: Lippincott Williams & Wilkins; 2001.
11. Short WH, Werner FW, Fortino MD, Palmer AK. Distribution of pressures and forces on the wrist after simulated intercarpal fusion and Kienböck's disease. J Hand Surg Am. 1992;17(3):443–9.
12. Moy OJ, Peimer CA. Scaphocapitate fusion in the treatment of Kienböck's disease. Hand Clin. 1993;9(3):501–4.
13. Watson HK, Fink JA, Monacelli DM. Use of triscaphe fusion in the treatment of Kienböck's disease. Hand Clin. 1993;9(3):493–9.
14. Watson HK, Weinsweig J. Treatment of Kienböck's disease with triscaphe arthodesis. Proceedings of the 6th Congress of the International Federation of Societies for Surgery of the Hand, 1995: 347–49.
15. Yasuda M, Masada K, Takeuchi E, Ando Y. Scaphotrapeziotrapezoid arthrodesis for the treatment of Lichtman stage 3B Kienböck disease. Scand J Plast Reconstr Surg Hand Surg. 2005;39(4):242–6.
16. Watson HK, Hempton RF. Limited wrist arthrodeses. I. The triscaphoid joint. J Hand Surg Am. 1980;5(4):320–7.
17. Rhee PC, Lin IC, Moran SL, Bishop AT, Shin AY. Scaphocapitate arthrodesis for Kienböck disease. J Hand Surg Am. 2015;40(4):745–51.
18. Watson HK, Ryu J, DiBella A. An approach to Kienböck's disease: triscaphe arthrodesis. J Hand Surg Am. 1985;10(2):179–87.
19. Viegas SF, Patterson RM, Peterson PD, Pogue DJ, Jenkins DK, Sweo TD, et al. Evaluation of the biomechanical efficacy of limited intercarpal fusions for the

treatment of scapho-lunate dissociation. J Hand Surg Am. 1990;15(1):120–8.
20. Watson HK, Weinsweig J. Intercarpal arthrodesis. In: Green DP, Hotchkiss RN, Pederson NC, editors. Operative hand surgery. 4th ed. New York, NY: Churchill Livingstone; 1998.
21. Meier R, van Griensven M, Krimmer H. Scaphotrapeziotrapezoid (STT)-arthrodesis in Kienböck's disease. J Hand Surg Br. 2004;29(6):580–4.
22. Iwasaki N, Minami A, Miyazawa T, Kaneda K. Force distribution through the wrist joint in patients with different stages of Kienböck's disease: using computed tomography osteoabsorptiometry. J Hand Surg Am. 2000;25(5):870–6.
23. Stewart DT, Froelich JM, Shin AY. Intercarpal arthrodeses. J Hand Surg Am. 2014;139(2):373–7.
24. Watson HK, Goodman ML, Johnson TR. Limited wrist arthrodesis. Part II: Intercarpal and radiocarpal combinations. J Hand Surg Am. 1981;6(3):223–33.
25. Watson HK. Triscaphe fusion for chronic scapholunate instability. In: Gelberman RH, editor. Master techniques in orthopaedic surgery: the wrist. New York, NY: Raven; 1994. p. 183–94.
26. Krimmer H, Krapohl B, Sauerbier M, Hahn P. Posttraumatic carpal collapse (SLAC- and SNAC-wrist)--stage classification and therapeutic possibilities. Handchir Mikrochir Plast Chir. 1997;29(5):228–33.
27. Rogers WD, Watson HK. Radial styloid impingement after triscaphe arthrodesis. J Hand Surg Am. 1989;14(2 Pt 1):297–301.
28. Guidera PM, Watson HK, Dwyer TA, Orlando G, Zeppieri J, Yasuda M. Lunotriquetral arthrodesis using cancellous bone graft. J Hand Surg Am. 2001;26(3):422–7.
29. Kleinman WB, Carroll CT. Scapho-trapezio-trapezoid arthrodesis for treatment of chronic static and dynamic scapho-lunate instability: a 10-year perspective on pitfalls and complications. J Hand Surg Am. 1990;15(3):408–14.
30. Pisano SM, Peimer CA, Wheeler DR, Sherwin F. Scaphocapitate intercarpal arthrodesis. J Hand Surg Am. 1991;16(2):328–33.
31. Sennwald GR, Ufenast H. Scaphocapitate arthrodesis for the treatment of Kienböck's disease. J Hand Surg Am. 1995;20(3):506–10.
32. Gislason MK, Stansfield B, Bransby-Zachary M, Hems T, Nash DH. Load transfer through the radiocarpal joint and the effects of partial wrist arthrodesis on carpal bone behaviour: a finite element study. J Hand Surg Eur Vol. 2012;37(9):871–8.
33. Iwasaki N, Genda E, Barrance PJ, Minami A, Kaneda K, Chao EY. Biomechanical analysis of limited intercarpal fusion for the treatment of Kienböck's disease: a three-dimensional theoretical study. J Orthop Res. 1998;16(2):256–63.
34. Lee JS, Park MJ, Kang HJ. Scaphotrapeziotrapezoid arthrodesis and lunate excision for advanced Kienböck disease. J Hand Surg Am. 2012;37(11):2226–32.
35. Luegmair M, Saffar P. Scaphocapitate arthrodesis for treatment of late stage Kienböck disease. J Hand Surg Eur Vol. 2014;39(4):416–22.
36. Nakamura R, Horii E, Watanabe K, Nakao E, Kato H, Tsunoda K. Proximal row carpectomy versus limited wrist arthrodesis for advanced Kienböck's disease. J Hand Surg Br. 1998;23(6):741–5.
37. Weinzweig J, Watson HK, Herbert TJ, Shaer JA. Congenital synchondrosis of the scaphotrapeziotrapezoidal joint. J Hand Surg Am. 1997;22(1):74–7.
38. Hohendorff B, Mühldorfer-Fodor M, Kalb K, van Schoonhoven J, Prommersberger KJ. STT arthrodesis versus proximal row carpectomy for Lichtman stage IIIB Kienböck's disease: first results of an ongoing observational study. Arch Orthop Trauma Surg. 2012;132(9):1327–34.

# Radioscapholunate Fusion in Kienböck's Disease

# 22

Ngoc Buu Ha, Joideep Phadnis, and Gregory Ian Bain

## Introduction

Radioscapholunate (RSL) fusion is a partial wrist fusion for localized disease with an intact midcarpal articulation. It is indicated for degenerative, inflammatory, post-traumatic, and Kienböck's arthritis [1]. The midcarpal joint is preserved, which is responsible for the dart thrower's motion, which is essential for daily use of a functional hand [2, 3].

N.B. Ha, MBBS
Department of Orthopedics and Trauma, Royal Adelaide Hospital, North Tce, Adelaide, SA 5000, Australia

J. Phadnis, FRCS (Tr & Orth)
Department of Trauma and Orthopedics, Brighton and Sussex University Hospitals, NHS Trust, Eastern Road, Brighton, East Sussex BN1 6AG, UK

G.I. Bain, MBBS, FRACS, FA(Ortho)A, PhD (✉)
Professor, Upper Limb and Research, Department of Orthopedic Surgery, Flinders University and Flinders Medical Centre, Bedford Park, Adelaide, SA, Australia
e-mail: greg@gregbain.com.au

## Preoperative Assessment

### Indications

If conservative modalities, such as modification of activities, analgesics, and use of a splint, have failed, surgical management may be considered. It is essential to identify which joints are involved in the disease process. An absolute prerequisite for this procedure is a functional midcarpal articulation (Fig. 22.1), to achieve painless motion following the fusion [4]. In Kienböck's disease, the RSL fusion can be performed where the cartilage deformities are limited to the proximal lunate and/or lunate facet. That is, cases with a Bain and Begg grade 1 or 2a (Fig. 22.2) [5].

### Imaging

Plain radiographs should be performed to determine the diagnosis and to assess the extent of the disease, including the status of the midcarpal joint. Computed tomography (CT) scan and magnetic resonance imaging are also of value in determining the extent of the disease in the lunate, and the remainder of the carpus. Arthroscopy is the gold standard to determine the integrity of the articular surfaces. Intraoperative direct visualization of the articular cartilage can be the final decision as to whether or not to proceed with the limited fusion.

© Springer International Publishing Switzerland 2016
D.M. Lichtman, G.I. Bain (eds.), *Kienböck's Disease*, DOI 10.1007/978-3-319-34226-9_22

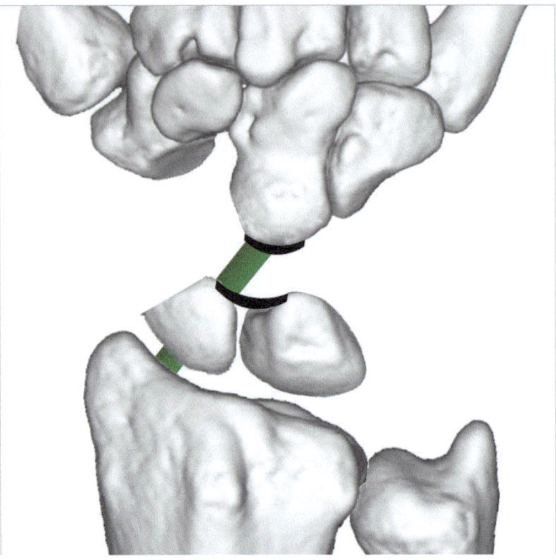

**Fig. 22.1** Prerequisite for radioscapholunate fusion: a functional scaphoid, lunate, and capitate articulation. The radioscaphocapitate ligament is important to maintain stability. Copyright Dr. Gregory Bain

### Fixation

There are many described methods of fixation for RSL fusion. These include K-wires, staples, plates, and screws [1, 6–9]. We used a set of principles when performing limited wrist fusions (Table 22.1) [1]. The insertion of K-wires allows for simple and accurate positioning to avoid impingement, however they do not offer compression. Non-locking plates have been associated with dorsal impingement, loss of fixation, and nonunion [8, 9]. We have used memory staples (Depuy International Ltd., Leeds, UK) as they are low profile and provide dynamic compress across the fusion site (Fig. 22.3a–c) [10]. Fixation devices with greater stability allow for earlier mobilization of the wrist.

## Types of Fusion

### Radioscapholunate Fusion

#### Surgical Technique

A dorsal approach via the third extensor compartment is used to expose the carpus. Some authors recommend excision of the posterior interosseous nerve, however we prefer to leave it intact to optimize proprioception. Using hand held curettes and rongeurs, the joint surfaces of the proximal scaphoid, lunate, and distal radius are thoroughly debrided. We avoid power instruments that may burn the bone. Using a closing fusion technique the radiocarpal fusion mass is stabilized (Fig. 22.4). That is, the full thickness of the articular surfaces are excised to allow the osseous structures to close [1]. To obtain a good long-term outcome, it is important to create a "stand-alone joint" which can potentially obtain a good long term outcome. Therefore the midcarpal joint surface of the scaphoid and lunate are perfectly aligned. We reduce the scapholunate interval, and stabilize it with 2 × 1.1 mm K-wires. Bone graft from the iliac crest is used to supplement the fusion mass.

The radiocarpal joint is then stabilized in 15° of extension, in order to achieve maximum extension and grip strength. The fusion site is stabilized using one of the methods described earlier (see Fig. 22.3a). Intraoperative fluoroscopy is used to confirm the position of the fusion mass and the internal fixation.

A plaster slab is then applied and the patient encouraged to elevate the arm and mobilize the fingers. At 1 week, a full cast or removable splint is applied, depending upon patient factors and the fixation. At 6 weeks the wrist is mobilized with graduated wrist strengthening and motion exercises.

#### Results

Variable rates of nonunion have been recorded between 0 and 25 % [4, 11, 12]. This is thought to be due to the scaphoid acting as a long lever and increasing pressure through the fusion mass [1].

The patients usually obtain good pain relief; however, there is a reduction in wrist range of motion. Normally the scaphoid flexes during wrist flexion and radial deviation. Thus, a fused radioscaphoid joint will mostly affect wrist movement in these two directions. The range of motion is 33–40 % of the normal wrist [12, 13], with a 40–50° flexion–extension (F-E) arc, and 21–28° radial–ulnar (R-U) arc [8, 14, 15].

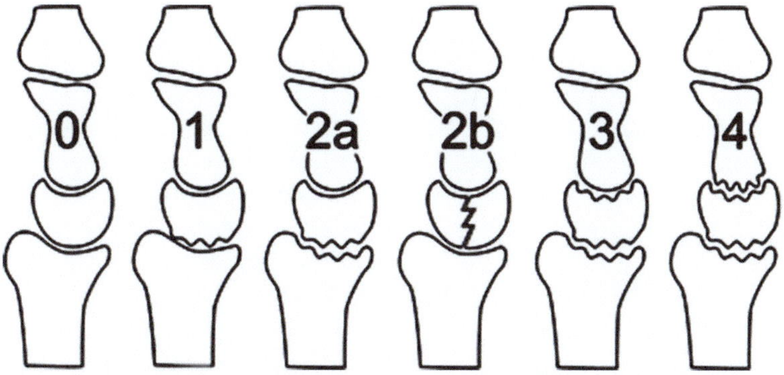


**Fig. 22.2** Bain and Begg arthroscopic classification for Kienböck's disease [1]. The grade is determined by the number of nonfunctional articular surfaces. The grading system assists the surgeon to determine the surgical treatment, based on the pathoanatomic findings. RSL fusion is indicated for grade 1 or 2a. Reproduced with permission Bain GI, Begg M. Arthroscopic assessment and classification of Kienböck's disease. Tech Hand Up Extreme Surg. 2006, 10(1): 8–13

**Table 22.1** Principles of limited wrist fusion[a]

| |
|---|
| Localized disease |
| Stand-alone joint |
| Mechanical debridement |
| Surface area of fusion mass |
| Respect the grid |
| Containment (e.g., triquetrum excision) |
| Closing fusion |
| Bone graft augmentation |
| Aim at extension |

[a]Modified with permission Bain GI, McGuire DT. Decision making for partial carpal fusions. J Wrist Surg. 2012, 1(2): 103–114. Copyright © 2012, Rights Managed by Georg Theime Verlag KG Stuttgart, New York

A long-term study by Nagy and Büchler reported an undesirable high complication rate with RSL fusion. Five of their 15 patients (33 %) required a full wrist fusion at a mean of 8 years. Average range of motion was 18° flexion, 32° extension, 25° ulnar, and 3° radial deviation. More than half developed midcarpal arthritis and 27 % had a nonunion. Good results were reported for only seven (47 %) of their patients [8].

Shin and Jupiter reviewed a series of five patients with two angled 2.4 mm distal radius locking plates across the fusion mass to achieve complete union in all patients. Functional outcome was not reported [11].

## RSL with Distal Scaphoid Excision

RSL fusion can be performed with excision of the distal scaphoid (see Fig. 22.3b), which can be used as bone graft. Clinical studies have reported that adding excision of the distal scaphoid improved motion [13], lowered the rate of nonunion [6] and midcarpal arthritis [16].

A cadaveric study by McCombe et al. demonstrated that excision of the distal scaphoid increased in the mean F-E arc from 60° to 122° and R-U deviation from 34° to 43° [13]. A similar study by Bain et al. reported that excision of the distal scaphoid reduced the long lever arm of the scaphoid and unlocked the midcarpal joint to increase wrist flexion and radial deviation (Table 22.2) [17].

Garcia-Elias et al. completed a review of 16 patients with RSL fusion and distal scaphoidectomy and reported improvement in pain, flexion, and radial deviation compared to previous studies with RSL fusions only. They reported no nonunions and a lower rate of midcarpal arthritis [12].

## RSL with Distal Scaphoid and Triquetrum Excision

Excision of the triquetrum decreases the containment of the midcarpal joint, and therefore increases the joint motion (see Fig. 22.3c and

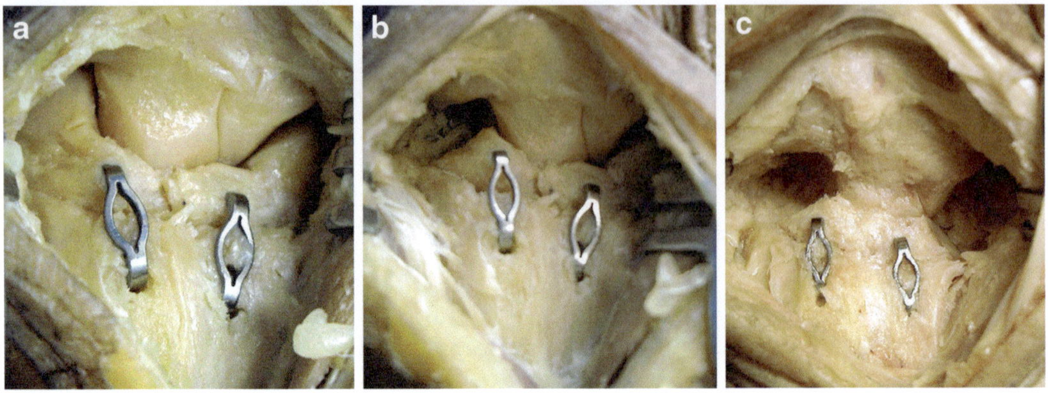


**Fig. 22.3** (**a**) Cadaveric model of RSL fusion using memory staples. (**b**) Excision of the distal scaphoid increases flexion and radial deviation. (**c**) Excision of the distal scaphoid and triquetrum increases extension and ulnar deviation. Reproduced with permission Bain GI, Sood A, Yeo CJ. RSL Fusion with excision of distal scaphoid and triquetrum: a cadaveric study. J Wrist Surg. 2014; 3(1): 37–41. Copyright © 2014, Rights Managed by Georg Theime Verlag KG Stuttgart, New York

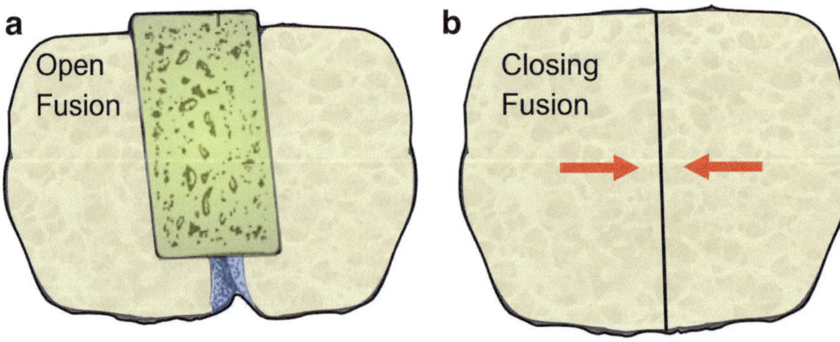


**Fig. 22.4** (**a**) Open fusion technique maintains height. (**b**) Closing fusion allows for bony apposition, stability, and increased union rate. Reproduced with permission from Bain GI, McGuire DT. Decision making for partial carpal fusions. J Wrist Surg. 2012, 1(2): 103–114. Copyright © 2012, Rights Managed by Georg Thieme Verlag KG Stuttgart, New York

**Table 22.2** Measured wrist motion of RSL fusion; cadaveric study[a]

| Procedures | Flexion | Extension | F-E arc | %[b] | RD | UD | R-U arc | %[c] |
|---|---|---|---|---|---|---|---|---|
| Capsulotomy | 59 | 57 | 116 | – | 22 | 24 | 46 | – |
| RSL fusion | 36 | 38 | 74 | 64 | 14 | 18 | 32 | 70 |
| Distal scaphoid excision | 49 | 50 | 99 | 85 | 22 | 21 | 43 | 93 |
| Triquetrum excision | 56 | 56 | 11 | 97 | 23 | 29 | 52 | 113 |

Data are expressed as the mean measured ROM in degrees
[a]Modified with permission from Bain GI, Sood A, Yeo CJ. RSL fusion with excision of distal scaphoid and triquetrum: A cadaveric study. J Wrist Surg. 2014; 3(1): 37–41. Copyright © 2012, Rights Managed by Georg Theime Verlag KG Stuttgart, New York
[b]Percentage from the baseline F-E arc
[c]Percentage from the baseline R-U arc

Table 22.2) [17, 18]. The triquetrum is the best bone graft as the scaphoid is often sclerotic.

Cadaveric studies have been published on the effect of additional triquetrectomy to RSL fusion and distal scaphoid excision. Bain et al. reported that excision of the triquetrum will improve the R-U arc by a further 21 % compared to RSL and distal scaphoidectomy alone (Table 22.3) [17].

**Table 22.3** Percentage change in ROM at each stage of the procedure[a]

| Procedures | Flexion | Extension | F-E arc | RD | UD | R-U arc |
|---|---|---|---|---|---|---|
| RSL fusion | −39 | −33 | −36 | −36 | −25 | −30 |
| Distal scaphoid excision | 36 | 32 | 34 | 57 | 17 | 34 |
| Triquetrum excision | 14 | 12 | 13 | 5 | 38 | 21 |

[a]Modified with permission from [17]. Copyright © 2012, Rights Managed by Georg Theime Verlag KG Stuttgart, New York

Berkhout et al. reported that the RSL fusion decreased the range of motion in all directions [14]. They reported excision of the scaphoid typically improves the F-E arc, while R-U deviation is most improved after excision of the triquetrum.

We have performed a minimum 10-year follow-up study of our RSL fusions, which include excision of the distal scaphoid and triquetrum in 24 patients. A mean follow-up of 14.7 years found these patients to have a strong trend toward a greater R-U arc than RSL fusion alone and RSL fusion with scaphoidectomy. There were no nonunions and radiological results showed preservation of the midcarpal joint. Pain scores progressively improved from pre-operation, to 2 years to 10 years following surgery. Patient satisfaction rate was 94 %.

## Long-Term Follow-Up of RSL Fusion in Kienböck's Disease

Of the 24 patients who had a RSL fusion, three patients had Kienböck's disease. They were all either Bain and Begg grade 2a or 1. One patient underwent RSL fusion, while two had RSL fusion with distal scaphoidectomy.

### Patient 1

Patient 1 is a 61-year-old female who had a RSL fusion with K-wires and staples to her nondominant wrist. Preoperatively, she had visual analogue scale (VAS) pain score of 4/10.

Six months post-operatively, plain radiographs demonstrated union of the fusion. At 18.4 years she was satisfied, with VAS pain score 0/10. Quick DASH score 6.8/100 and Mayo wrist score 85/100, which is graded as a good.

### Patient 2

Patient 2 is a 55-year-old male who had a RSL fusion with excision of the distal scaphoid. Once the necrotic part of the lunate was excised, the remaining lunate was thought to be too small for staples, and was therefore stabilized with K-wires. The K-wires were removed at 15 weeks. By 7 months he had return to full-time work with restricted duties.

At 17.7 years he was satisfied with VAS score 0/10, Quick DASH 11.4/100, and Mayo Wrist score 65 was satisfactory. Plain radiographs demonstrated a solid fusion and preservation of the midcarpal joint (Fig. 22.5).

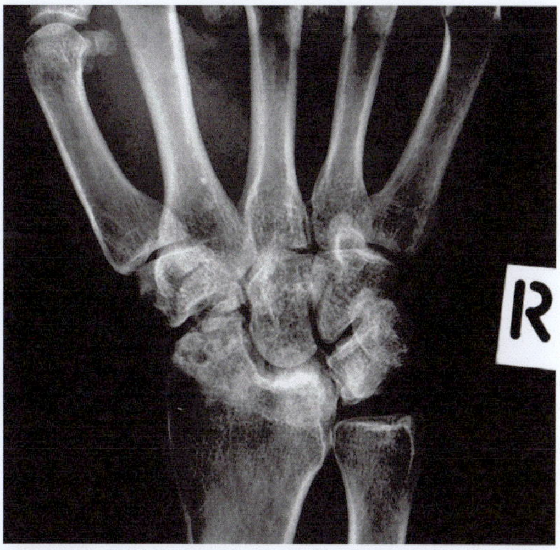


**Fig. 22.5** Patient 2: Plain radiograph demonstrating solid fusion and preservation of the midcarpal joint at 17.7 years follow-up. Copyright Dr. Gregory Bain

## Patient 3

Patient 3 is a 72-year-old male who also had a RSL fusion with excision of his distal scaphoid on his dominant wrist, using staples. In view of the associated ulnar wrist pain symptoms, a matched hemiresection of the distal ulna was also performed.

At 17.5 years follow-up he was satisfied with VAS pain score 1/10, Quick DASH 29.5/100 and Mayo wrist score 60. Plain radiographs confirmed union with preservation of the midcarpal articulation (Fig. 22.6a) and normal alignment (see Fig. 22.6b).

For the three Kienböck's patients, the mean F-E arc was 46.6° and R-U deviation arc 20.8°. There were no nonunions or other complications and none of them required a full wrist fusion. The mean scaphocapitate and lunocapitate joint spaces measured 2.0 mm and 1.7 mm respectively, reflecting negligible progression to midcarpal arthritis.

Clearly this is a small cohort; however, with such a long follow-up these results are certainly pleasing. We attribute the good results to:

1. Closely applied indications for surgery, in particular a well-preserved midcarpal joint.
2. Following the principles of limited wrist fusion (see Table 22.1) [1].
3. That a perfect reduction of the midcarpal joint is obtained.
4. Good stability of the radiocarpal joint until union.

As the reader would note, we began performing the RSL fusion for Kienböck's disease many years ago, in this very specific patient cohort. Since then newer methods of investigation have been introduced, such as gadolinium-enhanced MRI, which may further narrow the indication for this procedure.

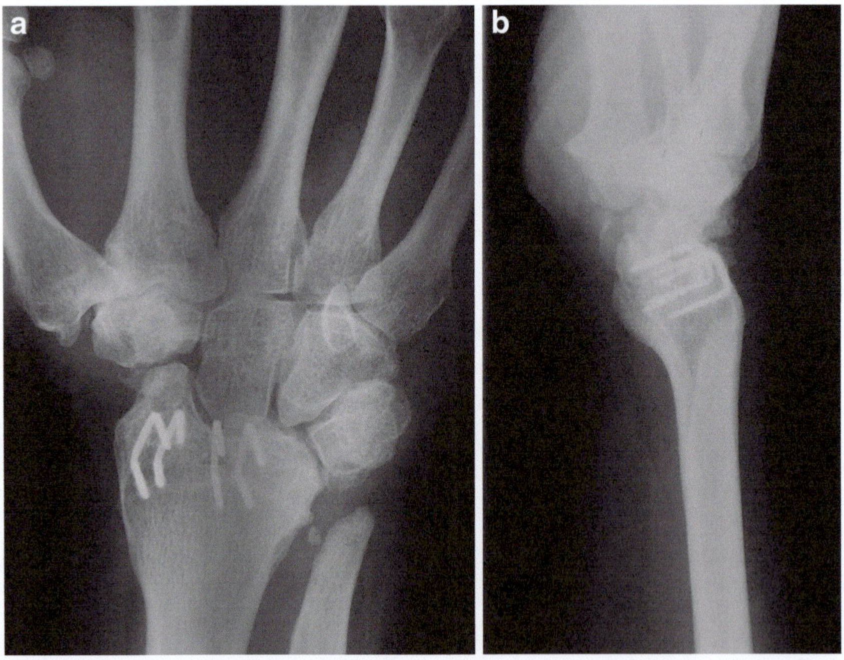

**Fig. 22.6** (**a**) Patient 3: Plain radiograph demonstrating solid RSL fusion with distal scaphoid excision and ulnar hemiresection. There is preservation of the midcarpal joint. (**b**) Patient 3: Plain lateral radiograph demonstrating normal radiocarpal alignment. Copyright Dr. Gregory Bain

## Conclusion

RSL fusion is indicated for patients with localized arthritis of the wrist with an intact midcarpal articulation. This procedure can include excision of the distal scaphoid and triquetrum, which increases the motion and union rate. Long-term outcome studies have shown RSL fusion to be sustainable with good clinical and radiological outcomes in those patients in which the midcarpal joint is anatomically reduced and fusion mass well stabilized.

## References


1. Bain GI, McGuire DT. Decision making for partial carpal fusions. J Wrist Surg. 2012;1(2):103–14.
2. Crisco JJ, Coburn JC, Moore DC, Akelman E, Weiss SP, Wolfe SW. In vivo radiocarpal kinematics and the dart thrower's motion. J Bone Joint Surg Am. 2005;87:2729–40.
3. Wolfe SW, Crisco JJ, Orr CM, Marzke MW. The dart-throwing motion of the wrist: is it unique to humans? J Hand Surg Am. 2006;31:1429–37.
4. Bain GI, Ondimu P, Hallam P, Ashwood N. Radioscapholunate arthrodesis - a prospective study. Hand Surg. 2009;14(2–3):73–82.
5. Bain GI, Begg M. Arthroscopic assessment and classification of Kienböck's disease. Tech Hand Upper Extrem Surg. 2006;10(1):8–13.
6. Mühldorfer-Fodor M, Ha HP, Hohendorff B, Löw S, Prommersberger KJ, Van Schoonhoven J. Results after radioscapholunate arthrodesis with or without resection of the distal scaphoid pole. J Hand Surg Am. 2012;37(11):2233–9.
7. Ishikawa H, Murasawa A, Nakazono K. Longerm follow-up study of radiocarpal arthrodesis for the rheumatoid wrist. J Hand Surg Am. 2005;30:658–66.
8. Nagy L, Buchler U. Long-term results of radioscapholunate fusion following fractures of the distal radius. J Hand Surg Br. 1997;22(6):705–10.
9. Mulford JS, Ceulemans LJ, Nam D, Axelrod TS. Proximal row carpectomy vs four corner fusion for scapholunate (Slac) or scaphoid nonunion advanced collapse (Snac) wrists: a systematic review of outcomes. J Hand Surg Eur Vol. 2009; 34:256–63.
10. Bain GI, Watts AC. The outcome of scaphoid excision and four-corner arthrodesis for advanced carpal collapse at a minimum of ten years. J Hand Surg Am. 2010;35(5):719–25.
11. Shin EK, Jupiter JB. Radioscapholunate arthrodesis for advanced degenerative radiocarpal osteoarthritis. Tech Hand Up Extrem Surg. 2007;11(3):180–3.
12. Garcia-Elias M, Lluch A, Ferreres A. Treatment of radiocarpal degenerative osteoarthritis by radioscapholunate arthrodesis and distal Scaphoidectomy. J Hand Surg Am. 2005;30:8–15.
13. McCombe D, Ireland DCR, McNab I. Distal scaphoid excision after radioscaphoid arthrodesis. J Hand Surg Am. 2001;26:877–82.
14. Berkhout MJ, Shaw MN, Berglund LJ, An KN, Berger RA, Ritt MJ. The effect of radioscapholunate fusion on wrist movement and the subsequent effects of distal scaphoidectomy and triquetrectomy. J Hand Surg Eur Vol. 2010;35(9):740–5.
15. Bach AW, Almquist EE, Newman DM. Proximal row fusion as a solution for radiocarpal arthritis. J Hand Surg Am. 1991;16(3):424–31.
16. Hug U, Guggenheim M, Kilgus M, Giovanoli P. Treatment of radiocarpal degenerative osteoarthritis by radioscapholunate arthrodesis: long-term follow-up. Chir Main. 2012;31(2):71–5.
17. Bain GI, Sood A, Yeo CJ. RSL fusion with excision of distal scaphoid and triquetrum: a cadaveric study. J Wrist Surg. 2014;3(1):37–41.
18. Bain GI, Sood A, Ashwood A, Turner PC, Fogg G. Effect of scaphoid and triquetrum excision on limited arthrodesis of the wrist: a laboratory study. J Hand Surg Eur Vol. 2009;34:614–7.

# 23 Lunarectomy and Progressive Capitate Lengthening (Modified Graner–Wilhelm Procedure)

Frédéric A. Schuind and Fabian Moungondo

Kienböck's disease predominantly affects young adults, between 20 and 40 years of age, usually male manual workers. The condition is most often unilateral [1, 2]. Many patients seek medical advice with an already advanced Lichtman stage III disease as defined by the presence of lunate collapse. Actually, stage III is subdivided into stage III-A, with preserved carpal height, and stage III-B, with diminished carpal height and fixed palmar flexion of the scaphoid [3–5]. Unlike the scaphoid malposition seen in advanced scapholunate lesions, no dorsal translation of the scaphoid proximal pole is observed in stage III-B [6], which may explain why stage III Kienböck's does not always progress to stage IV (with osteoarthrosis) and, when it does, why there is frequently a long delay between the two stages.

The treatment of stage III Kienböck's disease remains controversial, and the literature provides no evidence to support one therapeutic option over another. It is well known that symptoms are not correlated with the radiographic stage [7]. Asymptomatic patients should probably be conservatively treated, except for carpal tunnel release in the presence of an associated median nerve compression [1]. But symptomatic patients may benefit from an operation. The goals of surgery are to lower the load applied on the lunate, to preserve carpal height in stage III-A or restore it in stage III-B, to maintain hand strength and to prevent degenerative osteoarthrosis. This is usually achieved by intercarpal fusion by either scapho-trapezio-trapezoidal or scapho-capitate arthrodesis. However, intercarpal fusions cause marked loss of wrist range of motion and may be complicated by non-union or late osteo-arthrosis [2, 8]. Procedures indicated for stage II cases (no lunate collapse) like capitate shortening, forearm levelling or lunate revascularization may still be used in selected stage III cases. Another quite simple option is wrist denervation, without attempting to change the natural evolution of the lunate osteonecrosis, but to diminish the painful symptoms.

The morphology of the capitate head is relatively similar to the proximal pole of the lunate, making it well suited to articulate with the lunate fossa of the radius. This is what occurs after proximal carpal row resection [9]. Thus, another option for treating stage III Kienböck's disease is to replace the lunate by the head of the capitate. This is done by lunate resection and capitate lengthening, displacing the head of the capitate from the midcarpal joint to articulate with the lunate fossa of the radius, between the scaphoid and the triquetrum. This concept was originally proposed in 1966 by Graner [10], who performed capitate lengthening along with intercarpal fusion [10–12]. His patients obtained rel-

F.A. Schuind, MD, PhD (✉) • F. Moungondo, MD
Department of Orthopedics and Traumatology, Erasme University Hospital, Université libre de Bruxelles (ULB), 808 route de Lennik, Brussels 1070, Belgium
e-mail: Frederic.Schuind@Erasme.ulb.ac.be

© Springer International Publishing Switzerland 2016
D.M. Lichtman, G.I. Bain (eds.), *Kienböck's Disease*, DOI 10.1007/978-3-319-34226-9_23

atively good wrist motion and grip strength, but many ultimately developed radio-carpal osteo-arthrosis [13]. The Graner procedure has been criticised for this reason, and also because of the potential for devascularization of the head of the capitate with subsequent osteonecrosis. Indeed, the head of the capitate has a retrograde blood flow across the capitate waist, similar to the blood supply of the scaphoid [14]. Other complications were also reported, including non-union of the lengthened capitate [15]. Because of these problems use of the classical Graner operation was almost abandoned. In 1997, however, Wilhelm et al. [16] proposed progressive lengthening of the capitate by external fixation (callus distraction), thereby reducing the risks of osteonecrosis and non-union. However, they did not advocate performing an associated pan carpal arthrodesis. Wilhelm et al. [16], and later Hierner and Wilhelm [17], reported good long term results using this method, particularly in regard to grip strength and the absence of degenerative osteo-arthrosis. The only problem mentioned was some palmar flexion of the proximal capitate fragment caused by traction by the palmar ligaments, which potentially could lead to long-term degenerative changes at the radio-capitate joint. De Smet and Degreef [8] criticised the Wilhelm operation, believing its advantages were relatively limited compared to a simple proximal carpal row resection, and fearing that it could result in impingement between the radial styloid and the scaphoid. According to Fontaine [1], however, the results of proximal carpal row resection were not particularly good in Kienböck's cases. This opinion was controversial and not shared by others [20] but proximal row resection has been reported to result in long-term osteo-arthrosis of the new radio-capitate joint [1, 18–20]. This appears not to be the case after progressive capitate lengthening because the scaphoid and triquetrum are preserved and the carpal load is not exclusively applied to the lunate fossa.

This chapter presents the technique of lunarectomy and progressive capitate lengthening, as we have used it at our Institution (Fig. 23.1a–i).

## Indications

The modified Graner procedure with progressive capitate lengthening by external fixation is indicated in Lichtman stage III-A or III-B cases, without chondral lesions at either lunate fossa of the distal radius or head of capitate, that is in Bain–Begg Kienböck's grades 0 or 1 [21]. The status of the joints should therefore be assessed before the operation by either dedicated MR sequences, arthro-CT or by arthroscopy, as there is no relationship between the Lichtman stage and the Bain–Begg grade [1, 7, 21, 22]. The Bain–Begg grade is correlated to age [7], however, so the modified Graner procedure is in fact usually performed in relatively young patients.

## Surgical Technique

A dorsal arciform incision is performed, avoiding the future location of the external minifixation pins. The Berger ligament-preserving dorsal approach is used to expose the lunate and capitate bones, keeping some dorsal capsule inserted on the capitate. This allows partial denervation by resection of the distal dorsal interosseous nerve, if desired. After local synovectomy, the next step is the atraumatic resection of the necrotic, and usually fragmented, lunate. The cartilage of the lunate fossa and capitate head is inspected. Through separate stab wounds, two external minifixation pins (2 mm) are then implanted in the head of the capitate and two identical pins implanted in the corpus of the bone. Using an oscillating saw and cooling irrigation, a transverse osteotomy is then performed at the junction of the middle and the distal third of the capitate (more distal than at the neck). The surgeon makes sure that the osteotomy is complete but does not lengthen the capitate at this time in order to preserve the blood supply to the head of the capitate. The external mini-fixation lengthening device (Hoffmann II Micro Lengthener, Stryker Trauma®, Selzach, Switzerland) is then mounted on the pins. Contrary to the technique described by Wilhelm et al. [16], we do not temporarily transfix the scapho-capitate or

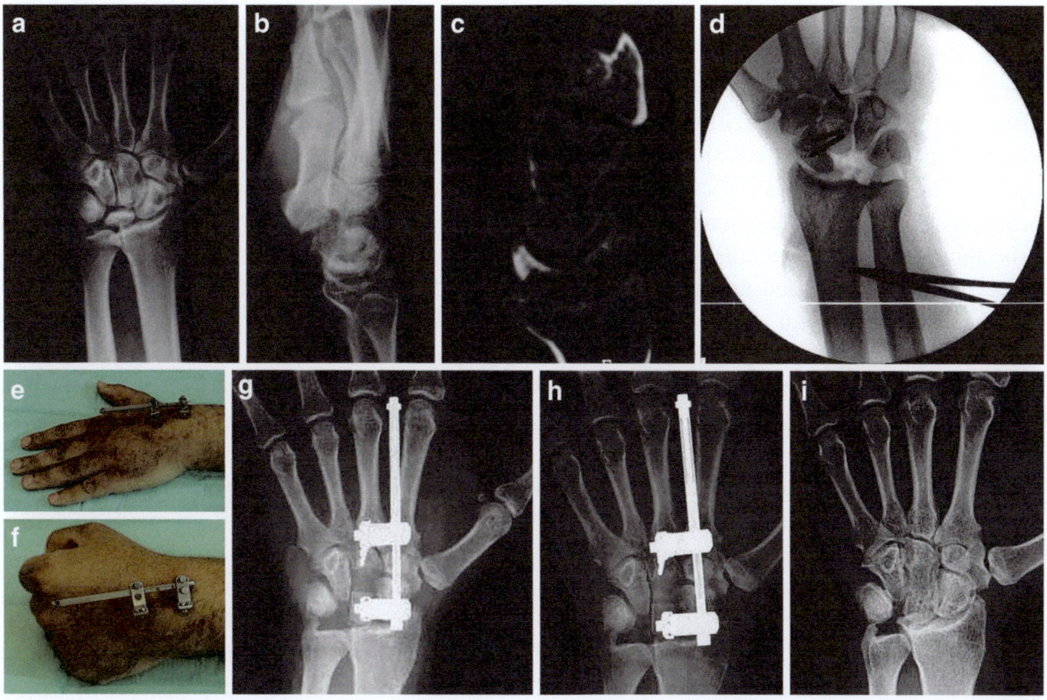


**Fig. 23.1** Graner–Wilhelm progressive lengthening of the capitate after lunarectomy for the treatment of a patient with stage III-B Kienböck's disease of the left wrist. (**a**, **b**) Preoperative X-rays. Note the existence of a lunate distal medial facet for articulation with the hamate (Viegas type II lunate). (**c**) Preoperative CT scan, demonstrating fragmentation of the necrotic lunate. (**d**) After resection of the lunate by dorsal approach, 39/2 mm external minifixation half pins are implanted in the head and corpus of the capitate. An osteotomy was then performed at the capitate's corpus, distal to the capitate neck. (**e–g**) Progressive distraction is applied after 7 days without wrist/hand immobilisation. (**h**, **i**) X-rays 32 days 46 days (**h**) and 4 years (**i**) after the initial operation with solid healing of the capitate and restoration of the carpal height. There is no evidence of osteo-arthrosis but the scaphoid is still moderately palmarly flexed. Note the space between capitate and triquetrum. At 4 years follow-up, the patient had slight persistent pain (VAS 1/10). His wrist joint motion was acceptable but somewhat reduced compared to the preoperative measurements. Parts (**a**) through (**h**) are from Schuind F, Eslami S, Ledoux P. Kienböck's disease. *J Bone Joint Surg* [*Br*] 2008;90:133–9. (Figures 1a, 1b, 2, 3, 2a, 4b, 5a, 5b and 5c). Reproduced with permission and copyright © of the British Editorial Society of Bone and Joint Surgery

scapho-trapezio-trapezoidal joints. Closure is done over suction drainage. No splint is used (see Fig. 23.1) and the patient is encouraged to actively mobilise the wrist and fingers.

After 7–10 days, progressive distraction is begun three times each day; 0.25 mm in the morning, 0.25 mm at noon, and 0.50 mm in the evening for a total of 1 mm/day. The distraction is not particularly painful and does not require the prescription NSAIDs, which are potentially harmful to bone distraction osteogenesis. Gentle cleansing of the pin's skin exit sites is performed twice a day. The distraction period is quite short, as the total lengthening required is only about 10–12 mm, at which point the capitate head reaches the distal radius joint surface and the carpal height is regained. The fixator is kept in place until bone healing is complete. After radiological confirmation of a solid bridge between the head and the corpus of the capitate, the fixator is removed under light anaesthesia.

## Discussion

As noted by Facca et al. [23], several related techniques are known by the name of Graner. What is usually referred to as the "Graner II" operation consists of lunate resection, intraoperative capitate lengthening with interposition of cancellous bone chips, and intercarpal bone arthrodesis leaving the trapezium un-fused. The Graner II procedure was subsequently modified by Fenollosa and Valverde [24], who limited the arthrodesis to the capitate–hamate joint. The procedure was further modified by Wilhelm et al. [16], who proposed progressive capitate lengthening. Finally, Lu et al. reported proximal transposition of the capitate on a vascularized pedicle as a replacement for the necrotic lunate [9, 25].

We believe that the progressive callus distraction of the capitate is an excellent procedure in Lichtman stage III Kienböck's cases without chondral lesions at the lunate fossa or the capitate head. The duration of capitate lengthening is relatively limited, about 10 days. The osteogenesis in this highly cancellous bone is relatively quick, so that the external minifixator can be removed within 3 months (to shorten the external fixation period, Hierner and Wilhelm [17] suggested replacing the minifixator—after lengthening—by percutaneous Kirschner wires). The procedure seems less painful than the classical Graner II procedure, and no immobilisation is necessary limiting the risks of CRPS and stiffness. The risks of devascularisation of the capitate head and of capitate non-union are reduced because the head is not forcefully mobilised but slowly displaced proximally and because the osteotomy is performed distal to the neck [17, 26]. There is no additional morbidity for bone graft harvesting. The procedure preserves hand strength by restoring carpal height. However, there is loss of wrist motion subsequent to bridging of the mid carpus [12, 24], analogous to the decrease seen following luno-capitate fusion. Finally, in theory there should be less degenerative changes at the radio-capitate joint than after a proximal carpal row resection because the scaphoid continues to transmit most of the carpal load. Indeed, after an in vitro simulation of the operation, Jia et al. [27] measured unchanged distribution of articular stresses.

The operation has limitations and risks. The patient will perform the actual lengthening; therefore good patient cooperation is mandatory. Wrist infection from the external fixation pins is a possibility. Toward the end of the lengthening period the proximal pin may impinge on the dorsal rim of the distal radius, limiting the possibility of wrist extension exercises. When the capitate head is narrower than the lunate, as in Viegas type II lunates [28], some gap between the lengthened capitate and the triquetrum is usual, however, this has been an inconsequential finding in our practice (see Fig. 23.1i). Owing to the good stability of the Stryker® minifixator distraction device we have not experienced the flexion deformity of the capitate head as reported by Hierner and Wilhelm [17].

## Conclusion

There are several different operations under the name of Graner. The technique presented in this chapter combines resection of the necrotic fractured lunate, osteotomy within the distal corpus of the capitate and implantation of an external minifixator with subsequent progressive lengthening of the bone until the carpal height is restored. This modified Graner–Wilhelm operation necessitates excellent cooperation from the patient and imposes about 3 months of external minifixation. It is indicated as an alternative to an intercarpal arthrodesis in stage III Kienböck's, in selected cases without cartilage degeneration at the head of the capitate and/or lunate fossa. It is not indicated in stage I and stage II disease, where radial shortening or lunate revascularization is indicated and stage IV disease.

## References

1. Fontaine C. Kienböck's disease. Chir Main. 2015; 34(1):4–17.
2. Schuind F, Eslami S, Ledoux P. Kienböck's disease. J Bone Joint Surg Br. 2008;90(2):133–9.
3. Goldfarb CA, Hsu J, Gelberman RH, Boyer MI. The Lichtman classification for Kienböck's disease: an assessment of reliability. J Hand Surg Am. 2003; 28:74–80.
4. Jafarnia K, Collins ED, Kohl HW, Bennett JB, Ilahi OA. Reliability of the Lichtman classification of

Kienböck's disease. J Hand Surg Am. 2000;25: 529–34.
5. Lichtman DM, Mack GR, MacDonald RI, Gunther SF, Wilson JN. Kienböck's disease. The role of silicone replacement arthroplasty. J Bone Joint Surg Am. 1977;59:899–908.
6. Kawanishi Y, Moritomo H, Omokawa S, Murase T, Sugamoto K, Yoshikawa H. In vivo 3-dimensional analysis of stage III Kienböck disease: pattern of carpal deformity and radioscaphoid joint congruity. J Hand Surg Am. 2015;40(1):74–80.
7. Tatebe M, Hirata H, Shinohara T, Yamamoto M, Okui N, Kurimoto S, et al. Arthroscopic findings of Kienböck's disease. J Orthop Sci. 2011;16(6):745–8.
8. De Smet L, Degreef I. Treatment options in Kienböck's disease. Acta Orthop Belg. 2009;75(6): 715–26.
9. Lu L, Gong X, Liu Z, Zhang Z. Capitate transposition to replace necrotic lunate bone with a pedicle for Kienböck's disease: review of 30 cases. Chin Med J (Engl). 2003;116(10):1519–22.
10. Graner O, Lopes EI, Carvalho BC, Atlas S. Arthrodesis of the carpal bones in the treatment of Kienböck's disease, painful ununited fractures of the navicular and lunate bones with avascular necrosis, and old fracture-dislocations of carpal bones. J Bone Joint Surg Am. 1966;48(4):767–74.
11. Nonnenmacher J, Naett R, Ben Abid M. Arthrodèse intracarpienne de revascularisation avec transposition du grand os (Graner type II). Ann Chir Main. 1982;1(3):256–9.
12. Takase K, Imakiire A. Lunate excision, capitate osteotomy, and intercarpal arthrodesis for advanced Kienböck disease. Long-term follow-up. J Bone Joint Surg Am. 2001;83(2):177–83.
13. Bartelmann U, Richter N, Landsleitner B. Operation nach Graner zur Therapie der Lunatumnekrose. Literaturübersicht und eigene Ergebnisse. Handchir Mikrochir Plast Chir. 1998;30(3):165–74.
14. Vander Grend R, Dell PC, Glowczewskie F, Leslie B, Ruby LK. Intraosseous blood supply of the capitate and its correlation with aseptic necrosis. J Hand Surg Am. 1984;9(5):677–83.
15. Ehall R, Pierer G, Neubauer W, Stampfel O. Interkarpale Pseudarthrose als Komplikation der Granerschen Operation. Handchir Mikrochir Plast Chir. 1989;21(5):257–61.
16. Wilhelm K, Hierner R, Brehl B. Kallusdistraktion zur progressiven Verlängerung des Os capitatum nach Resektion des Os lunatum bei Lunatummalazie im Stadium III. Operationstechnik und Eijjahres-Ergebnisse. Handchir Mikrochir Plast Chir. 1997; 29(1):10–9.
17. Hierner R, Wilhelm K. Long-term follow-up of callotasis lengthening of the capitate after resection of the lunate for the treatment of stage III lunate necrosis. Strat Trauma Limb Reconstr. 2010;5(1):23–9.
18. Croog AS, Stern PJ. Proximal row carpectomy for advanced Kienböck's disease: average 10-year follow-up. J Hand Surg Am. 2008;33(7):1122–30.
19. De Smet L, Robijns P, Degreef I. Proximal row carpectomy in advanced Kienbock's disease. J Hand Surg Br. 2005;30(6):585–7.
20. Lumsden BC, Stone A, Engber WD. Treatment of advanced-stage Kienböck's disease with proximal row carpectomy: an average 15-year follow-up. J Hand Surg Am. 2008;33(4):493–502.
21. Bain GI, Begg M. Arthroscopic assessment and classification of Kienböck's disease. Tech Hand Up Extrem Surg. 2006;10(1):8–13.
22. Watanabe K, Nakamura R, Imaeda T. Arthroscopic assessment of Kienböck's disease. Arthroscopy. 1995;11(3):257–62.
23. Facca S, Gondrand I, Naito K, Lequint T, Nonnenmacher J, Liverneaux P. Graner's procedure in Kienböck disease: a series of four cases with 25 years of follow-up. Chir Main. 2013;32(5):305–9.
24. Fenollosa J, Valverde C. Résultat des arthrodèses intracarpiennes dans le traitement des nécroses du semi-lunaire. Rev Chir Orthop Reparatrice Appar Mot. 1970;56(8):745–54.
25. Lu LJ, Gong X, Wang KL. Vascularized capitate transposition for advanced Kienböck disease: application of 40 cases and their anatomy. Ann Plast Surg. 2006;57(6):637–41.
26. Kerschbaumer F, Andree W, Poisel S. Lunatum-Malazie: Vergleich von Kapitatum –Verschiebeplastik und Silastic-Prothese. Orthopade. 1981;10(1):52–3.
27. Jia XY, Gong X, Lu LJ. Contact pressures in radiocarpal and triquetrohamate joints after vascularized capitate transposition. Ann Plast Surg. 2011;67(5):534–8.
28. Viegas SF, Wagner K, Patterson R, Peterson P. Medial (hamate) facet of the lunate. J Hand Surg Am. 1990;15(4):564–71.

# Arthroscopic Reconstructive Procedures for Kienböck's Disease: Arthroscopic Assisted Bone Grafting

24

Andrea Atzei and Loris Pegoli

## Introduction

Initial applications of wrist arthroscopy for the treatment of Kienbock's avascular necrosis were introduced at the end of 1990s, mainly for diagnostic purposes. In 1999, Menth-Chiari and colleagues [1] advocated the use of arthroscopy to assess the quality of the articular surfaces. The advantage of direct arthroscopic assessment is that it allows the surgeon to visually inspect and palpate the articular surfaces with no further threat to lunate vascularity. In addition, they reported that arthroscopic synovectomy and debridement of the necrotic fragmented lunate produced significant improvement in pain and wrist function for Lichtman grade IIIA or IIIB patients [3].

Accurate and specific arthroscopic assessment of the articular surface of the lunate and its adjacent articulations, form the basis of Bain and Begg's arthroscopic classification system [2]. In addition to classic staging, it has become a standard reference in the decision-making process for the treatment of Kienbock's disease. Since then, scant literature has been published regarding the use of arthroscopic reconstructive procedures for the treatment of Kienbock's disease. Exceptions include arthroscopic assisted drilling (forage) of the lunate [12], and more recently arthroscopic bone grafting of the lunate [11]. The aim of this paper is to describe the authors' experience with arthroscopic assisted bone grafting of the lunate in early Kienbock's disease.

A. Atzei, MD
Sezione di Chirurgia della Mano, Casa di Cura "Giovanni XXIII", Via Giovanni XXIII, 7, Monastier di Treviso 31050, Italy

L. Pegoli, MD (✉)
Hand and Reconstructive Microsurgery Unit, Humanitas San Pio X Clinic, Via F. Nava 31, Milan 20159, Italy
e-mail: info@drpegoli.com

## Methods

### Indications and Patient Selection

Patients affected by Lichtman's stage 1 Kienbock's disease, in which wrist pain showed no improvement after at least 3 months of conservative treatment, were considered eligible for arthroscopic assisted bone grafting. Kienbock's disease was diagnosed according to plain radiographs and MRI imaging that showed neither significant lunate collapse nor loss of its rotational alignment. Presence of diffuse MRI signal changes involving the whole lunate are considered pathognomonic of avascular necrosis, thus allowing differential diagnosis with other pathological conditions such ulnar–carpal abutment or intraosseous ganglion cysts. Intraoperative arthroscopic findings of significant chondral changes on either the midcarpal or the radiocarpal surfaces of the lunate, or both, were considered contraindications for the procedure.

© Springer International Publishing Switzerland 2016
D.M. Lichtman, G.I. Bain (eds.), *Kienböck's Disease*, DOI 10.1007/978-3-319-34226-9_24

## Surgical Technique

### Diagnositic Arthroscopy

Wrist arthroscopy is performed under regional anesthesia with the patient in the supine position, using standard wrist arthroscopic technique [4]. The arm is suspended by Chinese finger traps with about 3.5 kg of traction. A pneumatic tourniquet is used. Standard midcarpal and radiocarpal exploration is performed to confirm the absence of lunate chondropathy and associated lesions, confirming Lichtman's stage 1 and Bain and Begg's stage 0. The 3–4 and 6 R portals are used for scope and instrumentation, respectively.

### Lunate Drilling

The site of lunate drilling is localized on the dorso-ulnar aspect of the lunate in the less important load-bearing area, as close as possible to the proximal insertion of the lunotriquetral ligament. In order to confirm correct positioning of the drilling site, a needle is inserted under fluoroscopy (Fig. 24.1). A standard 3.0 mm motorized burr is used to remove the cartilage and the subchondral bone (Fig. 24.2a). Then, the burr's protection sleeve is shortened about a 1.5 cm, so that the burr's tip can be advanced into the lunate (Fig. 24.2b). This surgical step is performed under both arthroscopic and fluoroscopic control. Further advancement of the burr may require switching portals between the scope and the burr.

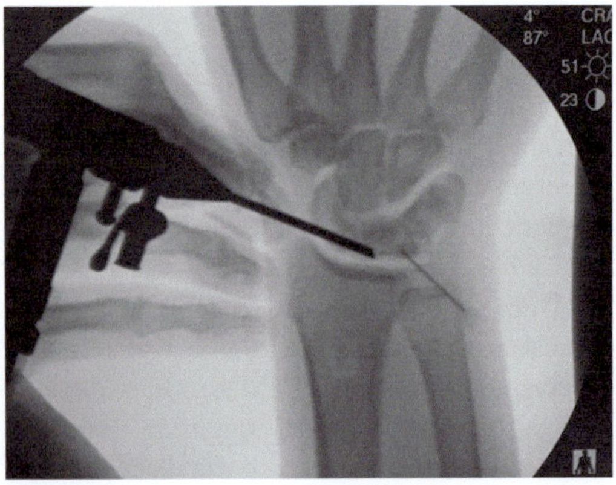

**Fig. 24.1** Intraoperative fluoroscopic view uses a needle to locate the drilling site on the dorso-ulnar aspect of the lunate

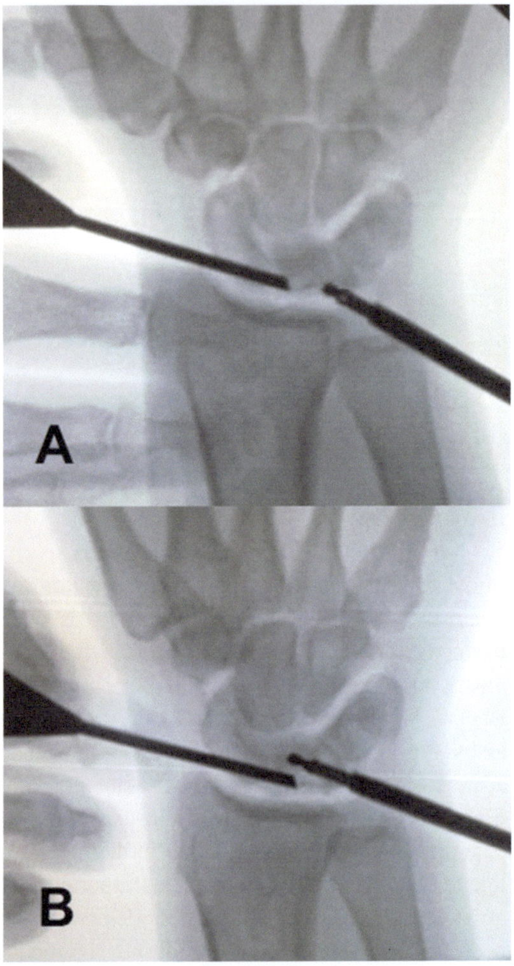


**Fig. 24.2** Intraoperative fluoroscopic view shows the scope in the 3–4 portal and the motorized burr in the 6R portal. The burr is positioned on the subchondral bone on the dorso-ulnar aspect of the lunate (**a**). It is then advanced into the lunate, to perform a core decompression (**b**)

When fluoroscopy confirms appropriate depth of the lunate cavity (Fig. 24.3), a 3-mm motorized shaver is introduced to debride the intraosseous cavity from the remaining soft tissues. To confirm the adequacy of the debridement and thorough soft tissues removal, the arthroscope can be introduced into the intraosseous cavity (Fig. 24.4), through the 6R portal.

### Bone Graft

Cancellous bone graft is then harvested from the volar aspect of the distal radius. A longitudinal incision is made on the volar aspect of the wrist,

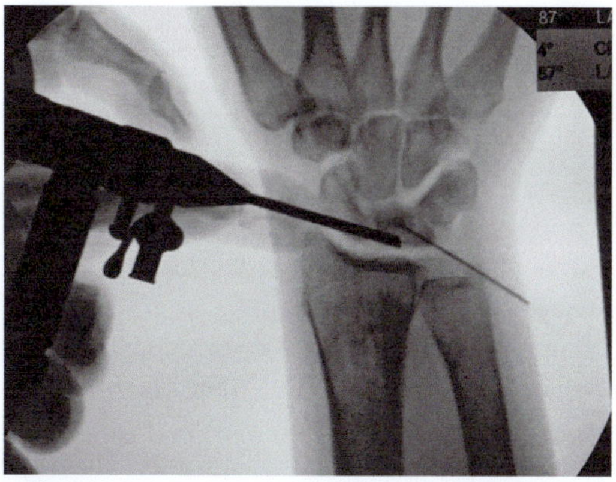

**Fig. 24.3** A needle is advanced into the lunate cavity and fluoroscopy is used to check proper drilling depth

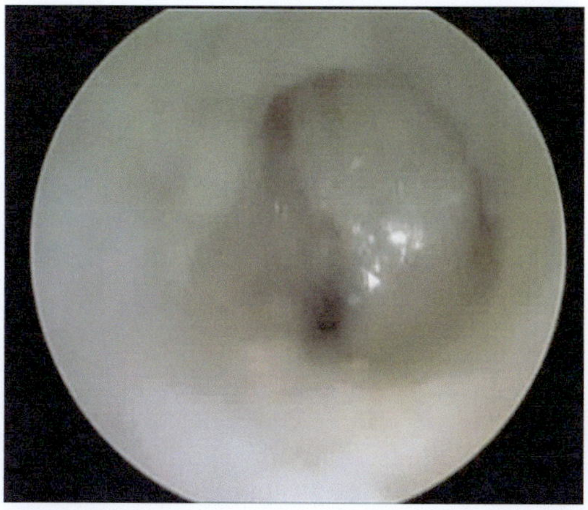

**Fig. 24.4** Arthroscopic view of the dorsal lunate, looking into the cavity, which has been created with a burr (scope in 6R portal)

along the radial margin of the flexor carpis radialis tendon sheath. The radial artery is separated with blunt dissection and protected. The pronator quadratus is divided along its fibers in order to expose the palmar cortex of the radius (Fig. 24.5). Through a small cortical window, the desired amount of bone is harvested by wide curettage of the radial metaphysis. At the end of the procedure, the skin of the forearm is closed with an intradermic suture. Then, a 3-mm cannula is advanced into the hole of the lunate, via 6-R portal. Fluoroscopy is used to confirm adequate positioning (Fig. 24.6). The harvested bone graft is inserted through the cannula (Fig. 24.7) and

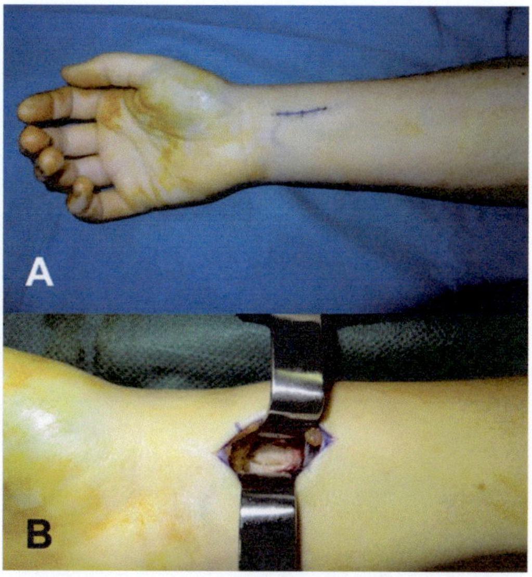


**Fig. 24.5** Planned skin incision on the palmar forearm (**a**) to access the metaphysis of the distal radius and create a cortical window for graft harvest (**b**)

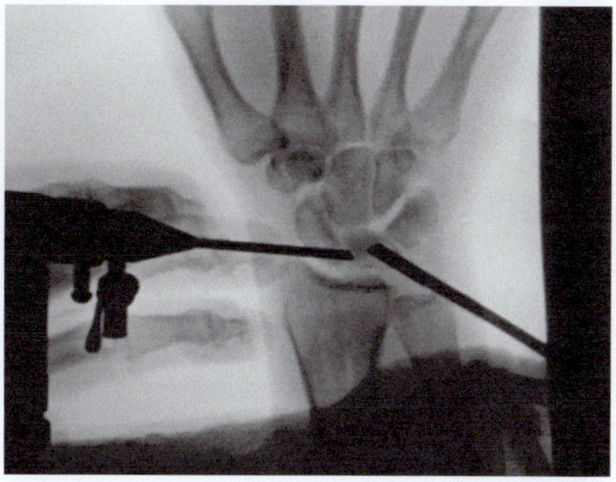

**Fig. 24.6** Fluoroscopy is used to confirm adequate positioning of a 3-mm cannula into lunate cavity. Note the defect in the metaphyseal radius, from where the bone graft was harvested

impacted into the lunate using a small tamping rod. This reduces the risk of any graft falling into the joint. The cavity is filled to the margin of the cortical bone, rather than to the level of the articular cartilage. The lunate is finally assessed arthroscopically (Fig. 24.8) and fluoroscopically to ensure correct positioning of the graft. The joint is irrigated and the portals closed with steristrips.

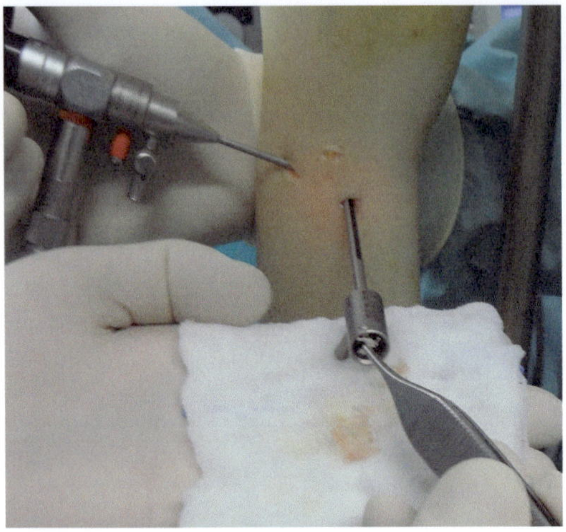

**Fig. 24.7** The bone graft is introduced into the cannula, then impacted into the lunate using a small tamping rod

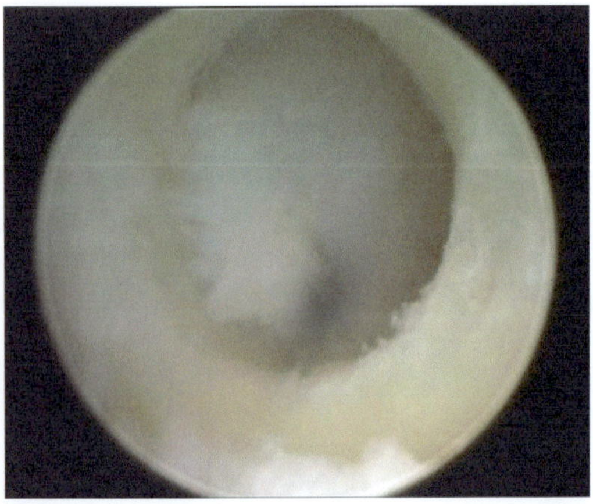

**Fig. 24.8** Graft filling of the lunate cavity is assessed with the scope

### Rehabilitation

A thermoplastic splint is applied for 4–6 weeks, according to radiological appearance of callus formation.

## Patient Series

From May 2008 to January 2011, arthroscopic assisted bone grafting of the lunate was performed in five patients. All patients were female, with an average age of 44 years (range: 25–59). The diagnosis of Kienbock's disease was made using standard radiographs and MRI according to the above eligibility criteria, so that all five patients were in Lichtman's stage 1. Indications for surgery were persistence of pain, restricted motion and function after 3 months of conservative treatment, consisting in physical therapy and wearing of a removable splint.

Intra-articular chondral involvement was also evaluated according to Bain and Begg's arthroscopic classification system [2], and all patients were classified as grade 0. The right (dominant) wrist was involved in three cases. Patients were assessed before the operation, after 1, 3, and 6 months and at final follow-up using the Mayo wrist score, Disability of Arm Shoulder Hand evaluation questionnaire (DASH), and Patient Related Wrist Evaluation (PRWE). Grip strength was measured using JAMAR® Hydraulic Hand Dynamometer and pinch strength using a JAMAR® Hydraulic Pinch Gauge. Pain was evaluated according to Visual Analogic Scale (VAS). Plain X-rays were evaluated at 1 week, 1 month, and 2 months after operation.

## Results

At an average follow-up of 32 months (12–46) all patients reported an improvement of symptoms and range of motion (Fig. 24.9). Mayo wrist score showed 4 excellent and 1 good result.

At final follow-up, there was improvement in the average of all the following outcome measures compared to the preoperative values:

DASH score improved from 88 (80–102) to 55 (45–70),
PRWE score from 71 (68–75) to 50 (36–60),
Grip strength 11 kg (8–13) to 19 kg (10–24),
Pinch strength 3 kg (3–4) to 5.2 kg (5–6),
VAS pain score at rest 5.6 (5–6) to 2.5 (2–3)
VAS pain score under load 7.4 (6–9) to 5 (3–8).

In all patients the X-rays showed an increase of lunate bone density and MRI showed an increase in the lunate vascular pattern.

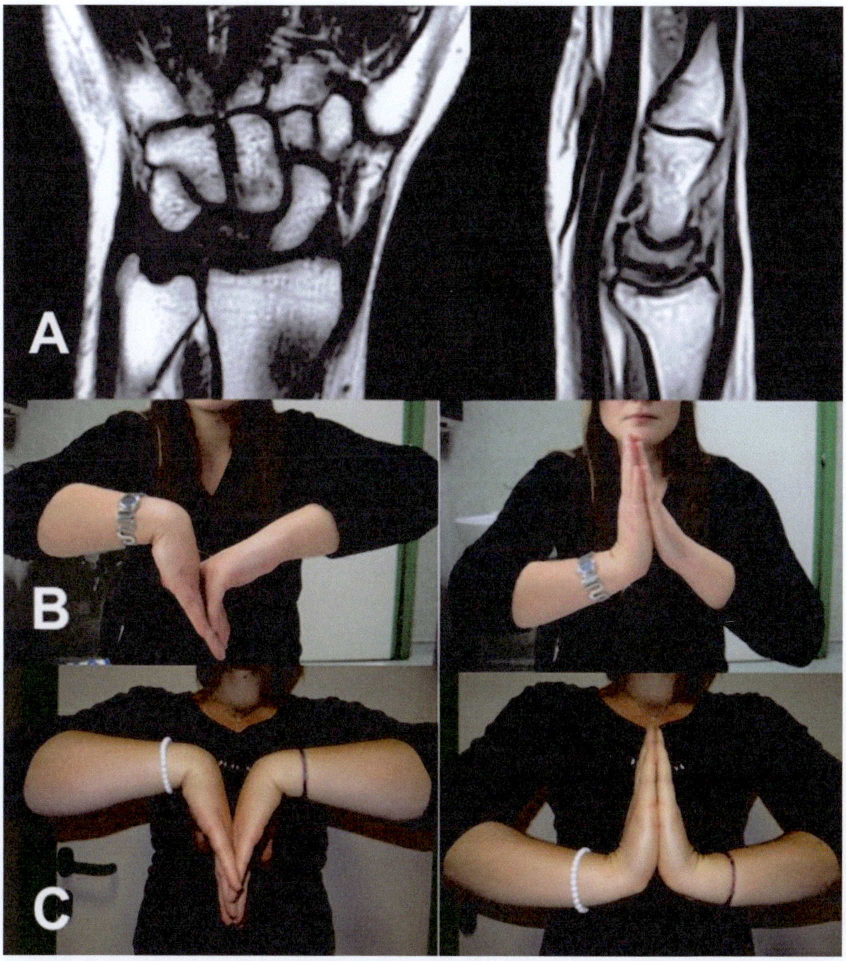


**Fig. 24.9** Clinical case: (**a**) Preoperative MRI imaging of a 24-year-old female diagnosed as Lichtman's stage 1. (**b**) Restricted preoperative flexion–extension range of motion. (**c**) Range of motion 3 years following surgery

## Discussion

Treatment of Kienbock's disease remains a challenge even for experienced wrist surgeons. Since the etiology of the disease is still poorly understood, there is no clear rationale to define which is the most appropriate treament option.

Provided that the disease is detected at early stages, traditional procedures aiming to unload the lunate, such as radial [5, 6] or capitate [7] shortening osteotomy or joint distraction by external fixation [8], show good results. Advanced cases may benefit from salvage procedures, such as proximal row carpectomy, radioscapholunate fusion, hemiarthroplasty, wrist fusion, or wrist replacement. However these procedures are rather aggressive, have more unpredictable results and potentially significant complications. More sophisticated procedures, such as vascularized transfers from the pisiform or distal radius or direct metacarpal artery implantation, are expected to have a greater potential. However, their value is being questioned due to the increasing importance attributed to intraosseous venous congestion, compared to poor arterial blood supply, as possible primary etiologic factors for avascular necrosis of the lunate [9]. The latter theory may represent a sound explanation of the good results achieved by the distal radial core decompression technique described by Illarramendi et al. [10]. According to the authors, early pain relief and long-term revascularization of the lunate may be due respectively to the decrease of intraosseous blood pressure and to carpal hyperemia in response to surgical manipulation of the distal radial metaphysis.

The technique of arthroscopic assisted bone grafting combines many advantages:

1. Direct drilling of the lunate, which causes an immediate decrease in venous congestion;
2. Decompression of the distal radial metaphysis during the harvest of the bone graft, which produces hyperemic response of the carpal vascular environment thus enhancing long term revascularization of the lunate;
3. Improved quality of the cancellous bone of the lunate following bone grafting, thus accelerating bone healing;
4. Respect of the periarticular soft-tissues and vascular environment by using a minimally invasive arthroscopic technique.

In order to achieve a good outcome, there are a few important points:

1. Patient selection; the indications for arthroscopic assisted bone grafting are strictly limited to those cases in which lunate shape and height are maintained almost unchanged and articular surfaces do not show major changes, such in patients classified as stage 1 according to Lichtman's classification and grade 0 according to Bain and Begg's arthroscopic staging.
2. Surgical technique; The procedure requires the use of advanced arthroscopic techniques.

The authors were pleased with their initial short-term outcomes published in 2011 [11]. The results presented in this chapter represent a further review with an average follow-up of 32 months. This latest review indicates that the initial good short-term results have been maintained. However, this very promising technique still requires confirmation with a larger series and a longer term follow-up.

A final advantage of the procedure is that no bridges are burnt; in case of further lunate collapse or pain, all remaining reconstructive and salvage options remain open.

## Conclusion

The technique of arthroscopic assisted bone grafting of the lunate is a technically demanding procedure that should be performed after adequate training for both the surgeon and the OR personnel. Clinical results show that it may represent a valuable option for treatment of selected cases of early Kienbock's disease, when lunate shape and height are preserved and articular surfaces are intact.

## References

1. Bain GI, Begg M. Arthroscopic assessment and classification of Kienbock's disease. Tech Hand Up Extrem Surg. 2006;10(1):8–13.
2. Menth-Chiari WA, Poehling GG, Wiesler ER, Ruch DS. Arthroscopic debridement for the treatment of Kienbock's disease. Arthroscopy. 1999;15(1):12–9.
3. Lichtman DM, Alexander AH, Mack GR, Gunther SF. Kienbock's disease. Update on silicone replacement arthroplasty. J Hand Surg Am. 1982;7:343–7.
4. Atzei A, Luchetti R, Sgarbossa A, Carità E, Llusà M. Set-up, portals and normal exploration in wrist arthroscopy. Chir Main. 2006;25:S131–44.
5. Schuind F, Eslami S, Ledoux P. Kienböck's disease. J Bone Joint Surg Br. 2008;90:133–9.
6. Raven EE, Haverkamp D, Marti RK. Outcome of Kienböck's disease 22 years after distal radius shortening osteotomy. Clin Orthop Relat Res. 2007;460: 137–41.
7. Gay AM, Parratte S, Glard Y, Mutaftschiev N, Legre R. Isolated capitate shortening osteotomy for the early stage of Kienböck disease with neutral ulnar variance. Plast Reconstr Surg. 2009;124(2):560–6.
8. Lichtman DM, Roure AR. External fixation for the treatment of Kienböck's disease. Hand Clin. 1993;9: 691–7.
9. Jensen CH. Intraosseous pressure in Kienbock's disease. J Hand Surg Am. 1993;18:355–9.
10. Illarramendi AA, Schulz C, De Carli P. The surgical treatment of Kienböck's disease by radius and ulna metaphyseal core decompression. J Hand Surg Am. 2001;26:252–60.
11. Pegoli L, Ghezzi A, Cavalli E, Luchetti R, Pajardi G. Arthroscopic assisted bone grafting for early stages of Kienböck's disease. Hand Surg. 2011;16(2):127–31.
12. Bain GI, Smith ML, Watts AC. Arthroscopic core decompression of the lunate in early stage Kienbock disease of the lunate. Tech Hand Up Extrem Surg. 2011;15(1):66–9.

# Arthroscopic Reconstructive Procedures for Kienböck's Disease

# 25

Wing-lim Tse, Xiaofeng Teng, Bo Liu, Clara Wong Wing-yee, Pak-cheong Ho, and Gregory Ian Bain

## Introduction

In stage 3B Kienböck's disease (Fig. 25.1), the lunate fails to support the load across the wrist and so it collapses in height with fixed rotation of scaphoid [1]. Arthroscopy often reveals dissociation of the lunate cartilage from the softened bone and the cartilage, which can no longer withstand load and shear since its firm attachment to subchondral bone is disrupted. Arthroscopy provides a more precise assessment of the articular cartilage, which helps the surgeon to make an informed decision regarding the "functionality" of the articular surfaces around the lunate. As described by Bain in his classification [2, 3], arthroscopy can assist in interpreting the articular findings and guides treatment.

## An Articular-Based Approach to Assessment and Management

The authors have used an articular-based approach to assess Kienböck's disease and its involvement of the carpus and to determine the optimal surgical treatment [2, 3].

## Arthroscopic Assessment

A tourniquet is applied over the arm but not inflated unless bleeding obscures the visualization during the procedure. We recommend the

**Electronic supplementary material:** The online version of this chapter (doi:10.1007/978-3-319-34226-9_25) contains supplementary material, which is available to authorized users. Videos can also be accessed at http://link.springer.com/chapter/[10.1007/978-3-319-34226-9_25].

W.-l. Tse, FRCS, FRCSEd, FHKCOS (✉)
General Office, Department of Orthopedics and Traumatology, Prince of Wales Hospital, 5/F, Old Wing, Shatin, Hong Kong, SAR, China
e-mail: tse@ort.cuhk.edu.hk

X. Teng
Department of Hand Surgery, NingBo Sixth Hospital of Zhejiang, Zhongshan East Road no. 1059, Ningbo, Zhejiang 315040, China

B. Liu, MD, FRCS
Department of Hand Surgery, Beijing Ji Shui Tan Hospital, 31 Xin Jie Kou East Street, Beijing 100035, China

C.W. Wing-yee, MRCS, FRCSEd, FHKCOS
Department of Orthopedics and Traumatology, Prince of Wales Hospital, 5/F, Old Wing, Shatin, Hong Kong 999077, China

40E, Block 3, Sun Tuen Mun Center, Tuen Mun, N.T., Hong Kong, China

P.-c. Ho, MBBS, FRCS, FHKCOS
Department of Orthopedics and Traumatology, Prince of Wales Hospital, Chinese University of Hong Kong, Shatin, N.T., Hong Kong, China

G.I. Bain, MBBS, FRACS, FA(Ortho)A, PhD
Professor, Upper Limb and Research, Department of Orthopedic Surgery, Flinders University and Flinders Medical Centre, Bedford Park, Adelaide, SA, Australia

© Springer International Publishing Switzerland 2016

D.M. Lichtman, G.I. Bain (eds.), *Kienböck's Disease*, DOI 10.1007/978-3-319-34226-9_25

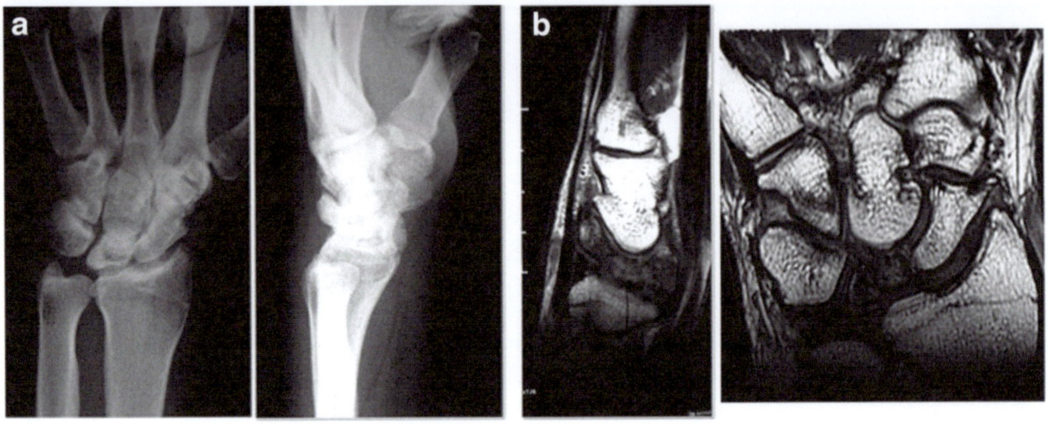


**Fig. 25.1** (**a**) A 22-year-old man with stage 3B disease on right wrist. Plain radiographs show lunate collapse with fixed flexion of scaphoid. (**b**) MRI showing low signal intensity on T1

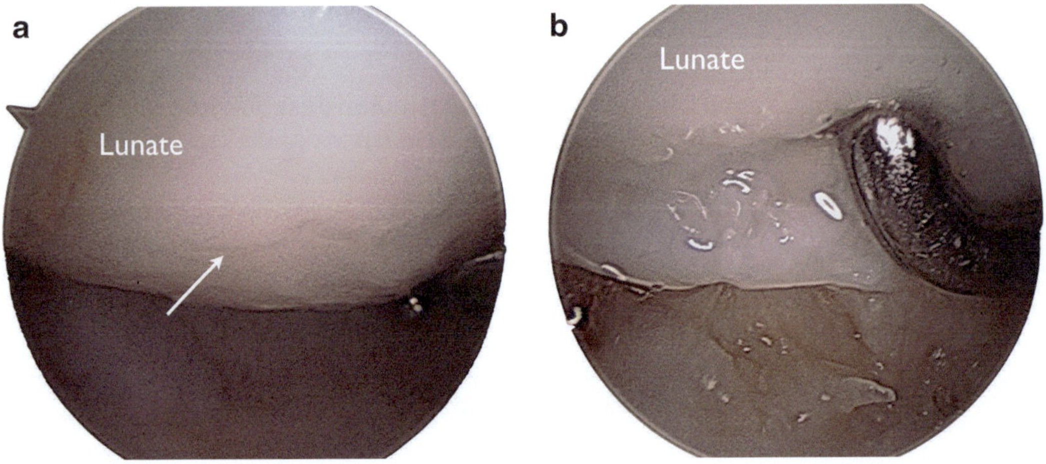


**Fig. 25.2** Arthroscopic view of a concealed fracture of the lunate. (**a**) Initially only an articular cartilage crease is seen (*arrow*). (**b**) With probing the fracture of the lunate can be identified. Copyright Dr. Gregory Bain

standard working portals in the RCJ (3–4, 4–5 and sometimes 6U) and MCJ (MCR and MCU) (Video 25.1). The lunate and adjacent articular surfaces are meticulously inspected for chondral integrity and fractures. The articular surfaces are probed to assess presence of softening, "floating" (unsupported) articular surface and degenerative changes [2]. A debridement of loose bony fragments, chondral flaps, and synovitis is performed.

## Classification

Bain and Begg developed an arthroscopic staging system based on the number of nonfunctional articular surfaces. The principle is to identify the articulations that are nonfunctional (compromised) and those that are functional [2]. **A functional articular surface** would have a normal arthroscopic appearance, which is smooth and glistening. The normal subchondral bone is firm to palpate without significant softening. Minor fibrillation is still considered a functional articular surface.

**Nonfunctional articular surface** would include those with extensive fibrillation, fissuring, localized or extensive loss, a floating articular surface, and fracture (Figs. 25.2 and 25.3).

The grade determined with the Bain and Begg classification depends upon the number of articulations involved (Fig. 25.4). Although arthroscopy is the gold standard method of

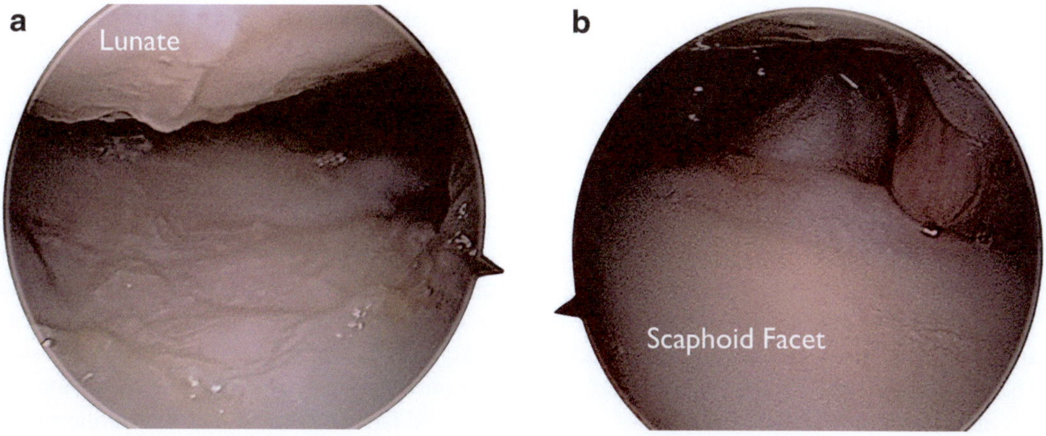


**Fig. 25.3** (**a**) Arthroscopic view of the irregular nonfunctional lunate facet and proximal lunate. (**b**) Arthroscopic view of the functional scaphoid facet. The patient is a candidate for a radioscapholunate or scaphocapitate fusion. Copyright Dr. Gregory Bain

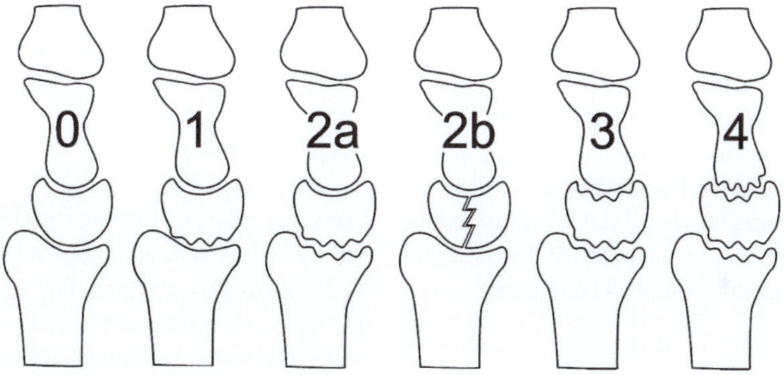


**Fig. 25.4** Bain and Begg arthroscopic classification of Kienböck's disease. The grade is determined by the number of nonfunctional articular surfaces. The grading system assists the surgeon to determine the best surgical option, based on the pathoanatomic findings. Reproduced with permission from Bain GI, Begg M. Arthroscopic assessment and classification of Kienböck's disease. Tech Hand Up Extrem Surg. 2006;10(1):8–13

assessment of the articular surface, it must be recognized that new imaging modalities that are non-invasive (e.g., MRI) will increasingly allow assessment of the articulation [4].

## Management Principles

1. Using an articular-based classification and treatment algorithm that respects the articular aspects of Kienböck's disease and uses it to guide treatment, based on patho-anatomical principles.
2. The aim of treatment is to reduce the pain while maintaining a functional wrist motion.
3. Wrist arthroscopy is a diagnostic modality that can be used to assess and classify the wrist.
4. Arthroscopic debridement in the form of synovectomy, removal of chondral flaps, and loose bodies can be helpful.
5. The principle of reconstructive surgery is to fuse, excise, or bypass the nonfunctional joint, and then mobilize the wrist through the remaining functional articulations.
6. The authors will often proceed directly to a reconstructive procedure.

7. Reconstructive procedures can now be performed using advanced arthroscopic techniques, which are described in detail in the manuscript.

## Selection of Reconstructive Procedure

The preferred treatment option is based on the arthroscopic findings and staging (Table 25.1). The following are the options, and they are usually applied in combinations:

1. *Debridement* of the synovitis and chondral flaps [3]
2. *Remove the nonfunctional* articular surfaces; examples include excision of the lunate or proximal row carpectomy. A prosthetic implant can be implanted to replace the lunate or proximal carpal row.
3. *Fuse the nonfunctional* articulations; examples include radioscapholunate (RSL), radiolunate (RL) and total wrist fusion.
4. *Bypass the nonfunctional* articulations; examples include scapho-capitate (SC) fusion and scaphotrapeziotrapezoid (STT) fusion.

**Table 25.1** Preferred reconstructive procedure based on arthroscopic findings and staging[a]

| Grade (Bain and Begg) | Nonfunctional surfaces | Recommendation |
|---|---|---|
| 1–2a | Proximal lunate and lunate fossa | RSL fusion |
| 2b | Proximal and distal lunate surfaces | PRC |
| 3 | Lunate fossa, proximal and distal lunate surfaces (radio-scaphoid articulation still functional) | SC fusion |
| 4 | All four surfaces (lunate fossa, proximal and distal lunate surfaces, proximal capitate) | Salvage (total wrist fusion or arthroplasty) |

[a]Modified from [2]

## Principles of Arthroscopic Inter-Carpal Fusion

The principle is to fuse the nonfunctional articular surfaces and allows motion across the functional articulations. Therefore, the prerequisite is to have a functional articular joint which can be used for mobilization. Accurate assessment of cartilage by arthroscopy is mandatory, followed by debridement of damaged articular surfaces and/or selected **carpal excision**. If bypass fusion is required (examples are STT or SC fusion for advanced Kienböck's disease), the cartilage over the opposing fusion surfaces is also debrided until there is bleeding from the subchondral bone (**preparation of the fusion surfaces**). The carpal malalignment is then corrected, followed by percutaneous fixation across the debrided articulation (whether damaged or as bypass) to achieve a limited wrist fusion (**fixation of fusion mass**).

## Carpal Excision

Excision of the any of the carpal bones requires a dedicated approach. Examples include excision of the lunate as part of the SC fusion, or resection of the entire proximal carpal row. Often the four working portals are needed and are interchanged for optimal efficiency. The joint is like a box, and the portals are introduced from various directions to obtain the ideal perspective for the scope and optimal position of the instrumentation (Fig. 25.5).

As an example, in arthroscopic excision of the lunate, the fragmented or degenerate cartilage is removed with an arthroscopic grasper and punch to expose the underlying fragmented bone. A motorized resector is positioned in the MCJ with the burr in the center of lunate and then proceeds radially (Video 25.2). The burr is re-positioned in the RCJ and directed distally. Once the center of the bone has been resected, there is usually a osteocartilaginous "shell" which remains attached to the intrinsic and extrinsic ligaments. These ligamentous attachments are released with radiofrequency ablation and grasped with a pituitary rongeur (Fig. 25.6). Visualization of the

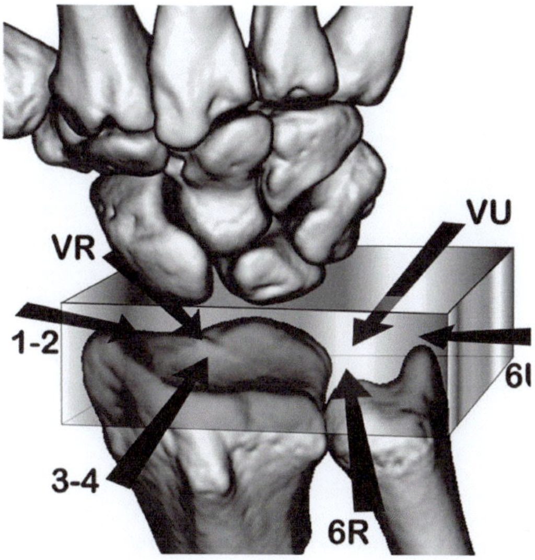


**Fig. 25.5** The box concept. The wrist can be thought of as a box, which can be visualized from almost any perspective. By interchanging the portals the optimal perspective can be obtained, and working instruments ideally positioned. Reprinted from Arthroscopy, 24(3), Bain GI, Munt J, Turner PC, New advances in wrist arthroscopy, 355–367, Copyright © 2008 Arthroscopy Association of North America. Published by Elsevier Inc. All rights reserved [5]

interval is now easier as the RCJ and MCJ now freely communicated.

## Preparation of the Fusion Surfaces

As an example, we will describe the technique of arthroscopic resection of the scaphocapitate surfaces. With the scope in the MCU and a 2.9 mm burr in the MCR the articular surfaces that require debridement are identified. For the SC fusion, the debridement is between the radial half of proximal capitate and scaphoid. We commence the resection at the inferior aspect, as the bleeding obscures the view of the dependent articulations. We progress upwards, removing the cartilage, and continue until there is punctate bleeding from the subchondral bone, which signifies adequate bone resection. The diameter of the burr serves as a reference for the depth of bone being resected.

## Fixation of Fusion Mass

There are many options for fixation of limited wrist fusions, but we prefer cannulated screws, as the guide wires can be positioned under arthroscopic and fluoroscopic guidance. Once the ideal position is obtained, bone graft or bone graft substitute is added if there is a void in the fusion mass.

For a SC fusion, we would have the arthroscope in the MCU portal and a 4.5 mm cannula in the MCR portal to introduce and impact bone graft or granules into the scaphocapitate interval. If lunate excision has been performed, a French 6 or 8 Foley catheter is inserted via the 4–5 portal and inflated with normal saline to fill the lunate void and prevent the graft spillage into the radiocarpal joint [6, 7].

The traction is removed from the arm, and the cannulated depth gauge is advanced over the guide wire. A screw is selected that is 4 mm shorter than measured, to allow for the countersinking and compression. Under fluoroscopic control, cannulated drills and 3.2 or 3.5 mm screws are then advanced over the guide wires to stabilize the fusion mass (Fig. 25.7).

Following the procedure, a plaster slab is applied for 7–10 days. Gentle active mobilization can be commenced at 10 days with a wrist brace for protection. Gentle passive mobilization can commence after 4 weeks and strengthening exercises after 3 months.

## Benefits of Arthroscopic-Assisted Fusion

1. Reducing surgical dissection of the soft tissue envelope, especially the extrinsic ligaments, to preserve the ligamentous support, intercarpal stability, and vascularity.
2. Precise cartilage and osseous debridement minimizes the osseous resection required to create congruent opposed bleeding fusion surfaces. Thus, carpal height is better maintained and utilization of bone graft is reduced and often avoided.
3. Percutaneous fixation with countersinking implants within the carpus minimizes the

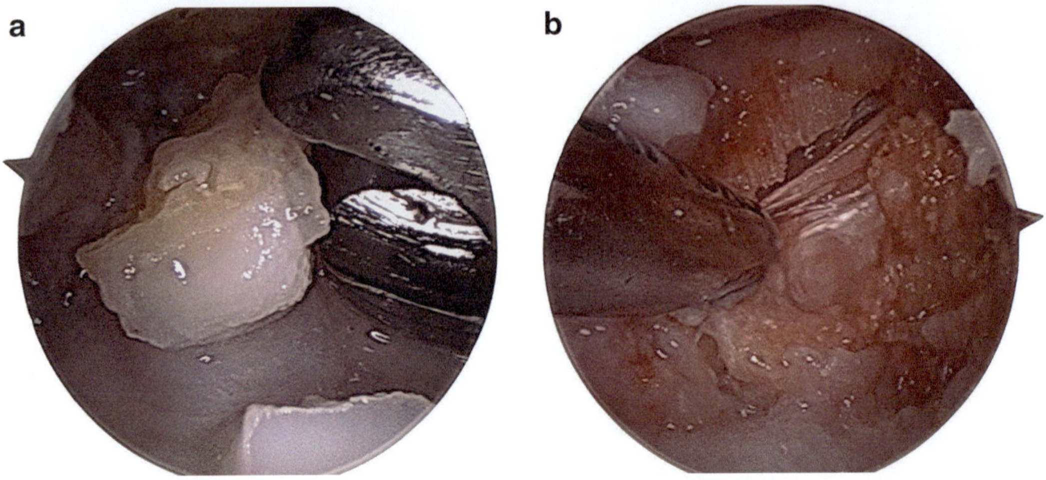


**Fig. 25.6** Arthroscopic excision of the lunate. (**a**) Use of the with pituitary rongeur, (**b**) arthroscopic resector. Copyright Dr. Gregory Bain

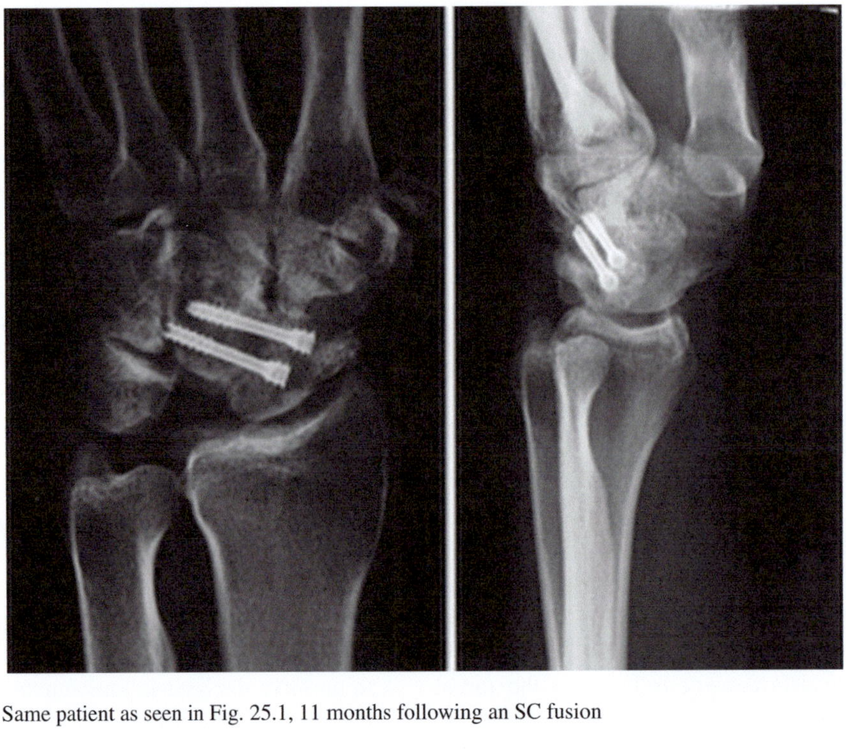

**Fig. 25.7** Same patient as seen in Fig. 25.1, 11 months following an SC fusion

implant-related complications such as impingement.

4. The minimally invasive techniques cause less soft tissue injury, postoperative pain, and swelling, to allow earlier rehabilitation and optimize outcome.
5. Provides a superior cosmetic outcome.

## Arthroscopic SC Fusion

SC fusion was first described by Sutro [8] for scaphoid nonunion in four patients, using an open technique. There are four clinical series of SC fusion for Kienböck's disease [8–11]. In general, pain improvement was observed, but nonunion remains a concern, with 10 and 12% reported in series by Luegmair [10] and Pisano [11], respectively. The results of SC fusion may be improved by modifying the techniques in ways that may increase the union rate and maintain the motion following surgery.

The STT and SC fusion both transfer the load from the central column to the radial column, therefore unloading the necrotic fragmented lunate which may in turn relieve the pain and progression of Kienböck's disease [12, 13]. Cadaveric studies [14, 15] have demonstrated no significant difference in wrist motion between an SC and STT fusion.

The authors developed the techniques of arthroscopic STT and SC fusion techniques [6, 7, 16]; however, we prefer SC fusion for stage 3B Kienböck's disease because the SC articulation is easier to arthroscopically access. The opposing surfaces of the capitate and the waist and proximal scaphoid need to be resected. The distal third of the scaphoid, trapezium and trapezoid do not need to be debrided. The percutaneous fixation across the SC articulation is more straightforward, and bone graft is not required.

We follow the standard principles of arthroscopic assessment, debridement, preparation and fixation as outlined above. The prerequisite is to have a functional scaphoid facet and proximal scaphoid. If the lunate is very fragmented we resect it. The opposing surfaces of the SC articulation are resected.

## Reduction of SC Angle and Fixation

We aim to stabilize the SC fusion in a position of normal alignment (e.g., SL angle between 30° and 57°, CL angle 0° ± 15°) [17]. We insert two guide pins across the SC interval. If lunate has been excised, the SC angle should be fixed between 30° and 57°. The position of scaphoid can be controlled by thumbing the scaphoid tubercle from the volar aspect. The first guide pin is advanced through the 1–2 portal. The guide pin should enter the scaphoid between the proximal and middle thirds. It should be inserted at 60° to the longitudinal axis of the wrist. In the lateral projection aim at the middle of scaphoid and capitate. Another guide pin should be inserted at least 5 mm distal and parallel to the first one, aiming to enter the scaphoid between the middle and distal thirds. The cannulated depth gauge, drill, and screws are advanced over the guide as described above.

## Results of Arthroscopic SC Fusion

Between August 2009 and October 2011 there were 18 patients with stage 3B Kienböck's disease managed with arthroscopic SC fusion in three centers (Prince of Wales Hospital, Hong Kong; 6th People's Hospital, Ningbo, China; Ji Shui Tan Hospital, Beijing, China). The mean age was 32.2 years (18–57), with 11 males and 7 females. Mean operating time was 90.2 min (120–360), and all fixations were achieved with two percutaneous cannulated screws (Fig. 25.8). Bone substitutes were used in two cases, but no supplement was used in the other 16 patients. A consolidated fusion was achieved in all 18 patients. There were no wound or neurovascular complications. One patient had persistent pain and was managed with a proximal row carpectomy and pyrocarbon Amandys interposition arthroplasty (Tornier).

In five of our cases, we excised the lunate, as there was significant widening of the lunate on the sagittal CAT scan, with impingement on the dorsal and/or volar aspect. In these cases we excised the lunate, which resulted in an increase in flexion, extension and ulnar deviation, but a loss of radial deviation [18, 19].

## Arthroscopic PRC

The prerequisite to perform a PRC is to have functional articular surfaces of the proximal capitate and lunate fossa. We reserve the arthroscopic PRC for patients with Lichtman's stage 3B and Bain's stage 2B disease. Patients who are lower demand and age >45 years will have better long-term outcomes [20].

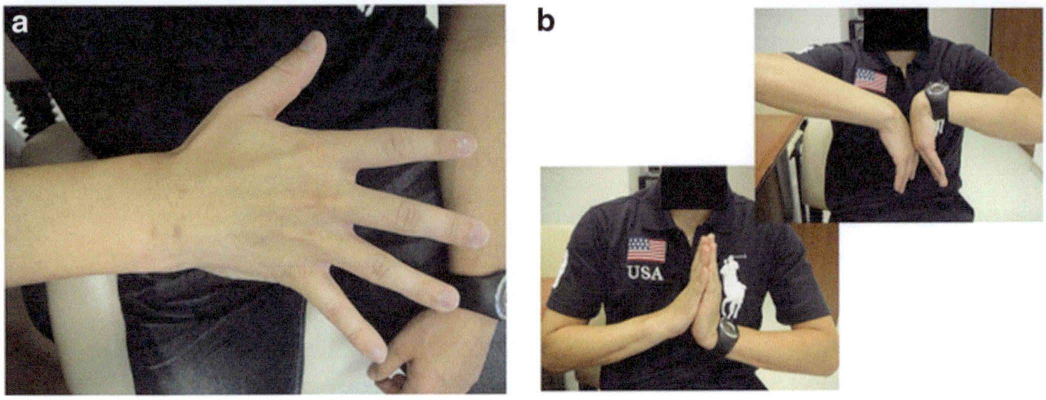


**Fig. 25.8** (**a**) Cosmetic scar after arthroscopic SC fusion. (**b**) Right wrist range of motion of same patient 11 months postoperatively

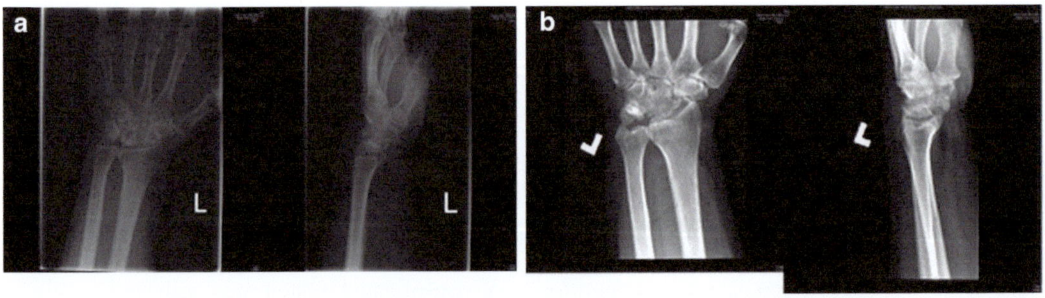


**Fig. 25.9** (**a**) Preoperative radiograph of 62-year-old man with stage 3B disease. (**b**) Postoperative radiograph 3 years after proximal row carpectomy

We perform a standard arthroscopy, debridement, and articular assessment [2, 3]. The four common working portals (3–4, 4–5, MCR and MCU) are all used as required. The central osseous portion of the lunate, scaphoid and triquetrum are removed first. The entire lunate and triquetrum are removed, but the distal one-third of scaphoid is retained for the attachments of STT and the dorsal intercarpal ligaments (Fig. 25.9).

Care is required to avoid the radial artery on the radial side of scaphoid and use meticulous hemostasis with radiofrequency. When using large burrs we maintain continuous irrigation to avoid overheating. The initial operating times were long, but since using larger burrs (3.2 mm or bigger), our operating times have markedly reduced.

## Arthroscopic RSL Fusion

The prerequisite for a RSL fusion is to have a functional midcarpal articulation. Therefore, it is limited to Bain stage 1 and stage 2A disease. With the scope in the 4–5 portal, and the burr in the 1–2 and 3–4 portals, we commence debridement of the dependent radial styloid and fossae, and then go to the overhanging proximal scaphoid and lunate surfaces. Because of the gross shape mismatch between the scaphoid/lunate and the corresponding radial fossae, bone graft or substitute filler is mandatory. The graft is delivered via the 4.5 mm cannula through the 1–2 and 3–4 portals, with the Foley catheter in the 4–5 portal. The graft is then compacted tightly from the radial and volar aspect, working towards the

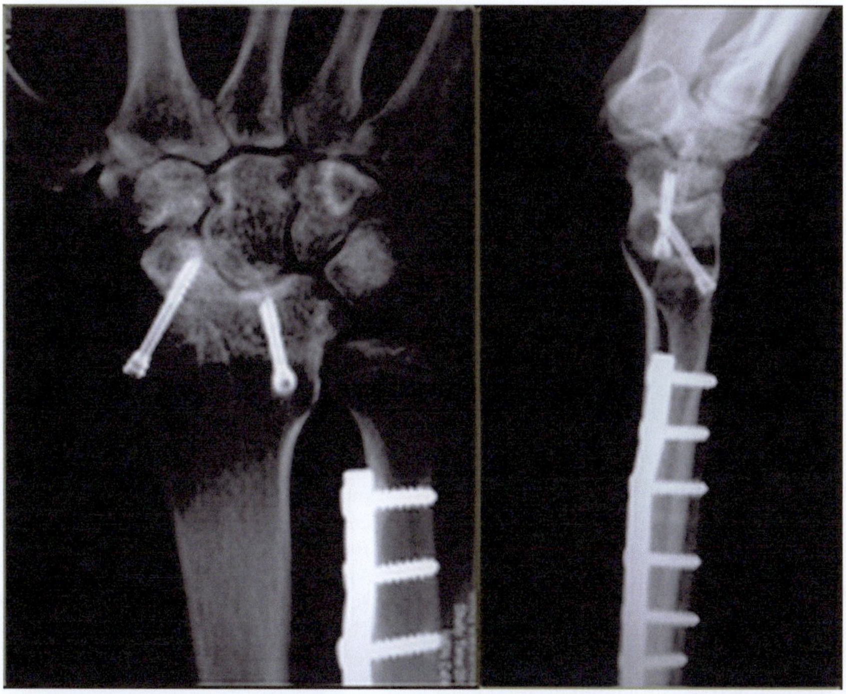

**Fig. 25.10** A 57-year-old man with an RSL fusion. Note the bone substitute at the radioscapholunate interval

dorsal and ulnar aspect. Under fluoroscopic control, a guide pin is advanced percutaneously through the middle column of distal radius to the lunate (RL pin) and another guide pin from the radial column to the scaphoid (RS pin). The RL pin is introduced 1 cm proximal to the dorsal rim of the radius and aimed at the volar horn of the lunate, to maximize lunate purchase, but avoid penetration, which may damage the medial nerve. The RS pin is introduced into the radial column towards the proximal scaphoid at 45° on the AP view. On the lateral view, the pin is aimed along the mid axis of radial styloid and proximal scaphoid. Then the cannulated compression screws are advanced as described above (Fig. 25.10).

## Discussion

In those cases in which the lunate has collapsed and there are articular abnormalities (e.g., Lichtman stage 3B and Bain 1, 2, and 3), reconstructive procedures are required to recreate a pain-free articulation. Examples include a proximal row carpectomy (PRC) or limited fusion (STT, SC). If the articular surfaces are all compromised (e.g., Lichtman stage 4 and Bain 4), a salvage procedure such as a total wrist fusion or arthroplasties is required [21–23].

The indications for the various procedures are strict; otherwise the results of surgery are unreliable. For example, a PRC with a pre-existing capitate articular lesion is known to do poorly, especially if the patient is younger than 45 years of age [20, 24]. We prefer the SC fusion, especially in the more advanced cases of Kienböck's disease, such as the Lichtman stage 3b and Bain grade 3, if the scaphoid and scaphoid fossa articulations are functional.

Reconstructive procedures using the arthroscopic approach as described in this article allow the following:

1. Accurate assessment of the articular surfaces to facilitate surgical decision making.
2. Cartilage and bone resection to be performed with precision, therefore maintaining better carpal height and reducing the need for bone

graft or substitute. The authors no longer use bone grafts or substitutes for the SC fusion, but do for the RSL fusion.

3. Reduces the soft tissue stripping, therefore maintaining better soft tissue attachments, stability and vascularity.
4. These factors reduce the postoperative pain and swelling, which facilitates recovery and rehabilitation, ultimately producing a better functional and cosmetic result.

There is a considerable learning curve with these advanced arthroscopic techniques. We have included many technical points to assist in overcoming some of the difficulties. Some of these are simple points, such as the use of larger burrs, which have enabled a more efficient resection of the sclerotic lunate. With the development of new techniques and instruments, we are expecting wider application of the arthroscopic approach in complex reconstructive procedures for wrist disorders.

## References


1. Lichtman DM, Lesley NE, Simmons SP. The classification and treatment of Kienböck's disease: the state of the art and a look at the future. J Hand Surg Eur Vol. 2010;35:549–54.
2. Bain GI, Begg M. Arthroscopic assessment and classification of Kienböck's disease. Tech Hand Up Extrem Surg. 2006;10(1):8–13.
3. Menth-Chiari WA, Poehling GG, Wiesler ER, Ruch DS. Arthroscopic debridement for the treatment of Kienböck's disease. Arthroscopy. 1999;15(1):12–9.
4. Bain GI, Durrant A. An articular-based approach to Kienbock avascular necrosis of the lunate. Tech Hand Up Extrem Surg. 2011;15(1):41–7.
5. Bain GI, Munt J, Turner PC. New advances in wrist arthroscopy. Arthroscopy. 2008;24(3):355–67.
6. Ho PC. Arthroscopic partial wrist fusion. Tech Hand Up Extrem Surg. 2008;12(4):242–65.
7. Ho PC. Arthroscopic partial wrist fusion. In: Geissler WB, editor. Wrist and elbow arthroscopy: a practical surgical guide to techniques. Berlin: Springer; 2014. p. 195–223.
8. Sutro CJ. Treatment of nonunion of the carpal navicular bone. Surgery. 1946;20:536–40.
9. Helfet AJ. A new operation for ununited fracture of the scaphoid. J Bone Joint Surg Br. 1952;34:329.
10. Luegmair M, Saffar P. Scaphocapitate arthrodesis for treatment of late stage Kienbock disease. J Hand Surg Eur Vol. 2014;39(4):416–22.
11. Pisano SM, Peimer CA, Wheeler DR, Sherwin F. Scaphocapitate intercarpal arthrodesis. J Hand Surg Am. 1991;16(2):328–33.
12. Garcia-Elias M, Cooney WP, An KN, Linscheid RL, Chao EYS. Wrist kinematics after limited intercarpal arthrodesis. J Hand Surg Am. 1989;14:791–9.
13. Horii E, Garcia-Elias M, Bishop AT, Cooney WP, Linscheid RL, Chao EY. Effect on force transmission across the carpus in procedures used to treat Kienböck's disease. J Hand Surg Am. 1990;15: 393–400.
14. Iwasaki N, Genda E, Barrance PJ, Minami A, Kaneda K, Chao EYS. Biomechanical analysis of limited intercarpal fusion for the treatment of Kienböck's disease: a three-dimensional theoretical study. J Orthop Res. 1998;16:256–63.
15. Viegas SF, Patterson RM, Peterson PD, Pogue DJ, Jenkins DK, Sweo TD, et al. Evaluation of the biomechanical efficacy of limited intercarpal fusions for the treatment of scapho-lunate dissociation. J Hand Surg Am. 1990;15(1):120–8.
16. Ho PC. Arthroscopic radiocarpal fusion for post-traumatic radiocarpal arthrosis. In: Pinel FD, Mathoulin C, Luchetti R, editors. Arthroscopic management of distal radius fractures. Berlin: Springer; 2010. p. 225–42.
17. Minamikawa Y, Peimer CA, Yamaguchi T, Medige J, Sherwin FS. Ideal scaphoid angle for intercarpal arthrodesis. J Hand Surg Am. 1992;17:370–5.
18. Lee JS, Park MJ, Kang HJ. Scaphotrapeziotrapezoid arthrodesis and lunate excision for advanced Kienböck's disease. J Hand Surg Am. 2012;37: 2226–32.
19. Matsuhashi T, Iwasaki N, Kato H, Minami M, Minami A. Clinical outcomes of excision arthroplasty for Kienbock's disease. Hand Surg. 2011;16(3):277–82.
20. Chim H, Moran SL. Long-term outcomes of proximal row carpectomy: a systematic review of the literature. J Wrist Surg. 2012;1(2):141–8.
21. Allan CH, Joshi A, Lichtman DM. Kienböck's disease: diagnosis and treatment. J Am Acad Orthop Surg. 2001;9:128–36.
22. Beredjiklian PK. Kienböck's disease. J Hand Surg Am. 2009;34:167–75.
23. Lutsky K, Beredjiklian PK. Kienböck disease. J Hand Surg Am. 2012;37(9):1942–52.
24. Iorio ML, Kennedy CD, Huang JI. Limited intercarpal fusion as a salvage procedure for advanced Kienbock disease. Hand. 2015;10:472. doi:10.1007/s11552-014-9705-z.

# Pyrocarbon Arthroplasty for Kienböck's Disease

**26**

Philippe Bellemère, Wisam Al-Hakim, Aude Le Corre, and Mark Ross

## Introduction

Ultimately, the goals for treatment of Kienböck's disease are to provide pain relief whilst maintaining as near normal function as possible. With these goals in mind, current outcomes for patients treated non-operatively can be poor. Moreover, outcomes for conventional surgical treatments generally remain unsatisfactory [1]. Longer-term studies suggest that early surgical intervention may not prevent collapse, with similar outcomes to non-operatively treated patients [2–5]. Pancarpal arthrodesis still remains the only reliable permanent solution to this debilitating disease, but the consequent functional deficit makes for a sombre compromise [6]. This key stimulus is what drives the search for an option that provides better functional outcomes for these patients. Joint replacements using more commonly used materials, such as metals with or without polyethylene, silicone, and ceramics, have all been used with varying success. Complications have included silicosis [7], cyst formation, osteolysis, aseptic loosening, chronic regional pain syndrome, reduced function, and a need for revision surgery. The challenges that must be considered include implant design, fixation, stability, joint bearings, and the techniques of surgical implantation. To date, no arthroplasty technique, implant design or implant material has been identified as a gold standard.

Pyrocarbon has been used in medicine for over 40 years [8]. Most notably it is one of the principle materials in cardiac valve replacement [9]. More recently it has seen a number of applications in the upper limb including humeral head resurfacing, radial head replacement, interposition arthroplasty of the radiocarpal joint, and hemi-, total or interposition arthroplasty of the first carpometacarpal (CMC), metacarpophalangeal (MCP), and proximal interphalangeal (PIP) joints [10]. Its material property profile suggests several potential benefits over other materials. These include excellent biocompatibility, optimal fatigue resistance, reduced osteolysis from stress shielding, and reduced rates of cartilage wear. Mid- and long-term results have been promising, particularly with regard to MCP joint

P. Bellemère, MD (✉) • A. Le Corre, MD
Institut de la Main Nantes Atlantique, Clinique Jeanne d'Arc, 21 rue des Martyrs, Nantes 44100, France
e-mail: Philippe.Bellemere@me.com

W. Al-Hakim, MBBS, BSc, PGDip, FRCS (Tr & Orth)
Department of Trauma and Orthopedics, The Royal London Hospital, Whitechapel Road, London E1 1BB, UK

M. Ross, MBBS, FRACS
Brisbane Hand and Upper Limb Research Institute, Brisbane Private Hospital, 9/259 Wickham Terrace, Brisbane, QLD, Australia

Department of Orthopedics, Princess Alexandra Hospital, Brisbane, QLD, Australia

School of Medicine, The University of Queensland, Brisbane, QLD 4072, Australia

© Springer International Publishing Switzerland 2016
D.M. Lichtman, G.I. Bain (eds.), *Kienböck's Disease*, DOI 10.1007/978-3-319-34226-9_26

arthroplasty [11]. Evolution and innovation in implant design and manufacture have allowed for increased use of pyrocarbon over time. Although very much in its infancy, pyrocarbon arthroplasty may become a mainstay option for treating Kienböck's disease in the future.

## What Is Pyrocarbon?

Carbon atoms are covalently bonded in different orientations to form several natural forms including diamond and graphite. Diamond has a tetrahedral molecular geometry where every carbon atom is covalently bonded to four others. This forms a rigid crystalline structure. Graphite consists of carbon atoms bonded to each other covalently to form macromolecular sheets. Weak Van Der Waal's forces hold these sheets together resulting in a high melting point. However, little energy is required to displace one sheet relative to another, meaning the material is very soft (hence its application in pencil lead). Stronger lattice structures can be synthesised artificially with stronger covalent bonds between layers, to form graphene. This artificial substance is pyrolytic carbon, which is very light, strong and has a small crystal grain sizes, giving it predictable isotropic characteristics. This uniform material can be polished to a very fine surface and although it is brittle, pyrolytic carbon is far less stiff than ceramics and metals.

A pyrocarbon implant is composed of a graphite core with a pyrolytic graphene outer coating, which is typically 1 mm thick [13]. It is this outer coating that confers the benefits of its material properties to the implant. The graphite core is usually impregnated with tungsten to make it radio-opaque. The outer layer is radiolucent, so radiologically it appears as a halo around the implant (which is sometimes mistaken for loosening). Precise machining fashions the implant shape and size from tungsten-impregnated graphite rods, which are then coated with pyrolytic carbon by a process known as chemical vapor deposition (CVD) [8, 10, 12].

## Material Properties of Pyrolytic Carbon

Pyrocarbon has a number of potentially advantageous material characteristics [10]. These include:

- Excellent wear characteristics, therefore creating minimal particulate debris.
- Good fatigue resistance [15].
- Excellent biocompatibility with peri-articular soft tissues.
- No soft tissue ingrowth, so prosthesis is press fit with non-cemented fixation via bone apposition.
- Young's modulus of 29.4 GPa±0.4, which is similar to the elasticity of cortical bone [14]. This may decrease wear of the pyrocarbon on the native cartilage or bone in hemiarthroplasty applications. It may result in minimization of stress shielding effects and bone reabsorption.

Cooke studied a canine hip model, in which the wear characteristics of a femoral hemiarthroplasty were compared with the normal hip over an 18-month period [11]. The wear results were compared for the pyrocarbon, cobalt chrome and titanium alloy. The pyrocarbon hemiarthroplasties had significantly lower rates of cartilage wear (Fig. 26.1) eburnation, fibrillation, glycosaminoglycan loss, and subchondral bone change compared to the other groups. Survivorship analysis showed that 92 % had preserved their cartilage in the pyrocarbon group compared to the 20 % in the other group. It is unclear why pyrocarbon has better wear properties against cartilage than other materials, but it may be due to surface-active phospholipids (SAPL), which adsorb to the implant surface [10, 16, 17].

In a laboratory study, identically shaped base of thumb and radial head implants made of pyrocarbon, cobalt chrome and ceramic all underwent cyclical laboratory testing against animal and cadaveric human specimens [18]. The volumetric cartilage and bone wear was 100 times greater in the metal group compared to the pyrocarbon group.

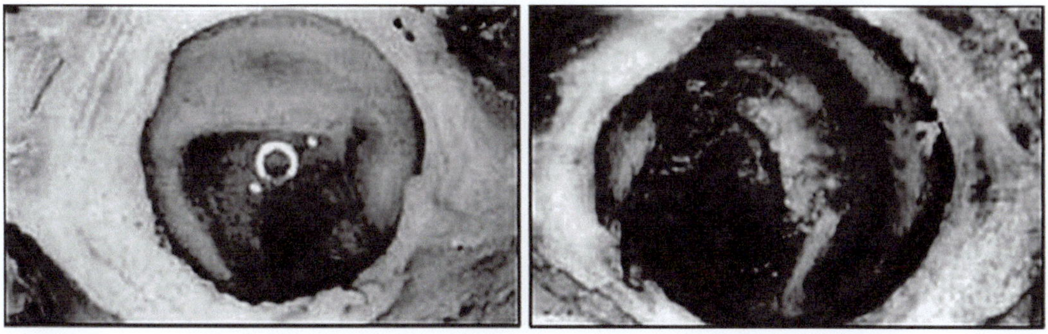

**Fig. 26.1** Canine acetabula macroscopic appearances following femoral head implantation using pyrocarbon versus cobalt chrome

Bone fixation of pyrocarbon implants is a subject of debate regarding the exact mechanism and its associated efficacy [10, 19]. Bony ingrowth has not been demonstrated in human subjects. Implants that are subjected to nonphysiological angular loads are more likely to demonstrate evidence of migration or loosening postoperatively. The MCP joint implants have less resorption than PIP joint implants. In addition, the authors have experience in shoulder hemiarthroplasty using stemmed pyrocarbon proximal humeral resurfacing implants in over 150 implants performed with up to 3-year follow-up [20]. We have found that, in spite of the higher loads seen in the shoulder, there has been virtually no implant migration observed. Therefore we have observed that implants with a spherical multi-plane articulation (e.g., humerus, MCP, capitate) have very little implant migration [20, 21], whereas in the PIP joint where there is a constrained uniplanar articulation [22], there is a far greater potential for malalignment and resorption.

When considering the bone-prosthesis interface at the time of implantation, the likelihood of migration also seems to be related to the quality of the residual bone in contact with the implant. We advise against high-speed powered instruments, which cause thermal damage to the adjacent bone.

Impaction bone grafting of any soft or deficient bone, prior to implantation may improve the quality of the initial press-fit. Bone graft is usually available locally in sufficient quantities from the "off-cuts" of the joint replacement or from PRC.

## Current Designs, Methods, and Results

Current designs on the market for clinical use of pyrocarbon to treat Kienböck's disease include the Amandys implant (Figs. 26.2 and 26.3) by Tornier (Grenoble, France); the Adaptive Proximal Scaphoid Implant (Figs. 26.4 and 26.5) by Tornier (Grenoble, France); the Pyrocarbon Lunate Replacement (Figs. 26.6 and 26.7) by Ascension (Austin, Texas, USA); and the Resurfacing Capitate Pyrocarbon Implant (Figs. 26.8 and 26.9a, b) by Tornier (Grenoble, France).

### Amandys

The Amandys is a good implant for use in stage 3 and 4 Kienböck's disease with mid-carpal arthritis. It can be used in primary surgery or after failure of other surgeries. It is an alternative to total wrist replacement or wrist fusion.

The Amandys is a free interposition pyrocarbon implant that provides an alternative surgical option to wrist fusion and total wrist arthroplasty. It is designed to replace the lunate, proximal one-third to two-thirds of the scaphoid and the proximal capitate. The implant has a quadri-elliptical shape with a convex proximal surface for congruent articulation with the radius, and a less convex distal surface for articulation with the distal carpal row (see Fig. 26.2). The minimal bone resection required allows for preservation of the

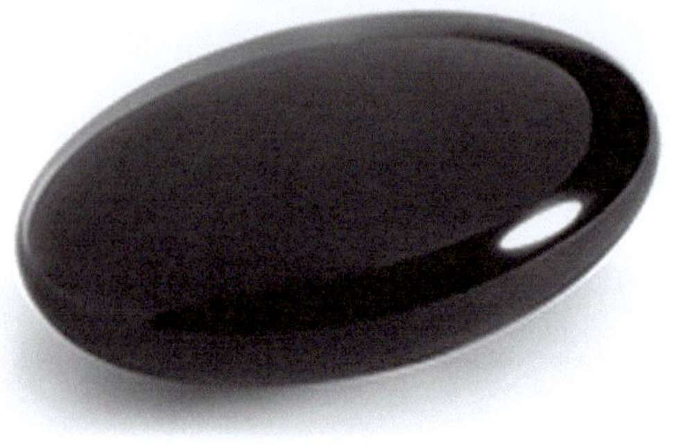

**Fig. 26.2** The Amandys prosthesis. Image courtesy of Tornier, Grenoble, France

important dorsal and volar extrinsic ligaments and motion at the radiocarpal and midcarpal joints. This allows in principle for a good range of stable movement whilst preserving the "dart-throwing motion" [23]. It has three axes of movement that allows it to act as a mobile and adaptive spacer which can slide, roll, and rotate, and is available in two lengths (24 and 26 mm) and four sizes.

The presence of bony cysts is not a contraindication (Fig. 26.10b) and can be managed well using bone grafts. The contraindications for this implant are the presence of radiocarpal and midcarpal instability, malalignment of the radial epiphysis, and the presence of infection.

The surgical technique can involve either a dorsal or radial approach. The dorsal approach is indicated when the procedure is being performed as a secondary surgery, when previous implants need to be removed or bone reconstruction is required. One of the primary authors (PB) has found the radial approach to be better in those patients undergoing primary surgery who do not have capsular deficiency with no significant osteophytes.

The surgical technique for the dorsal approach uses a dorsal longitudinal incision and division of the extensor retinaculum between the III and IV compartments. A flap of the retinaculum may be used later to strengthen the dorsal capsule if deficient. The posterior interosseous nerve is excised and a ligament sparing capsulotomy (Berger radially based flap [24]) is performed. A radial styloidectomy is performed with care taken to preserve the radio-scapho-capitate ligament, which is an important restraint of ulnar translation of the implant. The proximal scaphoid is then excised, preserving the distal one-third to two-thirds due to the ligament attachments. The lunate is carefully excised with a corkscrew to preserve the volar capsule and ligaments. The head of the capitate is then resected in the same line as the scaphoid. The radial carpal row articulations are contoured with an ovoid burr to remove the crest between the scaphoid fossa and the lunate fossa to obtain a homogenous concave ovoid surface along both the axes. On the carpal side, the new mid-carpal joint is smoothed and reamed to achieve a slightly concave sliding surface. Dorsal and volar radial osteophytes are excised taking care to preserve the ligament attachments. Other procedures are performed as required. These can include curetting the bone cavities and inserting bone graft; repairing a tear in the volar capsule, or plicating capsular distension with non-absorbable sutures. Various-sized implants are trialed until an implant of appropriate dimensions is selected that allows a good range of stable free motion without overstuffing the joint. Flexion and extension are tested with gravity. All movements are performed to check that the implant does not rotate. If the implant rotates on radial ulnar deviation such that the long axis becomes antero-posterior, this is a sign of insufficient bone excision mainly on the lateral aspect. Under fluoroscopy if the implant is anteriorly subluxated or the distal carpal row is subluxated dorsally, it requires anterior capsular plication. In the anterior view, the distance between the ulna and triquetrum reflects the thickness of the implant and ideally should be the same as prior to surgery. After fluoroscopic confirmation, the implant is correctly and congruently positioned. The capsule is repaired, as this preserves the stability of the implant. If the dorsal capsule is too thin, half of the extensor retinaculum pedicle flap is used to reinforce the capsule.

Postoperatively a custom-made thermoplastic splint is fabricated in neutral to slight wrist extension. A gentle wrist mobilisation program is initiated under the supervision of the hand therapist between first and 14 days. The splint is used for

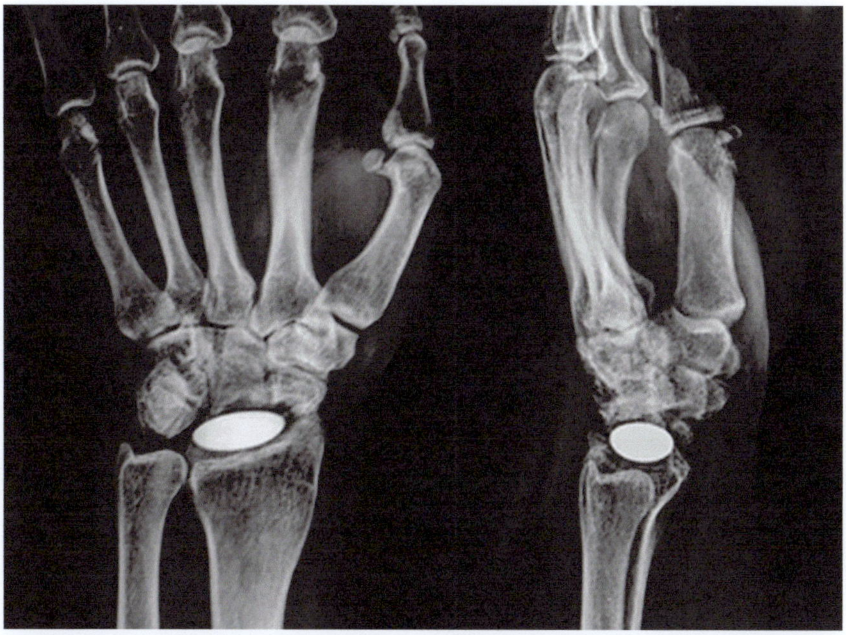

**Fig. 26.3** The Amandys interposition arthroplasty in situ. Pictures courtesy of Philippe Bellemère

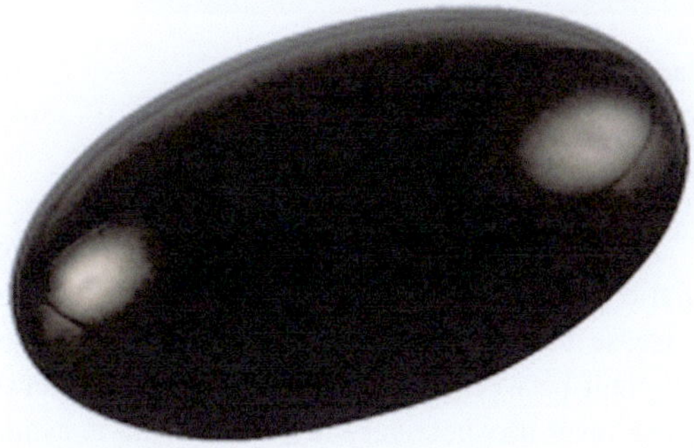

**Fig. 26.4** The APSI. Image courtesy of Tornier, Grenoble, France

up to 6 weeks following surgery before unrestricted movement is permitted.

Current literature examining the outcomes following pyrocarbon Amandys replacement is limited. Bellemère et al. have reported two different series. One of them showed 25 patients with a mean follow-up of 24 months [25]. Mean Visual Analogue Scale (VAS) reduced from 6.7 to 3.7. Mean grip strength was 16 kg (51 % contra-lateral side). Flexion-extension arc mean was 68°. Mean QuickDASH and Patient rated Wrist Evaluation (PRWE) scores improved from 63 to 36 and 61 to 32, respectively. Ninety-six percent of patients were satisfied or very satisfied. This series had no subluxations, dislocations or revision surgeries.

A series of six patients has also been reported in the literature [26]. They were followed up over an average of 16 months. Daruwalla and colleagues reported good results for their series of patients using the Amandys. However, all of these patients had evidence of carpal arthritis and the causative pathology was not Kienböck's disease. Hence, this should be considered when reviewing these outcomes.

One of the authors (MR) has treated seven patients with interposition arthroplasty using the Amandys implant. One of these patients had a primary diagnosis of Kienböck's disease. Mean age at surgery was 56.4 years (41–68). Five patients had surgery on the dominant size. The mean follow up was 12 months (9–36). Patients reported an average improvement in pain of 20 % using the VAS from 6 months after surgery. Mean QuickDASH and PRWE scores improved by 16 and 21 points, respectively. Mean grip improved from pre-operative grip 17.7–18.9 kg at 1 year. No adverse events such as infection, subluxation or dislocation have been reported.

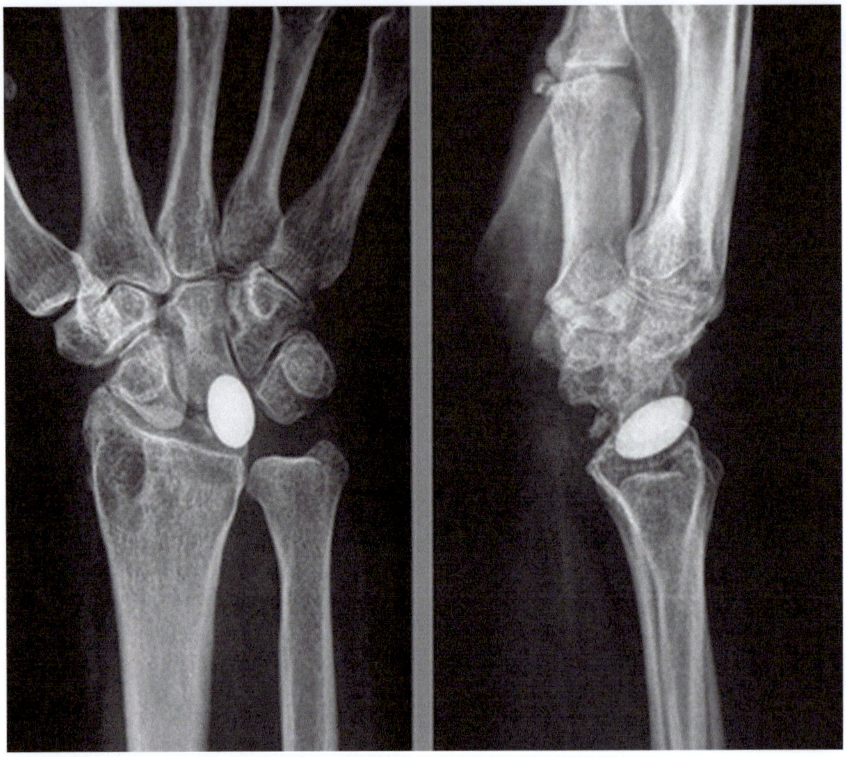

**Fig. 26.5** The APSI in situ. Picture courtesy of Philippe Bellemère

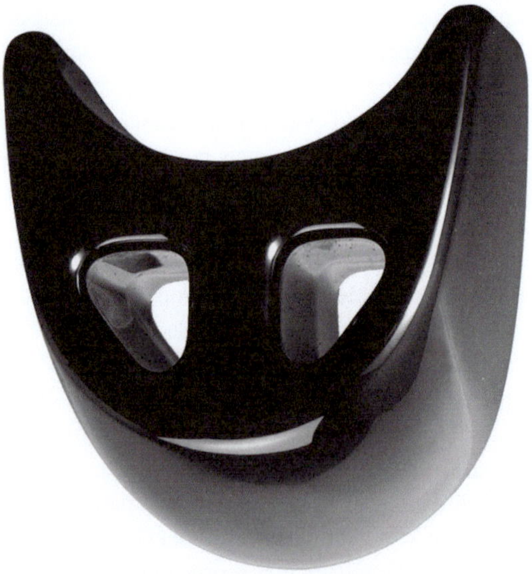

**Fig. 26.6** The lunate replacement implant. Image courtesy of Ascension, Austin, TX, USA

At one of the author's (PB) institution, 16 patients (11 male and 5 females) with Kienböck's disease have been managed with the Amandys implant between 2009 and 2014. These patients have been prospectively reviewed. Data is available for 14 of the 16 patients with one lost to follow-up and one patient deceased. Eight of the 14 patients had primary surgery for stage 4 Kienböck's disease. The remaining six patients had the surgery as a secondary procedure (three failed silicone lunate implants, two radial shortening and one Graner procedure). There were 13 treated with the dorsal approach, and one with a radial approach. Mean follow up was 33.3 months (5–60). Mean age at surgery was 51.9 years (37–70). Seven patients were "very satisfied" and seven patients were "satisfied". Wrist movement did not show an overall change following surgery. VAS had a mean reduction of 44/100 mm.

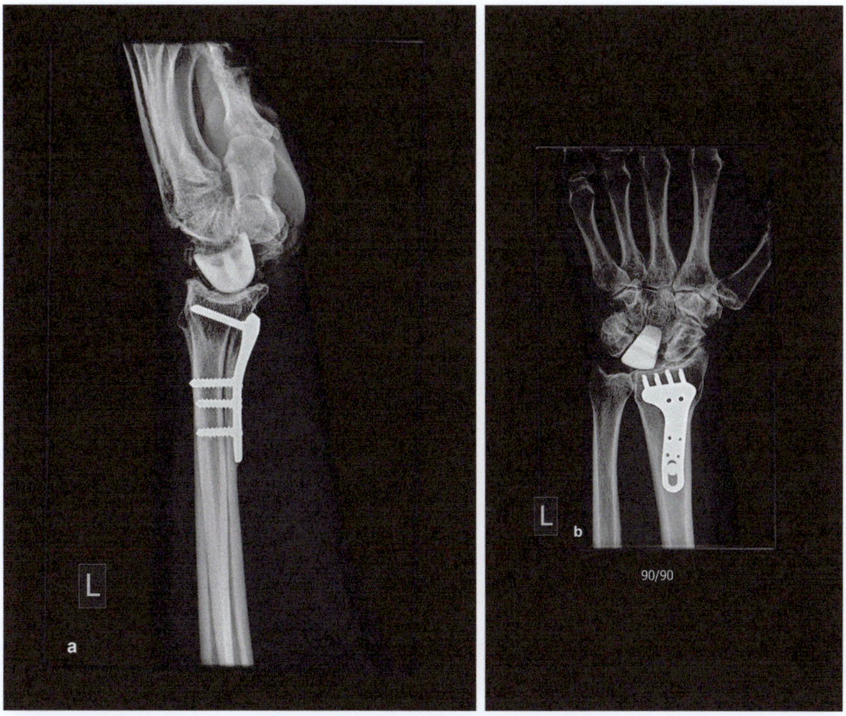


**Fig. 26.7** (**a**, **b**) The lunate replacement in situ. Pictures courtesy of Mark Ross

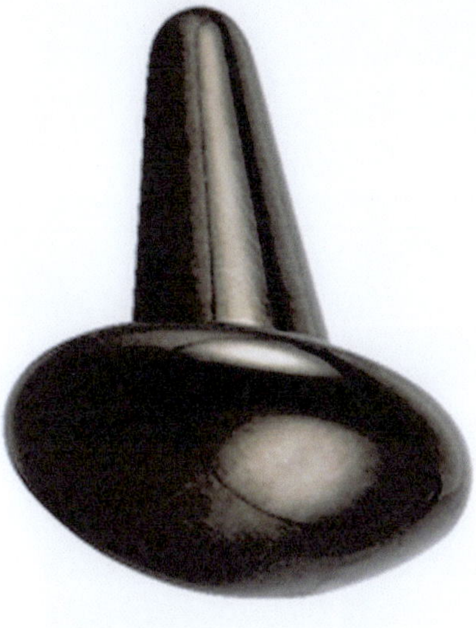

**Fig. 26.8** The RCPI. Image courtesy of Tornier, Grenoble, France

The PRWE score decreased from pre-op mean 60.8 to post-op mean 24.3 and the QuickDASH score decreased from pre-op mean 61.7 to post-op mean 31.9. Grip strength of the affected hand increased by a mean of 6 kg. Two patients had asymptomatic implant subluxation, however there were no dislocations or bone collapse. Three required revision surgery. One subluxated implant was replaced with a bigger implant. Another implant rotated and required a smaller implant and further bone resection because of lateral impingement. The third patient also had subluxation and underwent three revision surgeries. He first had an implant size increase, followed by plication of the anterior capsule. He finally required bone resection. This was the first patient to have surgery with the author (PB) and there may be a correlation with the learning curve of the technique. Two patients had associated bone graft in bone cavities due to inflammatory reaction around silicone implant. Both patients presented with normal X-rays at the last follow-up (see Fig. 26.10a–d).

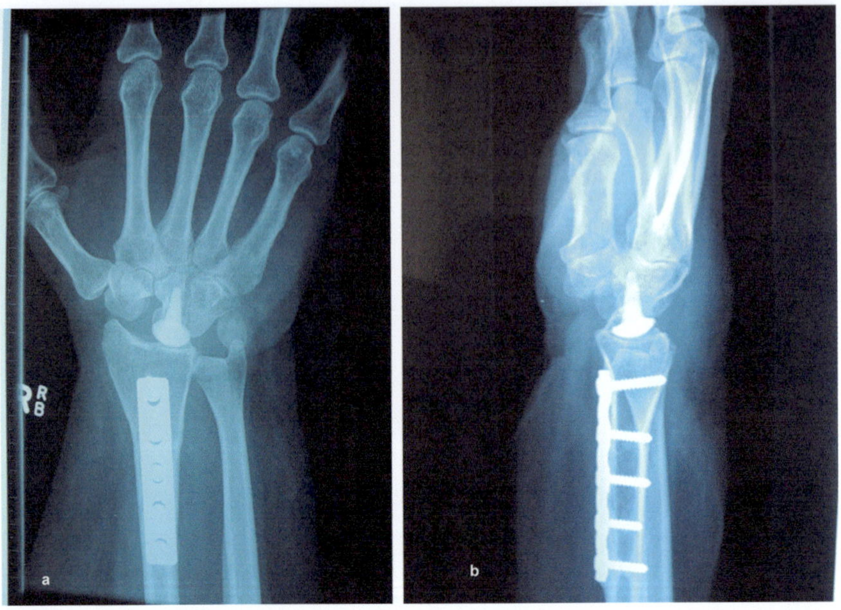


**Fig. 26.9** (**a**, **b**) Kienböck's patient who has had a radial shortening osteotomy, proximal row carpectomy and has an RCPI in situ. Pictures courtesy of Mark Ross

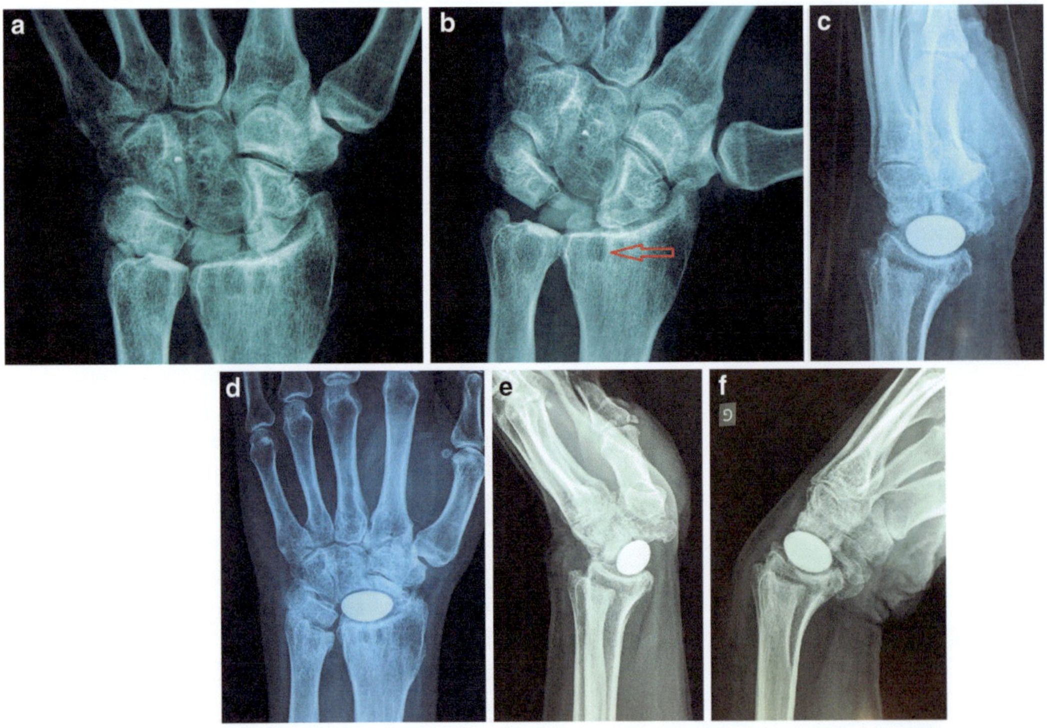


**Fig. 26.10** Silicone lunate implant inserted in 1992 for Kienböck's disease stage 3. Patients represent with pain and stiffness in 2009. (**a**) AP radiograph with silicone implant. (**b**) AP radiograph with radial inclination. *Red arrow* shows a bony defect. (**c**) Lateral radiograph, result at 1 year. (**d**) AP radiograph, result at 1 year. (**e**) Lateral radiograph, wrist in extension, result at 5 years. (**f**) Lateral radiograph, wrist in flexion, result at 5 years

## Adaptive Proximal Scaphoid Implant (APSI)

APSI (see Figs. 26.4 and 26.5) is another pyrocarbon implant that has similar design characteristics to the Amandys but it may be used as a lunate replacement. It is a dynamic spacer, which helps maintain the carpal height [27] and the coherence of the first row [23]. Being a nonfixed implant, it has 3D adaptability during wrist movement. This allows it to move and find its place depending on the forces applied to the implant [27]. The implant has two axes of movement; the long axis is anterior to posterior and the short axis is medial to lateral. The advantage of using the device is that it does not compromise bone stock for wrist fusion in the future [27]. The APSI is a good surgical option available for stage 3 and 4 Kienböck's disease. This implant is not recommended in the presence of radio-carpal or mid-carpal arthritis; bone cavity in the head of the capitate; in carpal instability or in the presence of infection. A prerequisite of using this device is that ligaments need to be intact in order to avoid implant dislocation. Implant dislocation has not occurred in our experience and has not been reported in the other published series [28, 29].

The articular approach is using a portion of the Berger flap [30] protecting the dorsal radiocarpal ligament. The lunate is partially removed, and the posterior horn is preserved because of its ligamentous attachments. The implant is tested in all planes of movement. The long axis of the implant is anterior to posterior (see Fig. 26.5). It is important that the implant moves as this indicates the size is correct. Dynamic X-ray is performed to confirm that the implant is correctly placed. The capsule is securely closed to preserve the stability of the implant. This implant does not require ligamentoplasty. If the posterior capsule is thin, the extensor retinaculum may be used as a flap to reinforce the capsule. It is very important not to oversize the implant so as to allow for it to have adaptable movement. A light dressing and a temporary plaster slab applied. Post-operatively a custom made thermoplastic splint is fabricated in neutral wrist position to be used for 2 weeks. A gentle wrist mobilization program is initiated under the supervision of the hand therapist at 2 weeks. The splint is used for 6 weeks following surgery before unrestricted movement is permitted.

The implant was originally developed in 2000 for use in patients with necrosis of the proximal scaphoid [27]. The implant has been used in Kienböck's disease for several years in France. Werthel et al. [29] reported two cases of Kienböck's disease treated with an APSI with an average follow-up of 36 months. These patients improved their mobility and grip strength. At a mean follow-up of 3 years, the average VAS pain score was 1/100 and the average DASH was 11.5.

Two patients with Lichtman's stage 4 Kienböck's disease have been treated using the APSI by one of the authors (PB). The first patient was a 44-year-old male manual worker (8-year follow-up) (see Fig. 26.5) and the second patient was a 56-year-old lady in an office-based occupation (3.4 year follow-up). VAS improved by 50 mm in the first patient and 54 mm in the second patient. Patients' flexion/extension increased by 10°/10° degrees and 5°/0° degrees, respectively. The PRWE score improved by 55 and 12 and the QuickDASH score improved by 55 and 9, respectively, in the two patients. Both patients were satisfied with their outcomes. The first patient presented with asymptomatic radiological signs of subluxation of the implant that did not warrant further treatment.

A third patient who also had stage 4 Kienböck's disease was treated with an Amandys implant used as an APSI. This was a 70-year-old retired manual worker with very large hands. Intraoperatively it was felt that the largest APSI was insufficient in size to preserve carpal height. The smallest-sized Amandys was used as an alternative as it has a similar design with two axes of movement and dynamic X-rays revealed that the Amandys was behaving similar to an APSI. The patient had a good outcomes with no pain, improvement in movement and all functional scores.

## Pyrocarbon Lunate Replacement

The Ascension Lunate Replacement (Ascension Orthopedics, Austin, Texas) (see Fig. 26.6) prosthesis differs significantly from the formerly described implants, as it is shaped like the lunate. It is flat on the radial and ulnar sides but wider ulnarly to mimic the articulation of the scapholunate and lunotriquetral joints. There are two holes in its center allowing for the passage of sutures and/or tendon grafts for stabilisation.

The lunate is excised and an appropriately sized implant is selected with care to avoid overstuffing. For suture anchor stabilisation alone, a template guide is used to place two suture anchors into the scaphoid and mark two drill holes through the triquetrum. The prosthesis is inserted after pulling the sutures through the two central holes of the implant, which are then passed through the triquetral drill holes and tied, stabilizing the implant (see Fig. 26.7a, b). Controlled mobilization may be introduced from the first few days post-op depending on the surgeons' assessment of the stabilization achieved. Up to 8 weeks of splint immobilization may be used.

The preferred technique of one of the senior authors (MR) is to utilise a transosseous partial FCR graft through the scaphoid, the dorsal hole in the implant and the triquetrum and a double barrel suture anchor with sutures passed from the scaphoid through the volar hole in the implant then through the triquetrum. The tendon portion of this stabilization is similar to the technique described for SLL reconstruction with scapholunate-triquetral tenodesis (SLT) [31].

The largest published series to date by Henry describes the results of the lunate replacement in 13 patients with late stage Kienböck's disease [32]. The mean age of the patients was 40 years with a mean follow-up of 30.3 months. Mean wrist flexion, extension and grip strength was measured on average as 29.2°, 24.2° and 12.3 kg preoperatively, which improved to 43.3°, 53.3° and 31.5 kg at follow-up. DASH scores improved from 39.1 to 7.7. Henry reported complications in three of his 13 patients [32]. One patient required conversion to a proximal row carpectomy during the primary surgery as the surgeon was not able to adequately position the implant in the sagittal plane. Another patient also did not comply with postoperative instructions and required re-operation to replace a migrated K-wire. A third patient developed osteonecrosis of the proximal pole of the scaphoid attributed to the drill holes made. This was revised to a proximal row carpectomy. Despite promising results, the author expressed concern over the implant design. In particular, he suggested that the two central holes were too close together which did not allow effective control of the sagittal balance of the prosthesis. These complications have lead to a modification of the technique by Henry [33]. He now recommends making only one drill hole in the scaphoid and triquetrum, and second pass of the graft is routed dorsal rather than through the implant.

Control of sagittal plane rotation of the implant remains the greatest challenge in implanting the pyrocarbon lunate.

## Case Example

A 27-year-old male safety advisor for the mining industry presented at one of the author's (MR) hospital with post-traumatic avascular necrosis of the lunate 1 year after a hyper-flexion injury to his right wrist (Fig. 26.11). This was treated with a pyrocarbon lunate replacement, stabilized with an FCR tendon transfer and suture anchor double suture (see Fig. 26.7a, b). Postoperatively he was immobilized in a splint for 6 weeks while performing only inner range flexion and extension exercises. Strengthening was commenced at 12 weeks. At his 12-month review, the patient had 90 % range of motion compared to the contralateral side (Fig. 26.12). At his 60-month review he reported a dull ache in his wrist (VAS 10 mm), and had a PRWE score of 18 and a QuickDASH score of 6.8.

## Resurfacing Capitate Pyrocarbon Implant

Proximal row carpectomy (PRC) is an established treatment option for unsalvageable Kienböck's disease when the lunate is irreversibly

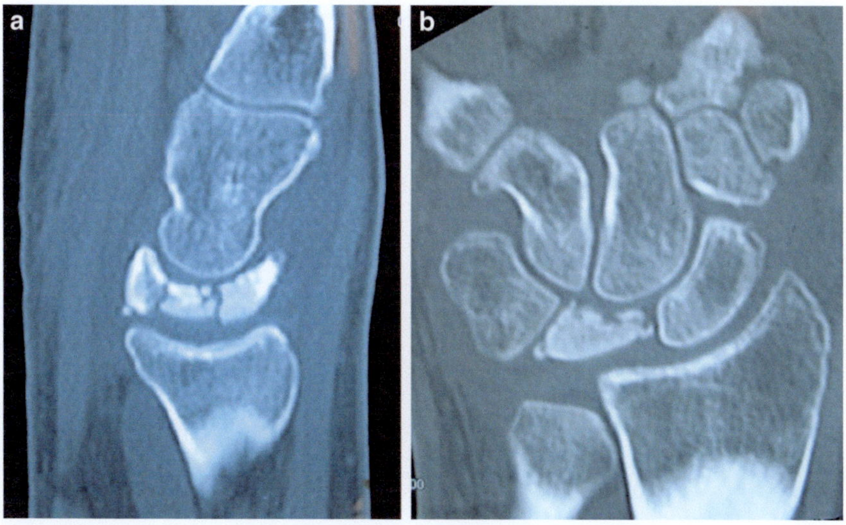


**Fig. 26.11** (**a**, **b**) Preoperative CT scans of Kienböck's wrist. Pictures courtesy of Mark Ross

damaged but the articular surfaces of the radius and distal carpal row remain healthy. However, these conditions are frequently not met (e.g., Bain, stage IV) and associated arthritis is present. In these circumstances, a PRC can be performed in combination with a Resurfacing Capitate Pyrocarbon Implant, or RCPI (Tornier, Grenoble, France). This is an asymmetric stemmed implant that is designed to sit with press fit fixation of the stem centrally within the capitate (see Fig. 26.8). A proximal convex surface is designed to articulate with the lunate fossa, even when the lunate fossa demonstrates cartilage damage or arthritis.

The surgical technique is simple and thus attractive for surgeons. A routine PRC is performed through a ligament sparing capsular approach, followed by excision of the proximal pole of the capitate with an oscillating saw. Reamers and rasps are then used to prepare the bone and either a 14- or 16-mm trial implant is inserted. The appropriate size is selected based on direct and radiologic observation of the congruence with the native lunate fossa. The wrist is immobilized for 1–5 days and then a removable thermoplastic splint is applied to allow early active range of motion exercises for the next 4 weeks.

Preliminary studies have been promising, although again these published case series are not exclusively Kienböck's patients [33, 34]. To date the largest series described by Marcuzzi et al. included 35 patients from a potential total of 41 (six lost to follow-up) with a median follow up of 34 months [35]. Thirty-two patients were satisfied with their operation. Mean VAS for pain improved from 8.4 to 1.4, DASH scores reduced from 56.9 to 11.4. Both grip strength and range of motion improved, contrary to the results from Goubier et al. [36]. Patients' mean flexion/extension increased from 25°/25° to 33°/34° and mean grip strength increased from 10 to 16.5 kg. Radiologically there were no issues with the 22 implants. In the remaining 13 patients, they identified a slight medial translation of the implant and in one patient a mild subsidence was described. They suspected that wrist laxity from the PRC and dorsal capsular incision in combination with the inclination of the distal radius attributed to this.

At one of the author's (MR) institution the RCPI was used in a series of 29 patients, with a mean follow-up of 35 months (6–113). Only three of these patients had Kienböck's disease but all had associated findings of mid carpal and/or radiocarpal arthritis. Mean VAS for pain and satisfaction were 30 and 77, respectively. Mean QuickDASH and PRWE scores were 35 and 36, respectively. Interestingly all three patients with

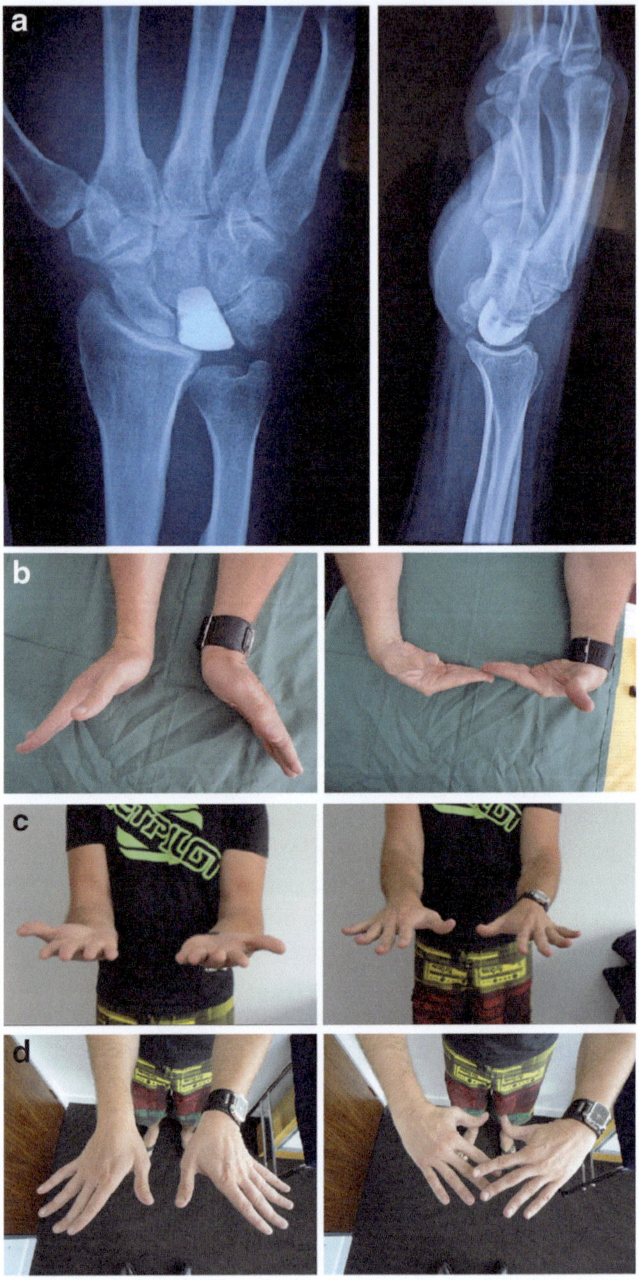


**Fig. 26.12** Postoperative images at 60 months, with pyrocarbon lunate replacement implant in situ. (**a**) Plain radiographs; (**b**) extension and flexion; (**c**) supination and pronation; (**d**) radial and ulnar deviation. Pictures courtesy of Mark Ross

Kienböck's disease scored very highly on satisfaction scores but all were ultimately revised to a total wrist fusion at 39, 33, and 14 months. Essentially this intervention was viewed as a holding therapy that allowed patients a good quality of life for a few years prior to total wrist arthrodesis.

## Conclusion

Current treatment outcomes for late stage Kienböck's disease remain far from satisfactory. Pancarpal arthrodesis is still the only permanent solution with an associated functional deficit that may be often unacceptable to the patient. Joint replacement surgery theoretically confers better function but traditional methods and designs have many shortcomings, some of which are related to the materials used. Pyrocarbon interposition arthroplasty uses a material that has many potential advantages that could give long-lasting satisfactory results. As with many of the current treatment strategies for Kienböck's disease, the patient may often undergo multiple operations throughout their life in an effort to obtain pain relief and maximise function before undergoing to a total wrist fusion. Whether the role of pyrocarbon arthroplasty becomes an efficacious treatment option with truly long-term satisfactory results currently remains unknown. Current evidence is limited due to small patient numbers and short length of follow-up. However, the early results are promising and further longer term studies with higher patient numbers are needed.

## References


1. Innes L, Strauch RJ. Systematic review of the treatment of Kienböck's disease in its early and late stages. J Hand Surg Am. 2010;35:713–7.
2. Koh S, Nakamura R, Horii E, Nakao E, Inagaki H, Yajima H. Surgical outcome of radial osteotomy for Kienböck's disease—minimum 10 years of follow up. J Hand Surg Am. 2003;28:910–6.
3. Raven EE, Haverkamp D, Marti RK. Outcome of Kienböck's disease 22 years after distal radius shortening osteotomy. Clin Orthop Relat Res. 2007;460:137–41.
4. Van den Dungen S, Dury M, Foucher G, Marin Braun F, Loréa P. Conservative treatment versus scaphotrapeziotrapezoid arthrodesis for Kienböck's disease: a retrospective study. Chir Main. 2006;25:141–5.
5. Watanabe T, Takahara M, Tsuchida H, Yamahara S, Kikuchi N, Ogino T. Long-term follow-up of radial shortening osteotomy for Kienböck disease. J Bone Joint Surg Am. 2008;90:1705–11.
6. Lin HH, Stern PJ. "Salvage" procedures in the treatment of Kienböck's disease. Proximal row carpectomy and total wrist arthrodesis. Hand Clin. 1993;9:521–6.
7. Roca J, Beltran JE, Fairen MF, Alvarez A. Treatment of Kienböck's disease using a silicone rubber implant. J Bone Joint Surg Am. 1976;58:373–6.
8. Bokros JC. Deposition, structure and properties of pyrolytic carbon used in medical applications. In: Walker PL, editor. Chemistry and physics of carbon. New York, NY: Marcel Dekker; 1969. p. 1–118.
9. Bokros JC, Haubold AD, Akins RJ, Campbell LA, Griffin CD, Lane E. The durability of mechanical heart valve replacement: past experience and current trends. In: Bodnar E, Frater RWM, editors. Replacement cardiac valves. New York, NY: Pergamon Press; 1991. p. 21–47.
10. Ross M, James C, Couzens G, Klawitter J. Pyrocarbon small joint arthroplasty of the extremities. In: Revell PA, editor. Joint replacement technology. 2nd ed. Cambridge: Woodhead Publishing; 2014. p. 628–73.
11. Cook SD, Beckenbaugh RD, Redondo J, Popich LS, Klawitter JJ, Linschied RL. Long-term followup of pyrolytic carbon metacarpophalangeal joints. J Bone Joint Surg Am. 1999;81:635–48.
12. Stanley J, Klawitter J, More R. Replacing joints with pyrolytic carbon. In: Revell PA, editor. Joint replacement technology. Cambridge: Woodhead Publishing; 2008. p. 631–56.
13. Kaae JL. The mechanism of deposition of pyrolytic carbon. Carbon. 1985;23(6):665–7.
14. Reilly DT, Burnstein AH. The mechanical properties of cortical bone. J Bone Joint Surg Am. 1974;56(5):1001–22.
15. Ritchie RO, Dauskardt RH, Yu W, Brendzel AM. Cyclic fatigue-crack propagation, stress corrosion and fracture toughness behaviour in pyrolite carbon coated graphite for prosthetic heart valve applications. J Biomed Mat Res. 1990;24:189–206.
16. Hills BA, Monds MK. Enzymatic identification of the load-bearing lubricant in the joint. Br J Rheumatol. 1998;37(2):137–42.
17. Qiu Y, Holland N, Ruegsegger M, Marchant R. Biomimetic engineering of non-adhesive glycocalyx-like surfaces using oligosaccharide surfactant polymers. Nature. 1998;392:799–801.
18. Strzepa P, Klawitter J. Ascension pyrocarbon hemisphere wear testing against bone. Poster 0897. In Proceedings of 51st Annual Meeting of the Orthopaedic Research Society, Washington, DC, 2005.
19. Thomas KA, Cook SD, Renz EA, Anderson RC, Haddad RJ, Haubold AD, et al. The effect of surface treatments on the interface mechanics of LTI pyrolytic carbon implants. J Biomed Mater Res. 1985;19:145–59.
20. Glasson JM, Duke P, Ross M. Pyrocarbon humeral resurfacing – an option in hemiarthroplasty. Paris International Shoulder Course 2013: Current concepts on shoulder arthroplasty 2013, pp. 97–101.
21. Wall LB, Stern PJ. Clinical and radiographic outcomes of metacarpophalangeal joint pyrolytic carbon arthroplasty for osteoarthritis. J Hand Surg Am. 2013;38(3):537–43.
22. Sweets TM, Stern PJ. Pyrolytic carbon resurfacing arthroplasty for osteoarthritis of the proximal interphalangeal joint of the finger. J Bone Joint Surg Am. 2011;93(15):1417–25.
23. Moritomo H, Apergis EP, Herzberg G, Werner FW, Wolfe SW, Garcia-Elias M. IFSSH committee report of wrist biomechanics committee: biomechanics of the so-called dart-throwing motion of the wrist. J Hand Surg Am. 2007;32(9):1447–53.

24. Berger RA, Bishop AT, Bettinger PC. New dorsal capsulotomy for the surgical exposure of the wrist. Ann Plast Surg. 1995;35(1):54–9.
25. Bellemère P, Maes-Clavier C, Loubersac T, Gaisne E, Kerjean Y. Amandys implant: novel pyrocarbon arthroplasty for the wrist. Chir Main. 2012;31(4):176–84.
26. Daruwalla ZJ, Davies KL, Shafighian A, Gillham NR. Early results of a prospective study on the pyrolytic carbon (pyrocarbon) Amandys for osteoarthritis of the wrist. Ann R Coll Surg Engl. 2012;94(7):496–501.
27. Pequignot JP, Lussiez B, Allieu Y. an adaptive proximal scaphoid implant. Chir Main. 2000;19:276–85.
28. Grandis C, Berzero F, Pasqualini M. Pyrocarbon A.P.S.I. prosthesis in Kien-bock's disease. J Hand Surg Eur Vol. 2006;31(Suppl):34–5.
29. Werthel JD, Hoang DV, Boyer P, Dallaudiere B, Massin P, Loriaut P. Treatment of Kienböck's disease using a pyrocarbon implant: case report. Chir Main. 2014;33(6):404–9.
30. Berger RA. A method of defining palpable landmarks for the ligament-splitting dorsal wrist capsulotomy. J Hand Surg Am. 2007;32(8):1291–5.
31. Ross M, Loveridge J, Cutbush K, Couzens G. Scapholunate ligament reconstruction. J Wrist Surg. 2013;2(2):110–5.
32. Henry M. Double bundle tendon graft for rotational stabilization of lunate implant arthroplasty. Tech Hand Up Extrem Surg. 2011;15(1):16–23.
33. Henry M. Outcomes assessment of lunate replacement arthroplasty with intrinsic carpal ligament reconstruction in Kienböck's disease. Hand. 2014; 9(3):364–9.
34. Szalay G, Stigler B, Kraus R, Böhringer G, Schnettler R. Proximal row carpectomy and replacement of the proximal pole of the capitate by means of a pyrocarbon cap (RCPI) in advanced carpal collapse. Handchir Mikrochir Plast Chir. 2012;44:17–22.
35. Marcuzzi A, Ozben H, Russomando A. The use of a pyrocarbon capitate resurfacing implant in chronic wrist disorders. J Hand Surg Eur Vol. 2013; 39(6):611–8.
36. Goubier JN, Vogels J, Teboul F. Capitate pyrocarbon prosthesis in radiocarpal osteoarthritis. Tech Hand Up Extrem Surg. 2011;15:28–31.

# 27 Wrist Hemiarthroplasty Combined with Proximal Row Carpectomy

Brian D. Adams

## Introduction

Although total wrist arthroplasty (TWA) has been used in select patients with advanced arthritis due to late Kienböck's disease, those with physically demanding lifestyles are infrequently considered appropriate due to a higher risk for implant loosening, particularly of the distal component. A wrist hemiarthroplasty may obviate the need for strict physical restrictions following TWA and thus provide another motion-preserving option for active patients with advanced wrist arthritis, especially those with distal radius or capitate articular degeneration. Wrist hemiarthroplasty combined with a proximal row carpectomy (PRC) has shown promising early clinical results in properly selected patients with arthritis for whom there are very limited options [1, 2].

In this chapter, a review of the concept of wrist hemiarthroplasty, including assessment in a cadaver study and the early clinical outcomes in a series of patients will be presented. Although hemiarthroplasty has shown promising early results, the procedure is relatively new and it is considered an "off-label" use of an implant system in the USA and some other countries.

B.D. Adams, MD (✉)
Department of Orthopedic Surgery, University of Iowa College of Medicine, Iowa City, Iowa, USA
e-mail: brian.adams@bcm.edu

## Surgical Technique

### Concept

The standard technique described for the Universal 2 (UNI 2) or Freedom wrist arthroplasty implant system (Integra Life Sciences, Plainsboro, NJ) is used. A PRC is performed, but only the radial component is implanted.

### Incision

In this technique, a dorsal longitudinal incision is made over the wrist in line with the third metacarpal, extending proximally from its midshaft to approximately 8 cm proximal to the wrist joint. The skin and subcutaneous tissue are elevated together off the extensor retinaculum, with care to protect the branches of the superficial radial nerve and the dorsal cutaneous ulnar nerve.

### Extensor Tendons

The EDQ extensor compartment is opened and the entire retinaculum is elevated radially, to the septum between the first and second extensor compartments. Each septum is divided carefully to avoid creating rents in the retinaculum, especially at Lister's tubercle. An extensor tenosynovectomy is performed if needed, and the tendons

© Springer International Publishing Switzerland 2016
D.M. Lichtman, G.I. Bain (eds.), *Kienböck's Disease*, DOI 10.1007/978-3-319-34226-9_27

are inspected. The ECRB must be intact or repairable (preferably the ECRL is also functional).

## Dorsal Capsule

A quarter inch Penrose tubing is used to retract the extensor tendons, with the EDQ and EDC tendons pulled ulnarly and the EPL, ECRB, and ECRL pulled radially.

The dorsal wrist capsule is raised as a broad distally based rectangular flap to the level of the mid-capitate. The capsule is raised in continuity with the periosteum over the distal ½ cm of the radius to create a longer flap for closure. The radial side of the flap is made in the floor of the second extensor compartment and the ulnar side extends from the radius to triquetrum. The first extensor compartment is elevated subperiosteally from the distal 1 cm of the radial styloid. The remaining dorsal wrist capsule is elevated ulnarly from the triquetrum. The wrist is fully flexed to expose the joint. If necessary, a synovectomy is performed. If the distal ulna is to be resected, a separate capsulotomy is made proximal to the triangular fibocartilage complex (TFCC).

## PRC

A proximal row carpectomy is performed with care to preserve the capitate head and volar wrist capsule. No further carpal preparation is required. The capitate head should not have any erosions or cysts that would lead to structural weakening. However, articular cartilage is not a requirement for a hemiarthroplasty.

## Trials

Using the radial trials, apply their articular surface against the capitate head to determine the appropriate size. The capitate head must fit easily into the articular surface of the radial trial and allow volar-dorsal translation throughout all ranges of motion.

## Implant

Although there is some difference in the radius preparation between the UNI 2 and Freedom implant systems, the UNI 2 technique is described here. Insert the radial intramedullary guide rod into radius, entering below Lister's tubercle and approximately 3 mm beneath the edge of the articular surface. Confirm the rod is entered in the radial canal using both PA and lateral fluoroscopic images. Apply the radial resection guide to the rod and adjust its position so as to remove on the dorsal rim of the radius; the cut need not remove the entire articular surface, particularly its volar portion. Secure the cutting guide with K wires, remove the guide rod, and then resect the radius without violating the sigmoid notch, triangular fibrocartilage or ulnar head. Reinsert the guide rod and sequentially broach to the planned implant size. Insert a trial radial component and perform a reduction to ensure the capitate head will easily fit and glide on the implant surface. Remove the trial and prepare three sets of paired holes along the dorsal rim of the distal radius and place three horizontal mattress sutures for later capsule closure. Insert the final implant using the impactor. Reduce the joint and close the capsule without imbrication. Repair the extensor retinaculum, leaving the radial wrist extensor tendons and extensor pollicis longus subcutaneous. Apply a dressing and plaster splint.

## Rehabilitation

Begin gentle range of motion exercises within a few days but do not allow excessive flexion until 4 weeks to protect the dorsal capsule repair. Advance to full available active motion and routine activities at 6 weeks. Long term restrictions include avoidance of impact loading such as using a hammer and forced wrist extension such as a push-up.

# Cadaver Study

A feasibility study focusing on joint alignment was undertaken in a cadaver study to determine if the concept of wrist hemiarthroplasty combined with a PRC should be considered for patients with wrist arthritis. The primary goal was to determine if wrist alignment remained similar to the natural wrist throughout a functional arc of motion. Because the articular shape of the radial component of the UNI 2 is designed to restore the natural loading axis of the wrist, which passes through the long axis of the third metacarpal, capitate, and lunate fossa, the expectation was that longitudinal alignment of the wrist would be maintained but some shortening of the wrist would occur due to the PRC. However, because only minimal resection of the radius is necessary, and there is some thickness of the radial component, the overall shortening of the wrist is minimal.

In this study, eight fresh-frozen specimens from eight donors, with an age range of 43–82 years, were amputated through the proximal forearm. Radiographs showed no preexisting arthritis or deformity. A radial component of the Universal 2 implant system was inserted using the standard described technique for this system.

Radiographic markers were placed in the base of the third metacarpal, in the capitate (near center of rotation) and in the distal radius to track changes in position of the capitate with respect to the radius. Fluoroscopic images were obtained for each specimen before component implantation and after the PRC with hemiarthroplasty (Fig. 27.1). These included; posterior-anterior (PA) images with the wrist in neutral, radial and ulnar deviation; and lateral images in neutral, 45° flexion and 45° extension.

The images were imported into AutoCAD 2002® (Autodesk, Inc, San Rafael, CA) and a pixilated two-dimensional Cartesian coordinate system was then constructed on each image. Projection error was calculated to range from 0.04 to 1.43 mm.

Changes in radial-ulnar alignment of the capitate ranged from 0.21 to 2.21 mm on the PA images and from 0.21 to 4.69 mm on lateral images. These were not significant. As expected, there was significant shortening due to the PRC, which was 4.36–5.43 mm on the lateral images and 5.72–6.10 mm on the PA images ($p<0.01$ in all wrist positions).

The results of these static measurements in this model demonstrated good wrist alignment in both the coronal and sagittal planes in all wrist positions following combined hemiarthroplasty with PRC (Figs. 27.2 and 27.3). Furthermore, although joint stability was not quantitatively assessed, none of the specimens were unstable during manipulation after the procedure.

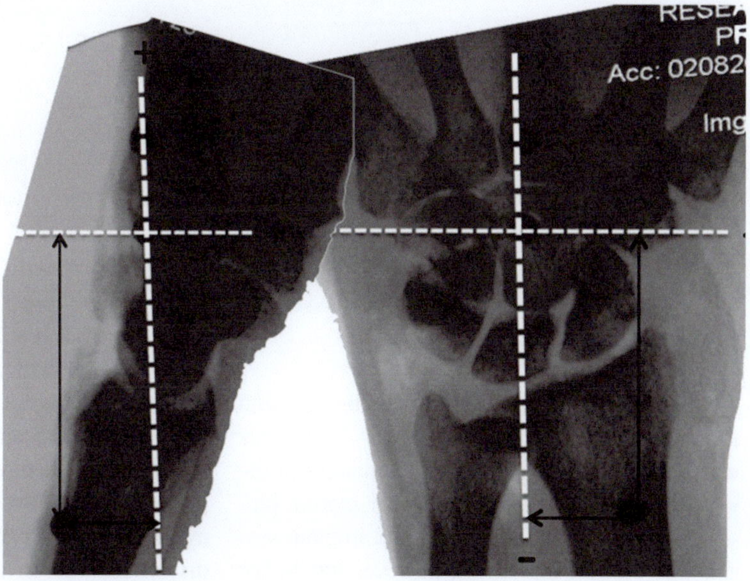


**Fig. 27.1** Cadaveric hemiarthroplasty study. Lateral and AP fluoroscopic images demonstrating the coordinate system used to perform measurements

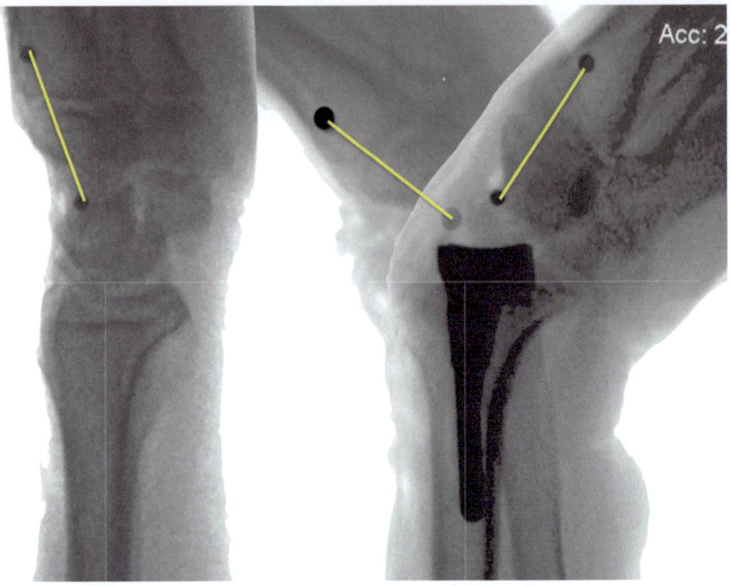

**Fig. 27.2** Lateral fluoroscopic image of the wrist. (*Left*) With markers in situ. (*Right*) Composite image following PRC and insertion of hemiarthroplasty (Universal 2, Integra Life Sciences, Plainsboro, NJ). Note the alignment throughout the flexion and extension range of motion

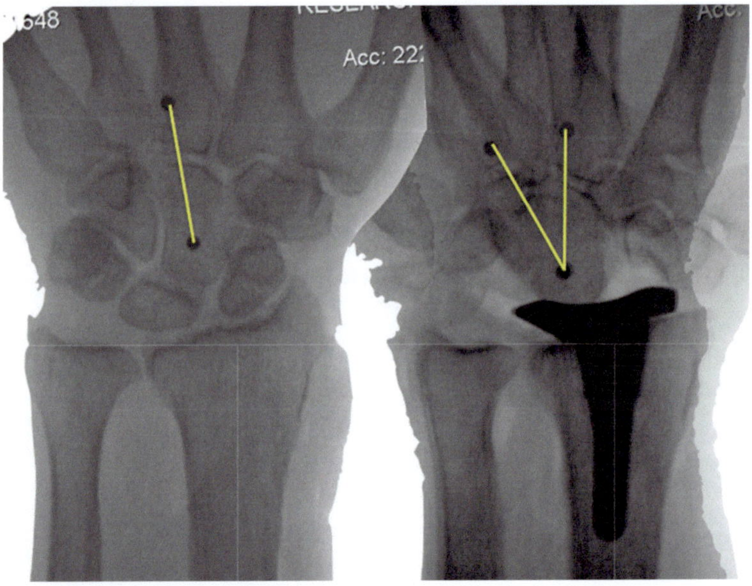

**Fig. 27.3** AP fluoroscopic image of the wrist. (*Left*) With markers in situ. (*Right*) Composite image following PRC and hemiarthroplasty (Universal 2, Integra Life Sciences, Plainsboro, NJ). Note the alignment throughout the range of radial and ulnar deviation

## Clinical Series

Twenty-six hemiarthroplasties combined with PRC were performed by the author in 23 patients who had a distribution of arthritic changes in the wrist that precluded the use of other motion preserving procedures. Only the UNI 2 implant system was used in this series, however the author converted to the use of the Freedom system when it became available. The surgical technique described above for the cadaver study was used in all patients. Indications initially included rheumatoid disease, osteoarthritis, post-traumatic arthritis and Kienböck's disease, however because some patients with active rheumatoid disease showed evidence of rapid carpal erosion the procedure was discontinued for these rheumatoid patients.

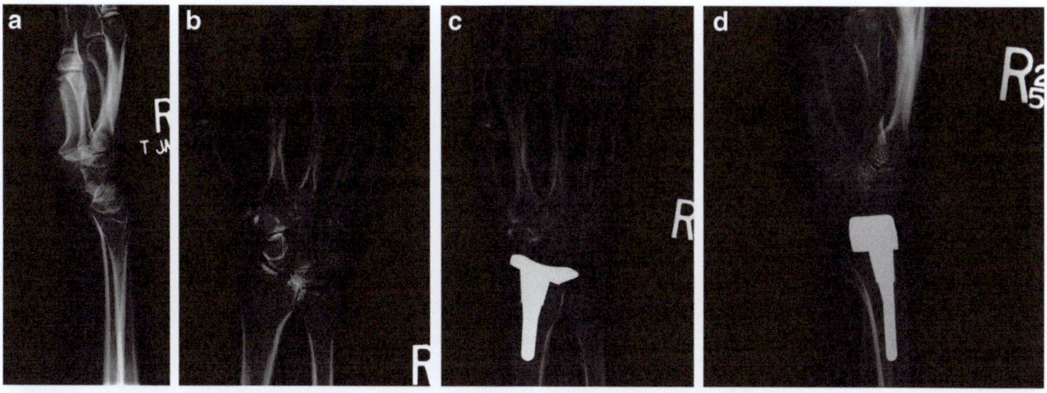

**Fig. 27.4** Preoperative posteroanterior and lateral views (**a**, **b**) of a patient with radiocarpal arthritis showing ulnar translocation of the carpus. Postoperative posteroanterior and lateral views (**c**, **d**) following treatment by hemiarthroplasty (Universal 2, Integra Life Sciences, Plainsboro, NJ) combined with PRC showing correction of ulnar translocation and reestablishment of the normal longitudinal loading axis across the wrist

Radiographic alignment measurements equivalent to those performed in the laboratory study were made in the first 15 wrists in 14 patients, at a range of follow-up of 1–2 years, to confirm the procedure was performing similarly in patients with arthritis who had some wrist deformity. The results showed maintenance of wrist alignment or realignment into a more normal position along the *x*-axis by improving preexisting ulnar translocation of the carpus; with the average change in the *x*-axis of 3.9 mm. Wrist shortening as measured on the *y*-axis averaged 4.8 mm, which occurred primarily due to the PRC.

Clinical and radiographic follow-up at a range of 3–6 years was performed for all 26 arthroplasties (Figs. 27.4 and 27.5). The average recorded results were: flexion 34° (range 22–53), extension 24° (18–44), radial deviation 12°, and ulnar deviation 21°. Change over time in wrist motion was assessed for the first 15 wrists in 14 patients who had measurements made at 1–2 years post-operative and again at 4–6 years post-operative. The average decrease in motion was flexion 11°, extension 9°, radial deviation 4°, and ulnar deviation 6°. This average loss of motion, however, was substantially influenced by three patients who lost considerably more motion than the other patients, retaining an average of only 11° of flexion and 9° of extension. These three patients had rheumatoid disease and showed obvious carpal erosion, and eventually went on to a complete arthrodesis. Following recognition of these impending failures, patients with rheumatoid disease were no longer treated by this procedure. The amount of capitate erosion that was measured in the non rheumatoid patients ($n = 20$) at follow up of 2–6 years, ranged from 1 to 5 mm, with the exception of one patient who had osteoarthritis and bilateral procedures showed 7 mm of erosion at 4 years in both wrists. This patient also had evidence of substantial preoperative capitate cystic changes and very active osteoarthritis involving multiple joints in other extremities. Based on this adverse outcome, caution should be exercised when considering this procedure in osteoarthritic patients who have substantial synovitis and cystic or erosive changes in the carpus, which likely indicates more advanced disease or compromised bone quality.

## Review of Literature

Boyer and Adams first described the procedure of combining a PRC with a distal radius hemiarthroplasty in a case study of two patients in 2010 [1]. The first patient was a 42-year-old rheumatoid patient who had bilateral wrist arthritis and the typical associated deformity and the second patient was a 52-year-old male with osteoarthritis of the right wrist and previous partial left fusion. The initial results were good in both patients but

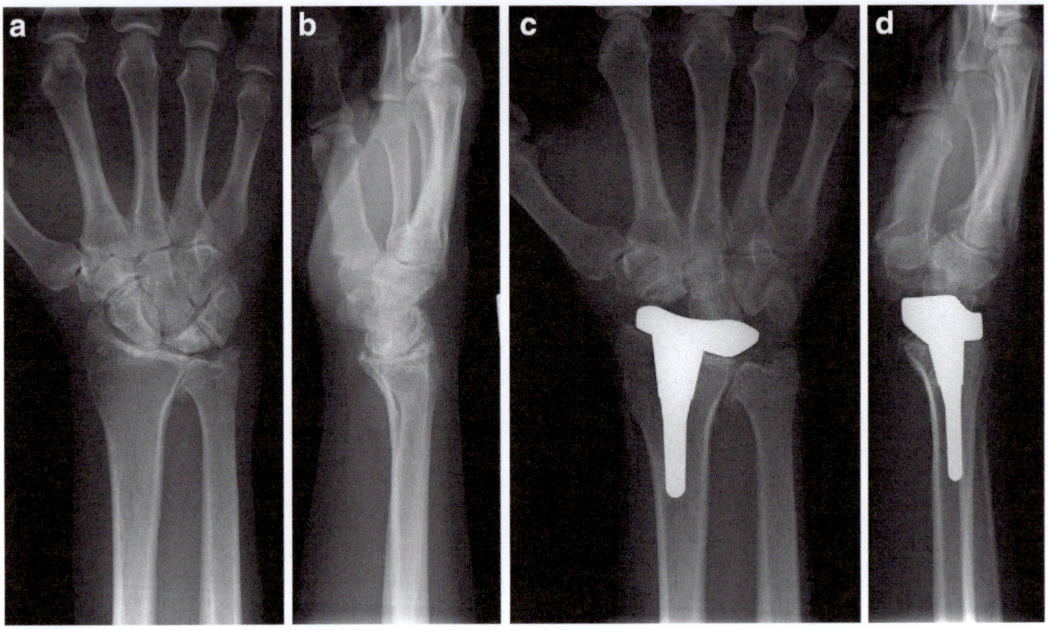


**Fig. 27.5** Preoperative posteroanterior and lateral views (**a**, **b**) of a wrist showing findings of Lichtman Stage 4 Kienböck's disease. Note that the capitate articular surface is preserved (Bain grade 3), making it a good indication for the hemiarthroplasty (Universal 2, Integra Life Sciences, Plainsboro, NJ). Postoperative posteroanterior and lateral views (**c**, **d**) after distal radius hemiarthroplasty combined with a PRC

the first patient developed the progressive carpal erosion described above while the second patient continues to have a good result at 6 years.

Culp et al. reported their results with this procedure using two different implants [2]. Their over all experience with the procedure included the use of the Maestro (Biomet, Warsaw, IN) radial implant that has polyethylene on its articular surface in the first 17 patients and the ReMotion (Small Bone Innovations, Morrisville, PA) that is made entirely of cobalt-chrome-molybdenum in the next 19 patients. They abandoned the use of the Maestro due to early osteolysis and reactive tenosynovitis from polyethylene wear of its articular surface. They had also stopped using the procedure in patients with inflammatory arthritis due to an apparent higher incidence of carpal erosion. Ten patients who did not have inflammatory arthritis and had proper medical records were reviewed in more detail at a follow up of 14–29 months. Post-operative wrist flexion and extension averaged 22° and 30°, respectively. Pain relief was often incomplete but improved following the procedure if there were no complications. They concluded the procedure provides a functional arc of motion and adequate grip strength in select patients but implant design likely plays a role an important role in outcome.

## Discussion

Active individuals with advanced Kienböck's disease often desire to maintain wrist motion so as to better perform tasks and activities that are important to their life style. However, due to the physical restrictions that are recommended following total wrist arthroplasty, those with physically demanding life styles are infrequently considered for total wrist replacement because of the risk for implant loosening, particularly of the distal component. A distal radius hemiarthroplasty may obviate the need for strict physical restrictions because of the durability typically found with radial component fixation.

Several criteria need to be satisfied before distal radius implant hemiarthroplasty is considered for routine use, including joint alignment and stability. The articular shape of the radial component of the UNI 2 and its successor, Freedom wrist system, conform well to the head of the capitate for optimum stability, but the shape also allows the necessary flexion–extension arc of motion as well as the important freedom of anterior-posterior and radial-ulnar translation to better replicate physiologic motion. Both the UNI 2 and Freedom systems are designed to restore the natural loading axis of the wrist, which passes through the long axis of the third metacarpal, capitate, and lunate fossa. In both the cadaver study and the clinical series, the UNI 2 design recreated the natural longitudinal loading axis in both the coronal and sagittal planes. Its successor, the Freedom system, maintains this important loading axis concept while providing a broader and shallower lunate fossa to allow increased capitate translation and increased wrist motion.

Despite the procedure including a PRC, which could potentially destabilize the joint, stability was not problematic in either the cadaver study or the clinical series. However, the UNI 2 and Freedom implant designs do not necessarily reflect the performance that will occur with other available radial implant designs. Furthermore, since none of the specimens and only a few of the wrists in the clinical series had severe deformity, the surgeon will need to exercise good judgment and proper caution when considering treatment in patients severe wrist deformity.

In clinical application, erosion of the carpus due to contact with the cobalt chrome surface is likely, but the rate of erosion will be difficult to predict. Erosion will probably depend on several factors including the initial condition of the carpus surface, bone density, and activity of the patient. In this series, some patients with rheumatoid arthritis showed rapid carpal erosion, which lead the author to discontinue this procedure in these patients. Additionally, patients who have substantial synovitis and cystic changes associated with active osteoarthritis are likely not good candidates. In the other patients, carpal erosion appeared to be acceptable and did not impact clinical results. Although pain relief will vary among patients due to variation in the response of the normal or arthritic joint surface against cobalt chrome. The results for up to 6.5 years indicate most patients can achieve good clinical and radiographic outcomes.

## Conclusion

Despite the potential disadvantages of hemiarthroplasty, it is an alternative for active patients with advanced wrist arthritis. This includes patients with Stage 4 Kienböck's disease who are not candidates for traditional motion preserving procedures due to distal radius or capitate articular degeneration. Our cadaver and clinical results indicate this technique has potential for a satisfactory clinical outcome in properly selected patients. However, the patient should fully understand the risks, including possibilities of incomplete pain relief, deterioration of outcome, and need for revision surgery.

## References

1. Boyer JS, Adams BD. Distal radius hemiarthroplasty combined with proximal row carpectomy: case report. Iowa Orthop J. 2010;30:168–73.
2. Culp RW, Bachoura A, Gelman SE, Jacoby SM. Proximal row carpectomy combined with wrist hemiarthroplasty. J Wrist Surg. 2012;1(1):39–46.

# Total Wrist Arthroplasty

# 28

Michel E.H. Boeckstyns and Guillaume Herzberg

## Introduction

Total wrist arthroplasty (TWA) is still a very controversial issue [1–6] and the reader should keep in mind that total wrist fusion (TWF) remains the gold standard for salvage of the severely destroyed, irreparable wrist. However, TWF may have an important negative impact on the health status of patients with osteoarthritis [7, 8] and TWA has become a challenger of TWF. It is more ambitious as patients usually prefer motion. On the other hand, failures do exist despite recent improvements [9] and periprosthetic osteolysis and loosening of the carpal component remain important problems. This chapter focuses on the most recent advances in TWA in terms of indications, recent design specifications and currently available results.

M.E.H. Boeckstyns, MD, PhD (✉)
Clinic for Hand Surgery, Gentofte Hospital/University of Copenhagen, Niels Andersens Vej 65, Hellerup 2900, Denmark

Kloeverbakken 11, 2830 Virum, Denmark
e-mail: mibo@dadlnet.dk

G. Herzberg, MD, PhD
Department of Orthopedic Surgery, Hopital Edouard Herriot, Pavillon T, Upper Limb Surgery, 5 Place d'Arsonval, Lyon 69437, France

## Indications

The indication for TWA in Kienböck's disease (KD) is painful arthritis in which TWF would be the only alternative option. This means a Lichtman stage IV (Kienböck's disease advanced collapse) but wrists destroyed by KD do not differ from other conditions leading to wrist degenerative arthritis in the context of surgical treatment. TWA has rarely been used for KD: according to a systematic review of the literature published between 1994 and 2013, it was the indication for TWA in less than 2 % of all cases [6]. Young age and high-demands are considered as contraindications. Active or latent infection after previous surgery always is a classic contraindication to any implant surgery.

## Specifications and Current Results of Recent TWA Designs

The latest generation of TWA is characterized by limited bone resection and limited fixation in the metacarpals compared with older designs. It is represented by the Maestro prosthesis (Biomet, Warsaw, IN, US), the UTW 1 (KMI, Carlsbad, CA, US), the UTW 2 (Integra LifeSciences, Plainsboro, NJ, US), the Freedom (Integra LifeSciences, Plainsboro, NJ, US), and the Remotion (Stryker Corporation, Kalamazoo, MI, US). They all are metal-on-polyethylene implants

© Springer International Publishing Switzerland 2016

D.M. Lichtman, G.I. Bain (eds.), *Kienböck's Disease*, DOI 10.1007/978-3-319-34226-9_28

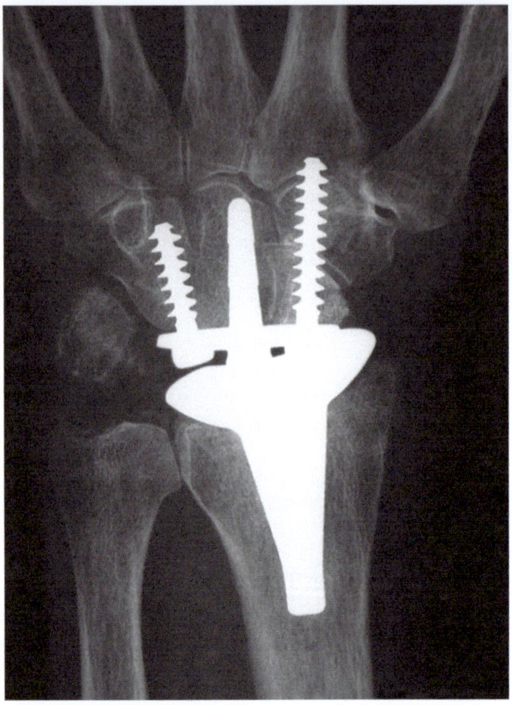

**Fig. 28.1** The Remotion TWA in a patient with idiopathic degenerative arthritis. Reprinted from ref. [13]

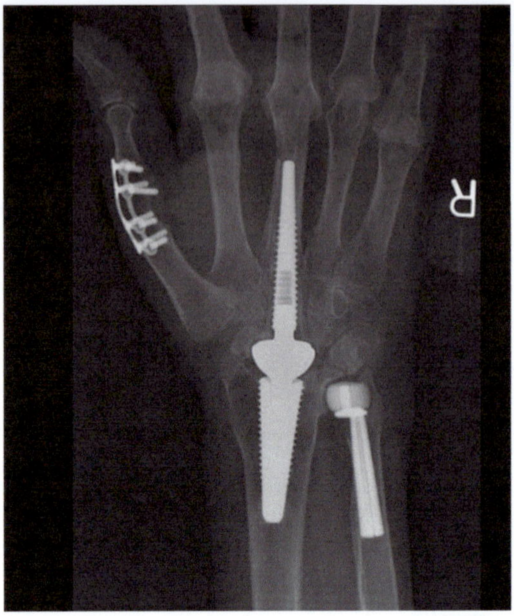

**Fig. 28.2** Motec TWA in a rheumatoid patient, combined with an Eclypse hemiarthroplasty in the distal radioulnar joint

and fixation of the carpal component is achieved by a central peg in the capitate augmented with screws in the hamate and scaphoid/trapezoid (Fig. 28.1). The screw on the radial side may cross the second carpometacarpal joint and penetrate the second metacarpal, although we do not recommend this as a general principle. With the implants currently available, infection and dislocation are rare complications [6] but the operation is challenging and requires advanced expertise in wrist surgery.

A very different recent design is the metal-on-metal Motec prosthesis with a long screw in the third metacarpal (Fig. 28.2).

Results have been published mainly as small series or series with a short follow-up.

The latest TWA-generation was introduced by Menon [10] with a series of 37 cases of UTW 1—the majority having rheumatoid arthritis (RA) and none specified as having KD—and an average follow-period of 6.7 years. Efficient pain relief was achieved. The revision rate was 8 %. The major problem was instability with a dislocation rate of 14 %. The UTW 1 has since been replaced by the UTW 2 and, very recently, the latest modifications have led to the freedom wrist arthroplasty. Using the UTW 2, Ferreres et al. [11] have published a series of 21 cases (mainly RA, two KD cases) with a follow-up period of at least 3 years (mean 5.5 years). Implant survival was 100 %. Van Winterswijk et al. have reported on 17 UTW 2-cases (16 RA, none with KD) with an average follow-up of 46 months and one revision of the carpal plate [12].

The Remotion has been reported in an early monocentric series by Herzberg in a series of 20 wrists (13 RA, none with KD) and an average follow-up of 32 months without the need of revisions [13]. In a larger multicenter series [14] with 112 cases with at least 2 years follow-up (average 4 years), Herzberg et al. reported no differences in clinical results or implant durability between RA and non-RA patients. The cumulated implant survival at 5 years was 92 % in RA as well as

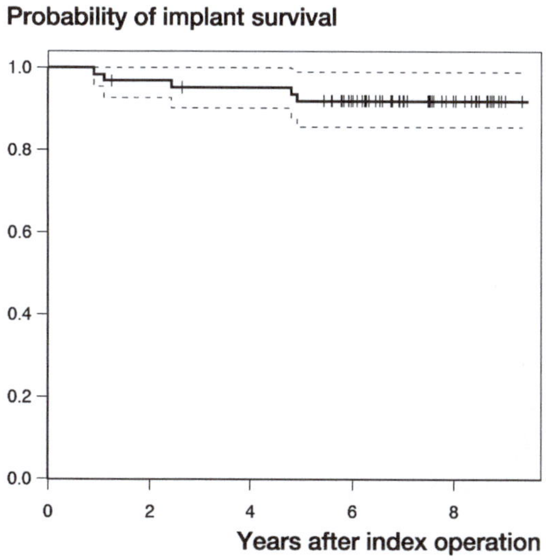


**Fig. 28.3** Cumulated implant survival of 65 Remotion prostheses. Reprinted from [13]

non-RA patients. A subsequent publication, including only patients with at least 5 years follow-up (one with KD) showed a cumulated implant survival of 90 % at 9 years [15] (Fig. 28.3). Radiological follow-up revealed that periprosthetic osteolysis was relatively frequently observed: 21 % showed osteolysis without frank loosening of the implant components and another 11 % of the implants—mainly the carpal component—seemed to be subsided, although clinically tolerated. In most cases, the osteolysis is localized to the bone adjacent to the prosthetic joint line, and tends to stabilize without frank loosening of the implant components [16] (Fig. 28.4). Nevertheless, a further decrease of the implant survival must be expected in younger patients.

Bidwai et al. published a small series of ten rheumatoid patients with Remotion and an average follow-up of 33 months. No implants were revised [17].

The Maestro TWA has been reported by Nydick et al. in a series of 23 cases (two KD), but follow-up time was short: 4–55 months (average 28) [18]. One of the 23 cases was revised for infection,

Sagerfors et al. have compared the outcomes of four implants 1 year after operation in a large series: Biax (no longer available), Remotion, UTW 2 and Maestro [19]; 177 of the 206 patients had RA.

Most series report an average postoperative range of flexion–extension of approximately 60–70° and radial–ulnar flexion of 25–30°, which is within the functional range of wrist motion, as defined by Palmer [20]. The Maestro series of Nydick shows somewhat better motion: 90° in flexion–extension and 43° of radial–ulnar flexion [18]. The study by Sagerfors et al. confirms the greater benefit in terms of motion with this implant [19]. Some series report clinically and statistically significantly improved motion at follow-up [17–19], but others do not [6, 13, 14]. It seems that the postoperative mobility is dependent on the preoperative mobility [15]. In all series, in which patient rated outcome measures (PROM) were recorded preoperatively and postoperatively, improvement in scores was reported (Table 28.1).

## Revision Surgery

For a failed TWA, a revision TWA or TWF can be considered (Figs. 28.5 and 28.6). Often TWF will be preferred, since it is most likely to be a final solution.

## Discussion

There has been a breakthrough regarding the use of TWA to treat wrist arthritis since 1998. The newer generations of arthroplasty have better results and survivorship, than their predecessors.

The main advantage of TWA over TWF is a higher degree of functionality. Most patients who have a TWA on one side and TWF on the other, would have preferred arthroplasty on both sides; but this is not always the case [21].

Murphy et al. compared TWA (24 RA, UTW 1) and TWF (27 RA) in a retrospective study [5]. The treatment groups were well matched by patient characteristics and radiographic staging. There were no statistically significant differences

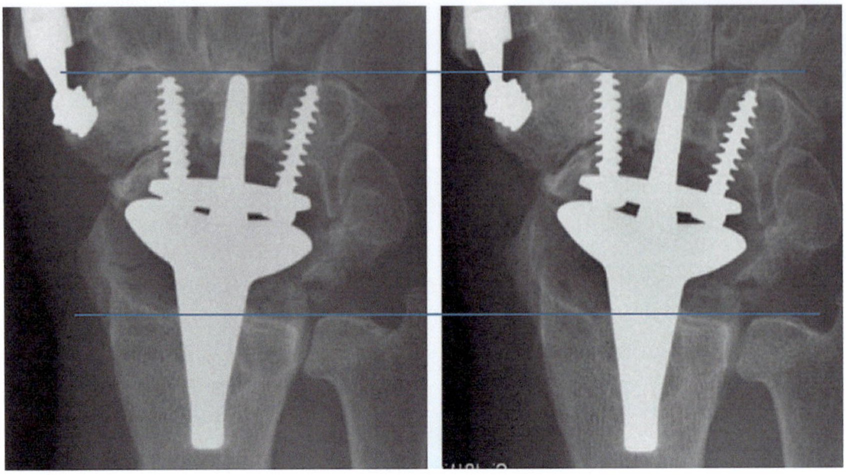

**Fig. 28.4** Osteolytic lesion 4 and 6 years after Remotion TWA. The osteolysis seems not to increase and the implant has not subsided

**Table 28.1** Functional improvement after TWA evaluated with Patient Rated Outcome Measures (PROM)

| Author/year | PROM | Mean improvement |
|---|---|---|
| Herzberg 2012 [14] | Quick DASH | 20 points |
| Van Winterswijk 2010 [12] | DASH | 24 points |
| Morapudi 2012 [23] | DASH | 10 points |
| | PRWE | 46 points |

between arthroplasty and arthrodesis in either DASH or PRWE scores.

Cavaliere and Chung performed a systematic review of the literature, in which they compared 18 TWA studies (503 procedures) with 20 TWF studies (860 procedures) in RA patients [2]. They concluded that the outcomes of TWF were comparable and possibly better than those for TWA. Unfortunately, major limitations of that study were the often weak methodology in the source publications, the fact the implants used were of older designs, and that the RA patients, often had multiple joint involvement. Nydick et al. found a statistically significant difference in PRWE-scores in favor of TWA compared to TWF in posttraumatic diagnoses, but not in DASH-scores [22]. The major flaw of that study was the very small number of cases and the question of how the patients were selected for the initial procedures.

## Conclusion

TWA may be a good surgical option for the low-demand elderly patient who requires a salvage procedure for advanced wrist disease and especially if there is bilateral involvement, The patient's and surgeon's decision-making should consider several factors. Firstly, TWF is the classic gold standard procedure with reliable long-term results for end-stage wrist arthritis. Secondly, the TWA is associated with significant complications and may require revision to TWF. Thirdly, patient compliance is paramount and should be carefully evaluated.

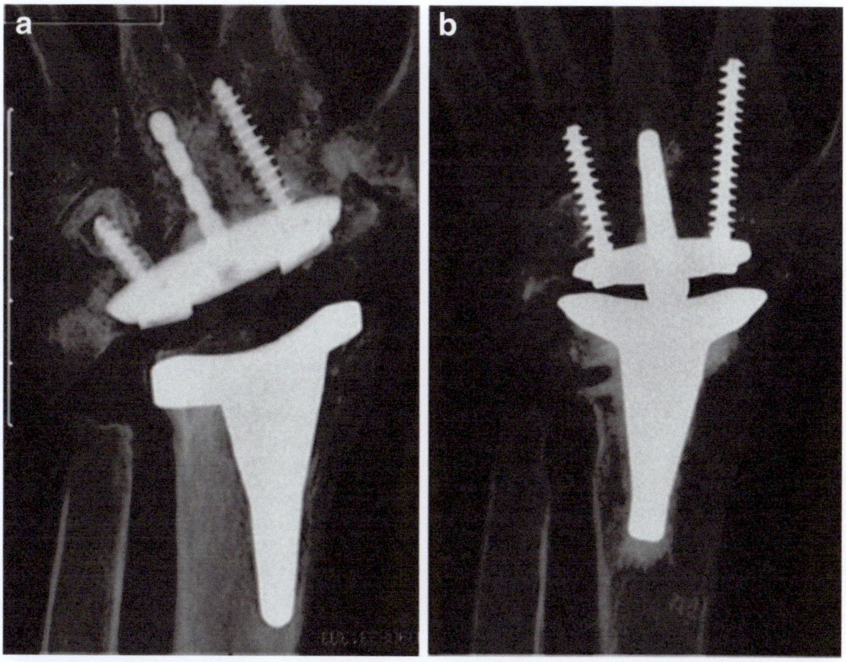

**Fig. 28.5** Revision of a UTW 1 implant that subsided 6 years after index operation (**a**) and replaced with a Remotion prosthesis, using a cemented bone-grafting technique. (**b**) Six years after revision. Because of resorption of the carpal bones, crossing the CMC joints was unavoidable

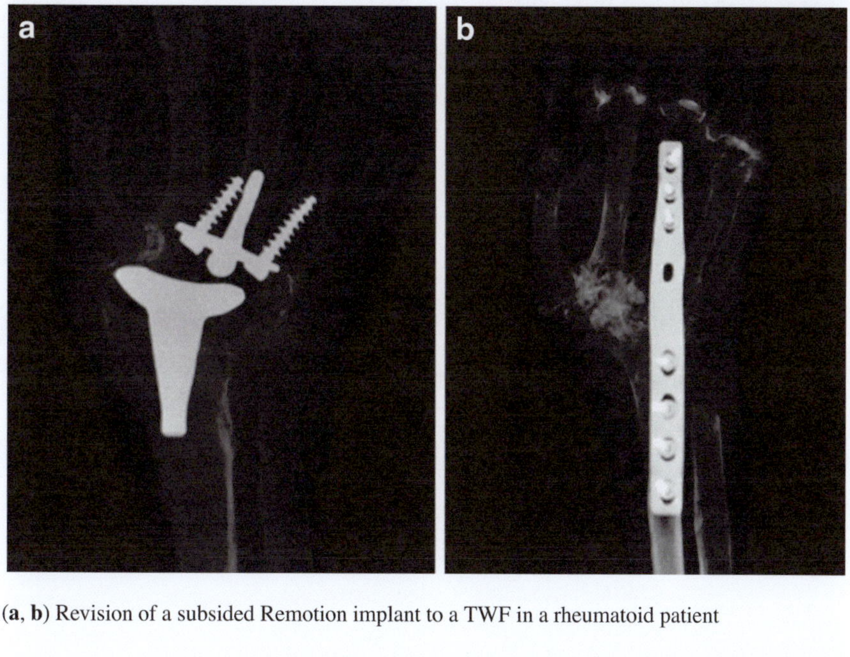

**Fig. 28.6** (**a**, **b**) Revision of a subsided Remotion implant to a TWF in a rheumatoid patient

## References


1. Cavaliere CM, Oppenheimer AJ, Chung KC. Reconstructing the rheumatoid wrist: a utility analysis comparing total wrist fusion and total wrist arthroplasty from the perspectives of rheumatologists and hand surgeons. Hand. 2010;5(1):9–18. doi:10.1007/s11552-009-9194-7.
2. Cavaliere CM, Chung KC. A systematic review of total wrist arthroplasty compared with total wrist arthrodesis for rheumatoid arthritis. Plast Reconstr Surg. 2008;122(3):813–25. doi:10.1097/PRS.0b013e318180ece3.
3. Cavaliere CM, Chung KC. Total wrist arthroplasty and total wrist arthrodesis in rheumatoid arthritis: a decision analysis from the hand surgeons' perspective. J Hand Surg Am. 2008;33(10):1744–55. doi:10.1016/j.jhsa.2008.06.022. 55.e1-2.
4. Trieb K. Treatment of the wrist in rheumatoid arthritis. J Hand Surg Am. 2008;33(1):113–23. doi:10.1016/j.jhsa.2007.09.011.
5. Murphy DM, Khoury JG, Imbriglia JE, Adams BD. Comparison of arthroplasty and arthrodesis for the rheumatoid wrist. J Hand Surg Am. 2003;28(4):570–6.
6. Boeckstyns ME. Wrist arthroplasty--a systematic review. Dan Med J. 2014;61(5):A4834.
7. Adey L, Ring D, Jupiter JB. Health status after total wrist arthrodesis for posttraumatic arthritis. J Hand Surg Am. 2005;30(5):932–6. doi:10.1016/j.jhsa.2005.06.004.
8. Sauerbier M, Kania NM, Kluge S, Bickert B, Germann G. Initial results of treatment with the new AO wrist joint arthrodesis plate. Handchir Mikrochir Plast Chir. 1999;31(4):260–5. doi:10.1055/s-1999-13536.
9. Adams BD. Complications of wrist arthroplasty. Hand Clin. 2010;26(2):213–20. doi:10.1016/j.hcl.2010.01.006.
10. Menon J. Universal total wrist implant: experience with a carpal component fixed with three screws. J Arthrop. 1998;13(5):515–23.
11. Ferreres A, Lluch A, Del Valle M. Universal total wrist arthroplasty: midterm follow-up study. J Hand Surg Am. 2011;36(6):967–73. doi:10.1016/j.jhsa.2011.03.034.
12. van Winterswijk PJ, Bakx PA. Promising clinical results of the universal total wrist prosthesis in rheumatoid arthritis. Open Orthop J. 2010;4:67–70. doi:10.2174/1874325001004020067.
13. Herzberg G. Prospective study of a new total wrist arthroplasty: short term results. Chir Main. 2011;30(1):20–5. doi:10.1016/j.main.2011.01.017.
14. Herzberg G, Boeckstyns M, Ibsen Sørensen A, Axelsson P, Kroener K, Liverneaux P, et al. "Remotion" total wrist arthroplasty: preliminary results of a prospective international multicenter study of 215 cases. J Wrist Surg. 2012;01(01):17–22.
15. Boeckstyns ME, Herzberg G, Merser S. Favorable results after total wrist arthroplasty: 65 wrists in 60 patients followed for 5-9 years. Acta Orthop. 2013;84(4):415–9. doi:10.3109/17453674.2013.823588.
16. Boeckstyns MEH, Herzberg G. Periprosthetic osteolysis after total wrist arthroplasty. J Wrist Surg. 2014;3(2):101–6.
17. Bidwai AS, Cashin F, Richards A, Brown DJ. Short to medium results using the remotion total wrist replacement for rheumatoid arthritis. Hand Surg. 2013;18(2):175–8.doi:10.1142/S0218810413500202.
18. Nydick JA, Greenberg SM, Stone JD, Williams B, Polikandriotis JA, Hess AV. Clinical outcomes of total wrist arthroplasty. J Hand Surg Am. 2012;37(8):1580–4. doi:10.1016/j.jhsa.2012.05.016.
19. Sagerfors M, Gupta A, Brus O, Rizzo M, Pettersson K. Patient related functional outcome after total wrist arthroplasty: a single center study of 206 cases. Hand Surg. 2015;20(1):81–7. doi:10.1142/S0218810415500112.
20. Palmer AK, Werner FW, Murphy D, Glisson R. Functional wrist motion: a biomechanical study. J Hand Surg Am. 1985;10(1):39–46.
21. Takwale VJ, Nuttall D, Trail IA, Stanley JK. Biaxial total wrist replacement in patients with rheumatoid arthritis. Clinical review, survivorship and radiological analysis. J Bone Joint Surg Br. 2002;84(5):692–9.
22. Nydick JA, Watt JF, Garcia MJ, Williams BD, Hess AV. Clinical outcomes of arthrodesis and arthroplasty for the treatment of post-traumatic wrist arthritis. J Hand Surg Am. 2013;38(5):899–903. doi:10.1016/j.jhsa.2013.02.013.
23. Morapudi SP, Marlow WJ, Withers D, Ralte P, Gabr A, Waseem M. Total wrist arthroplasty using the Universal 2 prosthesis. J Orthop Surg. 2012;20(3):365–8.

# Total Wrist Fusion in the Management of Kienböck's Disease

# 29

Mark Ross and Steven Marchalleck

## Introduction

The natural history of Kienböck's disease remains relatively unknown and this hinders effective decision-making regarding clinical management. Symptoms and clinical findings include varying levels of pain, decreased range of motion (ROM) and grip strength [1]. According to the radiologic classification system proposed by Lichtman [2], the disease progresses through five stages, which culminate in fragmentation of the lunate, progressive carpal collapse, altered kinematics of the wrist, and eventually chondral loss leading to pan-carpal osteoarthritis. There may be little correlation between symptomatology and radiologic changes. In this chapter we consider the management of the more advanced stages (3B and 4) of the disease.

M. Ross, MBBS, FRACS (✉)
Brisbane Hand and Upper Limb Research Institute, Brisbane Private Hospital, Brisbane, QLD, Australia

Department of Orthopedics, Princess Alexandra Hospital, Brisbane, QLD, Australia

School of Medicine, The University of Queensland, Brisbane, QLD 4072, Australia
e-mail: research@upperlimb.com

S. Marchalleck, BSc, BSc (Med Sci), MBBS
Department of Orthopedics, Princess Alexandra Hospital, Brisbane, QLD 4006, Australia

## Rationale for Management

The ultimate goal of any intervention is to provide a pain-free, stable, and functional wrist. In the advanced stages of the disease the lunate is not reconstructable and as symptoms and chondral wear progress, the options for surgical management become restricted to salvage procedures. Lunate excision, lunate arthroplasty, proximal row carpectomy (PRC), limited wrist arthrodesis (LWA), and total wrist arthrodesis (TWA) have been reported in several retrospective series in the literature [3–10].

While there is no evidence to support the use of one modality over another [11], the choice of procedure may be guided by the individual carpal joints found to be involved radiologically or arthroscopically. MRI is a noninvasive means of assessing the extent of cartilage loss [12] and is often employed in the pre-operative assessment. Of course, arthroscopy allows direct visualization of the affected joints. The disease can then be classified according to anatomical involvement and the severity of chondral loss. Synovectomy can be performed (where appropriate) and a definitive procedure planned [13]. The radiolunate joint is thought to be the first affected, then the capitolunate joint, followed by more global wrist involvement [13, 14]. Certainly in some reports, arthroscopy has identified chondral ulceration not indicated on plain radiographs in up to 61 % of cases [13, 14]. This has led some

© Springer International Publishing Switzerland 2016

D.M. Lichtman, G.I. Bain (eds.), *Kienböck's Disease*, DOI 10.1007/978-3-319-34226-9_29

surgeons to advocate an articular based approach for the planning of surgery for patients with Kienböck's disease [13–15].

## Motion-Sparing Surgery

The decision to proceed to a motion-sacrificing procedure (as opposed to a motion-sparing one) is based on the pattern of joint involvement, the patient's symptoms and expectations, and to some extent the surgeon's preference and experience. Some patients may decide to accept the risk of residual pain or requirement for further treatments to maintain some ROM.

Comparisons of the outcome of PRC and LWA have shown no statistically significant differences with respect to the average ROM, pain profile, or grip strength [7]. PRC is a technically straightforward operation without risk of nonunion and eliminates the diseased lunate entirely. A RSL fusion can be performed if the diseased articulation is restricted to the radiocarpal joint [14, 15]. However, if the proximal pole of the capitate and/or the lunate fossa is found to have chondral ulceration, then this procedure is likely to have a poor outcome [16]. PRC may be combined with pyrocarbon capitate resurfacing when chondral surfaces are not preserved (see Chap. 27).

Radiolunate arthrodesis ("Chamay" procedure) addresses the chondral area thought to be effected primarily as the disease progresses [17]. When arthroscopic assessment revealed isolated radiolunate arthrosis, Watanabe and colleagues suggested the use of the Chamay procedure [13]. There are very few reports on the outcomes of this procedure for Kienböck's disease, all with very small patient numbers. The nonunion rate can be as high as 50 %, which was thought to be due to trying to unite the small fragmented lunate [7, 11, 13].

## Total Wrist Arthrodesis

It is clear that once the disease has progressed to Lichtman Stage 4, Bain stage 4, or previous interventions have failed to relieve symptoms, a salvage procedure is indicated. In this case the most predictable surgical option is TWA. However, some arthroplasty techniques may still play a role. Contraindications for TWA include inadequate soft tissue coverage and active infection.

There are many surgical techniques and implants described to achieve union. Clayton described a technique of using an intramedullary Steinman pin inserted down the shaft of the third metacarpal and into the medullary canal of the radius [18]. Varying techniques using large corticocancellous iliac crest bone grafts with no internal fixation were employed for many years [19, 20]. In 1982, the AO Small Fragment Set manual outlined a technique of using a 3.5 mm dynamic compression plate for dorsal fixation with bone grafting [21]. Today, a variety of plates in varying contours and materials are available with locking and non-locking options. Low-profile, tapered, pre-contoured, dynamic compression plates have now been popularized by AO/Synthes (Fig. 29.1), and have led to the reduction of many of the well-known complications previously reported [22].

The optimal position for fusion of the wrist has been debated in the literature. Some authors previously have proposed that a neutral position is the best functional position, but the general consensus now is that 10–15° of extension with slight ulnar deviation is preferable for maintaining maximal grip strength [23–25]. When using a pre-contoured plate, the position of fusion is dictated by the contour of the plate and fixation to the radial metaphysis and shaft of the third metacarpal.

Bilateral Kienböck's disease is very rare. Yazaki et al. noted a rate of 4 % of cases over a 33 year period [26]. Bilateral TWA is controversial but not contraindicated. Jebson and Adams favored a motion-sparing procedure for the dominant hand and TWA for the nondominant hand [27]. If, after appropriate counseling to ensure realistic expectations, bilateral TWA is deemed appropriate, consideration should be given to fusing the nondominant wrist in 5–10° of flexion to facilitate perineal care [18].

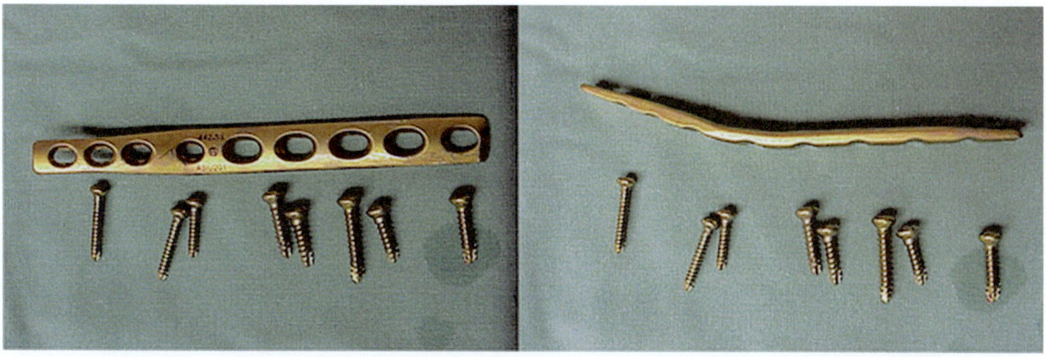

**Fig. 29.1** AO "straight plate" wrist fusion plate, which has been bent to provide some wrist extension for the patient

## Author's Preferred Surgical Technique of Dorsal Plating

A dorsal approach to the wrist is performed in a standard fashion. Extensor pollicis longus is released from its compartment and dissection is continued subperiosteally under the second and fourth compartments to expose the dorsal distal radius, the shaft of the third metacarpal, and the dorsal wrist capsule. The insertions of the wrist extensors (extensor carpi radialis longus and brevis) may occasionally be elevated to facilitate exposure, though they may also be used to facilitate soft tissue coverage at the end of the procedure. A dorsal ligament sparing capsulotomy is performed to develop a large radial based flap that can be used to cover hardware on layered closure. A broad osteotome is used to excise the ridge of bone on the dorsum of the distal radius in the region of Lister's tubercle. This allows for placement of the plate on a flat surface, keeping the plate profile low and further decreasing the risk of extensor tendon irritation postoperatively. Some of this bone is quite good quality and can be used as bone graft. Further bone graft is sourced from the triquetrum, which is routinely excised. If the lunate is severely fragmented and poor quality, it is excised and the triquetrum rotated into the lunate space to maintain carpal height. Not only is the triquetrum a generous source of graft, but also by excising or rotating it, there is a decreased risk of ulnar-sided wrist pain from the triangular fibrocartilaginous complex or ulnar carpal impingement (Fig. 29.2).

The joints to be incorporated into the fusion mass are identified and denuded of cartilage and subchondral bone to expose bleeding cancellous bone. The primary fusion mass is between the radius, proximal scaphoid, lunate (or interposed triquetrum), and capitate. The scapho-trapezio-trapezoid (STT) joint is not usually included unless there is clear arthrosis of the joint. The capitohamate joint is also not usually included as this joint is extremely stable. The third carpometacarpal (CMC) joint articular surfaces are excised and bone graft is packed in between the remaining cancellous surfaces as an 'open' fusion. The fusion mass is then spanned with a standard fusion plate with a bend that dips into the proximal carpal row. The plate is first fixed to the third metacarpal and then positioned on the flat surface created on the dorsal distal radius. The wrist is aligned and a compression screw is placed in the sliding hole of the plate. Bone graft is packed into the debrided joint surfaces before compression is applied. Fluoroscopy may be used to confirm alignment and to check screw lengths. Care is required to ensure that a screw in the capitate does not protrude into the carpal tunnel and irritate the flexor tendons. Meticulous soft tissue closure is beneficial to ensure adequate soft tissue coverage of the plate and to reduce extensor tendon irritation.

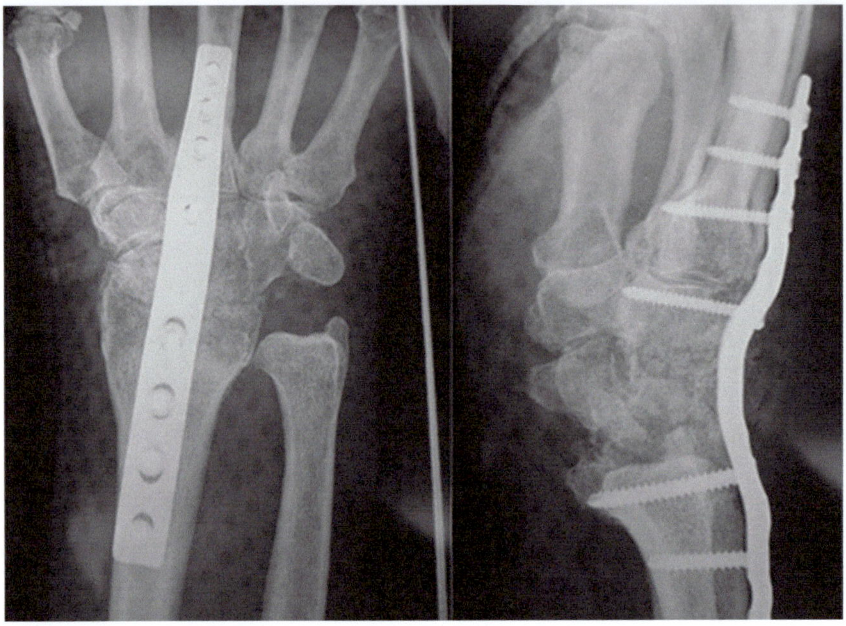

**Fig. 29.2** Wrist fusion with excision of triquetrum. The AO "standard bend" plate was used

## Conversion of Arthroplasty to Arthrodesis

When a previous interposition arthroplasty has been performed, certain technical issues arise that merit discussion. As discussed in a previous chapter in this textbook, we use three particular implant options.

1. Lunate replacement with a pyrocarbon lunate or Adaptive Proximal Scaphoid Implant (APSI), in which the proximal scaphoid is retained. In converting this to a TWA, there are two options. If the scaphoid remains in good shape, the triquetrum can be rotated in as an interposition graft, and fusion achieved as described previously. If the scaphoid is too damaged to incorporate, it can be excised and fusion performed as outlined for the Amandys implant below.
2. The Amandys replaces the lunate and proximal scaphoid. Therefore when this is converted to a TWA, the implant is removed, thereby essentially performing a PRC. The triquetrum is excised and used as bone graft. The capitate is apposed to the distal radius, resulting in loss of carpal height. In this case the AO "straight plate" has been bent to provide the wrist with a better profile and grip strength (Fig. 29.3).
3. The Resurfacing Capitate Pyrocarbon Implant (RCPI) presents similar issues to the Amandys, except that the triquetrum is not available. Distal radius bone graft is usually adequate, but the iliac crest should be prepared just in case (Fig. 29.4a, b).

## Discussion of Surgical Technique

Some surgeons advocate the incorporation of a proximal row carpectomy when performing a TWA, as this provides local bone graft and alleviates the need to harvest from a satellite position [22]. This results in a loss of carpal height, which may have implications for grip strength and hand function. For that reason we prefer to retain the lunate or interpose the triquetrum, to maintain the carpal height. If the necrotic lunate is left in situ, it may increase the risk of nonunion and act as a source of persistent pain, similar to that reported with the radiolunate fusion [11].

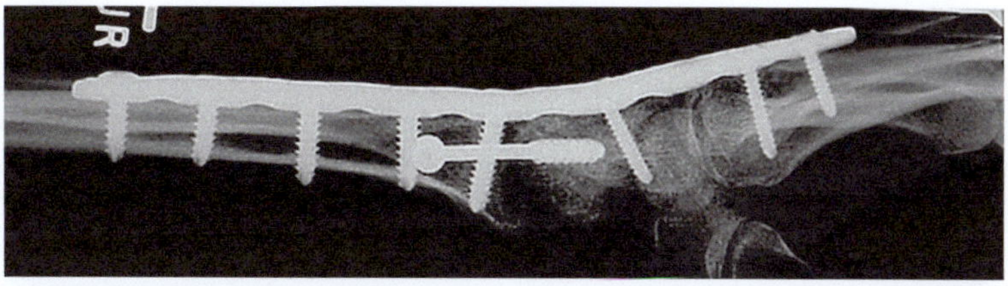

**Fig. 29.3** Wrist fusion with the AO "straight plate" wrist fusion plate, which has been bent to provide some wrist extension

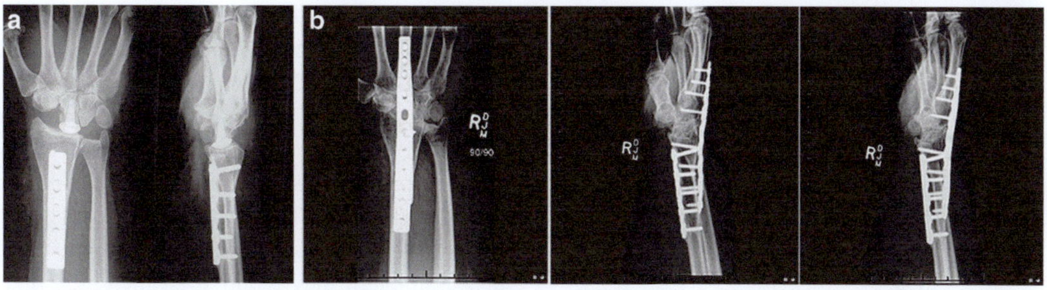


**Fig. 29.4** (**a**) Patient has had a previous radial shortening, proximal row carpectomy, and capitate resurfacing (RCPI). (**b**) Due to persistent pain a full wrist fusion was performed

A second controversy is the decision to include the third carpometacarpal (CMC) joint in the fusion mass. Nagy and Buchler showed less than 50 % radiographic fusion rates in the CMC joint when it was included in the index arthrodesis, and, upon plate removal, the CMC joint was more likely to be symptomatic if arthrodesis had been attempted than if it were simply bridged [28]. The senior author has found that an 'open' fusion technique with aggressive removal of joint surfaces and cancellous bone grafting reliably achieves third carpometacarpal fusion [29]. If the third CMC joint is not included in the fusion mass, most surgeons would advocate routinely removing hardware that crosses the joint to avoid the risk of implant fatigue and plate or screw breakage. We have occasionally used the Medartis plate (Medartis, Basel, Switzerland) at times, which has an expanded distal end to facilitate carpal fixation, thereby avoiding this issue. However, most of our fusions use a longer plate with third metacarpal fixation.

The distal radioulnar joint (DRUJ) is not usually involved in Kienböck's disease, but if concurrent arthrosis exists it can contribute to ongoing symptoms postoperatively and should therefore be addressed accordingly [24, 30]. Ulnar-sided pain is lessened by routine excision of the triquetrum.

See Table 29.1 for surgical tips.

## Rehabilitation

Due to the stability imparted by the plate, postoperative immobilization is not absolutely necessary, however a removable thermoplastic orthosis may be used at the surgeon's preference. A bulky bandage is applied and the limb is elevated. Rehabilitation can be divided into two phases. The early phase consists of digital ROM and forearm supination/pronation exercises. The late phase consists of strengthening exercises at about 6 weeks.

## Results

With the introduction of the modern low profile compression plates, TWA has a lower morbidity, with a highly predictable improvement in pain and grip strength. There is a high fusion rate (94–100 %) and patient satisfaction (80–100 %) [28, 31–33]. Most patients in previously reported

**Table 29.1** Surgical tips

| Surgical tip | Advantage |
|---|---|
| Excise triquetrum | Decreases risk of ulnar sided wrist pain |
| | Excellent source of bone graft |
| Excise lunate if markedly necrotic | Decrease risk of nonunion |
| | Triquetrum available as substitute |
| Include third CMC joint in the fusion mass | Avoids need for implant removal if using a spanning plate |
| Use an "open" fusion technique for third CMCJ | Avoids the "closing" fusion which requires greater soft-tissue stripping and is difficult to unite |
| If the third CMCJ is not included in the fusion mass but a spanning fusion plate is used, it is advisable to remove the plate at 12–18 months once a solid fusion is achieved | To avoid plate fatigue failure at the third CMCJ |
| Osteotomize dorsal distal radius and create a flat surface in the region of Lister's tubercle. | Allows the plate to sit with a low profile. |
| | Provides additional bone graft. |
| Raise ligament sparing capsular flap. | Provides a large radially based flap to cover the plate and protects the extensor tendons. |
| Ensure the capitate screw is not too long. | Avoid flexor tendon injury in the carpal tunnel. |

series had at least one prior surgical procedure and in fact many patients indicated that they would have preferred TWA earlier in their management [33, 34].

TWA addresses the primary concern for most patients, which is pain. However, by no means does it restore normal wrist function. Perineal care and working in small spaces where the shoulder and elbow can't compensate are difficult. However, subjectively patients reported little to no functional disability and good adaptation [27, 35, 36].

The senior author reported on the outcome of 53 TWAs in 48 patients for a variety of diagnoses utilizing the AO wrist fusion plate [33]. 83 % of patients reported a subjective global improvement. 50 of the 53 wrists reviewed fused primarily, with the other patient requiring secondary grafting. The average DASH score was 34.6. The Buck-Gramcko and Lohmann classification was used to establish an overall score with points provided for wrist range of motion, functional, pain during function, grip strength and global subjective impression of improvement. The score is graded excellent 9–10 points; good 7–8; satisfactory 5–6 and poor <5 points. The average Buck-Gramcko and Lohmann score was 5.73 (i.e., satisfactory) with 13 % excellent, 27 % good, 37 % satisfactory and 23 % poor. Thus 77 % of patients tested scored "satisfactory" or above. The Jebsen Taylor functional assessment revealed the patients were able to complete most tasks, although they required an increased time compared to the reported normal values.

## Complications

Complications of TWA are fairly common, but most are minor and self-limiting (Table 29.2) [33]. Postoperatively, haematoma formation, wound dehiscence, and paraesthesia can be encountered. Good surgical technique can minimize major complications, which include nonunion, deep infection, neuroma formation, hardware irritation, intrinsic contracture of the middle finger and acute carpal tunnel syndrome.

Hardware irritation and intrinsic contracture requiring secondary procedures for plate removal and intrinsic release have reduced in incidence with the introduction of tapered AO plates [22]. Postoperative acute carpal tunnel syndrome may require surgical release [22, 37].

**Table 29.2** Complications of total wrist arthrodesis[a]

| Complication | Incidence (%) |
|---|---|
| Infection | 2 (4) |
| Pain | 11 (21) |
| Paraesthesia | 3 (6) |
| Nonunion | 3 (6) |
| Tendon irritation | 3 (6) |
| Plate/screw failure | 3 (6) |
| Plate removal | 11 (21) |

[a]Adapted from ref. [33]

## Case Studies

We have experience with two patients with Kienböck's disease who were initially treated with radial shortening, further revised with an RCPI pyrocarbon implant and finally underwent a total wrist fusion.

A 62-year-old female underwent a total wrist fusion of her dominant hand 39 months after receiving an RCPI implant (see Fig. 29.4a, b). A CT scan prior to TWA showed a well fixed pyrocarbon implant but some potential wear of the implant against radius contributing to pain. She was reviewed at 39 months following the TWA and rated satisfaction with her wrist as 87/100. Pain ranged from 18 to 68/100 with functional activities. Grip strength was 13 kg (contralateral nondominant 11 kg). QuickDASH score was 84.09. On a Global Rating of Change (GRC) Score since surgery ("A Very Great Deal Worse" −7 to +7 "A Very Great Deal Better"), she rated her symptoms +3 and function +1.

A 59-year-old male with Kienböck's disease underwent a total wrist fusion of his right dominant wrist 33 months following RCPI insertion. He returned to normal work duties within 3 months of surgery. He was most recently reviewed 22 months following the fusion. He rated his satisfaction with his wrist since fusion surgery as 75/100. He reported no pain with normal functional activity. Grip strength was 18 kg (contralateral nondominant 36 kg). Both the QuickDASH score (13.63) and PRWE (4) scores were excellent. His Global Rating of Change Score since surgery was symptoms +7 and function +4.

## Conclusion

Modern internal fixation techniques and application of specific hardware has made TWA a predictable intervention in the management of Kienböck's disease. Although the loss of ROM may impact heavily on functional scores, it may be a preferable intervention where joint surface compromise makes motion-sparing procedures unpredictable, especially in a patient with a strong desire for a single procedure.

**Potential Conflict of Interest** *Mark Ross*: Fees for consultancy from Integra; fees for lectures and speakers bureaus from Integra, AO; patents pending with Integra; royalties from Integra; and Director of the Brisbane Hand and Upper Limb Research Institute (BHULRI), which receives financial support through charitable donations from Medartis.

## References


1. Beckenbaugh RD, Shives TC, Dobyns JH, Linscheid RL. Kienböck's disease: the natural history of Kienböck's disease and consideration of lunate fractures. Clin Orthop Relat Res. 1980;149:98–106.
2. Lichtman DM, Mack GR, MacDonald RI, Gunther SF, Wilson JN. Kienböck's disease: the role of silicon replacement arthroplasty. J Bone Joint Surg Am. 1977;59:899–908.
3. Swanson AB, De Groot Swanson G, DeHeer DH, Pierce TD, Randall K, Smith JM, et al. Carpal bone titanium implant arthroplasty. 10 years' experience. Clin Orthop Relat Res. 1997;342:46–58.
4. Viljakka T, Vastamaki M, Solonen K, Tallroth K. Silicone implant arthroplasty in Kienböck's disease. Acta Orthop Scand. 1987;58:410–4.
5. Kawai H, Yamamoto K, Yamamoto T, Tada K, Kaga K. Excision of the lunate in Kienböck's disease. Results after long-term follow-up. J Bone Joint Surg Br. 1988;70:287–92.
6. Begley BW, Enderberger ED. Proximal row carpectomy in advanced Kienböck's disease. J Hand Surg Am. 1994;9:1016–8.
7. Nakamura R, Horii E, Watanabe K, Nakao E, Tsunoda K. Proximal row carpectomy versus limited wrist arthrodesis for advanced Kienböck's disease. J Hand Surg Br. 1998;23:741–5.
8. Rhee SK, Kim HM, Bahk WJ, Kim YW. A comparative study of the surgical procedures to treat advanced Kienböck's disease. J Korean Med Sci. 1996;11:171–8.
9. Takase K, Imakiire A. Lunate excision, capitate osteotomy and intercarpal arthrodesis for advanced Kienbock's disease. Long-term follow up. J Bone Joint Surg Am. 2001;83:177–83.
10. Voche P, Bour C, Merle M. Scapho-trapezio-trapezoid arthrodesis in the treatment of Kienböck's disease, a study of 16 cases. J Hand Surg Br. 1992;17:5–11.
11. Tambe AD, Trail IA, Stanley JK. Wrist fusion versus limited carpal fusion in advanced Kienböck's disease. Int Orthop. 2005;29:355–8.
12. Tsou IY, Yegappan M, Ong WS, Goh PO, Tan JL, Chee TS. Cartilage injury and repair: assessment with magnetic resonance imaging. Singapore Med J. 2006; 47:80–7.

13. Watanabe K, Nakamura R, Imaeda T. Arthroscopic assessment of Kienböck's disease. Arthroscopy. 1995;11:257–62.
14. Bain GI, Begg M. Arthroscopic assessment of Kienböck's disease. Tech Hand Up Extrem Surg. 2006;10:8–13.
15. Bain GI, Durrant A. An articular-based approach to Kienböck avascular necrosis of the lunate. Tech Hand Upper Extrem Surg. 2011;15(1):41–7.
16. Lin HH, Stern PJ. "Salvage" procedures in the treatment of Kienböck's disease. Proximal row carpectomy and total wrist arthrodesis. Hand Clin. 1993;9:521–6.
17. Chamay A, Della Santa D. Radiiolunate arthrodesis in rheumatoid arthritis. Ann Hand Surg. 1991;10:197–206.
18. Clayton ML. Surgical treatment at the wrist in rheumatoid arthritis: a review of thirty-seven patients. J Bone Joint Surg Am. 1965;47:741–50.
19. Haddad RJ, Riordan DC. Arthrodesis of the wrist. A surgical technique. J Bone Joint Surg Am. 1967;49:950–4.
20. Carroll RE, Dick HM. Arthrodesis of the wrist for rheumatoid arthritis. J Bone Joint Surg Am. 1971;53:1365–9.
21. Heim U, Pfeiffer KM. Small fragment set manual. Technique recommended by the ASIF Group. 2nd ed. Berlin: Springer; 1982.
22. Green DP, Henderson CJ. Modified AO arthrodesis of the wrist (with proximal row carpectomy). J Hand Surg Am. 2013;38:388–91.
23. Brumfield RH, Champoux JA. A biomechanical study of normal functional wrist motion. Clin Orthop. 1984;187:23–5.
24. Rayan GM, Brentlinger A, Purnell D, Gracia-Moral CA. Functional assessment of the bilateral wrist arthrodesis. J Hand Surg Am. 1987;12:1020–4.
25. Clayton ML, Ferlic DC. Arthrodesis of the arthritic wrist. Clin Orthop Relat Res. 1984;55:1026–34.
26. Yazaki N, Nakamura R, Nakao E, Iwata Y, Tatebe M, Hattori T. Bilateral Kienböck's disease. J Hand Surg Br. 2005;30:133–6.
27. Jebson PJ, Adams BD. Wrist arthrodesis: a review of current techniques. J Am Acad Orthop Surg. 2001;9:53–60.
28. Nagy L, Buchler U. AO–wrist arthrodesis: with and without arthrodesis of the third carpometacarpal joint. J Hand Surg Am. 2002;27:940–7.
29. Bain GI, McGuire DT. Decision making for partial carpal fusions. J Wrist Surg. 2012;01(02):103–14.
30. Zachary SV, Stern PJ. Complications following AO/ASIF wrist arthrodesis. J Hand Surg Am. 1995;20:339–44.
31. Hastings H, Weiss AP, Quenzer D, Wiedeman GP, Hanington KR, Strickland JW. Arthrodesis of the wrist for post-traumatic disorders. J Bone Joint Surg Am. 1996;78:897–902.
32. Hayden RJ, Jebson PJ. Wrist arthrodesis. Hand Clin. 2005;21:631–40.
33. Mackay C, Couzens G, Cutbush K, Duke P, Hodder M, Copely M, Ross M. Wrist arthrodesis with the AO/ASIF wrist fusion plate. In: Proceedings of the 9th Congress of the International Federation of Societies for Surgery of the Hand. Budapest, Hungary, pp. 379–82, 2004.
34. Sagerman SD, Palmer AK. Wrist arthrodesis using a dynamic compression plate. J Hand Surg Br. 1996;21:437–41.
35. Weiss AP, Hastings H. Wrist arthrodesis for traumatic conditions: a study of plate and local bone application. J Hand Surg Am. 1995;20:50–6.
36. Herard J, Cohen G, Bacle G, Laulan J. Results of total wrist arthrodesis for degenerative disease. A review of 30 cases to 5 years. Chir Main. 2008;27:283–4.
37. Meads BM, Scougall PJ, Hargreaves IC. Wrist arthrodesis using a Synthes wrist fusion plate. J Hand Surg Br. 2003;28:571–4.

# The Future of Kienböck's Disease: A New Algorithm

# 30

David M. Lichtman, William F. Pientka II, and Gregory Ian Bain

## Introduction

Throughout this unique book on Kienböck's disease, there are extensive descriptions on the finer points of the etiology, pathology, natural history, diagnosis, and treatment. This knowledge has evolved over more than one hundred years since Robert Kienböck published his manuscript on osteomalacia of the lunate in 1910 [1]. The purpose of this chapter is to amalgamate much of this information, particularly the newer advances in diagnosis and treatment, into a practical, yet highly granular algorithm for the management of this disorder.

D.M. Lichtman, MD (✉)
Rear Admiral (Retired), US Navy Adjunct Professor, Department of Surgery, Uniformed Services University of the Health Sciences, Bethesda, MD, USA

Adjunct Professor, Department of Orthopedic Surgery, University of North Texas Health Sciences Center, Fort Worth, TX, USA
e-mail: RADML@ATT.NET

W.F. Pientka II, MD
Department of Orthopedic Surgery, John Peter Smith Hospital, 1500 S. Main St, Fort Worth, TX 76104, USA

6155 Highwoods Ct., Fort Worth, TX 76112, USA

G.I. Bain, MBBS, FRACS, FA(Ortho)A, PhD
Professor, Upper Limb and Research, Department of Orthopedic Surgery, Flinders University and Flinders Medical Centre, Bedford Park, Adelaide, SA, Australia

## Natural History

The natural history of untreated Kienböck's disease has been described in terms of the progression of clinical findings and serial changes on standard X-rays [2–5]. The Lichtman osseous classification scheme, devised in 1977, identifies these changes. The presentation of Kienböck's disease in pediatric patients is similar to that in adults, with dorsal tenderness, synovitis, and swelling, coupled with a decreased range of motion and grip strength [5, 8, 15]. However, the prognosis in the pediatric and elderly patients is better than the typical 20- to 40-year-old patient (Chap. 9) [8].

Irisarri [16] subdivided pediatric Kienböck's disease into infantile (12 years and younger) and juvenile (13 years to skeletal maturity) (Chap. 9). All patients in the infantile group were treated nonoperatively, and at final follow-up all had excellent outcomes, with lunate revascularization seen on MRI. However, in the juvenile group, which was also treated with immobilization, 30 % had progression requiring a joint leveling procedure. Irisarri recommended immobilization for patients under 15, and reserves joint leveling procedures for the older patient with disease progression despite immobilization.

Kienböck's disease behaves differently in the elderly when compared to the pediatric and adult cohorts [18–22]. Taniguchi reported that in Kienböck's patients older than 70 years, there

© Springer International Publishing Switzerland 2016

D.M. Lichtman, G.I. Bain (eds.), *Kienböck's Disease*, DOI 10.1007/978-3-319-34226-9_30

was less negative ulnar variance and a higher prevalence of women, who had more advanced radiological changes at presentation [19]. However, at a mean follow-up of 5.6 years, all 15 patients had progressed to stage IV disease, but had good to excellent clinical outcomes without surgical intervention.

## Clinical Assessment

To provide a more complete understanding of the lunate and carpus and enable detailed management decisions, Schmitt has recommended the following combination of imaging procedures [10, 11] (Chap. 11).

1. Plain radiographs of the wrist.
2. A high-resolution CT scan to provide the best understanding of the osseous components, which supports the previous published work of Quenzer [42].
3. An MRI to assess the articular cartilage.
4. MRI with gadolinium enhancement, to assess the perfusion of the lunate.

## Plain Radiographs

Plain radiographs have been used to diagnose and monitor the progression of Kienböck's disease, using the osseous Lichtman classification for almost 40 years [6] (Table 30.1, Fig. 30.1). It has evolved with time, with the addition of subclasses based on an increased understanding of the condition. The hypothetical stage 0 disease is analogous to stage 0 of the ARCO International classification of hip osteonecrosis [9], where patients have intermittent pain but normal radiographs and MRI. Theoretically, there is the potential to abort the onset of osteonecrosis by correcting the etiological or risk factors [8]. Stage IIIC disease has a coronal fracture or fragmentation of

**Table 30.1** Lichtman osseous classification [7, 8][a]

| Stage | X-ray | MRI | Treatment |
|---|---|---|---|
| 0 | Normal | Normal | Immobilization |
| I | Normal | T1 Signal: Decreased<br>T2 Signal: Variable | Immobilization |
| II | Lunate sclerosis | T1 Signal: Decreased<br>T2 Signal: Variable | Radial shortening (-ve UV)<br>Capitate shortening (+UV) |
| IIIA | Lunate collapse | T1 Signal: Decreased<br>T2 Signal: Variable | Same as Stage II, and/or:<br>Revascularization with dorsal pedicle |
| IIIB | Lunate and carpal collapse<br>Scaphoid rotation (RSA>60°) | T1 Signal: Decreased<br>T2 Signal: Usually Decreased | Reconstructive procedure<br>STT or SC fusion +/– lunate excision (if fragmented), or PRC |
| IIIC | Lunate coronal fracture | T1 Signal: Decreased<br>T2 Signal: Variable | PRC |
| IV | KDAC (Kienböck's disease advanced collapse) | T1 Signal: Decreased<br>T2 Signal: Decreased | Salvage Procedure (TWF, TWA, or PRC) |

*-ve UV* negative ulnar variance, *+ve UV* positive ulnar variance

[a]It is important to note how the classification simply divides the radiological findings, and defines the osseous state of the lunate

Stage 0—Lunate potentially threatened
Stage I and II—Lunate intact, but threatened
Stage III A—Localized lunate collapse
Stage III B—Lunate collapse and secondary wrist collapse
Stage III C—Lunate fragmentation, unreconstructable
Stage IV—KDAC, total wrist arthritis

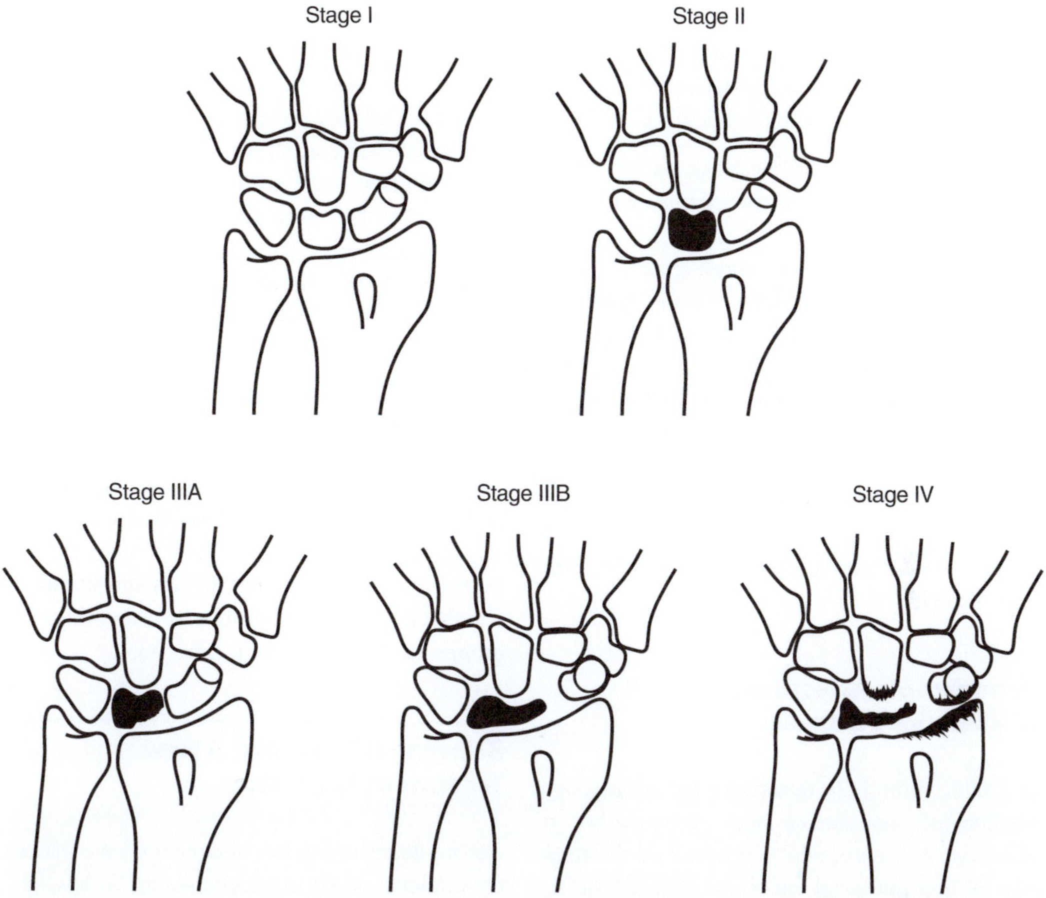


**Fig. 30.1** Modified Lichtman classification [7, 8]

the lunate, which in the authors' personal experience, has a poor prognosis for lunate revascularization.

## MR Imaging

In recent years, both T1- and T2-weighted MRI images have been used to evaluate viability of bone marrow [10]. On T1 images, normal viable marrow will have homogenous high signal intensity. Loss of this signal can be caused by anything that replaces viable marrow (edema, neovascularization, space occupying lesions, bone necrosis, or sequestrum). T2-weighted images have traditionally been used in Kienböck's disease to distinguish between fluid containing tissue (which provides a high T2 signal) and nonvascular or desiccated tissue, such as a sequestrum. However, T2-weighted images cannot distinguish between edema and neovascularization, which have different prognostic values.

Schmitt has highlighted how gadolinium perfusion techniques enhance T1-weighted FSE fat-saturated sequences (Chap. 11) [10]. He was able to distinguish low signal edema from enhanced high signal of neovascular repair tissue. Using these techniques, he was able to identify three zones or patterns of enhancement of the necrotic lunate: The proximal necrotic lunate with no enhancement, intermediate hyper-vascular repair zone, and the distal normal lunate. The hyper-enhancement in the reparative zone indicates areas with a good healing prognosis, whereas low signal indicates a poor prognosis due to nonviable marrow.

Based upon these findings, Schmitt [11] described a classification that depends on lunate signal changes after administration of IV gadolinium contrast (Fig. 30.2, Table 30.2).

1. In MRI stage A, homogenous lunate enhancement indicates marrow edema and intact perfusion.
2. MRI stage B shows inhomogenous signal with contrast enhancement of the reparative zone and viable distal bone with a necrotic proximal lunate.
3. MRI stage C has no enhancement corresponding to complete lunate osteonecrosis.

This work is most impressive, but it assumes that these perfusion studies correlate with lunate revascularization potential, and the clinical outcome.

## Arthroscopic Assessment of Kienböck's Disease

In 2006, Bain [12] described an arthroscopic method of assessment and classification of Kienböck's disease, which is based on the number of nonfunctional articular surfaces of the lunate (Fig. 30.3) [12, 13].

*A functional articular surface* has a normal smooth arthroscopic appearance and is firm to palpation without significant softening.

*A nonfunctional articular surface* has at least one of the following: extensive fibrillation, fissuring, localized or extensive loss, a floating articular surface or fracture. Synovitis was identified in all of our cases; therefore, it was not used for grading

Plain radiographs often underestimate the severity of articular changes and arthroscopic findings commonly change the recommended treatment. Interestingly, 82 % of cases had at least one nonfunctional articulation, and 61 % had at least two nonfunctional articulations [13].

From the spectrum of arthroscopic findings, an articular based approach was created where the distribution of functional articular surfaces determines treatment (Table 30.3) [12, 13]. The principle is to identify the articulations that are nonfunctional (compromised), and either excise or fuse or bypass them, to allow the wrist to then be mobilized with the remaining functional articulations. Then the remaining articulations are all functional surfaces, so it is more likely to result in a pain-free wrist with a functional range of motion [14]. However, performing a radial shortening osteotomy or vascularized bone graft would leave the wrist with a nonfunctional articular surface in 82 % of cases.

## Management

The management section of this book is extensive, and we are pleased that we have been able to bring together a group of quality authors, who have presented a wide spectrum of treatment options for Kienböck's disease. These can be categorized into groups, as demonstrated in Table 30.4.

## Bringing It Together: A New Treatment Algorithm

Before determining the treatment of the patient, the clinician needs to understand the following:

1. Patient's age.
2. Lunate Stage: How does the disease affect the lunate?
3. Wrist Stage: How does the disease affect the wrist?
4. What can the surgeon offer?
5. What does the patient want?

To demonstrate the synergy of the three separate classification systems, we have placed them side-by-side in Table 30.5 to see how their amalgamation can lead to a more nuanced treatment protocol. The new classification system takes this amalgamation several steps further: It aims to respect the importance that age has on prognosis, the revascularization potential of the lunate, the pathoanatomical aspects of the lunate disease and the secondary effects that the disorder has had on the entire wrist. The preferred treatment recommendations are based on all of these factors, including the status of remaining intact articulations, and are listed in Table 30.6.

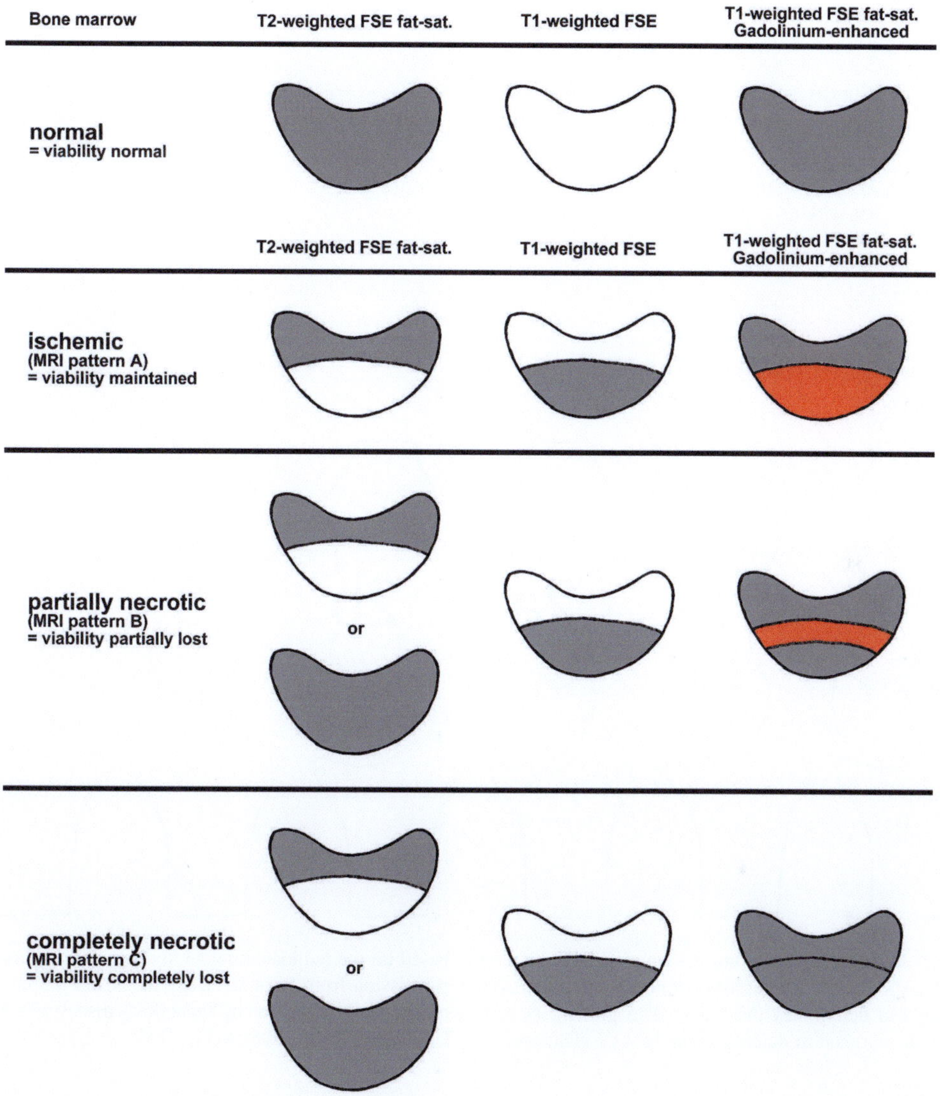


**Fig. 30.2** Schmitt's schematic diagram of bone-marrow viability in Gadolinium-enhanced MRI. **Normal marrow (viability unaffected)**, *first row*: The signal height is homogeneously dark in fat-saturated T2-w FSE, and homogeneously bright in T1-w FSE. No contrast-enhancement within a homogenously dark lunate is characteristic in fat-saturated T1-w FSE after intravenous Gadolinium. **Ischemic marrow (viability maintained)**, *second row*: The proximal pole of the lunate is hyperintense in fat-saturated T2-w FSE, and hypointense in T1-w FSE due to bone-marrow edema. In fat-saturated T1-w FSE, there is a homogeneous Gadolinium enhancement pattern of the entire proximal zone indicating maintained perfusion. **Partially necrotic marrow (viability partially lost)**, *third row*: The proximal pole of the lunate is hyperintense in fat-saturated T2-w FSE, and hypointense in T1-w FSE. Both necrotic and repairing zones are present. Differentiation is possible only with Gadolinium enhancement: The repairing zone has intense enhancement, which absent in the necrotic zone. **Completely necrotic marrow (viability completely lost)**, *fourth row*: Independent of present or missing bone-marrow edema in fat-saturated T2-w FSE, no enhancement on fat-saturated T1-w FSE after Gadolinium, when compared to plain T1-w FSE. Image reproduced with permission from Prof. Rainer R. Schmitt, Chap. 11

**Table 30.2** Schmitt classification of lunate vascularity/viability[a]

| Pattern | MRI findings | Prognosis |
|---|---|---|
| N | Normal lunate perfusion | n/a |
| | Normal signal | |
| A | Intact lunate perfusion | Good |
| | Homogenous enhancement of lunate with marrow edema. | |
| B | Partial osteonecrosis | Intermediate |
| | Inhomogenous signal with necrotic proximal lunate, reparative mid-zone enhancement and viable distal bone. | |
| C | Complete osteonecrosis | Poor |
| | No contrast enhancement. | |

[a]Table modified and reproduced from Schmitt (Chap. 11)

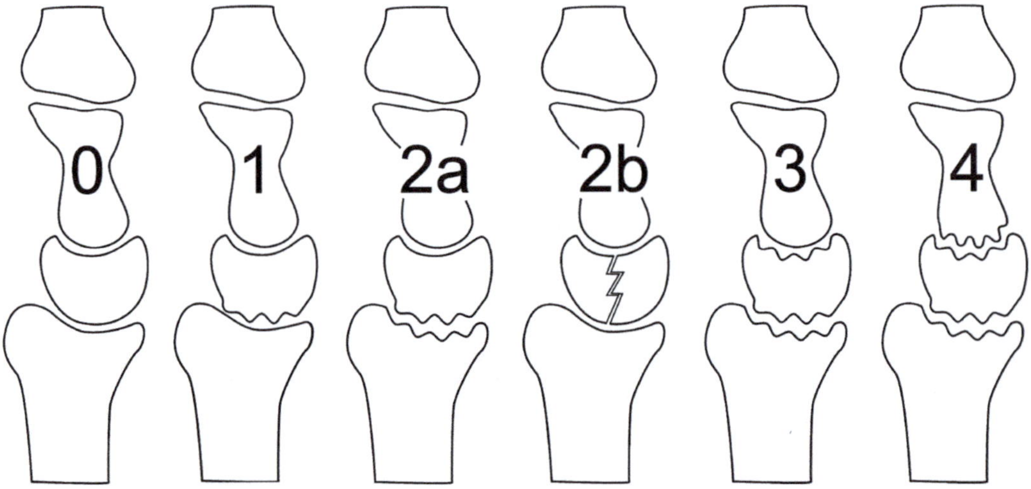


**Fig. 30.3** Bain and Begg arthroscopic classification of Kienböck's disease. The number of nonfunctional articular surfaces determines the grade. The grading system assists the surgeon to determine the best surgical option, based on the pathoanatomical findings. Reproduced with permission from Bain GI, Begg M. Arthroscopic assessment and classification of Kienböck's disease. Tech Hand Up Extrem Surg. 2006;10(1):8–13

The age of the patient and the staus of the lunate and wrist underpin the management of patients with Kienböck's disease. **The first three questions are the essential components** of the new combined classification system and are presented in Table. 30.6 with the associated treatment recommendations. The last two concern the capabilities of the surgeon and the needs of the patient and will also help guide the final management decision.

## Patient's Age

The age at time of presentation is important, with the "Teen-bock" and elderly patient having a better prognosis. As these are fundamentally different prognostic groups, we have separated them from the start. The treatment recommendations for these populations are:

*A1< 15 years*: Treat nonoperatively. Consider minimally invasive procedure if symptoms persist after 6 months.

*A2 16–20 years*: Trial of nonoperative management. Consider unloading procedure if no improvement in symptoms after 3 months.

*A3 >70 years*: Usually responds to nonoperative management. If symptoms persist beyond 6 months, consider synovectomy or treat as if the patient was younger than 70 years of age.

For patients between the ages of 21 and 69 proceed to sections B or C, as appropriate.

**Table 30.3** Bain/Begg articular-based classification for Kienböck's disease[a]

| Grade | Description | Recommendation |
|---|---|---|
| 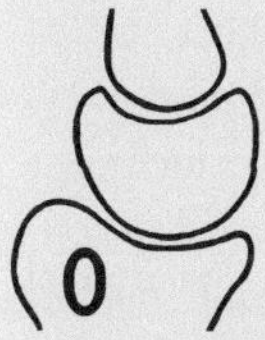 | *Grade 0*<br>0 Nonfunctional surface | Joint leveling procedure<br>Forage +/– bone graft<br>Vascularized bone graft |
| 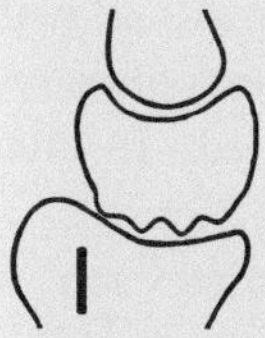 | *Grade 1*<br>1 Nonfunctional surface<br>– Proximal lunate | RSL fusion<br>PRC<br>Osteochondral grafting |
| 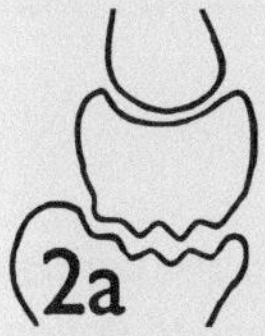 | *Grade 2a*<br>2 Nonfunctional surfaces<br>– Proximal lunate and lunate facet of radius | RSL fusion |
| 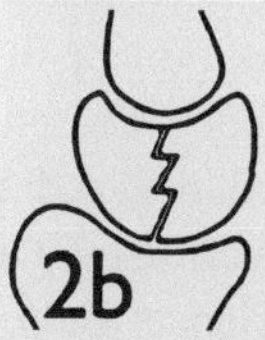 | *Grade 2b*<br>2 Nonfunctional surfaces<br>– Proximal and distal lunate | PRC<br>Lunate replacement<br>Capitate lengthening |
| 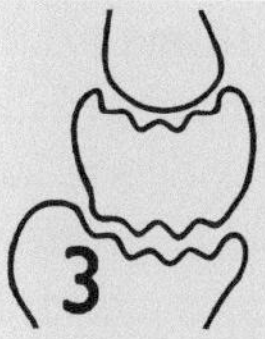 | *Grade 3*<br>3 Nonfunctional surfaces<br>– Capitate surface usually preserved | Hemiarthroplasty<br>(SC fusion if radial column intact) |
| 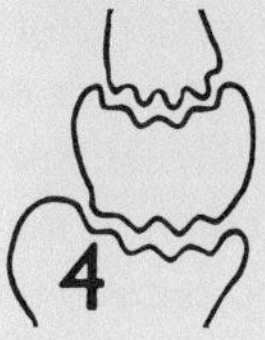 | *Grade 4*<br>All four articular surfaces are nonfunctional | Total wrist fusion<br>Total wrist arthroplasty<br>(SC fusion if radial column intact) |

Synovectomy is performed in all patients

SC fusion = scaphocapitate fusion, can be considered if the central column is nonfunctional, but the radial column is intact

[a]Articular-based approach to Kienböck's disease. The Bain/Begg arthroscopic classification system is derived from the number and location of nonfunctional articular surfaces in the central column. Treatment algorithm is based on the principle to excise, fuse, or bypass the nonfunctional articular surfaces. Modified from Bain GI, Begg M. Arthroscopic assessment and classification of Kienböck's disease. Tech Hand Up Extrem Surg 2006. Copyright Dr. Gregory Bain [12]

## Lunate Stage: How Does the Disease Affect the Lunate?

The lunate consists of osseous, vascular, and cartilaginous components. Each of these can be affected in different ways. There have been classification systems developed for each of these components. Osseous—Lichtman [6], Vascular—Schmitt [11], Cartilage—Bain [12].

We consider the lunate to be "intact" if it is not fractured and the articular surfaces are "functional". Lichtman stages 0, I and II, Schmitt stage A, Bain grade 0 all represent an intact lunate. A "compromised" lunate has localized areas of collapse or degeneration, but other areas that can be used to reconstruct and maintain a functional lunate. This coincides with the Lichtman Stage IIIA, Schmitt stage B and Bain grade 1. A lunate is "not recon-

**Table 30.4** Surgical options for Kienböck's disease

| Principle | Procedure | Chapter |
|---|---|---|
| Unloading | | |
| | Radial shortening | 16 |
| | Radial epiphysiodesis | 9 |
| | Capitate shortening | 15 |
| | External fixation | 14 |
| | STT joint pinning | 14 |
| | Opening and closing osteotomies | 17 |
| Revascularization | | |
| | Pedicle and free graft | 18 |
| | Radial forage (indirect vascularization) | 14 |
| Lunate reconstruction | | |
| | Medial femoral trochlear graft | 19 |
| Wrist reconstruction | | |
| | RSL fusion | 22 |
| | Lunate excision, capitate lengthening | 23 |
| | PRC | 20 |
| | STT, SC fusion | 21 |
| | Arthroscopic assisted reconstruction | 13, 24, 25 |
| | Interposition (pyrocarbon) arthroplasty | 26 |
| | Hemi-arthroplasty | 27 |
| Salvage | | |
| | Total wrist arthrodesis | 29 |
| | Total wrist arthroplasty | 28 |

structable" when it is fragmented, collapsed, or has completely lost its vascular supply. Lichtman stage IIIC, Schmitt stage C, and Bain grade 2b are examples of lunates that are not reconstructable.

## Lunate Intact: Lunate Protection

By definition, this group has a lunate that has not collapsed (Lichtman Stage 0, I, II), has functional articular surfaces (Bain 0), and has a positive prognosis for revascularization (Schmitt Stage A). There are three aims for treatment of this group:

1. Decrease the patient's pain and improve function.
2. Protect the vulnerable lunate before it collapses.
3. Set the stage for spontaneous revascularization.

## Nonoperative Management

In the earliest stages, patients are managed nonoperatively for at least 3 months. Short arm cast or splint immobilization is the usual treatment of choice; however, minimally invasive techniques may be appropriate as well. Patients are asked to avoid all strenuous activity involving, pushing, pulling, twisting, or lifting over 5 kg (10 lb) with the affected extremity. Medical causes of osteonecrosis are managed, if identified. If after 3 months, the patient is still symptomatic or imaging demonstrates disease progression, a lunate unloading or revascularization procedure is appropriate.

## Lunate Unloading Procedures

Lunate unloading is the next option for patients with intact lunates who do not respond to nonoperative measures. These procedures protect the lunate and set the stage for spontaneous revascularization. The most common procedure is radial shortening osteotomy, which is effective for the patient with a negative ulnar variance and/or abnormal radial inclination (Chaps. 16 and 17). If the physis is still intact, a radial epiphysiodesis is a possible surgical alternative, as it restricts radial growth, while allowing the short ulna to grow preferentially [17] (Chap. 9). If there is a neutral or positive ulnar variance, then a capitate shortening osteotomy can be performed. Patients with early Lichtman stage IIIA (minimal collapse) with functioning articular surfaces (Bain 0) may still be candidates for unloading procedures if the lunate has viable bone present (Schmitt A, early B).

## Lunate Decompression

Another option is lunate forage, which involves drilling the lunate to decompress the venous hypertension (Chaps. 13, 14, and 24). This can be performed arthroscopically, in conjunction with a synovectomy (Chap. 13) [12, 14, 35, 38] and cancellous bone grafting [35–37, 39] (Chap. 24).

## Revascularization Procedures

Core decompression of the distal radius is thought to provide an indirect revascularization of the lunate, due to the increased regional vascular

**Table 30.5** Amalgamation of the osseous, vascular, and cartilage classification systems for the assessment and treatment of Kienböck's disease

| Assessment | | | | Treatment | |
|---|---|---|---|---|---|
| Osseous (Lichtman) | Vascular (Schmitt) | Cartilage (Bain) | Description | Principle | Procedure |
| B1—Lunate Intact | | | | Lunate Protection | |
| 0, I, II | A | 0 | Intact lunate | Unload the lunate | Immobilization, Unloading procedures |
| | | | | Venous decompression | Lunate decompression |
| | | | | Revascularization | Vascularized bone graft[a] |
| B2—Lunate Compromised | | | | Lunate Reconstruction | |
| IIIA | B | 1 | Proximal lunate collapse | Lunate reconstruction | MFT graft[a], PRC (RSL Fusion, Lunate replacement[a]) |
| B3—Lunate Unreconstructable | | | | Lunate Salvage | |
| III C | C | 2b | Lunate collapse | Lunate excision | PRC (Lunate replacement[a], Capitate lengthening) |
| C1-2—Wrist Compromised | | | | Wrist Reconstruction | |
| IIIA | B | 2a | Radiocarpal joint compromised | Fuse or bypass radiolunate joint | RSL fusion[a], SC fusion |
| IIIA or C | B | 3, 4 | Radiocarpal and midcarpal joint compromise | Bypass central column | SC fusion, (Hemiarthroplasty if capitate intact[a]) |
| IIIB | B | 2–4 | Carpal collapse (RSA>60°) | Stabilize the radial column | SC fusion |
| C3—Wrist Not Reconstructable | | | | Wrist Salvage | |
| II, IV (KDAC) | C | 4 | Pan—OA | Salvage | Wrist fusion, Wrist arthroplasty[a] |

*SC* scaphocapitate, *MFT* medial femoral trochlear

*Better prognosis*: Age <15 years nonoperative, 16–20 consider unloading, >70 consider synovectomy or unloading procedure

*Lunate unloading procedures*: Negative ulnar variance—Radial shortening osteotomy; Physis intact—Radial epiphysiodesis; Neutral or positive ulnar variance—Capitate shortening

[a]Alternative procedures—Used in specialist clinics or in selected cases where patient has failed less invasive procedures

Adjunctive procedures—Synovectomy, STT pinning

**Table 30.6** Recommended treatment

| |
|---|
| A. Child/elderly |
| A1. <15 years—non-operative |
| A2. 16–20 years—non-operative (consider unloading procedure) |
| A3. >70 years—non-operative (consider synovectomy) |
| B. Adult—limited to lunate |
| B1. Lunate intact—radial shortening for ulnar –ve; capitate shortening for ulnar +ve variance (lunate forage +/– bone graft for Schmitt A; revascularization for Schmitt B and C[a]) |
| B2. Lunate compromised—MFT reconstruction[a] (SC fusion for higher demand; PRC for lower demand patient) |
| B3. Lunate not reconstructable—SC fusion with lunate excision for higher demand; PRC for lower demand patient (lunate replacement[a]) |
| C. Adult—wrist affected |
| C1a. Central column RL articulation compromised—RSL fusion (SC fusion for Schmitt C) |
| C1b. Central column RL and MC articulation compromised—SC fusion with lunate excision |
| C2. Carpal collapse with intact radioscaphoid articulation—SC fusion w or w/o lunate excision[b] |
| C3. Wrist not reconstructable—total wrist arthrodesis (arthroplasty[a]) |

Alternative procedures in parentheses are appropriate based on surgeon/patient preference
[a]Complex procedure to be used only with appropriate equipment/training
[b]Lunate excision for fragmented lunate with reactive synovitis

response [34]. Direct revascularization of the lunate has been performed for many years, with both pedicle and free vascularized bone graft (Chap. 18). Pedicle graft procedures are appropriate for patients with an intact, partially viable lunate (Schmitt B). It is also used as an alternative to unloading in patients with a positive ulnar variance.

### Lunate Compromised: Lunate Reconstruction (Lichtman Stage IIIA, Schmitt Stage B, and Bain Grade 1)

The lunate has localized disease, including areas of nonfunctioning proximal articular cartilage, but other areas are intact. Ideal treatment would involve localized reconstruction of the lunate.

#### Vascularized Medial Femoral Trochlea (MFT) Graft [23, 24]

The vascularized medial femoral trochlea (MFT) graft is indicated for reconstruction of the proximal osseous and articular lunate, and can also be used to restore carpal height (Chap. 19). As this is a demanding and time-consuming procedure, we need to have other treatment options available, such as lunate salvage (PRC or lunate replacement), RSL fusion, or SC fusion. Note that all of these alternative procedures are more destructive than an isolated lunate reconstruction.

### Lunate Not Reconstructable: Lunate Salvage (Lichtman IIIC, Schmitt C, Bain 2b)

The lunate is not reconstructable if there is advanced lunate collapse, there is no revascularization potential or the lunate articular surfaces are nonfunctional. Therefore, a salvage procedure of the lunate is required. Once the lunate has reached this level of destruction, it is common for the adjacent articulations to have degeneration and for the carpus to collapse as well. Once the disease process extends beyond the lunate, and involves the wrist, proceed to the section C of the algorithm.

#### Lunate Replacement

If the lunate is not reconstructable, it needs to be excised. Lunate replacement with silicone [6, 26], autogenous tendon, metallic spheres and the pisiform [25] have all had inconsistent or poor results [26]. If the capitate head and adjacent joint surfaces are intact, a lunate excision and capitate lengthening with interposition graft is a possible solution (Chap. 23). Recently, pyrocarbon implant replacement has been advocated. However, instability remains an issue, and further work is required to ascertain whether reliable clinical outcomes are possible [27, 28] (Chap. 26).

### Proximal Row Carpectomy

Proximal row carpectomy is a simple and reliable technique that is indicated for the unreconstructable lunate (Chap. 20). However, the articular surfaces of the lunate facet and the capitate must be functional (Bain 2b). The PRC is a good choice in those patients who have a low demand for the wrist. In high demand patients other options, such as a limited wrist fusion is preferred.

## Wrist Stage: How Does the Disease Affect the Wrist?

The secondary effects of the collapsing lunate are a "compromised" wrist, including degeneration of the central column at the radiolunate and midcarpal articulations, collapse of the central and radial columns and finally degeneration of the radial column as well.

Fractures of the lunate subchondral bone plate produce irregularity of the lunate articular surfaces. If the fracture settles and heals in a stable configuration then the prognosis is likely to be good. There may secondary "kissing lesions" of the lunate facet and capitate, and then progression to articular degeneration (nonfunctional cartilage) [12, 13]. If the fracture propagates, there will be continued loss of lunate height, which affects the kinematics of the perilunate ligaments and the central column. Comminution, disruption of the spanning trabeculi, or a coronal lunate fracture will result in collapse of the lunate, which will allow proximal migration of the capitate, and therefore collapse of the entire central column. Laxity of the scapholunate ligaments may also contribute to proximal migration and collapse of the central column.

In collapse due to lunate comminution, interposition of the capitate head between fragments appears on sagittal X-rays as a widening or elongation between the volar and dorsal lunate poles; or if the major fragments are pushed dorsally, the lunate will appear to be in flexion (VISI). On the other hand, A DISI deformity may occur if the capitate head migrates into a gap formed by scapholunate ligament disruption or if the major fragments are pushed anteriorly. In almost all instances, however, the mechanical effects of proximal migration of the capitate (and distal row) cause excessive flexion of the scaphoid (Lichtman stage IIIB), as manifested by a radioscaphoid angle >60° [40]. For a short time this scaphoid flexion is correctable but eventually the prolonged flexion will cause erosive degeneration of radioscaphoid articular cartilage and that joint, too, will become nonfunctional. The wrist has now reached its final stage of degeneration, or Kienböck's Disease Advanced Collapse (KDAC)

Prior to carpal collapse, the wrist with nonfunctional wrist areas can be reconstructed with motion preserving procedures by excising, fusing, or bypassing the nonfunctional aspects and maintaining the functional articulations. The specific recommended procedure will depend upon the extent of osseous collapse, but more importantly the remaining functional articular surfaces. The surgeon needs to match the remaining functional articular surfaces with the prerequisites.

After carpal collapse the radial column deformity is initially correctable, so lunate reconstructive procedure could theoretically be effective (e.g., lunate replacement). However, once there is a fixed deformity and central column articular degeneration, a limited wrist fusion is required. The scaphocapitate (or STT) fusion is a good surgical option at this stage, as it bypasses the diseased central column, stabilizes the radial column, and articulates through the intact radioscaphoid articulation. This is the same concept as the SLAC wrist procedure, which excises the radial column, stabilizes the central column, and mobilizes through the intact radiocarpal articulation.

Once the radioscaphoid articulation is also compromised (nonfunctional), the wrist is unreconstructable and a salvage procedure is required. This is only seen in very late Kienböck's disease (KDAC-Lichtman IV) or following failed reconstructive surgery.

### Central Column Compromised; Central Column Fusion or Bypass (Lichtman IIIA or C, Schmitt B, Bain 2a, 3, or 4)

(a) *Radiolunate articulation* nonfunctional (*Lichtman IIIA, Schmitt B, Bain 2a) and the midcarpal joint surfaces functional.* In this case a RSL fusion can be performed (Chap. 22).

If the lunate is not viable (MRI grade C), then bypassing the central column and performing a scaphocapitate fusion should be considered

(b) *Radiolunate and midcarpal articulations nonfunctional* (*Lichtman IIIA or C, Schmitt C, Bain 4*). The central column is not reconstructable and needs to be bypassed with a scaphocapitate fusion. As the proximal and distal lunate articular surfaces are compromised, the diseased and fragmented lunate is excised. *In the occasional case where the capitate articular surface is intact* (Lichtman IIIA or C, Schmitt C, Bain 3) a hemiarthroplasty can be performed (Chap. 27).

### Carpal Collapse; Wrist Stabilization (Lichtman IIIB, Schmitt B, Bain 2–4)

With collapse and/or degeneration of the central column, it is common for the radial column to also collapse, which has been reported to be present if the radioscaphoid angle is greater than 60° [40, 42]. Fortunately, the radioscaphoid articulation is usually functional. In this case, we recommend a scaphocapitate fusion, although STT fusion is an alternative (Chaps. 21 and 25). The lunate can be left in situ if it is not inciting a local synovitis.

In the early stages of carpal collapse, the lunate can be reconstructed, as described in B3. However, this is limited to those cases in which the articulations are intact, and there is not a fixed deformity. We do not recommend a lunate prosthesis in those cases with associated carpal collapse, as it is technically demanding to obtain stability.

#### Scaphocapitate Fusion

As part of the scaphocapitate fusion we recommend excising the lunate, if there is advanced disease with extensive lunate collapse and fragmentation. These changes frequently cause mechanical symptoms and incite an extensive synovitis of the wrist. Tse recommends excising the lunate if there was significant widening of the lunate seen on the sagittal CT scan (Chap. 25). He performed this as an arthroscopic procedure, and reported a resultant increase in range of motion. When performing an open excision of the volar lunate fragments, the surgeon needs to be cautious of not violating the volar carpal ligaments, that are intimately attached to the volar fragments. Otherwise ulnar translocation of the carpus will occur.

#### Arthroscopic Reconstructive Procedures

Most of the motion preserving procedures can now be performed arthroscopically, as expertly described by Tse (Chap. 25). However, the prerequisites of each procedure must still be respected.

### Wrist Not Reconstructable; Wrist Salvage (Lichtman Stage 4, Schmitt C, Bain Grade 4)

Once the radioscaphoid articulation also becomes nonfunctional, the wrist is no longer reconstructable. This is commonly termed Kienböck's advanced collapse (KDAC), which is due to late disease or failed previous reconstructive surgery. As there are no longer any functional articulations, a salvage procedure is required, such as total wrist fusion or total wrist arthroplasty (Chaps. 28 and 29). The specific recommended procedure will usually depend upon the demands of the patient. Total wrist arthroplasty should only be performed in those patients who will use the extremity in a controlled manner and not overload the wrist.

#### Adjuvant Procedures

There are a number of surgical procedures that can be considered adjunctive procedures, which can be performed as an independent procedure, or added to other procedures. These include:

*Synovectomy*. Synovitis of the wrist is a common finding in Kienböck's disease [12] and a frequent source of pain. Synovectomy and joint debridement can be performed as an open or arthroscopic [38] (Chap. 13) adjunctive procedure whenever indicated.

*STT Pinning*. Temporary pinning of the scaphotrapezio-trapezoid (STT) joint unloads the lunate, and allows time for revascularization [29–33]. The STT joint is pinned with the scaphoid in the extended position. This is a reasonable option as a primary treatment in the "Teenbock" patient (Chap. 9) or can be used to protect the lunate in conjunction with a vascularized bone graft [29] (Chaps. 9 and 14).

*PIN Neurectomy*. There are some authors who recommend posterior interosseous neurectomy to provide pain relief for patients with carpal pathology [41]. However, we are concerned that the concomitant loss of proprioception will negatively affect function and self-protection of the wrist.

## What Can the Surgeon Offer?

Because surgeons have different abilities, training, and experience, these factors must be taken into consideration after assessing the patient's age, status of the lunate, and condition of the wrist. Some treatment options require special equipment or advanced skills in microsurgery or arthroscopy, which may be beyond the capabilities of some surgeons or their operative facilities. We have identified these highly specialized procedures within the algorithm (*). With worldwide technical advances, most of these procedures will eventually become mainstream.

## What Does the Patient Want?

Ultimately, medical decision-making comes down to satisfying the needs and desires of the informed, competent patient. The patient's general health, lifestyle, and future demands on the wrist need careful consideration. Each patient is different, and personal considerations will affect all levels of the proposed algorithm. Unfortunately, constraints outside of the control of the doctor and patient, such as financial restrictions imposed by the insurer or governing bodies, also affect the final decision.

No treatment algorithm will cover every possible contingency, especially when addressing an enigmatic disease like Kienböck's that affects such a broad spectrum of the population. Armed with the information provided here, we feel that the treating physician can make an evidence-based decision that is tailored to the unique needs of the patient.

## Finale

The algorithm presented here is based on the accumulation of knowledge of Kienböck's disease currently available. We know, however, that there will be further advances in the understanding of the etiology, pathoanatomy, biomechanics, demographics, imaging, natural history, and treatment. These advances will need to be incorporated into the algorithm, and will aid in defining the definitive management of this fascinating disorder.

Finally, we thank all of the contributors of this book for permitting us to bring together their vast breadth of information. We trust that their efforts have advanced the management well beyond what Robert Kienböck could have ever imagined.

## References

1. Kienböck R. Über traumatische Malazie des Mondbeins und ihre Folgezustände: Entartungsformen und Kompressionsfrakturen, Fortschritte a.d. Gebiete d. Röntgenstrahlen, 1910; XVI(2):77–103
2. Lutsky K, Beredjiklian PK. Kienbock disease. J Hand Surg Am. 2012;37(9):1942–52.
3. Keith PP, Nuttall D, Trail I. Long-term outcome of nonsurgically managed Kienböck's disease. J Hand Surg Am. 2004;29(1):63–7.
4. Salmon J, Stanley JK, Trail IA. Kienböck's disease: conservative management versus radial shortening. J Bone Joint Surg Br. 2000;82(6):820–3.
5. Beckenbaugh RD, Shives TC, Dobyns JH, Linscheid RL. Kienböck's disease: the natural history of Kienböck's disease and consideration of lunate fractures. Clin Orthop Relat Res. 1980;149:98–106.
6. Lichtman DM, Mack GR, MacDonald RI, Gunther SF, Wilson JN. Kienböck's disease: the role of silicone replacement arthroplasty. J Bone Joint Surg Am. 1977;59(7):899–908.
7. Lichtman DM, Degnan GG. Staging and its use in the determination of treatment modalities for Kienböck's disease. Hand Clin. 1993;9(3):409–16.
8. Lichtman DM, Lesley NE, Simmons SP. The classification and treatment of Kienböck's disease: the state of the art and a look at the future. J Hand Surg Eur Vol. 2010;35(7):549–54.
9. Arco News. Association research circulation osseous (ARCO): committee on terminology and classification. ARCO News. 1992;4:41–6.
10. Schmitt R, Kalb KH. Imaging in Kienböck's disease. Handchir Mikrochir Plast Chir. 2010;42:162–70.

11. Schmitt R, Heinze A, Fellner F, Obletter N, Strühn R, Bautz W. Imaging and staging of avascular osteonecroses at the wrist and hand. Eur J Radiol. 1997; 25(2):92–103.
12. Bain GI, Begg M. Arthroscopic assessment and classification of Kienböck's disease. Tech Hand Up Extrem Surg. 2006;10(1):8–13.
13. Bain GI, Durrant A. An articular-based approach to Kienbock avascular necrosis of the lunate. Tech Hand Up Extrem Surg. 2011;15(1):41–7.
14. Bain GI, McGuire DT. Decision making for partial carpal fusions. J Wrist Surg. 2012;1(2):103–14.
15. Fontaine C. Kienböck's disease. Chir Main. 2015;34(1):4–17.
16. Irisarri C, Kalb K, Ribak S. Infantile and juvenile lunatomalacia. J Hand Surg Eur Vol. 2010;35(7):544–8.
17. Jorge-Mora A, Pretell-Mazzini J, Marti-Ciruelos R, Andres-Esteban EM, Curto de la Mano A. Distal radius definitive epiphysiodesis for management of Kienböck's disease in skeletally immature patients. Int Orthop. 2012;36(10):2101–5.
18. Geutjens GG. Kienböck's disease in an elderly patient. J Hand Surg Am. 1995;20(1):42–3.
19. Taniguchi Y, Yoshida M, Iwasaki H, Otakara H, Iwata S. Kienböck's disease in elderly patients. J Hand Surg Am. 2003;28(5):779–83.
20. Yoshida T, Tada K, Yamamoto K, Shibata T, Shimada K, Kawai H. Aged-onset Kienböck's disease. Arch Orthop Trauma Surg. 1990;109(5):241–6.
21. Giunta R, Lower N, Wilhelm K, Keirse R, Rock C, Muller-Gerbl M. Altered patterns of subchondral bone mineralization in Kienböck's disease. J Hand Surg Br. 1997;22(1):16–20.
22. Thomas AA, Rodriguez E, Segalman K. Kienböck's disease in an elderly patient treated with proximal row carpectomy. J Hand Surg Am. 2004;29(4):685–8.
23. Higgins JP, Bürger HK. Osteochondral flaps from the distal femur: expanding applications, harvest sites, and indications. J Reconstr Microsurg. 2014;30(7): 483–90.
24. Burger HK, Windhofer C, Gaggl AJ, Higgins JP. Vascularized medial femoral trochlea osteocartilaginous flap reconstruction of proximal pole scaphoid nonunions. J Hand Surg Am. 2013;38(4):690–700.
25. Saffar P. Vascularized pisiform transfer in place of lunatum for Kienböck's disease. Chir Main. 2010;29 Suppl 1:S112–8.
26. Roca J, Beltran JE, Fairen MF, Alvarez A. Treatment of Kienböck's disease using a silicone rubber implant. J Bone Joint Surg Am. 1976;58:373–6.
27. Werthel JD, Hoang DV, Boyer P, Dallaudière B, Massin P, Loriaut P. Treatment of Kienböck's disease using a pyrocarbon implant: case report. Chir Main. 2014;33(6):404–9.
28. Bellemère P, Maes-clavier C, Loubersac T, Gaisne E, Kerjean Y, Collon S. Pyrocarbon interposition wrist arthroplasty in the treatment of failed wrist procedures. J Wrist Surg. 2012;1(1):31–8.
29. Yajima H, Ono H, Tamai S. Temporary internal fixation of the scaphotrapezio-trapezoidal joint for the treatment of Kienböck's disease: a preliminary study. J Hand Surg Am. 1998;23(3):402–10.
30. Yasuda M, Okuda H, Egi T, Guidera PM. Temporary scapho-trapezoidal joint fixation for Kienböck's disease in a 12-year-old girl: a case report. J Hand Surg Am. 1998;23(3):411–4.
31. Shigematsu K, Yajima H, Kobata Y, Kawamura K, Nakanishi Y, Takakura Y. Treatment of Kienbock disease in an 11-year-old girl with temporary fixation of the scaphotrapeziotrapezoidal joint. Scand J Plast Reconstr Surg Hand Surg. 2005;39(1):60–3.
32. Kazuki K, Uemura T, Okada M, Egi T. Time course of magnetic resonance images in an adolescent patient with Kienböck's disease treated by temporary scaphotrapezoidal joint fixation: a case report. J Hand Surg Am. 2006;31(1):63–7.
33. Ando Y, Yasuda M, Kazuki K, Hidaka N, Yoshinaka Y. Temporary scaphotrapezoidal joint fixation for adolescent Kienböck's disease. J Hand Surg Am. 2009;34(1):14–9.
34. Illarramendi AA, Schulz C, De Carli P. The surgical treatment of Kienböck's disease by radius and ulna metaphyseal core decompression. J Hand Surg Am. 2001;26(2):252–60.
35. Bain GI, Smith ML, Watts AC. Arthroscopic core decompression of the lunate in early stage Kienbock disease of the lunate. Tech Hand Up Extrem Surg. 2011;15(1):66–9.
36. Mehrpour SR, Kamrani RS, Aghamirsalim MR, Sorbi R, Kaya A. Treatment of Kienbock disease by lunate core decompression. J Hand Surg Am. 2011;36(10): 1675–7.
37. Leblebicioğlu G, Doral MN, Atay öA, Tetik O, Whipple TL. Open treatment of stage III Kienböck's disease with lunate revascularization compared with arthroscopic treatment without revascularization. Arthroscopy. 2003;19(2):117–30.
38. Menth-Chiari WA, Poehling GG, Wiesler ER, Ruch DS. Arthroscopic debridement for the treatment of Kienböck's disease. Arthroscopy. 1999;15(1):12–9.
39. Pegoli L, Ghezzi A, Cavalli E, Luchetti R, Pajardi G. Arthroscopic assisted bone grafting for early stages of Kienböck's disease. Hand Surg. 2011;16(2):127–31.
40. Gelberman RH, Bauman TD, Menon J, Akeson WH. The vascularity of the lunate bone and Kienböck's disease. J Hand Surg Am. 1980;5(3):272–8.
41. Wilhelm A. Partial joint denervation: wrist, shoulder and elbow. Plast Reconstr Surg. 2010;126(1):345–7.
42. Quenzer DE, Dobyns JH, Linscheid RL, Trail IA, Vidal MA. Radial recession osteotomy for Kienböck's disease. J Hand Surg Am. 1997;22(3): 386–95.

# Index



© Springer International Publishing Switzerland 2016
D.M. Lichtman, G.I. Bain (eds.), *Kienböck's Disease*, DOI 10.1007/978-3-319-34226-9